Urogynecology

For Churchill Livingstone

Commissioning Editor: Sheila Khullar
Project Controller: Anita Sekhri
Copy editor: Frances Lewis
Indexer: Nina Boyd
Design Direction: Roger Fletcher

Urogynecology

The King's Approach

Edited by

Linda Cardozo MD FRCOG

Professor of Urogynaecology,
King's College, London, UK;
Consultant Gynaecologist
King's Healthcare Trust, London, UK

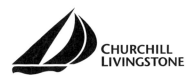

CHURCHILL
LIVINGSTONE

NEW YORK EDINBURGH LONDON MADRID MELBOURNE SAN FRANCISCO AND TOKYO 1997

The ICS has defined incontinence as, 'a condition of involuntary urine loss that is a social or hygienic problem and is objectively demonstrable'. This definition suggests a certain severity of urinary leakage rather than just any incontinence.

Prevalence studies have evaluated the presence of *any* incontinence or of *severe* incontinence, although only one has specifically evaluated the presence of socially problematic or unhygienic urinary leakage.[3] Severity has been assessed in a number of ways but most often with reference to the frequency of leakage, varying from 'daily' to 'weekly' to 'once or twice a month'. Unfortunately, in no study to date has the severity measure been validated against any known clinical parameter or quality of life measure!

Wyman et al[4] assessed the subjective impact and frequency of urinary leakage using the 'Incontinence Impact Questionnaire' (an unvalidated disease-specific quality of life measure) and a urinary diary. They found only a modest correlation between the two. These findings suggest that severity cannot be measured in terms of the frequency of incontinence alone and other severity criteria must be addressed.

The prevalence of any incontinence amongst adults

Age appears to be a major factor in the etiology of urinary incontinence and data are therefore usually presented accordingly. 'Elderly' has no absolute definition and for most studies refers to persons over 60 or 65 years of age. It should be remembered, however, that in studies conducted by geriatricians 'elderly' may refer to women over 70 or even 80 years of age.[5] The prevalence of incontinence amongst women living independently in the community is less than that among nursing home residents, and incontinence is often a major reason for nursing home placement. Unless otherwise stated the figures presented refer to women residing independently in the community. There is great variation between studies in the estimated prevalence of 'any incontinence' (Table 1.1) which can only partially be explained by the different study populations and methodologies used. Incontinence is likely to be under-reported rather than over-reported and therefore higher figures are likely to be more accurate. A prevalence of 30% for 'any incontinence' may be close to the truth.

Table 1.1   Prevalence of 'any incontinence' amongst women residing independently in the community

Study	Prevalence (%)
Milne et al (1972)[6]	34
65 + years	
Thomas et al (1980)[7]	
25–64 years	18
65 + years	23
Yarnell et al (1981)[8]	
25–64 years	46
65 + years	49
Vetter et al (1981)[9]	
61 years	14
Diokno et al (MESA) study (1986)[10]	
65 + years	30
Market Opinion Research[1] International (MORI) poll (1990)	
All women ($n = 2980$)	14

Prevalence of severe urinary incontinence

Although prevalence studies have not attempted to validate their measures of severity, estimates of 'severe incontinence' are more consistent than those for 'any loss' (Table 1.2). They range from 3 to 11%, with the majority being between 4 and 6%, and are therefore considerably lower than those of 'any urinary leakage'.

Table 1.2 Prevalence of severe urinary incontinence

Study	Prevalence (%)
Milne et al (1972)[6]	5
Yarnell and St Leger (1979)[11]	11
Thomas et al (1980)[7]	10
Vetter et al (1981)[9]	5
Campbell et al (1985)[12]	3
Diokno et al (MESA) study (1986)[10]	4

Although incontinence is common amongst adults residing independently in the community, studies have estimated that almost 50% of nursing home residents are incontinent of urine.[13] These figures are undoubtedly higher as they include the frailest elderly women who may have been admitted to nursing home care because of their incontinence.

Prevalence of incontinence which is a social or hygienic problem

Mäkinen et al[3] carried out a postal survey of 5247 Swedish women participating in a mass cervical screening programme. The aim of their study was to determine the prevalence of involuntary urine loss which was a 'social or hygienic' problem. Their questionnaire prompted women who considered their urinary leakage to be a social or hygienic problem to answer further questions. Incontinence was reported by 20.1% of respondents, with an overall response rate of 71%. Unfortunately, due to the nature of the parent study, women over 55 years were not included in the survey. Surprisingly, only 37% of women reporting incontinence felt they needed treatment, and less than one-fifth had sought medical help for their condition.

Prevalence of stress and urge incontinence

The complex symptomatology of lower urinary tract dysfunction and the common presentation of predominantly mixed symptoms must inevitably question the validity of studies designed to assess the prevalence of urge and stress incontinence alone. A diagnosis based on urinary symptoms alone often correlates poorly with urodynamic findings. Versi et al[14] analyzed the value of urinary symptoms for the prediction of genuine stress incontinence (GSI) in 252 patients, and correctly diagnosed 81% of cases with a false positive rate of 16%. Bergman & Bader,[15] however, evaluated 122 incontinent patients and found that a detailed urinary symptom questionnaire had a positive predictive value of 80% for GSI, and only 25% for detrusor instability (DI)!

gesterone level affects the ureters, bladder and urethra. During pregnancy physiological hydroureter is attributable to both the smooth muscle relaxant effects of progesterone[31] and the obstructive effects of the gravid uterus. This inevitably increases the risk of pyelonephritis secondary to lower urinary tract infection.

Cystometry during pregnancy has shown an increase in bladder capacity and compliance,[32] and these changes have also been demonstrated during the luteal phase of the menstrual cycle.[33]

Pregnant women commonly complain of stress incontinence, and this has been attributed to the high level of progesterone during pregnancy. However, Van Geelen et al[34] performed urethral pressure profilometry on 43 pregnant women and found no change in the maximum urethral closure pressure despite high levels of 17-hydroxyprogesterone. In contrast, Benness et al[35] evaluated 14 postmenopausal women on continuous estrogen and cyclical progestogen hormone replacement therapy and found an increased incidence of positive pad tests and worsening of GSI during the progestational phase of the cycle.

The clinical value and possible detrimental effects of progesterone in patients with urinary complaints await further evaluation. Progesterone may be of benefit to women with DI through its smooth muscle relaxant effects, and it may worsen GSI, although neither effect has been conclusively proven.[35,36]

Race

Racial differences in the prevalence of urinary incontinence are difficult to quantify as cultural factors alter the perception and presentation of urinary complaints. Although few epidemiological data are available incontinence appears to be least common amongst Chinese, Eskimo and Black women.

An anatomical study involving the dissection of Chinese female cadavers showed that the general anatomic relationship of the levator ani muscles and urethra was similar to that found in Western women. The levator ani muscle bundles of the Chinese cadavers were, however, judged to be thicker and to extend more laterally on the arcus tendineus than is seen in White cadavers. In addition the fascia of the pelvic diaphragm extending from the levator ani muscles to the posterior pubourethral ligaments was particularly dense in Chinese cadavers.[37]

Bump[38] compared clinical and urodynamic parameters of 200 Black (54) and White (146) women referred for evaluation of incontinence (154) and severe prolapse (46). He found the proportion of Black and White patients with severe prolapse to be the same, but showed the causes of urinary incontinence to be significantly different between the two groups (Table 1.4).

Childbirth

Thomas et al[7] reported a significant relationship between incontinence and parity (Fig. 1.1). Incontinence was less common amongst nulliparous women of all ages, but no difference in the prevalence of incontinence was noted for women who had had one, two or three vaginal deliveries.

Table 1.4   Cause of incontinence and racial origin[38]

Variable	Race	
	Black (%)	White (%)
Symptoms of incontinence		
Stress incontinence	7	31
Urge incontinence	56	28
Mixed incontinence	37	41
Cause of incontinence		
GSI	27	61
DI	56	28
Mixed incontinence	17	11

From Bump 1992[38]

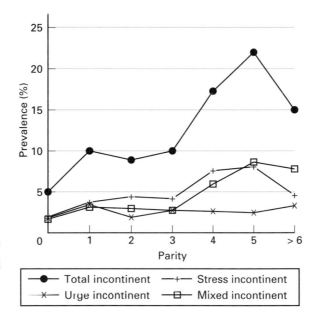

Fig. 1.1 Prevalence of stress, urge and mixed incontinence by parity. (From Thomas et al 1980. Prevalence of urinary incontinence. Br Med J 281: 1243–1245, with permission.)

Women who had had four or more vaginal deliveries were more likely to report regular incontinence. The association of parity and incontinence is mainly due to an increase in the incidence of stress incontinence, whereas postpartum DI appears to be little affected by pregnancy or childbirth. Cutner et al[39] have shown an increased incidence of DI during pregnancy, possibly related to physiologically elevated serum progesterone levels, although it appears that the majority of these cases resolve post partum. Many of the irritative bladder symptoms of pregnancy do not appear to correlate with urodynamic diagnoses, and therefore urodynamic investigations are essential to determine the true incidence of lower urinary tract dysfunction in pregnancy.

Injury during childbirth has been implicated as the major etiologic factor in GSI, and there is histological[40] and electromyographic[41,42] evidence of injury to the pelvic floor following vaginal delivery. Women delivered by Caesarean section without labour have greater pelvic muscle strength post partum and a lower incidence of urinary incontinence. Urethral pressure profilometry has shown a reduction in functional urethral length, urethral closure pressure and maximum urethral pressure following vaginal delivery, changes which are not observed following Caesarean section.[34]

Wilson et al[43] have shown that a program of intensive postpartum pelvic floor exercises can reduce the incidence of stress incontinence 1 year following delivery. Genuine stress incontinence cannot, however, be wholly explained by the effects of vaginal delivery and urinary incontinence does not appear to be a necessary consequence of childbirth.

Connective tissue factors

Bo & Stien[44] reported stress incontinence in 13 of 37 fit healthy nulliparous physical education students, and demonstrated significantly lower resting urethral pressures and stress profiles in this group compared to continent nulliparous controls.

Although it would be expected that such young nulliparous women would be at low risk for developing GSI, research has suggested that the collagen of women with prolapse and stress incontinence may be different from that of women who do not develop these conditions. Landon & Smith[45] found that abdominal wall collagen was stiffer in women with stress incontinence than in continent controls, and Sayer et al[46] showed that the collagen of the pubocervical fascia of stress incontinent women was weak due to an abnormal cross-linking of collagen fibrils. The composition of collagen in women with stress incontinence may therefore be abnormal and predispose them to urethral sphincter incompetence.

Type I collagen forms thick strong fibre units whereas Type III collagen forms thin, weak and isolated fibres. Keane et al[47] performed periurethral biopsies on 30 nulliparous women with urodynamically proven GSI. They found a decrease in Type I compared to Type III collagen, as well as a reduction in the total amount of collagen in GSI sufferers compared to continent controls. Norton et al[48] and Bergman et al[49] had similar findings in parous women with genital prolapse and GSI.

Smoking, obesity and chronic constipation

Any condition resulting in chronically elevated intra-abdominal pressure is likely to increase the risk of developing or exacerbating stress incontinence. Obesity, chronic constipation and smoking have been suggested as important predisposing factors in the causation of GSI, although insufficient data exist to refute or confirm these assumptions.

Dwyer et al[50] found that obesity (> 20% above average weight for height and age) was significantly more common in women with GSI and DI than in the normal population. There were, however, no significant differences between obese and non-obese incontinent women with respect to any urodynamic variables. Bump et al[51] studied 13 morbidly obese women before and after surgically induced weight loss. Weight loss resulted in a significant improvement in continence, obviating the need for treatment of incontinence in the majority of women.

Surgery for GSI may be technically more difficult in obese patients and the risks of operative and postoperative complications greater. Obesity may also increase the risk of recurrent incontinence although again this is unproven and further research is required.

In a large case-controlled study, Bump & McClish[52] noted a two-to threefold increase in the incidence of all forms of urinary incontinence amongst cigarette-smokers. Although the increased incidence of chronic chest complaints is likely to exacerbate stress incontinence, the effects of nicotine on the bladder require further evaluation.

Spence Jones et al[53] investigated 23 women with stress incontinence, 23 with uterovaginal prolapse and 27 control women using a detailed medical history, anal manometry and pudendal and perineal nerve terminal motor latencies. Straining at stool and an increased bowel frequency were significantly commoner amongst women with stress incontinence and prolapse than amongst controls. The findings of anal manometry and pudendal and perineal terminal motor latencies were normal for women with stress incontinence.

Hysterectomy and urinary incontinence

Urinary incontinence may be a complication of hysterectomy. In a review of 131 women following abdominal hysterectomy, Petri[54] found post-operative urinary incontinence in 68% of patients all of whom were pre-viously asymptomatic. Stress incontinence (37%) was more common than urge incontinence (29%). These results were similar to those of Farghaly et al[55] (60%), who reviewed 98 women following abdominal and vaginal hysterectomy, and Parys[56] (47%), who reviewed 126 women following abdominal hysterectomy.

Unfortunately, all of these studies are retrospective, and in two prospective studies[57,58] there was no evidence to suggest increased bladder dysfunction following abdominal hysterectomy. There are many potential mechanisms of incontinence following hysterectomy, namely derangement of the bladder supports,[59] pelvic nerve damage[60,61] and estrogen deficiency resulting from concomitant oophorectomy. In addition, postoperative catheter care may be suboptimal, and prolonged overdistension of the bladder resulting from urinary retention can lead to chronic bladder hypotonicity. At present the evidence is inconclusive and large detailed prospective studies are required.

Prolapse and anterior repair

Genital prolapse and urinary incontinence are common conditions and it is therefore not surprising to find both in some women. Unfortunately, clinical preoccupation with cystocele repair may overlook coexistent urinary problems and result in inappropriate treatment. Cystocele may be the cause of voiding difficulties,[62,63] and Rosenzweig et al[64] have shown almost 60% of women with severe genital prolapse and no symp-toms of incontinence to have underlying urinary incontinence revealed by urodynamic testing. Forty-one per cent of their patients had GSI following reduction of the prolapse with a ring pessary. Grady et al[62] showed that 30% of women with either small or large cystoceles had DI on urodynamic testing, and a higher percentage had symptoms of urge incontinence.

Although there have been several reports of the association of genital prolapse and urinary incontinence, the problem of stress incontinence following anterior repair has received little attention. Thomas et al[65] and Meyhoff et al[66] reported stress incontinence in 19% and 25% of continent women following anterior colporrhaphy for prolapse, and Iosif & Ulmsten[67] and Walter et al[68] reported a decrease in urethral closure pressure following similar surgery. Old age and previous pelvic surgery increase the risk of postoperative incontinence. This subject is thoroughly reviewed by Borstad.[69]

Radiotherapy and urinary incontinence

Radiotherapy is still frequently used for the treatment of locally invasive bladder cancer[70] and subsequent frequency and urgency of micturition affects as many as 50% of patients.[71] This is partly attributable to fibrotic bladder damage, and partly to denervation supersensitivity.[72] The characteristic urodynamic findings are a reduced bladder capacity and low compliance.

Urinary tract infection

Urinary tract infection is one of the most common reasons for general practitioner consultation by women, and it is has been estimated that 20% of women will experience UTI symptoms in any one year and that half of these will seek medical help.[73] It has been further estimated that between 10% and 20% of women experience recurrent episodes of cystitis or acute uncomplicated UTI,[74] although Mabeck[75] estimated that one-sixth of sufferers account for 70% of recurrences.

Many factors contribute to the frequency of UTI. Structural and functional abnormalities of the urinary tract and nephropathies associated with various diseases such as diabetes may lead to severe and complicated infection. Although the risk of UTI is relatively low for intermittent and short-term catheterization, it is a common consequence of long-term catheterization. Even with impeccable hygiene, and with or without anti-biotics, the incidence of catheter-associated bacteriuria is 3–10% per day. Thus by the end of 30 days' catheterization, the majority of patients are bacteriuric.[76]

Urinary tract infections are common in postmenopausal women as a result of estrogen deficiency. Withdrawal of estrogen and urogenital atrophy alter the vaginal flora and a subsequent increase in vaginal pH encourages colonization by Gram-negative uropathogens. There is evidence that these estrogen-dependent changes can be resolved with the use of hormone replacement therapy.[77]

Sexual intercourse is commonly implicated in the causation of UTI. Buckley et al[78] have shown that 30% of intercourse episodes are followed by a transient but significant increase in bacterial colony counts in urine.

Several behavioral factors have been shown to enhance the risk of recurrent UTIs. These include deferred voiding after sexual intercourse,[79] frequency of intercourse, low fluid intake and use of a contraceptive diaphragm.[80] The latter increases urethral pressure, reduces the urinary flow rate and may result in incomplete bladder emptying. Additionally, diaphragm use has been shown to increase vaginal pH, reduce colonization by lactobacilli, and increase colonization of the vagina and introitus by *Escherichia coli*.[81] Additionally, spermicidal cream containing nonoxynol-9 can kill lactobacilli and other vaginal flora, whilst most uropathogens and *Candida* thrive in its presence.[82]

Nocturnal enuresis

By 4 years of age 20–40% of normal children still wet the bed, with a spontaneous resolution rate of approximately 15% of cases each year; 1–2% retain the problem until adulthood, and in many cases lifelong (Fig. 1.2). Boys are more commonly affected than girls and heredity appears important.[83]

Rittig et al[84] investigated 15 enuretic children and 11 controls without nocturnal enuresis. Enuretic patients were found to lack the normal diurnal rhythm of vasopressin secretion and therefore suffered nocturnal polyuria. Bladder capacities of normal and enuretic children were similar and sleep patterns as judged by EEGs were similar in the two groups. Clinical trials of DDAVP (desmopressin) have revealed a second pathology, namely a nephrogenic receptor failure in which the renal collecting system is unresponsive to endogenous antidiuretic hormone (ADH) or exogenous DDAVP. What is unclear is why the enuretic child does not wake up when the bladder is full and needs emptying.

THE CLASSIFICATION OF LOWER URINARY TRACT DYSFUNCTION

The lower urinary tract comprises the bladder and urethra. Each has two functions, the bladder to store and void, and the urethra to control and convey. In addition the bladder and urethra have a complex synergistic

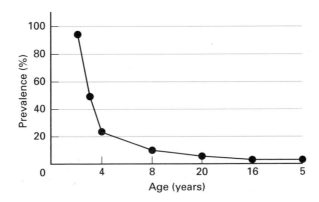

Fig. 1.2 The prevalence of nocturnal enuresis by age. (From Djurrhus et al. 1992. Nocturnal enuresis: a new strategy for treatment against a physiological background. Scand J Urol Nephrol Suppl 143: 7, with permission.)

relationship, of paramount importance for the preservation of normal lower urinary tract function. Together they form a single functional unit under complex neurological control, and dysfunction of one or both can result in urinary incontinence.

Assuming the absence of inflammation, infection and neoplasm, lower urinary tract dysfunction can be caused by:

- disturbances of neurological or psychological control
- disorders of muscle function
- structural abnormalities.

The International Continence Society classifies lower urinary tract dysfunction into disorders of the storage and voiding phases of the micturition cycle (Tables 1.5 and 1.6 respectively).

Urinary incontinence

For continence to exist urethral pressure must exceed intravesical pressure at all times except during voluntary micturition. Urinary incontinence is defined as the involuntary loss of urine which is a social or hygienic problem and is objectively demonstrable.[2]

Symptoms of urinary incontinence

Stress incontinence is the commonest symptom with which women present to a gynecologist, and indicates the involuntary loss of urine during physical exertion. *Urge incontinence* is the involuntary loss of urine associated with a strong desire to void. *Unconscious incontinence* is urinary leakage in the absence of urgency and without conscious recognition of the urine loss. *Enuresis* denotes any involuntary loss of urine, although it is usually used to describe incontinence during sleep (nocturnal enuresis). *Post-micturition dribble* and *continuous incontinence* are other symptomatic

Table 1.5   Lower urinary tract dysfunction during the storage phase of the micturition cycle (Abrams et al 1990)[2]

Bladder	
Detrusor activity	Normal
	Overactive (DI hyperreflexia)
Bladder sensation	Normal
	Increased (hypersensitive)
	Reduced (hyposensitive)
	Absent
Bladder capacity	$\triangle$ V/$\triangle$ P (Normally $\leq$ 15 cmH$_2$O pressure rise for filled volume $\leq$ 500 ml)
Urethra	
Urethral function	Normal
	Incompetent (urethral sphincter incompetence)

Table 1.6   Lower urinary tract dysfunction during the voiding phase of the micturition cycle

Detrusor	Acontractile (atonic bladder)
	Underactive (hypotonic bladder)
	Normal
Urethra	Obstructive (mechanical; urethral stricture; or
	Overactive; detrusor sphincter dyssynergia)

forms of urinary leakage often associated with prolapse, or a urethral diverticulum/fistula respectively.

Causes of urinary incontinence

The major causes of urinary incontinence may be listed as follows:

- GSI
- DI (detrusor hyperreflexia)
- overflow incontinence
- fistulae (vesicovaginal, ureterovaginal, urethrovaginal)
- congenital (e.g. epispadias/ectopic ureter)
- urethral diverticulum
- temporary (e.g. UTI, fecal impaction, drugs)
- functional (e.g. immobility).

GSI and DI can coexist (mixed incontinence).

Genuine stress incontinence This is a diagnosis made by urodynamic assessment. It is defined as the involuntary loss of urine when intravesical pressure exceeds the maximum urethral closure pressure in the absence of detrusor activity.[2] It occurs because the urethra is incompetent. This can be due to weakness in any component of the urethral sphincter mechanism as detailed below:

1. Supporting structures
   a. Pubourethral ligaments
   b. Pubovesical ligaments
2. Intrinsic sphincter mechanism
   a. Rhabdosphincter
   b. Collagen
   c. Urethral vascularity (smooth muscle)
3. Extrinsic sphincter mechanism
   a. Pelvic floor musculature.

The proximal urethra is normally maintained in an intra-abdominal position by its supporting structures. Weakness or damage to the pubourethral ligaments and the levator ani muscles results in descent of the proximal urethra such that it is no longer an intra-abdominal organ under the control of intra-abdominal pressure variations.

Damage to the rhabdosphincter or a scarred fibrosed urethra which cannot occlude properly will also result in GSI. Electromyographic studies have demonstrated denervation of both the intrinsic and extrinsic sphincter musculatue in women with GSI.[42,85] In addition, loss of urethral folds and the inability to form a watertight seal (due to loss of hermetic closure properties) will predispose to GSI.

Various factors are thought to predispose to the development of GSI and these may be listed as follows:

1. Raised intra-abdominal pressure due to
   a. Pregnancy
   b. Chronic bronchitis
   c. Abdominal/pelvic mass

    d. Ascites

    e. (Obesity)

2. Damage to the pelvic floor due to

    a. Childbirth

    b. Radical pelvic surgery

    c. (Menopause?)

3. Scarred 'drainpipe' urethra due to

    a. Vaginal surgery

    b. Surgery for GSI

    c. Urethral dilatation

    d. Recurrent urethritis

    e. Radiotherapy.

Detrusor instability The unstable detrusor is one that is shown objectively to contract, spontaneously or on provocation, during the filling phase of cystometry whilst the patient is attempting to inhibit micturition.[2] These contractions may result in the leakage of urine. The incidence increases with age and DI is the most common cause of urinary incontinence in the elderly.[5] Detrusor contractions may be either phasic or systolic, where they mimic the normal voiding reflex, or the bladder may demonstrate low compliance.

Urodynamic assessment is required to make a diagnosis. Women usually present with multiple symptoms, most commonly urgency, urge incontinence, frequency and nocturia. A list of the common causes of frequency and urgency of micturition is shown in Table 1.7.

The pathophysiology of DI is poorly understood, and an underlying cause for the condition is rarely found. In the majority of cases therefore the term idiopathic DI is used. Detrusor instability and urethral sphincter incompetence (GSI) can occur together, and DI can arise de novo following surgery for stress incontinence.

Phasic detrusor instability The cortical inhibition of detrusor contractions is part of the normal process of toilet training, and the most common form of DI, known as idiopathic DI, is thought to be an

Table 1.7   The causes of frequency and urgency of micturition

Type	Example
Gynecological/urological	UTI
	DI
	Inflammation (e.g. interstitial cystitis)
	Fibrosis (radiation)
	Atrophy (menopause)
	Intravesical lesion (e.g. calculus)
	Urethral pathology (e.g., urethral syndrome)
	External pressure (e.g. pelvic mass/fibroids)
	Pregnancy
Medical/psychological	Drugs (e.g., diuretics)
	Diabetes
	Neurological disease (e.g., multiple sclerosis)
	Excessive fluid intake
	Habit

unlearning, or poor initial learning, of this process. Research from Oxford[86] has suggested that DI may be a result of a functional denervation injury of the detrusor muscle. Experiments in pigs where partial urethral obstruction as piglets results in bladder hypertrophy, DI, supersensitivity of detrusor muscle to applied agonists with decreased response to transmural stimulation have confirmed this suspicion. Additionally histological evidence of denervation injury has been demonstrated.

Various authors have studied similar effects on the detrusor muscle of humans. Sibley[87] demonstrated supersensitivity to applied agonists in the detrusor muscle of women with DI and Kinder & Mundy[88] have also shown increased spontaneous activity in the detrusor muscle of these women. An excess of non-cholinergic neurotransmitters has been reported as the cause of this increased spontaneous activity.[89,90] Other studies have suggested the presence of inhibitory neurotransmitters which are decreased in cases of DI.[91]

Any neurological condition which interrupts the cortical inhibition of reflex detrusor contractions will result in unstable detrusor contractions. This is known as detrusor hyperreflexia and causes include multiple sclerosis and spinal cord lesions.

Irritation of the bladder epithelium may result in unstable detrusor contractions but more commonly causes the symptoms of urgency and frequency without actual detrusor contractions.

Urethral outflow obstruction can lead to incomplete bladder emptying which may result in the symptoms of urgency and frequency.

Low compliance In this condition there is an excessive rise in detrusor pressure associated with bladder filling. There are a variety of causes which include radiotherapy, radical pelvic surgery, recurrent UTI, pelvic masses and interstitial cystitis. These patients are often symptomatically the same as those with DI and low compliance may be difficult to distinguish from systolic detrusor contractions on cystometry. The different types of DI may be summarized as follows:

1. Idiopathic
2. Psychosomatic
3. Neurological
   a. Spinal cord injury
   b. Multiple sclerosis
   c. Diabetic neuropathy
4. Low compliance
5. Outflow obstruction
6. Postsurgical.

Sensory urgency This is diagnosed when there are intense irritative bladder symptoms in the absence of unstable detrusor contractions. Patients have a reduced functional bladder capacity (usually <400 ml), daytime frequency, nocturia, and sometimes incontinence. It may be caused by inflammatory conditions of the bladder or urethra (e.g. interstitial cystitis, atrophic urethritis), which can sometimes be diagnosed by cystoscopy and bladder biopsy.

Overflow incontinence This is a condition in which the bladder becomes a large flaccid bag with little or no detrusor activity. Occasionally, where there is chronic outflow obstruction the bladder becomes small and trabeculated due to fibrosis but again there is little or no detrusor activity. The woman fails to void and the bladder merely leaks each time it becomes full. In addition, due to the very small functional bladder capacity, she may develop frequency of micturition and recurrent lower and indeed upper urinary tract infections. Such injury can occur following epidural anesthesia used for obstetric delivery. Invariably poor catheter management means that overdistension occurs a number of times following the initial insult, compounding the original problem. If left unrecognized or inappropriately treated the detrusor may fail to work again, even after the initial cause has resolved.

The long-term sequelae include hydroureter and hydronephrosis with chronic reflux nephropathy and deteriorating renal function. Retention of urine of this sort can occasionally result secondary to detrusor–sphincter dyssynergia where, in addition to outflow obstruction, the bladder is hyperreflexic secondary to neurological bladder dysfunction and high detrusor pressures can predispose to rapidly deteriorating renal function.

The female bladder is particularly sensitive to overdistension and even one episode of acute retention of urine can result in a chronically atonic bladder and often the need for long-term clean intermittent self-catheterization. The diagnosis is made when the urinary residual is in excess of 50% of the bladder capacity. The different causes of overflow incontinence are shown in Table 1.8.

Overflow incontinence is the extreme of conditions which result in voiding difficulties and any of the conditions listed may cause a poor stream and incomplete bladder emptying without the development of incontinence.

Genuine stress incontinence, DI and overflow incontinence are the most common causes of urinary incontinence in women. Genuine stress in-

Table 1.8   The causes of overflow incontinence of urine

Acute retention	Secondary to surgery (any operation particularly gynecological and rectal surgery)
	Secondary to pain (e.g. *Herpes genitalis*)
Drugs	Tricyclic antidepressants
	Anticholinergic agents
	Alpha-adrenergic agonists
	Epidural analgesia
UTI	
Urethral Stricture	Surgery for GSI
	Urethral surgery (e.g. dilatations)
	Vaginal surgery
	Recurrent urinary tract infections
	Radiotherapy
Pelvic mass	Fibroids
	Fecal impaction
Cystocele	
Detrusor hypotonia	Lower motor neurone lesions (e.g. diabetes mellitus)
Psychogenic	Dementia

continence accounts for 50% of cases and DI 40%. Overflow incontinence accounts for most of the remaining 10%.

Fistulae secondary to obstetric trauma are a common cause of incontinence in developing countries and often a reason why women are abandoned by their husbands and cast out of their community. In the developed world fistulae are usually secondary to gynecological surgery although they are fortunately rare.

ECONOMIC ISSUES AND URINARY INCONTINENCE

Urinary incontinence is one of the most common chronic conditions experienced by women, affecting at least 14% of women over 30 years of age, and as many as 50% of nursing home residents. Studies of the economic impact of urinary incontinence are scarce, however, primarily because of the varying results of prevalence studies, the absence of reliable risk factor analysis and cost data and wide diversification of treatment strategies. Most of the available data have been collected in the USA and Scandanavia, and have focused on the cost of caring for incontinent people in nursing homes.

In 1986 Hu[92] studied the direct and indirect costs of urinary incontinence in the USA. Direct costs include those required to diagnose, treat, care for, and rehabilitate incontinent patients. Indirect costs include lost productivity of patients and unpaid carers and other expenses due to ill health. Based on multiple assumptions regarding incontinence prevalence rate and cost information, Hu estimated that the entire economic cost in 1984 of urinary incontinence was $8.1 billion; $6.6 billion direct costs and $1.5 billion indirect costs in the USA. Costs incurred by nursing homes, which are all direct costs, totalled $1.8 billion, which represents about 10% of nursing home expenditure.

Whether the investigation and treatment of urinary incontinence actually decreases the economic burden of urinary incontinence is unproven but likely to be the case. Ouslander & Kane[93] showed that active evaluation and treatment of nursing home residents resulted in considerable cost savings. Irrespective of direct financial incentives, the effective treatment of urinary incontinence considerably improves the quality of life of sufferers, the cost of which is difficult to quantify.

CONCLUSION

In October 1988 an expert panel of urogynecologists, urologists, geriatricians, epidemiologists, nurses, basic scientists and members of the public met at the National Institute of Health in America to consider the current state of our knowledge on all aspects of urinary incontinence.[94] A number of central issues were discussed.

1. What are the prevalence and the clinical, psychological and social impact of urinary incontinence among persons living at home and in institutions?

2. What are the pathophysiological and functional factors leading to urinary incontinence?
3. What diagnostic information should be obtained in the assessment of the incontinent patient, and what criteria should be employed to determine which tests are indicated?
4. What are the efficacies and limitations of behavioral, pharmacological, surgical and other treatments for urinary incontinence? What sequences or combination of these interventions are appropriate, and what management techniques should be employed when they fail or are not indicated?
5. What strategies are useful in improving public and professional knowledge about urinary incontinence?
6. What are the needs for future research related to urinary incontinence?

Many questions raised at the conference remained unanswered and the relevant chapters of this book attempt to cover these important issues. Although further advances have been made since that time the conclusions of this conference are still relevant to our current state of knowledge.

1. Although prevalent, urinary incontinence is never normal, and is always a symptom of an underlying problem(s).
2. Regardless of age, cognitive capacity or residential status, incontinence can often be cured, usually improved and always managed.

REFERENCES

1 Health Survey Questionnaire: Market and Opinion Research International (MORI). 1990; 95 Southwark Street, London SE1 OHX.
2 Abrams P, Blaivas JG, Stanton SL, Andersen JT. The standardisation of terminology of lower urinary tract function. Br J Obstet Gynaecol 1990; 97: (Suppl 6) 1–16.
3 Mäkinen JI, Grönroos M, Kiilholma PJA et al. The prevalence of incontinence in a randomised population of 5247 adult Swedish women. Int Urogynecol J 1992; 3(2): 110–113.
4 Wyman JF, Harkins S, Choi S, Taylor J, Fantl JA. Psychosocial impact of urinary incontinence in women. Obstet Gynaecol 1987; 70: 378–380.
5 Malone Lee J. Lower urinary tract function in late life. In Handbook of Neurourology ed D. Rushton Marcel Dekker. New York. 1994; pp 349–368.
6 Milne JS, Williamson J, Maule MM. Urinary symptoms in older people. Modern Geriatrics. 1972; 2: 198.
7 Thomas TM, Plymat KR, Blannin J, Meade TW. Prevalence of urinary incontinence. Br Med J 1980; 281: 1243–1245.
8 Yarnell J, Voyle G, Richards C, Stephenson T. The prevalence and severity of urinary incontinence in women. J Epidemiol Community Health 1981; 35: 71–4.
9 Vetter NJ, Jones DA, Victor CR. Urinary incontinence in the elderly at home. Lancet 1981; 2: 1275.
10 Diokno AC, Brock BM, Brown MB et al. Prevalence of urinary incontinence and other urological symptoms in the non institutionalised elderly. J Urol 1986; 136: 1022.
11 Yarnell JWG, St Leger AS. The prevalence, severity, and factors associated with urinary incontinence in a random sample of the elderly. Age Ageing 1979; 8: 81.
12 Campbell AJ, Reinken J, McCosh L. Incontinence in the elderly, prevalence and prognosis. Age Ageing 1985; 14: 65.
13 Ouslander JG. Urinary incontinence in nursing homes. JAGS 1990; 38: 289–291.

14 Versi E, Cardozo L, Anand D, Cooper D. Symptoms analysis for the diagnosis of genuine stress incontinence. Br J Obstet Gynaecol 1991; 98 (8): 815–819.

15 Bergman A, Bader K. Reliability of the patient's history in the diagnosis of urinary incontinence. Int J Gynaecol Obstet 1990; 32: 255–259.

16 Svanborg A. The gerontological and geriatric population study in Göteborg, Sweden. Acta Med Scand 1977; Suppl 611: 1–37.

17 Gjorup T, Hendriksen C, Lund E, Stromgard E. Is growing old a disease? A study of the attitudes of elderly people to physical symptoms. J Chron Dis 1987; 40(12): 1095–1098.

18 Herzog AR, Fultz NH. Prevalence and incidence of urinary incontinence in community dwelling populations. JAGS 1990; 38: 273–281.

19 Cardozo LD. Role of estrogens in the treatment of female urinary incontinence. JAGS 1990; 38: 326–328.

20 Iosif S, Batra S, Ek A, Astedt B. Oestrogen receptors in the human female lower urinary tract. Am J Obstet Gynaecol 1981; 141: 817–820.

21 Batra SC, Fosil CS. Female urethra, a target for estrogen action. J Urol 1983; 129: 418–420.

22 Batra SC, Iosif LS. Progesterone receptors in the female lower urinary tract. J Urol 1987; 138: 1301–1304.

23 Van Geelen JM, Doesburg WH, Thomas CMG, Martin CB. Urodynamic studies in the normal menstrual cycle: the relationship between hormonal changes in the menstrual cycle and urethral pressure profiles. Am J Obstet Gynaecol 1981; 141(4): 384–392.

24 Tapp AJS, Cardozo LD. The postmenopausal bladder. Br J Hosp Med 1986; 35: 20–23.

25 McCallin PE, Stewart Taylor E, Whitehead RW. A study of the changes in cytology of the urinary sediment during the menstrual cycle and pregnancy. Am J Obstet Gynaecol 1950; 60: 64–74.

26 Solomon C, Panagotopoulous P, Oppenheim A. Urinary cytology studies as an aid to diagnosis. Am J Obstet Gynaecol 1958; 76: 57–62.

27 Iosif CS. Bekassy Z. Prevalence of genito-urinary symptoms in the later menopause. Acta Obstet Gynecol Scand 1984; 63: 257–260.

28 Jolleys JV. Reported prevalence of urinary incontinence in women in general practice. Br Med J 1988; 296: 1300–1302.

29 Kondo A, Kato K, Saito M, Otani T. Prevalence of hand washing urinary incontinence in females in comparison with stress and urge incontinence. Neurourol and Urodynam 1990; 9: 330–331.

30 Versi E, Cardozo LD. Estrogens and lower urinary tract function. In: Studd JWW, Whitehead MI (eds) The menopause 1988: pp 76–84, Blackwell Scientific Publications.

31 Van Wagenen G, Jenkins RH. An experimental examination of factors causing ureteral dilatation of pregnancy. J Urol 1939; 42: 1010–1020.

32 Youssef AF. Cystometric studies in gynaecology and obstetrics. Obstet Gynaecol. 1956; 8: 181–188.

33 Gritsch E, Brandsfetter F. Phasen Sphinktero-Zystometrie. Zentralbl Gunaekol 1954; 39: 1746–1750.

34 Van Geelen JM, Lemmens WAJG, Eskes TKAB, Martin LB Jr. The urethral pressure profile in pregnancy and delivery in healthy nulliparous women. Am J Obstet Gyneacol 1982; 144: 636–649.

35 Benness C, Gangar K, Cardozo LD, Cutner A, Whitehead M. Do progestogens exacerbate incontinence in women on HRT? Neurourol and Urodynam 1991; 10: 316–318.

36 Olah KJ, Bridges N, Farrer D. The conservative management of genuine stress incontinence. Int Urogynaecol J 1991; 2: 161–167.

37 Zacharin RF. 'A Chinese anatomy' the pelvic supporting tissues of the Chinese and Occidental female compared and contrasted. Aust NZ J Obstet Gynaecol 1977; 17: 1.

38 Bump RC. Racial comparisons and contrasts in urinary incontinence and genital prolapse. Neurourol and Urodynam 1992; 11(4): 357–358.

39 Cutner A, Cardozo LD, Benness CJ. Assessment of urinary symptoms in the second half of pregnancy. Int Urogynaecol J 1992; 3: 30–32.

40 Gilpin SA, Gosling JA, Smith ARB, Warrell DW. The pathogenesis of genitourinary prolapse and stress incontinence of urine; a histological and histochemical study. Br J Obstet Gynaecol 1989; 96: 15–23.

41 Snooks SJ, Badenoch D, Tiptaft R, Swash M. Perineal nerve damage in genuine stress incontinence: an electrophysiological study. Br J Urol 1985; 57: 422–426.

42 Smith ARB, Hosker GL, Warrell DW. The role of pudendal nerve damage in the aetiology of genuine stress incontinence in women. Br J Obstet Gynaecol 1989; 96: 29–32.

43 Wilson D, Herbison P, Borland M, Grant A. A randomised trial of physiotherapy treatment of post natal urinary incontinence. Proceedings of the 26th British Congress of Obstetrics and Gynaecology. Manchester, 1992: 162.

44 Bo K, Stien R. Pelvic floor muscle function and urethral closure mechanism in young nullipara subjects with and without stress incontinence symptoms. Neurourology and Urodynamics 1993; 12 (4): 432–434.

45 Landon CR, Smith ARB. Biomechanical properties of connective tissue in women with stress incontinence of urine. Neurourology and Urodynamics 1989; 8: 369–370.

46 Sayer TR, Dixon JS, Hosker GL, Warrell DW. A study of paraurethral connective tissue in women with stress incontinence of urine. Neurourol and Urodynam 1990; 9: 319–320.

47 Keane DP, Sims TJ, Bailey AJ, Abrams P. Analysis of pelvic floor electromyography and collagen status in pre-menopausal nulliparous females with genuine stress incontinence. Neurourol and Urodynam 1992; 11(4): 308–309.

48 Norton P, Boyd C, Mitchell MD, Deak S. Altered Type I: Type III collagen ratio in patients with genital prolapse. (Abstract 420) Presented to the 39th Annual meeting of the Society for Gynecologic Investigation, San Antonio, Texas. 18–21 March 1992.

49 Bergman A, Chung D, Perelman N, Nimni ME. Biochemical composition of collagen in continent and stress incontinent women (Abstract 418) Presented at the 39th Annual meeting of the Society for Gynecologic Investigation, San Antonio, Texas, 18–21 March 1992.

50 Dwyer PL, Lee ETC, Hay DM. Obesity and urinary incontinence in women. Br J Obstet Gynaecol 1988; 95: 91.

51 Bump RC, Sugarman HJ, Fantl JA, McClish DK. Obesity and lower urinary tract function in women. Effects of surgically induced weight loss. 1992 Am J Obstet Gynecol 167 (2): 392–397.

52 Bump RC, McClish DK. Cigarette smoking and urinary incontinence in women. Am J Obstet Gynaecol 1992; 167: 1213.

53 Spence-Jones C, Kamm MA, Hudson CN. Bowel dysfunction: a pathogenic factor in uterovaginal prolapse and urinary stress incontinence. Neurourol and Urodynam 1992; 11(4): 313–314.

54 Petri E. Bladder dysfunction after radical surgery. In Ostergaard DR (ed) Gynecologic urology and urodynamics. Theory and practice. Baltimore, Williams and Wilkins, 1985: pp 545–555.

55 Farghaly SA, Hindmarsh JA, Worth PHL. Post hysterectomy urethral dysfunction: evaluation and management. Br J Urol 1986; 58: 299–302.

56 Parys BT, Woolfenden KA, Parsons KF. Bladder dysfunction after simple hysterectomy: urodynamic and neurological evaluation. Eur Urol 1990; 17: 129–133.

57 Brown ADG, Weir J, Jequier ADM, Whiteside CG, Turner-Warwick R. A urodynamic study of the effect of hysterectomy on the bladder. In: Proceedings of the 4th Annual meeting of the International Continence Society, Mainz 3, 1974.

58 Langer R, Neuman M, Ron El R et al. The effect of total abdominal hysterectomy on bladder function in asymptomatic women. Obstet Gynaecol 1989; 74: 205–207.

59 Kikku P. Supravaginal uterine amputation versus hysterectomy with reference to subjective bladder symptoms and incontinence. Acta Obstet Gynecol Scand 1985; 64: 375–379.

60 Mundy AR. An anatomical explanation for bladder dysfunction following rectal and uterine surgery. 1989; Br J Urol 54: 501–504.

61 Parys BT. Lower urinary tract dysfunction after total hysterectomy. Int Urogynaecol J 1992; 12: 108–111.

62 Grady M, Kozminski M, Delancey J, Elkins T, McGuire EJ. Stress incontinence and cystoceles. 1991; J Urol 145: 1211–1213.

63 Rosenzweig BA, Soffici AR, Thomas S, Bhatia NN. Urodynamic evaluation of women with cystocele. 1992; J Reprod Med. 37: 162–166.

64 Rosenzweig BA, Pushkin S, Blumenfeld D, Bhatia NN. Prevalence of abnormal urodynamic test results in continent women with severe genitourinary prolapse. Obstet Gynecol 1992; 79: 539–542.

65 Thomas TM, Fischer AM, Walsh JM et al. Urinary incontinence before and after pelvic floor surgery. Proceedings of the 8th meeting of the International Continence Society, Oxford: Pergamon Press, 1978: pp 163–166.

66 Meyhoff HH, de Nully MB, Oleson KP, Lindahl F. The effects of vaginal repair on anterior bladder suspension defects. Obstet Gynecol Scand 1985; 64: 433–435.

67 Iosif S, Ulmsten U. Urodynamic studies of women with prolapse and stress incontinence before and after surgical repair. Zbl Gynecol 1979; 101: 1433–1437 (English Abstract).

68 Walter S, Oleson KP, Hald T et al. Urodynamic evaluation after vaginal repair and colposuspension. Br J Urol 1982; 54: 377–380.

69 Borstad E. The risk of urinary stress incontinence after anterior vaginal repair. Urogynecol J 1992; 3: 163–167.

70 Hendry WF. Diagnosis and management of primary bladder cancer: a British perspective. In: Raghaven D (ed) The management of bladder cancer, p 68–69. London: Edward Arnold, 1988: pp 68–69.

71 Parkin DE, Davis JA, Symonds RP. Urodynamic findings following radiotherapy for cervical carcinoma. Br J Urol 1988; 61: 213–217.

72 Vale JA, Trott KR, Whitfield HN. Post-radiotherapy bladder dysfunction-adenervation disorder? Neurourol and Urodynam 1991; 10(4): 349–350.

73 Sanfod JP. Urinary tract symptoms and infections. Ann Rev Med 1975; 26: 485–498.

74 Johnson JR, Stamm WE. Diagnosis and treatment of acute urinary tract infections. Infect Dis Clin North America 1987; 1: 773–791.

75 Mabeck CE. Treatment of uncomplicated urinary tract infection in non pregnant women. Ann Rev Med 1982; 26: 485–498.

76 Warren JW. Urine collection devices for use in adults with urinary incontinence. JAGS 1990; 38: 364–367.

77 Raz R, Stamm WE. A controlled trial of intravaginal oestriol in post menopausal women with recurrent urinary tract infections. New Engl J Med 1993; 329(11): 753–756.

78 Buckley RM, McGuckin M, MacGregor RR. Urine bacterial counts after sexual intercourse. N Engl J Med 1978; 298: 321–324.

79 Adatto K, Doebele KG, Galland L et al. Behavioural factors and urinary tract infection. JAMA 1979; 241, 2525–2526.

80 Leibovici L. Behavioural risk factors for urinary tract infections in women. Int Urogynecol J 1991; 12: 105–107.

81 Hooton TM, Fihn SD, Johnson C, Roberts PL, Stamm WE. Association between bacterial vaginosis and acute cystitis in women using diaphragms. Arch Int Med 1989; 1932–1936.

82 McGroarty JA, Chong S, Reid G, Bruce AW. Influence of the spermicidal compound Nonoxynol-9 on the growth and adhesion of urogenital bacteria in vitro. Curr Microbiol 1990; 21: 219–223.

83 Djurhuus JC, Norgaard JP, Hjälmäs K, Wille S. Nocturnal enuresis: a new strategy for treatment against a physiological background. Scand J Urol Nephrol 1992; (Suppl 143): 7

84 Rittig S, Knudsen UB, Norgaard JP et al. Abnormal diurnal rhythms of plasma vasopressin and urinary output in patients with enuresis. Am J Physiol 1989; 256: F664.

85 Allen RE, Hosker GL, Smith ARB, Warrell DW. Pelvic floor damage and childbirth: a neurophysiological study. Br J Obstet Gynaecol 1990; 97: 770–779.

86 Brading AF, Turner WH. The unstable bladder: towards a common mechanism. Br J Urol 1994; 73: 3–8.

87 Sibley GNA. An experimental model of detrusor instability in the obstructed pig. Br J Urol 1985; 57: 292–298.

88 Kinder RB, Mundy AR. Atropine blockade of nerve mediated stimulation of human detrusor. Br J Urol 1985; 57: 418–421.

89 Hindmarsh JR, Idowu OA, Yeates WK, Zar MA. Pharmacology of evoked contractions of human bladder. Br J Pharmacol 1977; 61: 115.

90 Sjogren C, Andersson KE, Husted S, Mattiasson A, Moller-Madsen B. Atropine resistance of transmurally stimulated isolated human bladder muscle. J Urol 1982; 128: 1368–1371.

91 Gu J, Blank MA, Huang WM et al. Vasoactive intestinal polypeptide in the normal and unstable bladder. Br J Urol 1983; 55: 645–647.

92 Hu TW. The economic impact of urinary incontinence. Clin Geriatr Med 1986; 2: 673.

93 Ouslander JG, Kane RL. The cost of urinary incontinence in nursing homes. Med Care 1983; 22: 69.

94 National Institutes of Health Consensus Development Conference. Urinary Incontinence in Adults. J Am Geriatr Soc 1990; 38: 265–272.

Section 2 Basic Science

2

Embryology and anatomy

INTRODUCTION

The lower urinary tract comprises the bladder and urethra. In association with supporting ligaments and muscles they act as a single functional unit with a dual role to store urine (passive) and to expel it (active). The male and female lower urinary tracts, although similar in many ways, have distinct differences and part of this may be due to their different embryological and fetal development.

EMBRYOLOGY

By the 12th day after fertilization the embryo has developed from a single ball of cells into a bilaminar structure containing ectoderm and endoderm. These layers subsequently become separated by the mesoderm at 17 days (Fig. 2.1).[1] The endoderm is initially a layer of cells

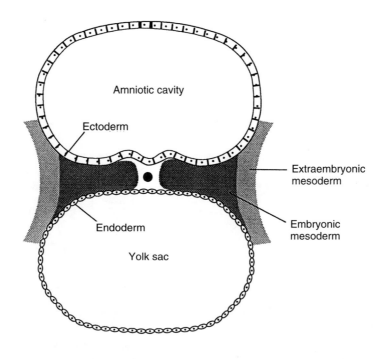

Fig. 2.1 Cross-section of a 17-day-old embryo

lining the embryonic yolk sac. Part of this invaginates into the embryo to form the foregut, midgut and hindgut by 4 weeks. The remainder comes to lie within the umbilical cord as the vitellointestinal duct. A diverticulum develops from the hindgut and is known as the allantois (Fig. 2.2).[1] That part of the hindgut which is connected to the allantois is called the cloaca (Fig. 2.3).[1] Division of the cloaca by a wedge of mesenchymal tissue called the urorectal septum, by 6 weeks, results in

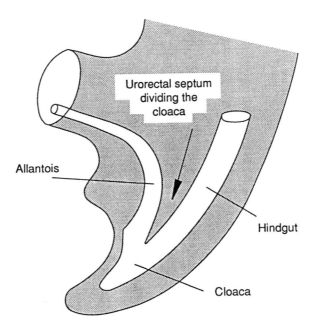

Fig. 2.2 Longitudinal section of a 4-week-old embryo

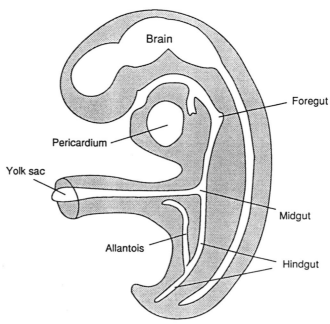

Fig. 2.3 Longitudinal section of a 5-week-old embryo

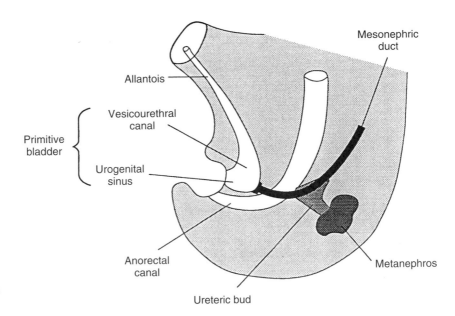

Mesonephric duct

Allantois

Vesicourethral canal

Primitive bladder

Urogenital sinus

Anorectal canal

Metanephros

Ureteric bud

Fig. 2.4 Longitudinal section of a 6-week-old embryo

an anterior part (the primitive bladder) and a posterior part (the anorectal canal).[2,3,4]

At the same time the kidneys are developing. The first stage is the pronephros but this disappears by 4 weeks. The mesonephros is derived from mesenchymal tissue and its developing tubules open into a single collecting duct on each side known as the mesonephric duct. The mesonephros functions initially as a primitive kidney but subsequently undergoes degeneration. This is largely complete by 12 weeks. The mesonephric duct develops an outgrowth, the ureteric bud, which will become the ureter. The distal end of the mesonephric duct enters the anterior part of the cloaca (primitive bladder) on each side.[2,3,4,5] The mesonephric ducts divide the primitive bladder into two parts: the area above is the vesicourethral canal and the area below is the urogenital sinus (Fig. 2.4).[1] The upper part of the vesicourethral canal dilates to form the bladder whilst the caudal portion remains narrow to form the upper urethra. The urogenital sinus forms the distal part of the urethra.

The caudal part of the mesonephric duct is absorbed by the bladder, thus drawing in the ureteric duct. With growth of the bladder the ureteric ducts move laterally and the mesonephric ducts come to lie more caudally close together at that part of the primitive bladder which will become the urethra. The area of the bladder derived from the mesonephric ducts will become the trigone and can be defined by 6 weeks (Fig. 2.5).[1] Thus the upper part of the bladder is derived from the yolk sac and lined by endoderm, and the trigone, derived from the mesonephric ducts, is lined by cells of mesodermal origin. It is generally believed that the trigonal surface is later replaced by cells of endodermal origin.[3,4,6]

The most caudal part of the cloaca is called the urogenital sinus and this forms the distal part of the urethra and vagina in the female. The fallopian tubes, uterus and cervix are formed from the paramesonephric ducts, which are an invagination of coelomic epithelium of mesodermal

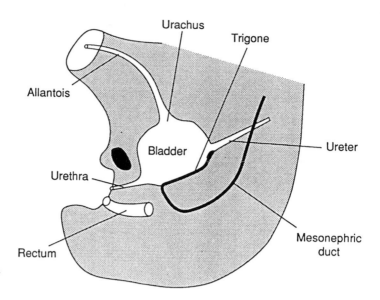

Fig. 2.5 Longitudinal section of an 8-week-old embryo

origin. Thus the fallopian tubes, uterus and trigone appear to have a common embryological origin and the upper bladder, the urethra and vagina another. In the male, part of the penile urethra is derived from the genital tubercles, which are ectodermal in origin. The membranous urethra and distal part of the prostatic urethra are formed from the urogenital sinus, and the proximal part of the prostatic urethra is derived from the mesonephric ducts. Full development occurs by the 12th week.

We have studied the development of the lower urinary tract in fetuses obtained at termination of pregnancy.[7] Its growth occurs in a linear fashion (Figs 2.6 and 2.7). The male and female bladder have obvious differences in the fetal stage; the verumontanum can be identified on the posterior surface of the male urethra as early as 10 weeks[5,7] (Fig. 2.8). The male urinary tract is longer than the female and this difference increases with fetal age. The difference is accounted for by the length of the urethra as there are no differences in the length of the bladder with fetal sex (Fig. 2.6). It is interesting that not only the external features grow in a linear manner but also the trigone. We have demonstrated linear growth of the interureteric distance and the side of the trigone and there were no sex differences present. In addition the trigone forms an equilateral triangle in all cases.[5,7]

Although cells may be derived from a common origin further differentiation occurs to correspond to function. Studies of both human and animal lower urinary tract epithelium have demonstrated this process of differentiation.[8,9] Thus the structure and function of the adult lower urinary tract is determined by its embryological origins and subsequent differentiation.

Bladder

The muscular development of the lower urinary tract has been described by several authors.[2,5,10,11] Some suggest that the smooth muscle of the

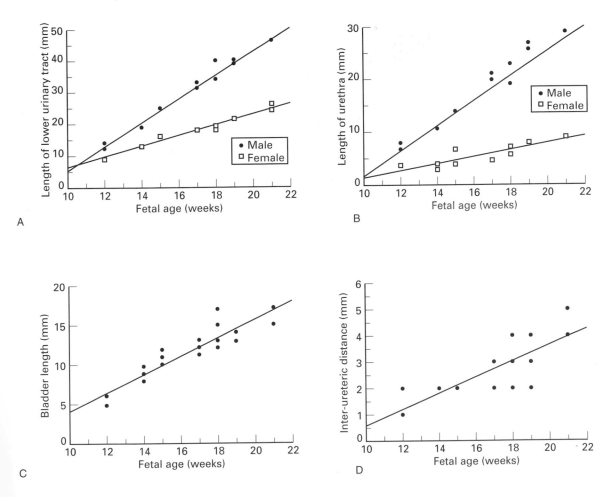

Fig. 2.6 Graphical representation of the growth of the human fetal lower urinary tract: **A** lower urinary tract; **B** urethra; **C** bladder; **D** interureteric distance. (From Cutner et al 1992. Growth of the normal human lower urinary tract from 12 to 21 weeks gestation. Anatom Rec 234(4): 568–574, with permission.)

Fig. 2.7 Growth of the lower urinary tract: **A** 12-week male bladder; **B** 15-week male bladder; **C** 19-week male bladder. (From Cutner et al 1992. Growth of the normal human lower urinary tract from 12 to 21 weeks gestation. Anatom Rec 234(4): 568–574, with permission.)

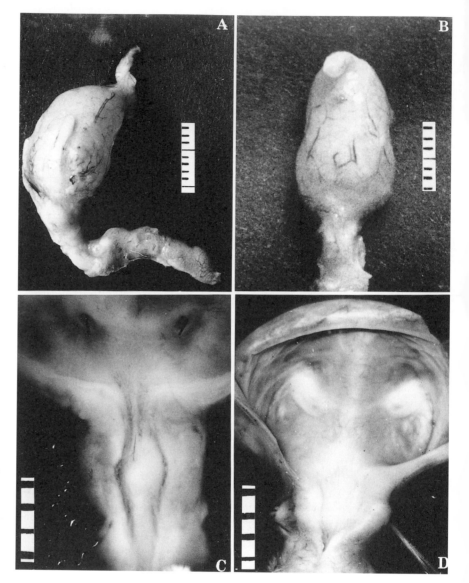

Fig. 2.8 **A** Right lateral view of a 19-week distended male bladder. **B** Anterior view of a 19-week distended female bladder. **C** The opened male bladder at the region of the trigone and proximal urethra. The uteric orifices have been probed with a hair. Note the presence of the verumontanum on the posterior wall of the urethra. **D** The opened female bladder. Note the absence of the verumontanum. (From Cutner et al 1992. Growth of the normal human lower urinary tract from 12 to 21 weeks gestation. Anatom Rec 234(4): 568–574, with permission.)

detrusor and urethra are of the same origin and form a continuous structure surrounding the bladder and urethra which can be considered as a single tube.[2,10] However, Droes[11] examined 5 male and 6 female fetuses. He showed that the lower urinary tract smooth muscle develops as three distinct systems: the detrusor muscle, the trigonal muscle system and the urethral smooth muscle. The detrusor muscle surrounds the whole bladder and consists of three layers. It is fixed to surrounding structures by longitudinal bundles of fibres. The trigonal muscle consists of an inner longitudinal layer and an outer circular layer and is continuous with the ureteral musculature. Its fibres pass between bundles of the detrusor muscle and completely encircle the proximal part of the urethra.

Urethra

The urethral smooth musculature consists of an outer circular layer and inner longitudinal layer surrounding the middle part of the urethra in a horseshoe shape. The intimate relationship of the muscle groups led to the original belief that they formed a single unit but their distinct nature explains some disorders of micturition.

The urethral striated muscle surrounds the smooth muscle and extends to the lower edge of the detrusor muscle. It is horseshoe-shaped, thickest anteriorly surrounding the proximal part of the urethra and inserting into the trigonal region. Caudally the fibres insert into the lateral vaginal wall and the perineal body. With development of the striated muscle, the urethral smooth muscle largely disappears in the female.

The development of receptors in animal bladders and the changes with increasing fetal age have been studied in animal models.[12,13] There is very little work on the human fetal lower urinary tract, but one group of investigators has studied autonomic receptors in human fetal material.[14] They discovered that cholinergic receptors were present on the detrusor and urethral sphincter as early as 4 months gestation, but although their density increases in the detrusor with increasing fetal age, there is a gradual reduction in the urethral sphincter. α-adrenergic receptors developed after 6 months but only in the urethral sphincter. β-adrenergic receptors were present only in the detrusor. Thus the fetus develops the adult arrangement of receptors although some differences are present early in development.

ANATOMY

The lower urinary tract is lined by transitional cell epithelium. The wall of the bladder is composed of a syncytium of smooth muscle fibres known as the detrusor. Contraction of this mesh of fibres results in simultaneous reduction of the bladder in all its diameters. The triangular area of the bladder bounded by the two ureteric orifices and the top of the urethra is known as the trigone. The smooth muscle of the trigone has two layers as in the fetal bladder.[11] This is less developed than the detrusor which extends behind it. The trigone is of different embryological origin[2,3,4,5] and this may account for the finding of stratified squamous epithelium in some women.[15,16]

The female urethra is about 4–5 cm long. At the bladder neck there is smooth muscle but this is not thought to be functionally important in the female. There is controversy as to whether this is continuous or distinct from the detrusor.[10,11,17,18,19,20] It was originally believed to be a distinct entity consisting of an inner longitudinal and outer oblique layer. However, more recently it has been referred to as the detrusor loop[20] (Fig. 2.9). This part of the detrusor has α-adrenergic innervation and its malfunction is believed to occur in women who have an open bladder neck. The significance of an open bladder neck remains doubtful.[21] However, it is more common in women with genuine stress incontinence.[22]

The functional anatomy of the bladder neck, urethra and pelvic floor and the mechanism by which continence is maintained is not fully

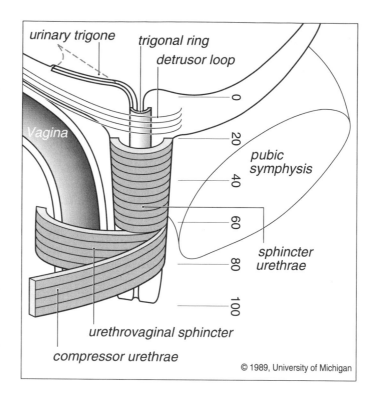

urinary trigone   trigonal ring
detrusor loop

0

Vagina

20

pubic
symphysis

40

60

sphincter
urethrae

80

100

urethrovaginal sphincter

compressor urethrae

© 1989, University of Michigan

Fig. 2.9 The component parts of the internal and external sphincteric mechanisms and their locations. The sphincter urethrae, urethrovaginal sphincter and compressor urethrae are all parts of the striated urogenital sphincter muscle. (With permission from John DeLancey.)

understood. Recently the original concepts have been challenged by DeLancey.[20,23,24]

Functional anatomy of the bladder neck and urethra

Original concept The original belief was that the urethral sphincter was divided into intrinsic and extrinsic portions[25] (Fig. 2.10), the intrinsic part consisting of epithelial, vascular, connective tissue and muscular elements. The muscular element is the rhabdosphincter, which is a circular ring of striated muscle. It is thickest anteriorly, thins laterally and is virtually absent posteriorly. The muscle contains mainly slow twitch fibres which are able to contract over long periods of time without fatiguing. This is important in the maintenance of continence at rest.

The extrinsic portion comprises the striated muscle of the levator ani through which the urethra passes. Its fibres run laterally to the urethra just inferior to the rhabdosphincter. The fibres are mainly of the fast twitch variety and are therefore able to contract more efficiently but over shorter periods of time. This is important during periods of exertion or sudden stress when there are increases in the intra-abdominal pressure.

The bladder neck is supported and maintained in the correct position by connective tissue supports. These are known as the pubovesical or pubourethral ligaments. Some authors have attributed a purely static role to these structures.[26,27] Others[28,29] have demonstrated active opening of the bladder neck on initiation of micturition, suggesting that the ligament is not merely supportive in nature. Indeed it is partly composed

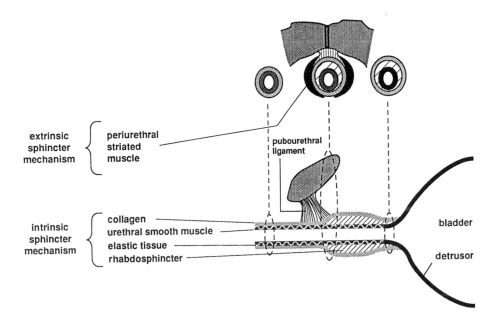

extrinsic sphincter mechanism { periurethral striated muscle

pubourethral ligament

intrinsic sphincter mechanism { collagen — urethral smooth muscle — elastic tissue — rhabdosphincter —

bladder

detrusor

Fig. 2.10 The bladder neck and urethra showing the components of the urethral sphincter mechanism

of smooth muscle. These supports maintain the proximal two-thirds of the urethra in an intra-abdominal position.

The final anatomical factor important in lower urinary tract function is the urethral mucosa. The urethra is lined by transitional cell epithelium but distally the lining becomes stratified squamous epithelium. The sub-mucosa contains a venous plexus which contributes to urethral resistance and helps it to form a watertight seal. However, there is conflicting opinion regarding the importance of the vascular plexus in the maintenance of continence.[30,31]

According to the above theory, continence during exertion depends on the correct position of the proximal urethra, an intact extrinsic urethral sphincter mechanism and the state of the urethral mucosa. Appropriate voiding relies on voluntary relaxation of the urethral sphincter.

New concept The concepts put forward by DeLancey[20,23,24] explain some of the apparent contradictions between anatomy and function. He suggests three factors in the maintenance of continence: correct support of the bladder neck and urethra, the internal sphincter and the external sphincter. If one mechanism fails then the others may be able to compensate. Thus all systems work in unison.

The original idea was that the intra-abdominal pressure needed to be transmitted to the proximal urethra, which was supposed to lie above the pelvic floor. This would not explain how some women with a large cystocele remain continent. The original explanation was that the cystocele caused kinking of the urethra and relative outflow obstruction, but not all continent women with a cystocele have voiding difficulties. DeLancey[20] suggests that raised intra-abdominal pressure causes downward pressure and descent of the urethra and the anterior vaginal wall. As long as the anterior vaginal wall is supported at any level, the downward pressure on the urethra against the fixed anterior vaginal wall will cause urethral compression and hence continence. Thus the important anatomical supports are not to the urethra but rather to the anterior vaginal wall. Indeed a colposuspension supports the paravaginal tissue rather than the urethra in a fixed position. Multiple operations are doomed to failure presumably because the urethra is scarred and unable to be compressed against the anterior vaginal wall.

The supports consist of the arcus tendineus fasciae pelvis (the white line), the levator ani muscles and the endopelvic fascia around the urethra

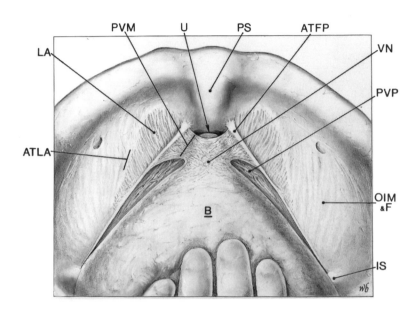

Fig. 2.11 Space of Retzius drawn from cadaver dissection. Pubovesical muscle (PVM) can be seen going from vesical neck (VN) to arcus tendineus fasciae pelvis (ATFP) and running over the paraurethral vascular plexus (PVP). ATLA = arcus tendineus levator ani, B = bladder, IS = ischial spine, LA = levator ani muscles, OIM&F = obturator internus muscle and fascia, PS = pubic symphysis and U = urethra. (With permission from John DeLancey.)

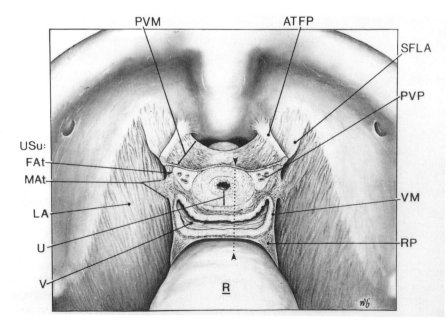

Fig. 2.12 Cross-section of the urethra (U), vagina (V), arcus tendineus fasciae pelvis (ATFP) and superior fascia of levator ani (SFLA) just below the vesical neck (drawn from cadaver dissection). Pubovesical muscles (PVM) lie anterior to urethra and anterior and superior to paraurethral vascular plexus (PVP). The urethral supports (USu) ('the pubourethral ligaments') attach the vagina and vaginal surface of the urethra to the levator ani muscles (LA) (MAt = muscular attachment) and to the superior fascia of the levator ani (FAt = fascial attachment). R = rectum, RP = rectal pillar and VM = vaginal wall muscularis. (With permission from John DeLancey.)

and vagina (Fig. 2.11 and 2.12). The arcus tendineus fasciae pelvis is a condensation of fibrous tissue extending from the lower part of the pubic bone to the ischial spine. The anterior part of the arcus tendineus fasciae pelvis lies on the inner surface of the levator ani. Anteriorly the levator ani arises from just above the arcus tendineus fasciae pelvis and posteriorly it inserts into another fibrous band known as the arcus tendineus levator ani. The arcus tendineus fasciae pelvis and the arcus tendineus levator ani fuse near the ischial spine. The endopelvic fascia attaches to the arcus tendineus fasciae pelvis and also the anterior vaginal wall at the position of the proximal urethra. In addition some fibres of the levator ani interdigitate with the anterior vaginal wall at the same position.

Contraction of levator muscle between the arcus tendineus levator ani and the white line will elevate the white line. This results in support of the anterior vaginal wall in the region of the bladder neck and maintains the proximal urethra in its correct position. This part of the levator is adapted to maintain constant tone and is of slow twitch variety. When the abdominal muscles contract as in a cough, the pelvic floor also contracts in unison. This causes downward pressure of the bladder neck against the anterior vaginal wall, which is supported by the levator ani, and thus the urethra is compressed.

In addition to these supports of the anterior vaginal wall, the bladder neck is attached to a portion of the arcus tendineus fasciae pelvis by the pubovesical muscle. This is smooth muscle of detrusor origin. When the pelvic floor is relaxed during voiding the direction of the pubovesical muscle is such that it tends to open the bladder neck. Thus straining by contracting the abdominal muscles and the anterior fibres of the levator ani increases urine flow. This would explain voiding difficulties after incontinence surgery, as the bladder neck would be unable to descend during voiding. Thus the pubovesical muscle may be more important in opening the bladder neck during voiding than in determining the correct position of the bladder neck as was originally believed.

Apart from these supports, DeLancey refers to the urethral sphincter, which he divides into the internal and external sphincter (see Fig. 2.9). The internal sphincter lies at the level of the urethrovesical junction, where closure is determined by the detrusor loop as already described.

The external sphincter consists of three different elements. The proximal part is a circular band of muscle. Distal to this the band of muscle attaches to the vaginal wall as the urethrovaginal sphincter. The most distal part attaches to the perineal membrane as the compressor urethrae. The muscle of this sphincter mechanism is striated and of slow twitch variety, and is important in maintaining continence at rest and as a back-up mechanism during periods of stress. Slow twitch muscles are capable of contraction over a prolonged period of time but have a slow response time. Conversely, fast twitch muscles respond rapidly but also fatigue quickly.

In addition to the muscular elements, the vascular plexus around the urethra is particularly prominent and tends to compress the urethra. During periods of stress there is engorgement of the veins, further compressing the urethra. The final element is the ability of the epithelial lining of the urethra to form a watertight hermetic seal.[32]

SUMMARY

Thus continence is maintained by connective tissue elements, the vascular plexus and the sphincteric mechanism. During periods of stress the supporting mechanism of the anterior vaginal wall is such that the urethra is compressed against the anterior vaginal wall, thus raising the intraurethral pressure. This explains why pelvic floor denervation results in genuine stress incontinence and explains the mechanism behind the success of colposuspension procedures.

REFERENCES

1 Cutner A. The lower urinary tract in pregnancy. MD thesis. University of London, 1993.
2 Tanagho EA, Smith DR. Mechanism of urinary continence. 1. Embryological, anatomic and pathologic considerations. J Urol 1968; 100: 640–646.
3 Hamilton WJ, Mossman HW. 1972; In: Human Embryology. Chapter 12: The urogenital system. Cambridge pp. 377–437.
4 Moore KL. In: The developing human. Clinically orientated embryology. Chapter 13: The urogenital system. 4th ed. Philadelphia, Saunders, 1988; pp 245–285.
5 Wesson MB. Anatomical, embryological and physiological studies of the trigone and neck of the bladder. J Urol 1920; 4: 279–315.
6 Gyllensten L. Contributions to the embryology of the urinary bladder. Part 1: The development of the definitive relations between the openings of the Wolffian ducts and the ureters. Acta Anatom 1949; 7: 305–344.
7 Cutner A, Moscoso G, Cardozo LD, Driver M, Cooper D. Growth of the normal human lower urinary tract from 12 to 21 weeks gestation. Anatom Rec 1992; 234(4): 568–574.
8 Ayres PH, Shinohara Y, Frith CH. Morphological observations on the epithelium of the developing urinary bladder of the mouse and rat. J Urol 1985; 133: 506–512.
9 Newman J, Antonakopoulos GN. The fine structure of the human fetal urinary bladder. Development and maturation. A light, transmission and scanning electron microscopic study. J Anat 1989; 166: 135–150.
10 Woodburne RT. The sphincter mechanism of the urinary bladder and the urethra. Anatom Rec 1901; 141: 11–20.
11 Droes JTPM. Observations on the musculature of the urinary bladder and the urethra in the human foetus. Br J Urol 1964; 46: 179–185.
12 Levin RM, Keating MA, Potter L, Wein AJ. Ontogeny of purinergic function in the rabbit bladder. Neurourol Urodyn 1989; 8: 386–387.
13 Saeki H, Okazaki T, Kadowaki H, Shimamoto T, Miyagawa I. The development of the autonomic innervation and contractile response of the rat urinary bladder. Neurourol Urodyn 1989; 8: 388.
14 Mitolo-Chieppa D, Schonauer S, Grasso G, Cicinell F, Carratu MR (1983). Ontogenesis of autonomic receptors in detrusor muscle and bladder sphincter of human fetus. Urol. 21: 599–603.
15 Tyler DE. Stratified squamous epithelium in the vesical trigone and urethra: findings correlated with the menstrual cycle and age. Am J Anat 1962; 111: 319–325.
16 Packham DA. The epithelial lining of the female trigone and urethra. Br J Urol 1971; 43: 201–205.
17 Tanagho EA, Smith DR. The anatomy and function of the bladder neck. Br J Urol 1966; 38: 54–71.
18 Hutch JA. The internal urethral urinary sphincter. A double-loop system. J Urol 1971; 105: 375–383.
19 Gosling J. The structure of the bladder and urethra in relation to function. Urol Clin North Am 1979; 6: 31–38.
20 DeLancey JOL. Anatomy and physiology of urinary incontinence. Clinical Obstet Gynecol 1990; 33(2): 298–307.
21 Versi E, Cardozo LD, Studd JWW, Brincat M, O'Dowd TM, Cooper DJ. Internal urinary sphincter in maintenance of female continence. Br Med J 1986; 292: 166.
22 Benness CJ, Cutner A, Cardozo LD. Bladder neck competence in women with lower urinary tract symptoms. International Urogynecology Journal. 1990; 1(3): 173. Abstract.

23 DeLancey JOL. Pubovesical ligament: a separate structure from the urethral supports ('pubo-urethral ligaments'). Neurourol Urodyn 1989; 8: 53–61.
24 Delancey JOL. Histology of the connection between the vagina and levator ani muscles. J Reprod Med 1990; 35: 765–771.
25 Gosling JA, Dixon JS. Light and electron microscopic observations on the human external urethral sphincter. J Anat 1979; 129: 216. Abstract.
26 Zacharin RF. The suspensory mechanism of the female urethra. J Anat 1963; 97: 423–427.
27 Milley PS, Nichols DH. The relationship between the pubo-urethral ligaments and the urogenital diaphragm in the human female. Anat Rec 1971; 170: 281–283.
28 Turner-Warwick R. Observations on the function and dysfunction of the sphincter and detrusor mechanisms. Urol Clin North Am 1979; 6: 13–30.
29 McGuire E. Urethral sphincter mechanisms. Urol Clin North Am 1979; 6: 39–49.
30 Rud T, Andersson K-E, Asmussen M, Hunting A, Ulmsten U. Factors maintaining the intraurethral pressure in women. Invest Urol 1980; 17: 343–347.
31 Gosling JA, Dixon JS, Humpherson JR. Functional anatomy of the lower urinary tract. Edinburgh: Churchill Livingstone, 1983.
32 Zinner NR, Ritter RC, Sterling AM. The mechanism of micturition. In: Williams DI, Chisholm GD (eds) Scientific foundations of urology. London: Heinemann, 1976: pp 39–51.

3

The neurology of the lower urinary tract: Innervation, neuropharmacology and neurophysiology

INNERVATION

The detrusor, bladder neck and urethra are innervated by branches of the pelvic plexus. The plexus is formed from trunks or branches of the pelvic (parasympathetic) and hypogastric (sympathetic) nerves. The pelvic nerve conveys efferent parasympathetic innervation to the bladder and urethra, derived from S_{2-4}. It arises from sacral ventral roots and consists of three or four trunks in humans. The hypogastric nerve conveys efferent sympathetic innervation to the bladder and urethra. Arising from T_{10-12}, nerves pass via the sympathetic chain to the preaortic plexus. The hypogastric nerve is the caudal subdivision of the superior hypogastric plexus (Fig. 3.1).

The distribution of cholinergic innervation is uniform throughout the bladder, but it is sparsely supplied with adrenergic innervation.[1] It is

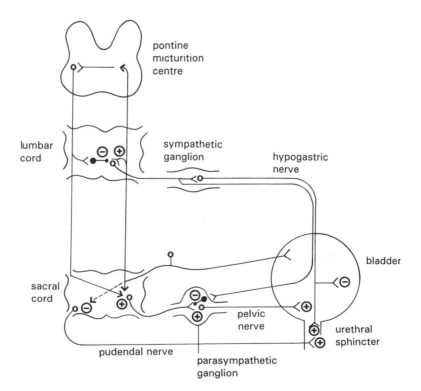

Fig. 3.1 Innervation of the lower urinary tract

likely, therefore, that sympathetic nerves do not act directly on the detrusor in humans but inhibit detrusor activity by modulating cholinergic activity at the level of the pelvic plexus.

Innervation of the bladder and urethra arises almost exclusively from peripheral ganglia which are adjacent to or within the target organ. The ganglia contain three cell types; cholinergic principal neurones, adrenergic principal neurones and small intensely fluorescent cells (SIF). These SIF cells modulate ganglionic transmission and vasomotor function. Some cholinergic and sympathetic fibers pass uninterrupted through urogenital ganglia, or may terminate there. Some efferent fibers synapse with sensory nerves to form neural circuits which bypass the spinal cord.

Afferent nerve fibers are conveyed by the pelvic, pudendal and hypogastric nerves. It has been suggested that sensation of bladder distension originates in tension receptors in the bladder wall and travels via the pelvic nerve, whereas other mechanoreceptor afferents are present in the hypogastric nerve.[2,3] Both hypogastric and pelvic nerves convey nociceptive afferents. Afferent pathways from the striated sphincter and urethra transmit sensation of temperature, pain, urethral wall distension and passage of urine and are conducted by the pudendal nerve. The main afferent pathway that triggers initiation of voiding consists of A-delta and C axons that are linked with vesical tension receptors. These axons are conveyed by the pelvic nerve.[3]

The urethral rhabdosphincter in the male cat has triple innervation: somatic, autonomic cholinergic and autonomic adrenergic.[4] Most authors, however, agree that both the intrinsic and extrinsic components of the human striated sphincter receive only somatic innervation. Disagreement exists as to the actual nerve which carries the fibers. Originally, both elements were thought to be innervated by the pudendal nerve.[5,6] Donker et al[7] suggest that the striated sphincter is predominantly innervated via the autonomic nervous system through the hypogastric plexus. Gosling et al[1], however, believe that the slow twitch fibers of both intrinsic and extrinsic sphincters are innervated by somatic fibers within the pelvic nerve.

NEUROPHARMACOLOGY AND NEUROPHYSIOLOGY OF THE BLADDER AND URETHRA

Cholinergic and adrenergic systems

Cholinergic (muscarinic) receptors have been found in the body and base of the human bladder.[8] Acetylcholine causes contraction of the smooth muscle of the bladder body and base, but only weak contraction of human urethral strips in vitro.[9] The predominant receptor type found in the body of both the rabbit and human bladder is the M2 variety.[10]

The smooth muscle of the body and base of the bladder and the proximal urethra contain β-adrenergic receptors. α-receptors predominate at the bladder base and in the proximal urethra.[11] Postjunctional α_1-receptors are believed to mediate urethral smooth muscle contraction in the human.[12]

It is generally believed that reflex activation of the pelvic nerve is responsible for bladder contraction in normal micturition; however, the role of the sympathetic nervous system is less clear and remains controversial. Its primary function is to facilitate the filling and storage phase of micturition. It may achieve this effect in three ways: by inhibition of bladder contractility by parasympathetic blockade at the level of the pelvic ganglia mediated by α-receptors, by direct stimulation of β-receptors in the bladder body and by increasing bladder outlet resistance by stimulation of α-receptors in the bladder base and proximal urethra.

During bladder filling afferent impulses in the pelvic nerves activate efferent sympathetic pathways in a spinal reflex.[13] Edvardsen[14] has shown that a similar reflex exists in the cat. Sympathectomy leads to increased bladder activity, decreased bladder capacity and a shift in the cystometric curve to the left in cats[15] and in dogs.[16]

Intravaginal electrical stimulation at low intravesical pressures induces bladder inhibition in cats via the hypogastric nerve.[17] This inhibition may be eliminated by β-adrenoceptor blockade. Pudendal nerve afferent stimulation was found to produce detrusor inhibition in the cat by the same mechanism.[18]

Bladder neck contraction in response to sympathetic stimulation has been reported in monkeys[19] and in dogs.[20] McGuire supported the concept of enhanced urethral smooth muscle activity during bladder filling mediated by α-adrenergic receptors. He also suggested that the adrenergic system is involved in the mechanism of bladder neck opening prior to the onset of voiding. Preganglionic parasympathetic stimulation which results in detrusor contraction is also believed to activate postganglionic adrenergic fibers which act upon β-adrenoceptors in the urethral smooth muscle. This view was endorsed by Elbadawi,[22] but other authorities do not believe the sympathetic nervous system is significantly involved in bladder filling/storage or emptying.

Nordling[23] suggested that α-adrenergic stimulation enhances urethral closure via action on urethral vessels rather than the smooth muscle and also via α-adrenergic receptors in the central nervous system which regulate striated sphincter tone.

Non-cholinergic, non-adrenergic neurohumoral influences

Several theories have developed to explain the relative resistance of detrusor contractility to atropine, following pelvic nerve stimulation.

Burnstock[24,25] proposed the presence of other neurotransmitters and the concept of a modulatory transmitter mechanism, including presynaptic inhibition or enhancement of transmitter release, postsynaptic modulation of transmitter action and the secondary involvement of locally synthesized hormones and prostaglandins. The co-transmitter may act directly on postsynaptic cells, facilitate action of the classical transmitter or act as an inhibitor of its release. The two transmitters may be stored in the same vesicles and released together or may be stored separately. This theory may explain why blockade of cholinergic receptors with atropine only partially abolishes the effects of nerve stimulation.

The phenomenon of 'atropine resistance' has been shown in field-stimulated bladder strips from rabbits and pigs. In humans, however, atropine produces effective blockade of the contractile response with only 1–7% persisting. This figure is not reduced significantly by tetrodotoxin, suggesting that it is not nerve mediated.[26]

A much reduced inhibitory effect of atropine was demonstrated by Sjögren et al[27] in field-stimulated bladder strips from patients with detrusor instability or hypertrophy. It is possible that the non-adrenergic, non-cholinergic component of detrusor contractility is more important in patients with bladder dysfunction than in normals.

The exact nature of the non-adrenergic, non-cholinergic innervation of the bladder remains to be defined, but neurokinin-2 receptors have been shown to exist in the human bladder, and stimulation of these with neurokinin-A results in contraction of isolated detrusor strips at concentrations 100 times less than acetylcholine.[28]

In the cat, bladder response to pelvic nerve stimulation has been shown to consist of two parts.[29] The first response was a transient spiked rise in pressure, followed by a secondary plateau phase. The first phase was partially antagonized by Arylazido Aminoprop ionyl Adenosine Triphosphate ANAPP$_3$, a blocker of adenosine 5' triphosphate (ATP), whereas atropine had no effect. This suggested that ATP was involved in the initial phase of bladder contraction. The second phase was atropine sensitive and produced by acetylcholine release.

This biphasic response was also shown by Levin et al.[30] Purinergic stimulation accounted for 50% of the initial phase of bladder contraction, but virtually all bladder emptying occurred during the plateau period. Thus purinergic stimulation may be important in the initiation of voiding, while bladder emptying appears to be a cholinergic phenomenon.

Prostaglandins of the type E and F result in contraction of detrusor strips in vitro.[31] It has been suggested that they are released during stimulation of the bladder and contribute to the atropine-resistant part of this response.[32] Others believe that prostaglandins are not involved in bladder emptying, but are responsible for maintaining tone or spontaneous activity in the detrusor. They may also act as modulators of transmitter release.[33]

Mechanical irritation of rabbit bladder epithelium was shown to increase basal tension and spontaneous activity in response to electrical stimulation of bladder muscle.[34] These effects were mimicked by prostaglandins of the E, F and I series. Pretreatment of the epithelium with prostaglandin synthetase inhibitors significantly reduced the effect. This study suggests a potential role of prostaglandins in the initiation of bladder hyperactivity following trauma to the bladder epithelium.

In rats, xylene-induced cystitis results in a reduction in cystometric capacity and the threshold at which reflex micturition occurs. These effects can be blocked by a thromboxane A$_2$ antagonist, GR 32191. Thromboxane A$_2$ may be a mediator of the micturition reflex in irritative disorders of the bladder.[35] Thromboxane A$_2$ elicits contraction of isolated strips of human detrusor muscle. It acts on specific receptors on the smooth muscle cell, mediating direct contraction, and also on intrinsic nerves, mediating potentiation of acetylcholine release.[36]

Substance P is a decapeptide originally detected in the gut and brain, which is found in small amounts in the human bladder. In vitro it causes bladder contraction in the dog which is atropine resistant.[37] Antagonists of substance P, however, have no effect on contractile responses to field stimulation and this suggests that substance P is not a mediator of non-cholinergic contraction.[38]

Substance P has been isolated from bladder afferents and may be a sensory transmitter. Capsaicin, derived from red chilli peppers, is known to deplete substance P and other peptides from small-diameter afferents and has been shown to depress the micturition reflex in rats resulting in urinary retention.[39] In cats, following spinal transection at the lower thoracic level, a spinal micturition reflex emerges which is mediated by C-fiber afferents. This reflex can be blocked by capsaicin in sub-cutaneously administered doses that do not affect the micturition reflex in intact animals.[40] In man, a pilot study of intravesical capsaicin for the treatment of intractable detrusor hyperreflexia has been reported with a good response in 4 out of 5 cases.[41] A clinical trial is currently being undertaken to further assess the efficacy of this substance.

Vasoactive intestinal peptide (VIP) contains 28 amino acids, and VIP-containing nerves are found in all layers of the bladder, beneath the epithelium, around blood vessels and in the muscle layers. The level of this peptide is higher in the region of the trigone than in the dome of the bladder. Of all the peptide-containing nerves, those containing VIP are the most abundant in the bladder. Vasoactive intestinal peptide has been shown to have an inhibitory effect on both bladder and urethral smooth muscle.[42] Decreased levels of VIP have been recorded in patients with detrusor instability,[43] but the role of VIP remains uncertain.

Neuropeptide Y is a 36-amino-acid peptide which is distributed within the bladder in a similar way to VIP. It may also act as an inhibitory agent and has been shown to induce a reduction of the non-cholinergic, non-adrenergic contractile response to field stimulation in the guinea pig bladder.

Histamine H_1 receptors have been identified in the human bladder[44] and activation of these receptors results in detrusor contraction. 5-Hydroxytryptamine (5-HT) produces a contractile response in the guinea pig, dog and cat bladder, and may act to potentiate reflex bladder excitation.

Gamma-amino butyric acid (GABA) is a central inhibitory neuro-transmitter. GABA receptors have been found in the dome of the guinea pig bladder, and GABA may transiently enhance excitatory neuro-transmission before evoking a more sustained inhibition of contractility.[45] In the mouse, GABA receptors are found presynaptically and when stimulated inhibit release of acetylcholine.[46] Gamma-amino butyric acid has been isolated from all areas of the human bladder but is in highest concentration in the body of the detrusor,[47] and it has been shown to produce a dose-dependent inhibition of contractions produced by nerve stimulation in isolated human detrusor muscle strips.[48] The maximal degree of inhibition was 40% and was blocked by the $GABA_B$ antagonist 2-hydroxysaclofen.

The action of the cholinergic and adrenergic systems in the control of normal bladder function is well established. The role of other neuro-transmitters and peptides in the mechanism of continence and the etiology of incontinence remains to be clarified. Increased understanding of bladder neuropharmacology and neurophysiology may result in the development of more efficacious drug treatments for detrusor instability. At present treatments consist primarily of non-specific, anticholinergic agents.

Central control of micturition

The ultimate control of lower urinary tract function lies within the central nervous system. The structures responsible for regulating micturition, together with their ascending and descending pathways, comprise a complex neurological system which is not fully understood.

Spinal cord

The spinal micturition center is localized to the sacral spinal cord segments S_{2-4} with S_3 being the most important. The motor innervation to the bladder arises from this region. Innervation to the striated muscle of the pelvic floor and the periurethral and anal sphincters arises from Onuf's nucleus. Sensation of pain, temperature and touch from the urothelium ascends in the spinothalamic tracts to synapse in the thalamus in the sensorimotor cortex.

Proprioceptive impulses pass from the detrusor and the rhabdosphincter into the posterior columns and synapse in the nucleus tegmentolateralis dorsalis in the pons.[49] This is termed 'long routing' and suggests only a minor role for a spinal micturition centre in normal individuals. Following spinal cord transection, however, vestigial spinal pathways may develop into a spinal micturition reflex.

Pudendal reflex pathways are organized at the spinal level. Proprioceptive impulses from the pelvic floor enter the spinal cord and divide. One part synapses with pudendal motor neurones, while the other ascends to the cerebellum.

Brain stem

The area called Barrington's center in the anterior region of the pons (nucleus lateralis dorsalis) is the site of origin of facilitatory impulses to the bladder.[50] Destruction of this center causes permanent voiding difficulties,[51] and transection above this level leads to detrusor hyperreflexia. This area receives input from the cerebellum, basal ganglia, thalamus and hypothalamus.

Cerebellum

The cerebellum acts as a modulator of information derived from other areas of the central nervous system. It receives sensory input from the bladder and pelvic floor and its efferent impulses are important in the maintenance of pelvic floor tone, and the strength and co-ordination of detrusor contraction and rhabdosphincter relaxation. Ablation of the cerebellar vermis causes detrusor hyperreflexia in experimental animals.

Basal ganglia

These subcortical nuclei are believed to have an inhibitory effect on spontaneous detrusor contraction.[52] Basal ganglia dysfunction often gives rise to detrusor hyperreflexia, e.g. in the case of Parkinson's disease.

Thalamus, hypothalamus and limbic system

The thalamus is a collection of nuclei which relay sensory axons to the cerebral cortex. The precise routing of pudendal and pelvic nerve afferents is unknown. The role of the hypothalamus is also unclear, but bladder distension causes firing in certain hypothalamic nuclei.[53] The limbic system is principally located in the temporal lobe and comprises the amygdala, hippocampus and cingulate gyrus. Electrical stimulation of specific nuclei has been shown to facilitate or depress bladder activity, but no specific bladder dysfunction occurs in people with temporal lobe disorders.

Cerebral cortex

The superomedial portion of the frontal lobes and the genu of the corpus callosum are concerned with bladder function.[54] Transection experiments show that these areas have an inhibitory effect on the detrusor and ablation of the cerebral cortex is usually characterized by detrusor hyper-reflexia. The neurotransmitters involved are generally unknown, but GABA and glycine are believed to be inhibitory central neurotransmitters. Sillen[55] has shown that excitatory dopaminergic and muscarinic and in-hibitory GABA-ergic receptors modulate the basic micturition reflex arising from the pontine-mesencephalic area.

Opioid peptides have been shown to exert tonic inhibition of the micturition reflex.[56] This may be achieved by inhibition at the level of the peripheral bladder ganglia, the sacral spinal cord or the pontine micturition centre. Naloxone, an antagonist of endogenous opioids, has been shown to decrease bladder capacity and to increase bladder pressure during cystometry in normal men and women.[57] Several types of opioid receptor exist at different sites. δ-receptors are found in bladder ganglia, on the preganglionic nerve terminal. δ-agonists are effective in blocking trans-mission at this level, by inhibition of acetylcholine release, whereas μ- and κ- agonists are ineffective.[3] It has been suggested that μ-receptors in the brainstem are involved in alteration of bladder capacity, whilst δ-receptors in the spinal cord modulate the strength and duration of detrusor contraction.

Historically, there has been controversy as to the site of the organization center for the micturition reflex. The idea of a sacral reflex which was modulated by higher centres in the central nervous system was supported by many workers.[58,59,60] More recently, evidence has suggested that the primary micturition centre lies in the pontine mesencephalic region of the brainstem.[61,62]

THE MECHANISM OF CONTINENCE

Filling phase

In order to maintain urinary continence, the intraurethral pressure must exceed intravesical pressure at all times except during voiding. During physiological bladder filling there is very little rise in intravesical pressure for a large increase in bladder volume. This high compliance is due to the viscoelastic properties of the bladder wall, together with inhibitory neuronal mechanisms that are activated during bladder filling. These include a spinal sympathetic reflex which activates β-receptors in the body of the bladder, and inhibits parasympathetic motor activity to the bladder at the level of the bladder ganglia. These reflex pathways may be initiated by pelvic nerve and pudendal nerve afferents. During normal bladder filling there is no involuntary contractile activity of the detrusor.

Urethral pressure gradually increases as the bladder fills. The nature of this pressure increase is unclear, but it is associated with increased pudendal and hypogastric activity in the cat.[63] Pelvic floor electromyogram (EMG) activity increases as the bladder fills, suggesting that increased activity of the striated sphincter is responsible for the rise in urethral pressure. The sympathetic reflex also leads to stimulation of the α-receptors in the urethral smooth muscle and further enhances urethral closure during bladder filling.

Passive properties of the urethra are also important in the maintenance of continence. The elastic and collagenous components of the urethra exert pressure on the soft submucosa to form a watertight seal.

During stress episodes, leakage of urine is prevented due to the transmission of increased intra-abdominal pressure to the bladder neck and proximal urethra.[64] This is achieved because the normal bladder neck is situated within the abdominal cavity, supported by the pubourethral ligaments, pubocervical fascia and the levator ani muscles. Active closure of striated or smooth muscle components of the urethral sphincter have been postulated, since the increase in urethral closure pressure seen during stress episodes may exceed the rise in intra-abdominal pressure.[65]

Voiding phase

During voiding there is a decrease in pelvic floor EMG activity and a decrease in urethral pressure which precedes the onset of detrusor contraction.[65,66] Intravesical pressure increases produce the sensation of distension which leads to voluntary initiation of micturition. The organizational center for the micturition reflex is in the brainstem, and co-ordinated bladder emptying relies on intact ascending and descending neural pathways. The spinal sympathetic reflex is suppressed, somatic efferent activity to the striated sphincter is inhibited, and parasympathetic activity to the detrusor via the pelvic nerve is enhanced. This results in a highly co-ordinated contraction of the detrusor muscle together with a decrease in outlet resistance involving both urethral smooth and striated muscle. Bladder neck descent and funnelling occurs and the flow of urine commences. When micturition is voluntarily brought to an end, the pelvic floor contracts to elevate and oppose the bladder neck to the symphysis pubis, the bladder neck closes and the detrusor pressure falls. Urine proximal to the mid-urethra is 'milked back' into the bladder and filling once again commences. Normal bladder control and voiding is a learnt phenomenon which requires normal anatomy and intact neurological pathways. Voluntary control of micturition is achieved at the time of 'potty training'. Maladaptive patterns of behavior learnt at this stage may persist and present with symptoms of lower urinary tract dysfunction in adult life. In certain conditions, e.g. dementia, voluntary control of the micturition reflex is lost and uninhibited voiding occurs.

The neurology, neuropharmacology and neurophysiology of the lower urinary tract are complex. Our understanding of the control of normal bladder function and the pathophysiology of incontinence is incomplete, and further advances in basic science research are awaited. Few pharmacological agents developed from animal or in vitro experiments have been found to be clinically effective in the treatment of lower urinary tract dysfunction. Lack of in vivo efficacy, problems with drug administration or the development of unacceptable side effects may prevent putative therapies from reaching clinical practice.

REFERENCES

1 Gosling JA, Dixon JA, Lendon RG. The autonomic innervation of the human male and female bladder neck and proximal urethra. J Urol 1977; 118: 302–305.
2 De Groat WC, Booth AM. Autonomic systems to the urinary bladder and sexual organs. In: Dyck PJ et al (eds) Peripheral neuropathy. Philadelphia: Saunders, 1984; pp 285–299.
3 De Groat WC, Kawatani M. Neural control of the urinary bladder: possible relationship between peptidergic inhibitory mechanisms and detrusor instability. Neurourol Urodyn 1985; 4: 285–300.
4 Elbadawi A, Schenck E. A new theory of the innervation of bladder musculature. 4. Innervation of the vesicourethral junction and external urethral sphincter. J Urol 1974; 111: 613–615.
5 Fletcher TF, Bradley WE. Neuroanatomy of the bladder-urethra. J Urol 1978; 119: 153–160.
6 Elbadawi A. A neuromorphologic basis of vesicourethral function I. Histochemistry, ultrastructure, and function of intrinsic nerves of the bladder and urethra. Neurourol Urodyn 1982; 1: 3–50.
7 Donker PJ, Droes JThPM, Van Ulden BM. Anatomy of the musculature and innervation of the bladder and urethra. In: Chisholm GD, Williams DI (eds) Scientific foundations of urology. Chicago: Yearbook, 1982; pp 404–411.
8 Levin RM, Shofer F, Wein AJ. The muscarinic cholinergic kinetics of the human urinary bladder. Neurourol Urodyn 1983; 2: 211.
9 Ek A. Adrenoceptor and cholinoceptor mediated responses of the isolated human urethra. Scand J Urol Nephrol 1977; 11: 97–102.
10 Ruggieri M. Muscarinic receptor subtypes in human and rabbit bladder. Neurourol Urodyn 1987; 6: 119–128.
11 Wein AJ, Levin RM. Comparison of adrenergic receptor density in the urinary bladder in man, dog, and rabbit. Surg Forum 1979; 30: 576–578.
12 Mattiasson A. On the peripheral nervous control of the lower urinary tract. Thesis, University of Lund, Sweden, 1984.
13 De Groat WC, Theobald RJ. Reflex activation of sympathetic pathways to vesical smooth muscle and parasympathetic ganglia by electrical stimulation of bladder afferents. J Physiol 1976; 259: 223–237.
14 Edvardsen P. Nervous control of the urinary bladder in cats: I The collecting phase. Acta Physiol Scand 1968a; 72: 157–171.
15 Edvardsen P. Nervous control of the urinary bladder in cats: III Effects of autonomic blocking agents in the intact animal. Acta Physiol Scand 1968b; 72: 183–193.
16 Nishizawa O. Role of the sympathetic nerve in bladder and urethral sphincter function during the micturition cycle in the dog evaluated by pressure flow EMG study. J Urol 1985; 134: 1259–1261.
17 Fall M, Erlandson BE, Carlsson CA, Lindstrom S. The effect of intravaginal electrical stimulation on the feline urethra and bladder. Neurological mechanisms. Scand J Urol Nephrol 1977; (Suppl) 44(2): 19–30.
18 Sundin T, Carlsson CA, Kock NG. Detrusor inhibition induced from mechanical stimulation of the anal region and from electrical stimulation of pudendal nerve afferents. Invest Urol 1974; 11(5): 374–378.
19 Elliot TR. The innervation of the bladder and urethra. J Physiol 1907; 35: 367–445.
20 Kleeman FJ. The physiology of the internal urethral sphincter. J Urol 1970; 104: 549–554.
21 McGuire EJ. Mechanisms of urethral continence and their clinical application. World J Urol 1984; 2: 272–279.
22 Elbadawi A. A neuromorphologic basis of vesicourethral function I. Histochemistry, ultrastructure, and function of intrinsic nerves of the bladder and urethra. Neurourol Urodyn 1982; 1: 3–50.

23 Nordling J. Influence of the sympathetic nervous system on lower urinary tract in man. Neurourol Urodyn 1983; 2: 3–26.

24 Burnstock G, Dumsday B, Smythe A. Atropine resistant excitation of the urinary bladder: the possibility of transmission via nerves releasing a purine nucleotide. Br J Pharmacol 1972; 44: 451–453.

25 Burnstock G. Nervous control of smooth muscle by transmitters, co-transmitters and modulators. Experientia 1985; 41: 869–874.

26 Sibley GN. A comparison of spontaneous and nerve mediated activity in bladder muscle from man, pig and rabbit. J Physiol 1984; 354: 431–443.

27 Sjögren C, Andersson KE, Husted S, Mattiasson A, Moller-Madsen B. Atropine resistance of transmurally stimulated isolated human bladder muscle. J Urol 1982; 128: 1368–1371.

28 Marshall I, Burt RP, Chapple CR, Andersson PO, Bojanic D, Wyllie MG. Neurokinin NK$_2$ receptors in human and pig urinary bladder. Neurourol Urodyn 1991; 10: 325–326.

29 Theobald RJ. The effect of ANAPP$_3$ on the inhibition of pelvic nerve induced contractions of the cat urinary bladder. Eur J Pharmacol 1986; 120: 351–354.

30 Levin RM, Ruggieri MR, Wein AJ. Functional effects of the purinergic innervation of the rabbit urinary bladder. J Pharmacol Exp Ther 1986; 236: 452–457.

31 Andersson KE, Sjögren C. Aspects on the physiology and pharmacology of the bladder and urethra. Prog Neurobiol 1982; 19: 71–89.

32 Johns A, Paton DM. Evidence for a role of prostaglandins in atropine resistant transmission in the mammalian urinary bladder. Prostaglandins 1976; 11: 595–597.

33 Andersson KE, Mattiasson A, Sjögren C. Electrically induced relaxation of the non-adrenaline contracted isolated urethra from rabbit and man. J Urol 1983; 129: 210–214.

34 Downie JW, Karmazyn M. Mechanical trauma to bladder epithelium liberates prostanoids which modulate neurotransmission in rabbit detrusor muscle. J Pharmacol Exp Ther 1984; 230: 445–449.

35 Pietra C, Bettelini L, Gaviraghi G, Trist DG. Effect of the thromboxane A$_2$ receptor antagonist GR 32191 in a model of experimental cystitis in the rat. Neurourol Urodyn 1993; 12(4): 354–355.

36 Palea S, Corsi M, Toson G et al. Activity of the thromboxane A$_2$ receptor antagonist GR 32191 on human isolated detrusor muscle. Neurourol Urodyn 1993; 12(4): 355–356.

37 Norlen LJ. Contractile effect of substance P on the canine urinary bladder in vivo. Neurourol Urodyn 1983; 2: 232.

38 Husted S, Sjögren C, Andersson KE. Substance P and somatostatin and excitatory neurotransmission in rabbit urinary bladder. Arch Int Pharmacodyn 1981; 252: 72–85.

39 Maggi CA, Santicioli P, Meli A. The effects of topical capsaicin on rat urinary bladder motility in vivo. Eur J Pharmacol 1984; 103: 41–50.

40 DeGroat WC, Kawatani T, Hisamitsu T et al. Mechanisms underlying the recovery of urinary bladder function following spinal cord injury. J Autonomic Nervous System 1990; 30: 71–78.

41 Fowler CJ, Beck RO, Betts CD, Lynn B, Fowler CG. Intravesical capsaicin for treatment of detrusor hyperreflexia. Neurourol Urodyn 1992; 11(4): 465–466.

42 Klarskov P, Gerstenberg T. Vasoactive intestinal polypeptide influence on lower urinary tract smooth muscle from human and pig. J Urol 1984; 131: 1000–1004.

43 Gu J, Restorick JM, Blank M. Vasoactive intestinal polypeptide in the normal and unstable bladder. Br J Urol 1983; 55: 645–647.

44 Van Buren GA, Anderson GF. Comparison of the urinary bladder base and detrusor to cholinergic and histaminergic receptor activation in the rabbit. Pharmacology 1979; 18: 136–142.

45 Maggi CA, Santicioli P, Meli A. Dual effect of GABA on the contractile activity of the guinea pig isolated urinary bladder. J Auton Pharmacol 1985; 5: 131–141.

46 Santicioli P, Maggi CA, Meli A. The postganglionic excitatory innervation of the mouse urinary bladder and its modulation by prejunctional GABA$_B$ receptors. J Auton Pharmacol 1986; 6: 53–66.

47 Chen TF, Doyle PT, Ferguson DR. Measurement of GABA in the human urinary bladder: evidence for GABA as a peripheral neurotransmitter. Neurourol Urodyn 1993; 12(4): 360–361.

48 Chen TF, Doyle PT, Ferguson DR. GABA an inhibitory neurotransmitter in the human urinary bladder. Neurourol Urodyn 1993; 12(4): 358–360.

49 Bhatia NN, Bradley WE. Neuroanatomy and physiology: innervation of the urinary tract. In: Raz S (ed) Female urology. Philadelphia: Saunders, 1983: pp 12–32.

50 Barrington FJF. The relation of the hindbrain to micturition. Brain 1921; 44: 23–53.

51 Bradley WE, Conway CJ. Bladder representation in the pontine mesencephalic reticular formation. Exp Neurol 1966; 16: 237–249.

52 Carlsson CA. The supraspinal control of the urinary bladder. Acta Pharmacol Toxicol 1978; 43(II): 8–12.

53 Hald T, Bradley W. The urinary bladder: neurology and dynamics. Baltimore: Williams and Wilkins, 1982.

54 Andrew J, Nathan PW. The cerebral control of micturition. Proc R Soc Med 1965; 58: 553–555.

55 Sillen U. Central neurotransmitter mechanisms involved in the control of urinary bladder function. Scand J Urol Nephrol 1980; (Suppl 58): 1–45.

56 Booth AM. Regulation of urinary bladder capacity by endogenous opioid peptides. J Urol 1985; 133: 339–342.

57 Murray KHA, Feneley RCL. Endorphins – a role in urinary tract function? The effect of opioid blockade on the detrusor and urethral sphincter mechanisms. Br J Urol 1982; 54: 638–640.

58 Denny-Brown D, Robertson EG. On the physiology of micturition. Brain 1933; 56: 149–190.

59 McClellan FC. The neurogenic bladder. Springfield, Illinois: Thomas, 1939.

60 Lapides J. Neuromuscular vesical and ureteral dysfunction. In: Chappell MF, Harrison JH (eds) Campbell's urology. Philadelphia: Saunders, 1970.

61 Bradley WE, Timm GW, Scott FB. Innervation of the detrusor muscle and urethra. Urol Clin North AM 1974; 1: 3–27.

62 DeGroat WC. Nervous control of the urinary bladder of the cat. Brain Res 1975; 87: 201–211.

63 DeGroat WC, Booth AM. Physiology of the urinary bladder and urethra. Ann Intern Med 1980; 92(2): 321–325.

64 Enhorning G. Simultaneous recording of the intravesical and intraurethral pressures. Acta Chir Scand (Suppl) 1961; 276: 1–68.

65 Tanagho EA. The anatomy and physiology of micturition. Clin Obstet Gynecol 1978; 5: 3–26.

66 McGuire EJ. Physiology of the lower urinary tract. Am J Kidney Dis 1983; 2: 402–408.

Section 3 Investigations

4 The principles of urodynamics

INTRODUCTION

The term 'urodynamics' was first used by D.M. Davis in the *Annals of Surgery* in 1954[1] and first appeared in the urological literature in 1962.[2] Initially, it referred to the hydrodynamics of the upper urinary tract but soon encompassed 'the physiology and pathophysiology of urine transport from the kidney to the bladder as well as its storage and evacuation'.[3] There are now many components to the complex dynamic investigations of both the upper and lower tracts, although in many cases the techniques developed independently. They were finally married in the sophisticated laboratory of Earl R. Miller in the University of San Francisco.[4] The combined techniques were popularized in Europe by Bates, Whiteside & Turner-Warwick.[5]

For most of the twentieth century surgical developments have far outstripped a real understanding of the pathophysiology of urinary tract dysfunction as demonstrated by urodynamic testing. Herein lies the continued failure of urodynamics to obtain universal acceptance. If cure rates for incontinence of 80% were possible in 1914[6] with patients selected solely on clinical grounds, what additional benefit can these tests supply if similar results are still seen even after testing?

HISTORICAL REVIEW

The development of uroflowmetry started in earnest with William Drake.[7] Before this, matters of timing, distance of urine projection[8] and urethral exit pressures had been advocated. With the use of electronics[9] and the combination of uroflowmetry with voiding cystometry, sophisticated voiding parameters can now be measured. The measurement of intravesical pressure goes back to Dubois[10] in 1876, but Mosso and Pellacani are credited with the significant early development. In 1927 Rose[11] coined the term 'cystometer' and advocated that it should be used to determine neurological vesical abnormality rather than the popular cystourethroscopy. Talbot in 1948[12] introduced the descriptive terms 'stable' and 'unstable' when referring to the cystometric recordings. With measurement of bladder pressure well recognized, Bonney[13] reported on the measurement of urethral pressure in 1923. Technology in this field advanced slowly until the seminal paper by Goran

Enhorning,[14] who simultaneously measured both urethral and bladder pressure and finally established the pathophysiology of genuine stress incontinence.

X-rays were introduced into urology in 1896 when John MacIntyre detected a urinary calculus. Fluoroscopy enabled functional studies of normal and abnormal micturition to be performed. When Earl R. Miller combined the available techniques videocystourethrography was developed.

PATIENT ASSESSMENT

Urodynamic studies are only part of the assessment of a patient with urinary symptoms and the potential for their misuse is great. History and examination are the foundation for this assessment. Examination may be supplemented by clinical testing of dubious value, such as the Q-tip test or the modified Bonney's test. Simple investigations may include a urinary diary, urine microscopy and culture, X-rays and pad testing. More complex or invasive investigations include ultrasound, computerized tomography amd magnetic resonance imaging as well as endoscopic techniques. Urodynamics forms part of this comprehensive patient assessment.

Normal storage and voiding is a dynamic process, with many parameters changing during the filling–emptying cycle. Physiological investigations of this function, therefore, have to be dynamic in nature and single measurements can only be of significance if interpreted in relation to the whole. Some pathology in such a dynamic process will inevitably relate to a breakdown in its integrated function (e.g. detrusor instability), whereas other pathology may arise as a consequence of a straightforward physical defect (e.g. vesicovaginal fistula). Urodynamics is the dynamic part of the investigation of lower urinary tract function and dysfunction. The overriding advantage of complex sophisticated investigations such as videocystourethrography is that they supply both structural information and functional data.

The diagnosis of disease relies on the three elements of history examination and investigation. The relative weight of each of these depends on the circumstances. A child who is mildly unwell with a fever and crops of vesicles and who perhaps has had recent contact with a similarly affected child clearly has chickenpox. Electron microscopy of the vesicular fluid or measurement of specific varicella IgM is unnecessary and wasteful. However, a manual laborer who has a pyrexia of unknown origin and splinter hemorrhages will require investigation including blood cultures and echocardiography to make the diagnosis of subacute bacterial endocarditis. In many practitioners' eyes, history and examination of a patient with urinary symptoms represent the most important elements in the diagnostic process with urodynamic testing having only a minor role. However, relying solely on history and examination results in significant diagnostic inaccuracy in many patients regardless of the experience of the interviewing physician.[15,16]

The function and dysfunction of the lower urinary tract are intensely personal and a patient's history is frequently confusing. Urodynamic investigations which reproduce the patient's symptoms — particularly incontinence — do not only supply a diagnosis but also confirm the presence of a particular symptom. With an accurate diagnosis appropriate treatment can be planned and the patient can be informed of the likely outcome of various treatment options. The efficacy of treatment may also be assessed with further appropriate testing. Our understanding of the pathophysiology of the various disease processes resulting in urinary tract symptoms is far from complete, but urodynamic testing in the research setting supplies useful data.

REPRODUCIBILITY

Urodynamic tests are not without their problems and pitfalls. Many of the recorded components of the test are subjective and dynamic in nature and are inevitably not reproducible. An example would be the volume at first sensation. Other components, while not being reproducible and having little relevance to actual events, supply valuable information to the investigator, such as the cystometric capacity in the supine position. Some parameters are more objective and have reproducible results such as the maximal urethral pressure measured at 3 o'clock in the supine position using microtipped transducers, although here the result may be of little diagnostic or therapeutic value.

CHOOSING THE RIGHT TEST

The investigations chosen must be relevant to the patient's symptoms and seen to be contributing to patient management. A young fertile woman with a watery loss mid-cycle which is misinterpreted as incontinence may simply require a pad test with urea and creatinine estimation on any fluid collected. However, an elderly woman with restricted mobility and a clear history of urge incontinence may be best served by a home assessment before a therapeutic trial of anticholinergics without urodynamic investigations.

The environment of many urodynamic laboratories can be far from conducive to the reproduction of physiological processes. With a radiographer, nurse, technician and perhaps two doctors present the patient may be asked to void erect with both rectal and bladder lines present and a female urinal clutched between her legs. It is important that efforts should be made to make the patient feel comfortable and relaxed and that the investigator regularly enquires if events recorded whilst the tests are being performed are similar to those outside the laboratory. If the test fails to reveal abnormality the test rather than the patient is probably at fault; however, modern technology and ingenuity usually overcome this problem. An example of this would be the use of ambulatory cystometry for the diagnosis of detrusor instability where provocative cystometry has failed to identify this disease. The artificial nature of the test may produce abnormality. Such matters must be clarified with the patient to avoid inappropriate and potentially harmful treatment. On the other hand, the endless quest for a diagnosis is a characteristic of the medical zealot and overtesting when the likelihood of significant pathology is low is of little advantage to the patient and a waste of resources. In such circumstances history, examination, urinary diary and pad testing will be helpful to clarify the severity of the situation if not the pathology.

URODYNAMICS IN CLINICAL PRACTICE

Urodynamic investigations must go through a rigorous process of assessment before they are accepted into common practice. The test should be based on a clear understanding of the physiology and pathophysiology of voiding disorders. It should be able to differentiate in absolute or relative terms between normality and abnormality. The test should produce reproducible results, be acceptable to patients and have low complication rates. Additional advantages for a test may be that it supplies further information to the pool of knowledge about a particular disease process and that it is useful for monitoring therapy. A test which failed to meet most of these criteria but which nevertheless gained popularity was the assessment of the posterior urethral angle.[17] For many years correction of this angle was the aim of surgical treatment and was justified on the basis of the association of the loss of the angle with stress incontinence. However, abnormal angles are seen in continent women and normal angles in incontinent women. More importantly, there was no convincing explanation as to why the angle was relevant in the first place. With Enhorning's[14] understanding of the pathophysiology of genuine stress incontinence this investigation disappeared from clinical practice.

Normal urodynamic values are elusive both as a consequence of the wide variation in normality and the effect of the test itself on the test result. Frequently, a single result or value is of little use but patterns of abnormality appear as the tests proceed. The elements of art and experience often engender criticism from those with little knowledge. This means that training is of vital importance if a particular unit is not going to fall into disrepute. Unfortunately, in many instances, despite an accurate urodynamic diagnosis, treatment that will have a dramatic effect on symptoms is not available. This inevitably adds to the skepticism of those who doubt the value of testing.

Urodynamic equipment has moved on from simple home-made devices to expensive, complex, computer-driven, all-encompassing machines which, in many circumstances, have superfluous facilities. The most common complication of urodynamic testing is urinary tract infection despite rigorous antisepsis. The risk of this may be reduced by antibiotic prophylaxis in all patients or alternatively only in those with a significant residual urine. Hematuria as a consequence of trauma is rarely seen and usually settles rapidly.

WHO NEEDS URODYNAMICS?

The indications for investigation will vary depending on the availability of equipment, the enthusiasm of the staff and the funds available. The application of the various investigation modalities will then have to be individualized depending not only on clinical findings but also on the circumstances of the patient. The most commonly cited indications for investigation are:

- persistence of urinary tract symptoms following simple treatments[18]
- intention to carry out surgical intervention for lower urinary tract symptoms[15]
- failure of the chosen treatment modality.[19]

Such guidelines leave considerable leeway for individual interpretation. However, as the problem of lower urinary tract dysfunction and incontinence is publicized and accepted by the community, the need for accurate diagnosis is imperative so that the opportunity to supply good medical care is not lost in a mass of inappropriate prescribing and treatment.

The demand for medical care is difficult to quantify, as all governments have found. If a new service is established it is used and grows because it is there. With between 2%[20] and 91%[21] of the female population incontinent, the potential demand is unknown but is likely to be large.

AVAILABILITY OF URODYNAMICS

The investigations used in both secondary and tertiary hospitals will vary depending upon demand from the population and the ability and interest of the local physicians. A moderate-sized District General Hospital should expect to be able to offer microbiology, pad testing, uroflowmetry, filling and voiding cystometry, videocystourethrography, urethral pressure profilometry, cystourethroscopy, intravenous pyelography and ultrasound. Tertiary referral centers should offer subspecialists in urogynecology where over half of the practitioner's time is spent carrying out this specialty. Additional investigative procedures available in the tertiary referral center should be elechomyographic studies, nerve conduction studies and ambulatory urodynamics. In each District General Hospital a service will inevitably be required, but the adequacy of this local service will depend on the application of sound principles.

REFERENCES

1 Davies DM. The hydrodynamics of the upper urinary tract (urodynamics). Ann Surg 1954; 140: 839–849.
2 Davies DM, Zimskind P. Progress in urodynamics. J Urol 1962; 87: 243–249.
3 Susset JG. Urodynamic Society Presidential Address. Urodynamics — a step forward in experimental urology. Neurourol and Urodynam 1985; 4: 147–160.
4 Miller ER. Techniques of simultaneous display of X-ray and physiological data. In: Boyarsky S (ed) The neurogenic bladder. Baltimore? and Wilkins, 1967; pp 79–85.

 5 Bates CP, Whiteside BM, Turner-Warwick R. Synchronous cine/pressure/flow/cysto-urethrography with special reference to stress and urge incontinence. Br J Urol 1970; 42: 714–723.
 6 Kelley HA, Dumm W. Urinary incontinence in women without manifest injury to the bladder. Surg Gynaecol Obstet 1914; 18: 444–450.
 7 Drake W. The uroflowmeter: an aid to the study of the lower urinary tract. J Urol 1948; 59: 650–658.
 8 Ballenger EG, Older OF, McDonald HP. Voiding distance decrease: an important early symptom of prostatic obstruction. South Med J 1932; 25: 863–864.
 9 von Garretts B. Analysis of micturition: a new method of recording the voiding of the bladder. Acta Chir Scand 1956; 112: 326–340.
10 Smith JC. Urethral resistance to micturition. Br J Urol 1968; 40: 125–156.
11 Rose DK. Determination of bladder pressure with the cystometer. J Am Med Assoc 1927; 88: 151–156.
12 Talbot HS. Cystometry, and the treatment of vesical dysfunction in paraplegia. J Urol 1948; 59: 1130–1148.
13 Bonney V. On diurnal incontinence in women. J Obstet Gynaecol Br Empire 1923; 30: 358–365.
14 Enhorning G. Simultaneous recording of intravasical and intraurethral pressure. Acta Chir Scand 1961; 276: 1–68.
15 Abrams PH, Feneley RCG, Torrens MJ. Urodynamics. Berlin: Springer-Verlag, 1983.
16 Jarvis GH et al. An assessment of urodynamic examination in incontinent women. Br J Obstet Gynaecol 1980; 87: 893–896.
17 Jeffcoat TN, Roberts H. Observations on stress incontinence of urine. Am J Obstet Gynaecol 1952; 64: 721–738.
18 Blavias JG et al. Urodynamic procedures: recommendations of the Urodynamic Society. 1. Procedures that should be available for routine urological practice. Neurourol and Urodynam. 1982; 1: 51–56.
19 De Bolla AR, Arkell DG. Urodynamic investigations in a District General Hospital. Annals of the Royal College of Surgeons of England 1983; 65: 173–175.
20 Halt T. Number of people with urinary incontinence in Denmark. Ugeskr Laeger 1975; 137: 3001–3063.
21 McLaren SM et al. Prevalence and severity of incontinence in hospitalised female psychogeriatric patients. Health Bulletin 1981; 39: 157–161.

5 Setting up a urodynamic clinic

INTRODUCTION

A urodynamic clinic is not merely a diagnostic facility but rather an advisory unit performing investigations in order that correct diagnoses can be made and appropriate clinical advice given. Medical, paramedical and non-medical staff are required to run an efficient service and the sophistication of the investigations will depend on the type of referrals received and the expertise of the unit.

A urodynamic clinic can perform relatively simple investigations for a local population and refer on complicated cases, or it can act as a tertiary referral center for complex situations. Also the type of investigation carried out will be further influenced by whether or not there is a research aspect to the unit. Some investigations, although very informative regarding the underlying pathophysiology, have little place in the clinical management of patients. Auditing the efficacy of prescribed treatments and operations performed is now an important part of clinical practice and this can only be accurately assessed by objective testing. A standard approach to patient investigation should therefore be adopted so that changes with time are meaningful.

An efficient unit requires secretarial support. Referral letters should initially be screened by one of the medical team, who will decide whether a clinic appointment is necessary prior to investigation. The secretary will arrange appointment times and include details of tests required, such as midstream urine sample (MSU), prior to the urodynamic investigations. Ideally there should be an information sheet explaining the test to be carried out. A contact number will enable cancellations to be made so that other patients can receive these appointments, thus reducing wasted clinic time.

Not only is the expertise of the investigator of importance but also the degree of non-medical support. For maintenance of equipment a medical physics department or a service contract with the urodynamic equipment manufacturers is of benefit, and for videocystourethrography X-ray facilities need to be available. Simple investigations are cheap and the cost will increase with greater sophistication. The cost of equipment is largely a 'one off' expense with relatively low running costs. The most expensive equipment is not necessarily the best. Complicated computer software incorrectly utilized may give misleading results, whereas a simple paper chart recorder may yield easily interpretable data.

A continence advisor is an essential part of a fully integrated unit. She/he will directly refer patients who have failed to improve on simple management and may help carry out some investigations. Where techniques such as intermittent self-catheterization are needed she/he will be able to teach the patient at the clinic. Her/his role in referring women who have failed to respond to pelvic floor exercises and bladder drill, and indeed teaching these treatments where indicated, will overlap with that of the physiotherapist. She/he will also be able to advise patients and medical staff about available appliances and correct waterproof protection for clothing.

In the ideal unit, there would also be a urodynamic nurse in addition to the continence advisor. This nurse would have a more active role in patient assessment and in particular the carrying out of pad tests and ambulatory urodynamics. This would prevent the need for patients to attend on more than one occasion for additional investigations.

SUBJECTIVE TESTING

When considering setting up a unit, one needs to look at all aspects of lower urinary tract pathophysiology. Patients present with symptoms and these must not be ignored in favour of the results of complex investigations. Initially, it may seem that taking a history is relatively straightforward, but different ways of doing this may yield different results and some may be more open to bias than others. The latter point is of particular importance when changes in symptoms in patients involved in a research project are being examined by different clinicians passing through a unit. Therefore a standard symptom questionnaire should be established. This must be carefully thought out, as changes over time will make the comparison with previous data difficult and possibly meaningless. In addition it is important to collect data in a form which is easily stored on computer for analysis. In some units staff question patients whilst sitting at a computer terminal, but this often leads to patient dissatisfaction as there is less patient–doctor interaction.

Subjective assessment of lower urinary tract symptoms can be undertaken using self-administered questionnaires, direct questioning or visual analog scores. Self-administered questionnaires are notoriously unreliable as they depend on the patient's full comprehension of the terms used. Direct questioning by an investigator eliminates this problem but the severity of symptoms cannot be ascertained and the method is time consuming. Visual analog scores have been extensively used in assessment of pain[1] but there have been few studies evaluating their use in determining the presence and severity of lower urinary tract symptoms.[2,3,4,] Their correlation with direct questioning has never been ascertained. The main advantage of visual analog scores lies in the fact that they not only enable the severity of symptoms to be determined but also make it possible to assess subsequent changes in the same patient.

The most common variety utilized is a straight line 10 cm long, where one end denotes absence of the symptom and the other end maximum severity of the symptom. The patient marks on the line the position of her symptom and a measurement is made to indicate its severity. A disadvantage of this technique is that very few patients will mark a cross at the zero position and therefore if this method is used to ascertain the presence of a symptom, a falsely high impression may be gained.

This can be overcome by the use of visual analog scores in which there are gradations along the line and the patient scores within each box. This, however, has its own limitations in that the patient is guided by the gradations. There is no standard number of these.

Prior to investigation, the doctor in our unit asks the patient directly about a large number of lower urinary tract symptoms (Fig. 5.1), and in

KCH — URODYNAMICS DEPARTMENT

To ALL women: Would you please fill in as much of the following information as you can while you are waiting for your investigation.
Fill in the FIRST page only.

NAME: ....
.... DATE ....
ADDRESS ....
....
PHONE NO. (H) .... (W) ....
HOSPITAL NO. (KCH) ....
DATE OF BIRTH .... AGE: ....
NAME AND ADDRESS OF FAMILY DOCTOR
....
NAME AND ADDRESS OF REFERRING DOCTOR OR CONSULTANT
....
....
What are the main urinary problems that concern you? How long present?
(1) .... Present for ....
(2) .... Present for ....
(3) .... Present for ....
Do you have any current medical problems?
(1) ....
(2) ....
(3) ....
Have you had any other medical problems in the past?
(1) ....
(2) ....
(3) ....
Have you had any operations in the past?
(1) .... What year? ....
(2) .... What year? ....
(3) .... What year? ....
Do you have any children? .... How many? ....
Did you have any caesarean sections? ....
What was the weight of the heaviest child? ....
Are you still having your periods? ....
What medications are you currently taking?
(1) ....
(2) ....
(3) ....
How many cigarettes do you smoke daily? ....
How many 'water' infections have you had in the past two years? ....
Have you had any treatment in the past for your urinary symptoms? ....
If so, what?   ....
....

Fig. 5.1a Symptom questionnaire used at King's College Hospital

URINARY SYMPTOMS – DIRECT QUESTIONING
(to be answered only with the doctor)

Frequency – day (no. of times): 1 = 7 2 = 4 – 6 3 = 3 4 = 2 5 = 1 – 2 6 = 1
– night (no. of times): 0, 1, 2, 3, 4, 5, 6, 7+

Other symptoms: (0 = no, 1 = occasionally, 2 = frequently)

Stress incontinence. ☐

Urgency. ☐

Urge incontinence. ☐

Wet at rest. ☐

Wet on standing. ☐

Wet at night. ☐

Unaware of wetness. ☐

Pads/pants? ☐

Poor stream? ☐

Unable to interrupt flow. ☐

Post-mict dribble. ☐

Strain to void. ☐

Incomplete emptying. ☐

Cough. ☐

Constipation. ☐

Leg weakness. ☐

Rectal soiling. ☐

Perineal discomfort/prolapse. ☐

Enuresis after school age. ☐

Pain on micturition. (0 = nil, 1 = urethral, 2 = perineal, 3 = s/pubic ☐
4 = loin)

Fig. 5.1b   *(Cont'd)*   Dyspareunia (0 = no, 1 = superficial, 2 = deep) ☐

addition the patient fills in visual analog scores for a select number of
lower urinary tract symptoms (Fig. 5.2). This combined approach enables
a full picture of the presence and severity of the patient's complaint to be
obtained and also allows for future changes in symptoms to be accurately
documented.

OBJECTIVE ASSESSMENT

Objective assessment is the cornerstone to accurate diagnosis and correc
treatment. Different levels of sophistication are available, each having it
appropriate place. A unit must decide the level to which it wishes to

VISUAL ANALOG SYMPTOM SCORE

Name _____

Number

Visit

Date

Frequency (Daytime)

Normal |_____| Very frequent

Nocturia (Night)

Normal |_____| Very frequent

Stress incontinence

Not a problem |_____| Very severe

Urgency

Not a problem |_____| Very severe

Urge incontinence

Not a problem |_____| Very severe

Bedwetting

Not a problem |_____| Very severe

Stream

Normal |_____| Very slow

Complete emptying

Always |_____| Never

Fig. 5.2 Visual analogue score used at King's College Hospital

investigate and therefore which tests to employ. The various investigations which are available may be summarized as follows:

1. Non-specialist investigations
   a. Midstream specimen of urine
   b. Frequency/volume chart
   c. Pad test

2. Specialist investigations
   a. Uroflowmetry
   b. Cystometry
   c. Imaging techniques
      i.   Videocystourethrography
      ii. Micturating cystography
      iii. Intravenous urography
      iv. Ultrasonography
   d. Ambulatory urodynamics
   e. Urethral pressure profilometry
   f. Urethral electrical conductance
   g. Electromyography
   h. Cystourethroscopy.

Midstream specimen of urine

This is mandatory for all patients presenting with lower urinary tract symptoms and relies on the services of the microbiology department. A pure growth of >10^5 organisms/ml of urine is taken to signify an infection if cultured from a clean midstream specimen of urine.[6]

Urinary tract infections are not a common cause of incontinence but they will certainly aggravate any symptoms which are present. In addition, the presence of a urinary tract infection may invalidate the results of any investigation performed.[7] If urodynamic investigations are to be performed it is of benefit to ask referring physicians to obtain the results of an MSU and enclose a copy with the referral letter. This avoids the need to give all patients prophylactic antibiotics or treat empirically those patients who appear to have a urinary tract infection at the time of investigation.

Frequency/volume charts

Frequency/volume charts can be used objectively to assess voiding patterns. They are also used to determine fluid intake and urine output and to document incontinent episodes.[8] There are no recommendations as to the duration of time that they should span. Several different types have been described with recordings from 2 to 7 days.[9,10,11]

It is particularly useful to have this information prior to the urodynamic investigation and consideration should be given to sending a chart together with simple instructions with the appointment time so that the patient presents to the urodynamic clinic with a completed chart. Further details on frequency/volume charts can be obtained in Ch. 7.

Pad tests

Pad tests are used to quantify the degree of urine loss. They are also useful for documenting urinary leakage when the results of other tests are negative. Apart from the purchase of suitable pads, the main expense is the purchase of an accurate weighing machine. Except for research purposes, the use of pad tests will be limited to those women in whom the findings of urodynamic investigations have proved negative and most hospitals will have an appropriate weighing device which can be

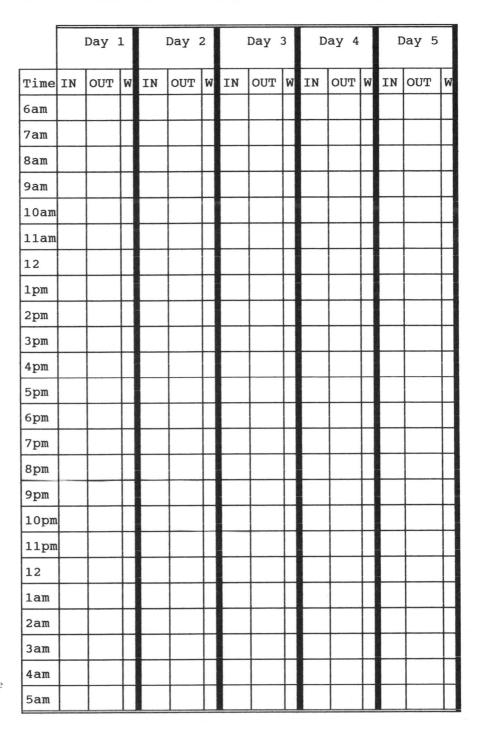

	Day 1			Day 2			Day 3			Day 4			Day 5		
Time	IN	OUT	W	IN	OUT	W	IN	OUT	W	IN	OUT	W	IN	OUT	W
6am															
7am															
8am															
9am															
10am															
11am															
12															
1pm															
2pm															
3pm															
4pm															
5pm															
6pm															
7pm															
8pm															
9pm															
10pm															
11pm															
12															
1am															
2am															
3am															
4am															
5am															

Fig. 5.3 Frequency/volume chart used at King's College Hospital

borrowed when required, thus reducing costs. If the urodynamic clinic is going to use pad testing to monitor improvement, then it is essential that the same mode of testing should be used for all patients in order to standardize results.

Urodynamic investigations

Although these are the investigations which are carried out in a urodynamic clinic, the criteria for history taking and simple investigations outlined above must be satisfied before consideration can be given to the investigations described below. The accuracy of any equipment used will not only depend on its inherent properties but also on correct usage, calibration and maintenance. The accuracy of commercially available systems will be predetermined, whereas locally constructed equipment will need to be checked to confirm that it conforms to the standards of commercial equipment. Home-made equipment by its nature tends to be much cheaper and will give roughly comparable results. The equipment used in the urodynamic unit at King's College Hospital was made from commercial components by the medical physics department. It is as accurate as commercial equipment and we perform over 1000 urodynamic investigations per year. The cost was a fraction of that of the commercial equipment and it has the advantage that it can be adapted for both clinical requirements and research projects as required.

The basic urodynamic equipment consists of uroflowmetry and cystometry components. The two may be purchased individually or as a complete system. The results may be displayed numerically, via a paper chart recorder, or stored on a computer disk from which a recording can be obtained.

Data presentation

Numeric read-outs will give clear numbers and at first would appear to result in more accurate data. However, inaccurate calibration or malfunction during the investigation, even if minor, will result in possibly undetected errors. Also there is no visual display and therefore the temporal concept of the urodynamic investigation is lost.

Paper chart recorders alone are used in the cheaper systems, with direct visualization of information as it is being generated. Malfunctions and operational errors will be evident as they happen and urodynamic events occurring in conjunction with the patient's symptoms are at once apparent. Measurements can be made from the gradations on the paper or with a ruler. Many machines will give digital read-outs which can be used in conjunction with the paper display.

The first generation of computerized systems uses the computer screen to give a visual display as the investigation is performed and the information is then stored on disk. The trace can be reviewed on the screen or printed out at a later date. In some systems there is the option of a real-time paper tracing in addition, so that the advantages of both recording methods may be enjoyed. Most of these systems require the cursor to be used to make measurements after the procedure is complete and this form of computerization is therefore only a more convenient method of paper storage. To the user it may seem that the fine measurements made with the computer cursor are preferable to the cruder measurements made with the ruler and paper print-out. However, the accuracy of the computer measurement largely exceeds the inherent accuracy of the urodynamic equipment itself and cannot therefore be fully utilized. Also, it is important to acknowledge that graphic storage entails a large amount of memory and therefore storage capabilities are limited and with time may in fact be less convenient than paper storage.

The most recent urodynamic systems offer complete computerization. Measurements are made from the recording each time an event marker is pressed and this can be automatically transferred into a patient database. This is useful in research where time spent inputting data by hand is thus saved. In clinical practice reports can be generated from the database and therefore reduce duplication of work. These systems are far more expensive and the numbers recorded should be checked against a visual display. As in the simple computerized systems, the apparent accuracy exceeds the accuracy of the test. Thus computerized systems are far more expensive than paper systems and the cost probably outweighs any advantage in clinical practice.

Uroflowmetry

Uroflowmetry is an essential part of any urodynamic assessment. The first flowmeter was described by von Garrelts in 1956.[12] The original design utilized a strain gauge weighing transducer placed under a cylindrical receptacle into which the patient voids. The weight of fluid is electronically converted to give a simultaneous flow rate. In addition the total volume of fluid can be measured. It is important to appreciate that the strain gauge is in fact measuring a change in mass, and for this reason it needs to be calibrated for fluid of the correct density. This method has been shown to be accurate for both clinical and experimental use.[13] Other commonly used devices include an electronic dipstick,[14] a rotating disc,[15] ultrasound[16] and the displacement of air from a container.[17]

Different commercial designs use different measuring devices, all claiming similar accuracies and durability. An independent assessment of five commercially available flowmeters[18] found the percentage error in measuring the flow rate to range from 4.5% to 15% and the error in the voided volume from 1.3% to 7.5%. The most accurate was the rotating disc device. This was followed by the electronic dipstick, with the strain gauge being the least accurate. However, all were accurate enough for clinical use as the variation in flow rate with the volume voided[19] is far greater than the variation in the accuracy between the different types of equipment. The strain gauge flowmeter, although possibly less accurate, has the advantage that it is easier to calibrate prior to use and easier to clean between patients (Fig. 5.4).

All commercial flowmeters record the peak flow rate and the volume voided. In addition most will give a visual demonstration of the shape of the flow curve. This is all the information that is required for making a clinical diagnosis of voiding difficulties. More sophisticated software will calculate the average flow rate, the time to peak flow, the voiding time and hesitancy. These parameters may be useful in the research setting but are not helpful in clinical practice. Variations in price reflect the different degrees of sophistication (Table 5.1). All commercially available flowmeters cost between £2500 and £3000.

Cystometry

Subtracted cystometry involves measurement of both the intravesical and intra-abdominal pressure simultaneously. Electronic subtraction of

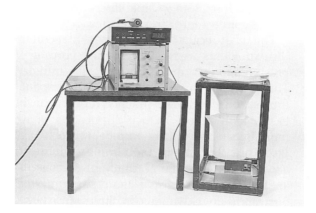

Fig. 5.4   A strain gauge flowmeter

Table 5.1   Different flowmeters commonly purchased

	Home-made	Albyn Medical (Gr100F)	Dantec (Urodyn 1000)	Lectromed (Uroflow)	Wiest (Ultracompact)
Measurement device	Strain gauge	Hydrostatic pressure	Spinning disk	Dipstick	Strain gauge
Print-out of flow curve	Yes	Yes	Yes	Yes	Yes
Peak flow rate	Measured from curve	Yes	Yes	Yes	Yes
Volume voided	Yes	Yes	Yes	Yes	Yes
Voiding time	No	No	Yes	Yes	Yes
Flow time	Measured from curve	Yes	Yes	Yes	Yes
Time to maximum flow rate	Measured from curve	Yes	Yes	Yes	Yes
Average flow rate	Measured from curve	Yes	Yes	Yes	Yes
Hesitancy	No	No	Calculated	Calculated	Yes

the latter from the former enables the detrusor pressure to be determined. A cystometrogram is necessary to make a diagnosis of detrusor instability, as this is a urodynamic diagnosis. Genuine stress incontinence may be diagnosed by exclusion. Cystometry is particularly useful in differentiating between cough-induced detrusor instability and genuine stress incontinence. Various factors in the equipment may affect results and a review of available information may determine the equipment and type of investigation performed in a particular unit.

Methods of testing Several studies have compared single-channel and subtracted cystometry with varying results.[20,21,22] However, repeated investigations in the same patient may have led to different results.[23]

Table 5.2 Studies comparing single- and multichannel cystometry

Study	n	Positive predictive value	Negative predictive value
Wheeler et al[20]	30	100%	89%
Sand et al[21]			
(single test)	100	74%	81%
(two tests)	100	69%	87%
Ouslander et al[22]			
(all cases)	171	85%	62%
(females)	139	84%	63%
Cutner et al[24]	107	98%	73%

More recently we have compared single- and multichannel cystometry in 107 women.[24] The patients had multichannel cystometry (video-cystourethrography) performed and reported by one doctor. The intra-vesical readings were fed into a single-channel chart recorder from which a second doctor made a diagnosis. Thus both tests were performed simultaneously, removing the possibility of errors due to repeated investigations in the same patient.[23] The positive and negative predictive values in the diagnosis of detrusor instability from simple cystometry when compared to subtracted cystometry in the above studies are shown in Table 5.2.

Thus it would appear that single-channel and subtracted cystometry give different results. The supposition of some of these authors that single-channel cystometry can be used as a screening test appears to be justified but this approach may cause overdiagnosis of detrusor instability. However, it may be that other factors have led to this discordance. The method of pressure measurement, the filling medium, the rate of filling and whether it was incremental or continuous and the effects of repeated tests may well have affected the results.

Pressure transducers Different types of pressure-measuring device have been described. The water manometer originally used does not facilitate a continuous pressure reading but provides incremental pressure measure-ments during filling (Mosso and Pellacani 1881) (Fig. 9.1). In 1921 Walker[25] described a new device for measuring incremental bladder pressures. This was a mercury manometer from which individual pressures were noted at different stages of filling and during voiding. Lewis[26] went further and measured bladder pressure continuously during filling via an aneroid barometer and recorded the results on a paper drum.

Two types of pressure transducer are used nowadays: fluid-filled catheters attached to an external pressure transducer (Fig. 5.5) and solid-state microtip pressure transducers mounted on a catheter. The fluid-filled catheters can have a balloon mounted on the end to prevent leakage of fluid when being used to measure intrarectal or intravaginal pressure. The advantages of fluid-filled pressure catheters are that they are less expensive and more durable. In addition they enable a zero reference to be utilized at the level of the symphysis pubis.[27] Pressure recordings are made either on a paper chart recorder or on to computer software. The advantage

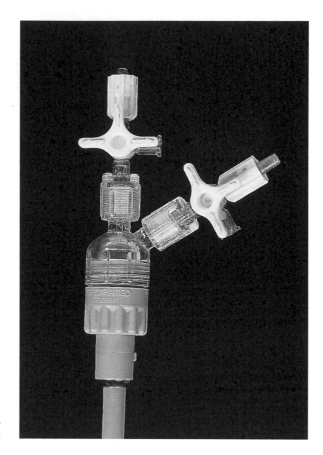

Fig. 5.5 External pressure transducer to which the fluid-filled pressure line is attached

of microtip pressure transducers is that they have a faster response time. A disadvantage is that after each patient the microtip pressure transducer catheter needs to be sterilized. In addition, microtip transducers are expensive and prone to mechanical failure if not used carefully.

Filling medium This can be either gas or liquid. Originally water was used, but nowadays 0.9% saline is the most commonly used filling medium. If simultaneous radiological screening is to be carried out, then a radio-opaque filling medium such as Urografin can be used. Gas cystometry is popular in North America. Air was the original gas used but has now been largely replaced by carbon dioxide. The disadvantages of gas cystometry are discussed in Ch. 9.

Mode of filling Other factors which may affect results are the rate of filling, the temperature of the fluid and whether filling is incremental or continuous. Again these are discussed in Ch. 9.

Due to the considerable variations outlined, the International Continence Society has recommended that tests should be performed in a standard manner and the techniques used described fully.[8] Parameters include: type of catheter, filling medium (including temperature and rate), type of pressure transducer and recording equipment. In addition the position of the patient during filling and the type of provocation tests used should be noted. Thus each unit should standardize its method of investigation so that comparisons can be made over time.

What equipment to purchase

One might assume that single-channel cystometry equipment is cheaper to purchase than that for subtracted cystometry; however, this is not the case with commercial systems. In the 'home-made' setting, a cheap system using a water manometer with incremental filling can be set up at very little expense, but this could only be used as a screening test and we would not recommend it as a routine investigation. Carbon dioxide as a filling medium is not recommended in the UK for reasons outlined in Ch. 9. We have found fluid-filled pressure transducers to be reliable over many years of use but with time it is possible that solid-state transducers will become more durable.

An independent survey of eight different commercially available systems was reported in 1991.[28] The authors outlined the problems with different makes of equipment and commented on the lack of advantage of computerized systems. They concluded that we are not in the age of automated urodynamics and warned of the dangers of not appreciating artefacts when using a computerized system.

They stated that the ideal urodynamic equipment should be compact, maneuverable, robust and user-friendly. There must be a pause mode for checking the system set up and for rechecking (if necessary) during an investigation. During the pause mode, a graphic display is an advantage. Realtime display and paper print-out, in addition to computer storage, enable rapid diagnoses to be made and safe-guard against hard disk failure. The ideal system would automatically analyze and store the results, but until recently this has not been possible. There are now urodynamic machines available whereby results denoted by event markers during the test are automatically transferred into a database on the computer. However, again results should be checked as the computer systems are unable to differentiate artefact from reality.

Different urodynamic systems

There are many systems available and below is a list of some of the popular makes and the cost for the basic equipment for subtracted cystometry with uroflowmetry. We have given the basic price and the final cost may be greater than that quoted if extra features are required. They have been set out in increasing order of complexity.

1. Home-made (Fig. 5.6)
Cost: £1500
Five-channel chart recorder. (secondhand)
Fluid-filled pressure lines.
Paper print-out.
All measurements made from printed trace.

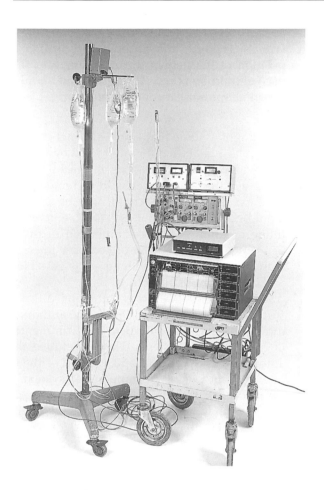

Fig. 5.6   Home-made urodynamic equipment used at King's College Hospital

2. Lectromed (5000 CA) (Fig. 5.7)
Cost: £6000
Now available as reconditioned model.
Paper print-out.
Event markers.
Five-channel chart recorder.

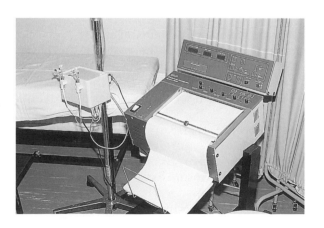

Fig. 5.7   Lectromed (5000 CA)

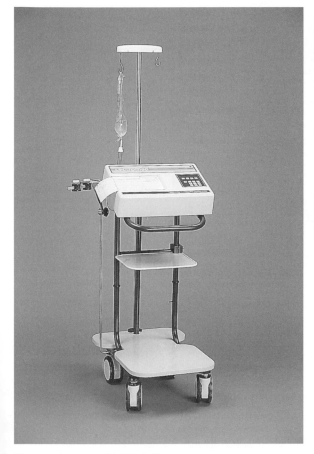

Fig. 5.8   Lectromed (6700 CA)

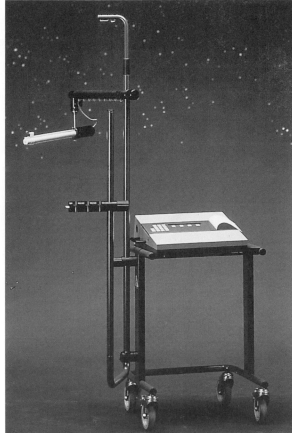

Fig. 5.9   Dantec (Etude)

Minimal data printed automatically on to paper print-out.
Most measurements recorded direct from paper print-out.

Now replaced by the Lectromed (6700 CA) (Fig. 5.8)
Cost: £7000.

3. Dantec (Etude) (Fig. 5.9)
Cost: £9000
Paper print-out.
Event markers.
Event markers and pressure measurements are automatically printed out.
Small amount of UPP data is also automatically calculated.

4. Wiest (Merkur) (Fig. 5.10)
Cost: £12 000
Can be operated via a remote control unit.
On-screen print-out and paper print-out possible.
Stores one hour of traces. Downloading is possible with the purchase of
additional software and a computer.

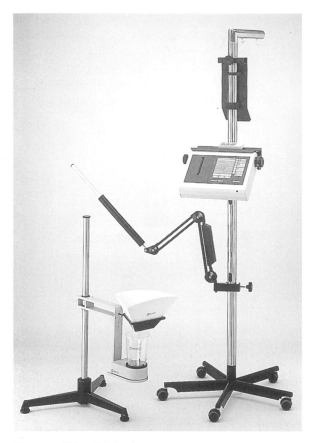

Fig. 5.10   Wiest (Merkur)

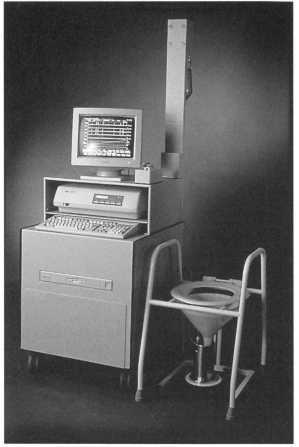

Fig. 5.11   Albyn Medical (Griffin)

Most clinical measurements are automatically recorded and printed out. Future potential to use as part of a fully integrated VCU system but this vastly increases the price.

5. Albyn Medical (Griffin) (Fig. 5.11)
Cost: £15 000
Computer-based.
Computerized reports can be generated.
Some results are automatically generated but many measurements involve on-screen analysis.
Results can be automatically transferred to a database.
Continuous paper print-out is an option.
Can download traces onto disk.

Computerized systems The following are some of the fully computerized systems which also include VCU integration. They all have paper print-out options and generate most data automatically. In addition parameters can be measured using a screen cursor. The data can be transferred into a database on most systems and the recordings can be stored on disk. The exact features of each system are similar and purchase will depend on individual requirements and preference for ease of use. Increased cost normally reflects the degree of complexity and versatility of the system. It may also reflect the options which are included in the basic set-up model. All are fairly complex to use and should not be purchased without full on-site demonstration.

Wiest (Jupiter) (Fig. 5.12)
Cost: £25 000

Albyn Medical (Phoenix) (Fig. 5.13)
Cost: £20 000

Dantec (Menuet) (Fig. 5.14)
Cost: £15 000

Lectromed (6000 CA) (Fig. 5.15)
Cost: £18 000

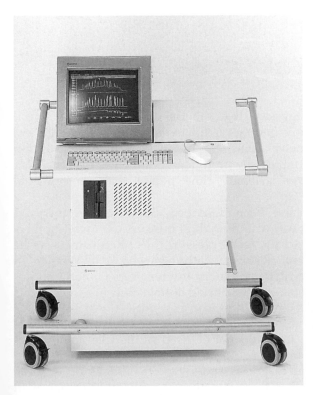

Fig. 5.12   Wiest (Jupiter)

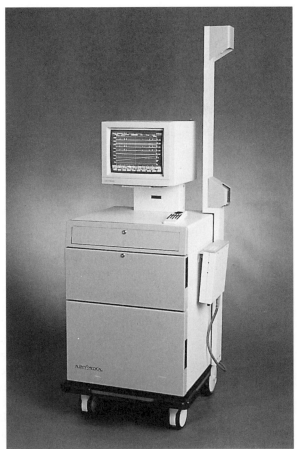

Fig. 5.13   Albyn Medical (Phoenix)

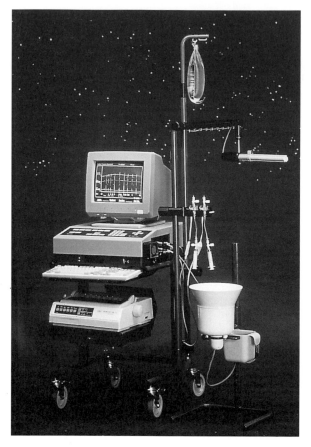

Fig. 5.14 Dantec (Menuet)

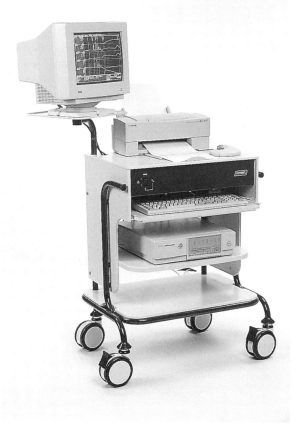

Fig. 5.15 Lectromed (6000 CA)

Ambulatory urodynamics

Recently it has been suggested that the lack of correlation between symptoms and urodynamic findings is due to the mode of investigation, with subtracted cystometry being too insensitive in the detection of detrusor instability. Ambulatory urodynamics involves the recording of bladder function over a longer time period than conventional urodynamics.

Different techniques have been described. Some studies involved measurement of the intravesical and urethral pressures,[29,30] whilst others have in addition measured the rectal pressure.[31,32,33] Recordings can be made on a 24-hr tape which is subsequently reviewed.[31,32,33] Workers in this field have suggested that ambulatory urodynamics is more physiological as the assessment takes place during normal daily activities and is more sensitive in the detection of detrusor instability.[30,31,33] However, as yet it is not a routine test in the assessment of lower urinary tract function or dysfunction. It should not be used as the sole mode of investigation and is really only used in the clinical setting in those women in whom the urodynamic diagnosis and symptomatology appear to be totally incongruous or when there is a normal result in a woman with persistent symptoms.

Urethral pressure profilometry

The first report of urethral pressure measurements was in 1923.[34] One early method involved measuring the intraurethral pressure via a balloon catheter.[54] This method has two main disadvantages. First there is distortion of the urethra, and secondly pressure recordings are from the whole length of the balloon and not at a discrete point.

Fluid perfusion techniques can be used to measure the intraurethral pressure.[37] Pressure changes along the length of the urethra are determined and the intravesical pressure is simultaneously recorded.[36,37,38] Although this method enables the urethral pressure profile at rest to be determined, the response time (known as the rise time) of the system is too slow to measure dynamic changes in pressure.

Both the above systems are still sold but their use in the urodynamic clinic, except possibly in research, is obsolete. The advent of solid-state microtransducers circumvented these problems. Simultaneous urethrocystometry was first popularized by Asmussen & Ulmsten.[39] A catheter with two pressure-tip transducers a set distance (usually 6 cm) apart is gradually withdrawn at a constant rate along the urethra enabling simultaneous recording of the intravesical and intraurethral pressures (Fig. 5.16). Electronic subtraction of these recordings can be made. Many different parameters of the resultant trace can be analyzed. The profile can be assessed both at rest and during stress.

Urethral pressure profilometry is a useful research tool in the investigation of lower urinary tract dysfunction. In clinical practice it is useful in cases of voiding difficulties and following previous incontinence surgery. It is particularly applicable to tertiary referral centers. Thus the expense of a double microtip pressure transducer catheter and mechanized withdrawal device has to be considered carefully in the routine clinical setting. The cost will depend on the make of equipment but will have to

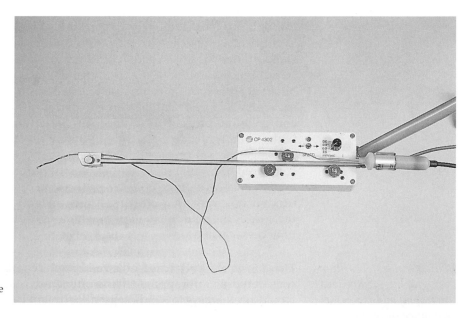

Fig. 5.16   Wiest urethral pressure profile withdrawal device with urethral pressure profile catheter attached

be compatible with the basic urodynamic set-up. Costs start at around £2500.

Urethral electrical conductance

Urethral electrical conductance has not achieved widespread acceptance even as a screening test. As it has little to offer in a unit performing subtracted cystometry, its use is not recommended.

Electromyography

This test is useful in those units with a large referral pattern from neurological centers as it enables testing of the integrity of a muscle and its nerve supply. Its use, however, is mainly as a research tool and routine purchase is not justified. Most commercial urodynamic equipment (especially computerized systems) have a port to which an electromyogram probe can be fed and therefore allows its use should the unit develop an interest.

The lower urinary tract can be visualized with X-rays, ultrasound, via a cystoscope and most recently with magnetic resonance imaging. X-ray screening as part of the urodynamic investigation enhances dynamic assessment of the lower urinary tract. Combined with cystometry it is known as videocystourethrography (VCU).[40]

Videocystourethrography

If radio-opaque medium is used to fill the bladder, the lower urinary tract can be visualized during cystometry using X-ray screening, usually with an image intensifier. Thus the unit must have access to a radiology department and in most hospitals this would involve setting up the equipment each time it is used. Movement (even of portable equipment) increases the incidence of breakages and therefore increases the running costs. In addition, in Europe any personnel involved with X-rays are required to have a certificate endorsing their safety to use them. Users need to wear a dose detection badge and this would be organized through the local radiology department. Videocystourethrography is a sophisticated mode of investigation and probably currently the 'gold standard' for the investigation of lower urinary tract function.[23,41] An on-screen representation of the urodynamic trace with the X-ray image can be set up for more meaningful video storage. However, VCU is more expensive and more cumbersome to perform than subtracted cystometry and therefore probably only necessary in tertiary referral centers dealing with complicated cases. In addition the running costs of each investigation are greater due to the cost of radio-opaque filling media compared to normal saline. Urodynamic equipment at the top end of the market enables storage of X-ray pictures on disk in conjunction with the urodynamic trace, thus creating a fully integrated system. This will make the cost of the equipment very much more expensive and is probably an unnecessary luxury.

Plain X-rays, micturition cystography, intravenous urography and magnetic resonance imaging

These tests are performed by a radiology department and would not be considered as appropriate to a urodynamic unit. However, such a unit would need access to a radiology department in certain cases.

Ultrasound

Ultrasound is a non-invasive technique. Both abdominal and vaginal ultrasound are routinely used for determining bladder volumes.[42,43,44] The bladder capacity and urinary residual can be estimated. Ultrasound is also employed to examine the upper tracts in search of ureteric dilatation and renal tumors.

The role of ultrasound in examining the lower urinary tract in the diagnosis of urinary incontinence has not yet been established. The use of vaginal ultrasonography to differentiate genuine stress incontinence from detrusor instability has been suggested by several authors.[45,46] Other workers have used rectal[47] and perineal ultrasound[48] to examine the anatomy of the lower urinary tract. It is important to appreciate that although ultrasound examination is able to detect morphological abnormalities of the lower urinary tract, it is unable to replace those investigations which assess dynamic pressure changes of the lower urinary tract. In addition, the image produced by ultrasound is really not as clear as that produced by radiological screening.

The cost of purchasing an ultrasound machine to measure urinary residuals is probably not justified in view of the relatively low cost of a catheter. However, many units may have access to an ultrasound machine used for other indications, thus making its use more attractive. There have recently appeared on the market small, cheap ultrasound machines solely designed to measure urinary residuals, which may make this technique a more viable proposition. In the research setting, the potential of ultrasound in assessing the dynamics of the lower urinary tract has not yet been fully realized.

Cystourethroscopy

This is normally carried out under general anesthesia but if a flexible cystoscope is used then local anesthesia can be employed. Improvements in fibre optics resulting in smaller-diameter scopes has enabled cystourethroscopy to be performed in the urodynamic clinic. It is, however, expensive equipment and the cost for sole use in a urodynamic clinic would be prohibitively high.

SUMMARY

There are many investigations of lower urinary tract dysfunction but subtracted cystometry remains the most useful in making an accurate diagnosis. It is important that any unit decides its requirements from its referral pattern and local expertise. The method of history taking should be standardized as should the mode of investigation. Uroflowmetry with subtracted cystometry is the baseline and the minimum requirement. Paper recorders will suffice and expensive and often complex computerized systems should not be considered until basic concepts have been fully grasped. Digital read-outs and smart graphic presentation are no substitute for the basic urodynamic trace.

REFERENCES

1 Huskisson EC. Measurement of pain. Lancet 1974; 2: 1127–1131.
2 Parkin DE, Davis JA. Use of a visual analogue scale in the diagnosis of urinary incontinence. Br Med J 1986; 293: 365–366.
3 Frazer MI Sutherst JR, Holland EFN. Visual analogue scores and urinary incontinence. Br Med J 1987; 295: 582.
4 Frazer MI, Haylen BT, Sutherst JR. The severity of urinary incontinence in women. Comparison of subjective and objective tests. Br J Urol 1989; 63: 14–15.
5 McLoughlin J, Abel PD, Shaikh H, Waters J, Williams G. Visual analogue scales distinguish between low urinary flow rates due to impaired detrusor contractility and those due to bladder outflow obstruction. Br J Urol 1990; 66: 16–18.
6 Kass EH. Bacteriuria and the diagnosis of infections of the urinary tract. AMA Archives Int Med 1957; 100: 709–714.
7 Bergman A, Bhatia NN. Urodynamics: effect of urinary tract infection on urethral and bladder function. Obstet Gynecol 1985a; 66: 366–371.
8 Abrams P, Blaivas JG, Stanton SL, Andersen JT. The standardisation of terminology of lower urinary tract function. Br J Obstet Gynaecol 1990; 97 (Suppl 6): 1–16.
9 Larsson G, Victor A. Micturition patterns in a healthy female population, studied with a frequency/volume chart. Scand J Urol Nephrol 1988; Suppl 114: 53–57.
10 Sommer P, Bauer T, Nielsen KK et al. Voiding patterns and prevalence of incontinence in women. A questionnaire survey. Br J Urol 1990; 66: 12–15.
11 Bailey R, Shepherd A, Tribe B. How much information can be obtained from frequency/volume charts? Neurourol Urodyn 1990; 9: 382–383.
12 von Garrelts B. Analysis of micturition: a new method of recording the voiding of the bladder. Acta Chir Scand 1956; 112: 326–340.
13 Nyman CR, Boman J, Gidlof A. Von Garrelts uroflowmeter, a technical and clinical evaluation. Proceedings of the 7th Annual Meeting of the International Continence Society, Portoroz, 1977: pp 88–90.
14 James ED. A novel 'dip-stick' type urine volume and flow rate monitor. Proceedings of the 7th Annual Meeting of the International Continence Society, Portoroz, 1977; p 85.
15 Rowan D, Mackenzie AL, McNee S, Glen E. A technical and clinical evaluation of the Disa uroflowmeter. Proceedings of the 6th (*Annual Meeting of the*) International Continence Society, Antwerp, 1976.
16 Rollema HJ. An ultrasonic volumeter for uroflowmetry. Proceedings of the 6th (*Annual Meeting of the*) International Continence Society, Antwerp, 1976.
17 Gierup J, Ericsson NO, Okmian L. Micturition studies in infants and children. Scand J Urol Nephrol 1969; 3: 1–8.
18 Christmas TJ, Chapple CR, Rickards D, Milroy EJG, Turner-Warwick RT. Contemporary flow meters: an assessment of their accuracy and reliability.
19 Haylen BT, Ashby D, Sutherst JR, Frazer MI, West CR. Maximum and average flow rates in normal male and female populations — the Liverpool nomograms. Br J Urol 1989b; 64: 30–38.
20 Wheeler Jr JS, Niecestro RM, Fredian C, Walter JS. Comparison of a simple cystometer with a multichannel cystometer in females with voiding dysfunction. Int Urogynecol J 1991; 2: 90–93.
21 Sand PK, Brubaker LT, Novak T. Simple standing incremental cystometry as a screening method for detrusor instability. Obstet Gynecol 1991; 77: 453–457.
22 Ouslander J, Leach G, Abelson S, Staskin D, Blaustein J, Raz S. Simple versus multichannel cystometry in the evaluation of bladder function in an incontinent geriatric population. J Urol 1988; 140: 1482–1486.
23 Benness CJ, Barnick CG, Cardozo L. Is there a place for routine videocystourethrography in the assessment of lower urinary tract function? Neurourol Urodyn 1989; 8: 299–300.
24 Cutner A, Wise BG, Cardozo LD, Burton G, Abbott D, Kelleher CJ. Single channel cystometry as a screening test for abnormal detrusor activity. Neurourol Urodyn 1992; 11(4): 455–456.
25 Walker G. Apparatus to aid differentiation between an obstruction in the urinary outlet and paralysis of the bladder. JAMA 1921; 77: 286–287.
26 Lewis LG. A new clinical recording cystometer. J Urol 1939; 41: 638–645.
27 Rowan D, James ED, Kramer AEJL, Sterling AM, Suhel PF. Urodynamic equipment: technical aspects. J Med Engineering and Technology. 1987; 11: 57–64.
28 Barnes DG, Ralph D, Lewis CA, Shaw PJR, Worth PHL. A consumer's guide to commercially available urodynamic equipment. Br J Urol 1991; 68: 138–143.

29 Bhatia NN, Bradley WE, Haldeman S, Johnson BK. Continuous monitoring of bladder and urethral pressures: new technique. Urol 1981; 18: 207–210.

30 Bhatia NN, Bradley WE, Haldeman S. Urodynamics: continuous monitoring. Urol 1982; 128: 963–968.

31 van Waalwijk van Doorn ESC, Zwiers W, Wetzels LLRH, Debruyne FMJ. A comparative study between standard and ambulant urodynamics. Neurourol Urodyn 1987; 6: 159–160.

32 Janknegt RA, van Waalwijk van Doorn ESC. Clinical experiences with advanced ambulatory urodynamics. Neurourol Urodyn 1989; 8: 402–404.

33 McInerney PD, Vanner TF, Harris SAB, Stephenson TP. Ambulatory urodynamics. Br J Urol 1991; 67: 272–274.

34 Bonney V. On diurnal incontinence of urine in women. J Obstet Gynaecol Br Emp 1923; 30: 358–365.

35 Simons I. Studies in bladder function. 2. The sphincterometer. J Urol 1936; 35: 96–102.

36 Enhorning G. Simultaneous recordings of the intravesical and intraurethral pressure. A study on urethral closure in normal and stress incontinent women. Acta Chir Scand 1961; Suppl 276: 1–68.

37 Toews HA. Intraurethral and intravesical pressures in normal and stress-incontinent women. Obstet Gynecol 1967; 29: 613–624.

38 Brown M, Wickham JEA. The urethral pressure profile. Br J Urol 1969; 41: 211–217.

39 Asmussen M, Ulmsten U. Simultaneous urethrocystometry with a new technique. Scand J Urol Nephrol 1976; 10: 7–11.

40 Enhorning G, Miller ER, Hinman F Jr. Urethral closure studied with cineroentgenography and simultaneous bladder–urethra pressure recording. Surg Gynecol Obstet 1964; 118: 507–516.

41 Turner-Warwick R. The valuation of urodynamic function. Urol Clin North Am 1979b; 6: 51–54.

42 Haylen BT. Residual urine volumes in a normal female population: application of transvaginal ultrasound. Br J Urol 1989a; 64: 347–349.

43 Haylen BT. Verification of the accuracy and range of transvaginal ultrasound in measuring bladder volumes in women. Br J Urol 1989b; 64: 350–352.

44 Benness CJ, Tapp AJS, Cardozo LD. Estimation of urinary residual volume in the puerperium by ultrasound. Neurourol Urodyn 1989b; 8: 329–330.

45 Koelbl H, Bernaschek G. A new method for sonographic urethrocystography and simultaneous pressure–flow measurements. Obstet Gynecol 1989; 74: 417–422.

46 Quinn MJ. Vaginal ultrasound and urinary stress incontinence. Contemp Rev Obstet Gynaecol 1990; 2: 104–110.

47 Bergman A, McKenzie CJ, Richmond J, Ballard CA, Platt D. Transrectal ultrasound versus cystography in the evaluation of anatomical stress urinary incontinence. Br J Urol 1988; 62: 228–234.

48 Gordon D, Pearce M, Norton P, Stanton SL. Comparison of ultrasound and lateral chain urethrocystography in the determination of bladder neck descent. Am J Obstet Gynecol 1989; 160: 182–185.

6

History and examination

INTRODUCTION

Symptoms are subjective observations resulting from an interaction between the disease process, the environment and the ability to modify behaviour. The environment and a woman's ability to cope with her disease can profoundly alter her quality of life. A woman who is always close to a toilet may not notice her urinary frequency but the same woman with no access to a toilet may have urinary incontinence, wear protective pads and be severely incapacitated.

Can the severity of urinary symptoms be modified by behavior? A woman can alter the volume of urine produced by changing the amount of fluid drunk.[1] A change in urine production can significantly alter symptoms. Women with severe detrusor instability may restrict their fluid intake to < 200 ml a day; on direct questioning the urinary problem may not appear severe since there is a normal diurnal urinary frequency, and it may be only with a frequency volume chart that a complete picture of the severity of the detrusor instability can be determined. The volume of urine excreted relies not only on fluid intake but also on the secretion of antidiuretic hormone, which is impaired in diabetes insipidus; moreover the circadian secretion of this hormone is reversed in some women[2] and children suffering nocturia and nocturnal enuresis.[3]

HISTORY

The history must be taken in the patient's own words; these are then clarified into an easily understandable list of graded symptoms for the clinician. A standard questionnaire is used see (Fig. 5.1), and when the symptoms and final urodynamic diagnosis are compared there is a marked overlap between diagnostic groups. The diagnosis based on history and examination is only correct in about 65% of women.[4,5] Mixed incontinence is found in a large proportion of women of all diagnostic categories, 55% of women with urethral sphincter incompetence and 35% of women with detrusor instability.[6] Symptom complexes have been used in an attempt to improve diagnostic accuracy. Wise et al[7] evaluated the diagnostic accuracy of visual analog scores and found that these did increase discrimination between women with genuine stress incontinence and detrusor instability but the separation on the visual analog scores was not sufficient for diagnosis.

If symptoms are not of diagnostic value why record them? Symptoms are valuable as a guide in determining treatment. In addition, symptoms should be taken into consideration during the urodynamic test as the provocative maneuvers should mimic conditions encountered by the woman in her normal daily activities and lead to her urinary symptoms. A 90-year-old woman with urgency and no stress incontinence is an inappropriate candidate for performing 'star jumps' with a full bladder!

When questioning women complaining of urinary symptoms, all symptoms complained of should be explained in a woman's own words. Stress incontinence is the term used to describe urinary leakage which occurs with a cough or sneeze or follows it by a few seconds even when considerable urgency is associated with the leakage.

The severity of each symptom and its effect on the woman's quality of life are noted, as cure can be achieved by directing treatment to relieve the troublesome symptoms. Determining the length of time that the symptoms have been present discriminates between transient and established incontinence and it should also be established whether the symptoms have changed over time. General enquiry should be made of all urinary symptoms, as the woman may not be able to describe them or may be too embarrassed to mention them. For this reason a questionnaire is a useful guide as it ensures that all symptoms are enquired about. The symptoms can be grouped as follows:

1. Abnormal storage
   a. Incontinence
      i. Urge
      ii. Stress
   b. Frequency/nocturia
   c. Nocturnal enuresis
2. Abnormal voiding
   a. Straining to void
   b. Hesitancy
   c. Incomplete emptying
   d. Poor stream
   e. Postmicturition dribble
3. Abnormal sensation
   a. Urgency
   b. Dysuria
   c. Absent sensation
   d. Painful bladder.

This classification of symptoms does not help in diagnosis as overflow incontinence can produce similar symptoms to detrusor instability. Urinary frequency in overflow incontinence is caused by incomplete bladder emptying resulting in a reduced bladder capacity, and in detrusor instability urinary frequency is caused by an overactive detrusor. The same symptom is thus produced by two different mechanisms.

SPECIFIC SYMPTOMS

Frequency

Frequency is the number of times a woman voids during waking hours; normal diurnal frequency is considered to be between 4 and 7 voids per day, but in a symptomatic population the range may be greater (Fig. 6.1). Frequency is not diagnostic for detrusor instability[8] or for genuine stress incontinence,[9] although women with detrusor instability do void more frequently. Clustering of voids during the day may suggest a cause such as diuretics prescribed for congestive cardiac failure, intake of large volumes of fluid or simply bad habit. Abnormal urinary frequency may occur for a number of reasons, which may be listed as follows:

1. Increased fluid intake and urine output: normal bladder capacity
   a. Osmotic diuresis, e.g. diabetes mellitus
   b. Abnormal antidiuretic hormone production, e.g. diabetes insipidus
   c. Polydipsia: often the woman enjoys a favourite beverage and only rarely is the behavior psychotic
2. Reduced functional bladder capacity
   a. Inflamed bladder increasing bladder sensation, e.g. acute bacterial cystitis, interstitial cystitis
   b. Detrusor instability
   c. Habit or fear of urinary incontinence
   d. Urinary residual secondary to detrusor hypotonia or outlet obstruction (rare)
   e. Increased bladder sensation of normal bladder, e.g. anxiety
3. Reduced structural bladder capacity
   a. Fibrosis after infection, e.g. tuberculosis
   b. Non-infective cystitis, e.g. interstitial cystitis, carcinoma
   c. Irradiation fibrosis, e.g. bladder or cervical carcinoma
   d. Post surgery, e.g. partial cystectomy
   e. Detrusor hypertrophy

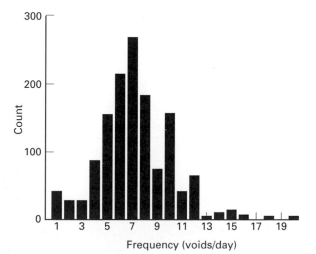

g. 6.1 Voiding frequency symptomatic women

4. Decreased urinary frequency
   a. Detrusor hypotonia
   b. Impaired bladder sensation, e.g. diabetic neuropathy
   c. Reduced fluid intake.

The diurnal frequency did not increase with age in the symptomatic population seen in our urodynamic clinic between January 1993 and September 1994 (Table 6.1).

Nocturia

Nocturia is the number of times a woman has to wake from sleep to pass urine; it is important to discriminate between this and a woman who is voiding because she is awake. The normal upper limit to the number of voids alters with age (Table 6.2). If a woman passes urine more than once a night up to the age of 70 years this is abnormal; voiding at night increases on average once every decade after the age of 70 in normal women. This change is probably due to changing sleep patterns in the elderly and postural effects due to daytime pooling of extracellular fluid in the lower limbs which returns to the vascular compartment at night. It is important to discriminate between the woman who is awake and therefore voids and the woman who is woken by the desire to void; the first group of women often have no increase in their diurnal urinary frequency.

Urinary incontinence

Urinary incontinence requires careful evaluation. This is involuntary urine loss which is a social or hygienic problem and is objectively

Table 6.1 Diurnal frequency in a symptomatic population (seen in urodynamic clinic, King's College Hospital, between January 1993 and September 1994)

Age (years)	Mean Frequency	n (total = 1893)
5–14	6.00	5
15–24	4.48	41
25–34	5.47	176
35–44	6.31	364
45–54	6.05	513
55–64	5.87	361
65–74	5.63	263
75–84	5.04	137
85–94	5.93	33

Table 6.2 Nocturnal voids and nocturia with age (seen in urodynamic clinic, King's College Hospital, between January 1993 and September 1994)

Age (years)	Mean voids per night	% Nocturia	n
5–14	0.8	0	5
15–24	1.24	17	41
25–34	1.79	27	176
35–44	1.83	38	364
45–54	1.53	30	513
55–64	1.94	31	361
65–74	2.20	47	263
75–84	2.55	46	137
85–94	2.69	58	33

demonstrable. Loss of urine through channels other than the urethra is extraurethral incontinence.[10] It is important that incontinence is regarded as a symptom or a sign and not a diagnosis. Severe urinary incontinence of any origin has overlapping symptoms associated with urethral sphincter incompetence and detrusor instability. The causes of urinary incontinence are many and can be classified as follows:

1. Urethral sphincter incompetence
   a. Sphincter dysfunction
   b. Abnormal bladder neck support
2. Detrusor overactivity
   a. Idiopathic detrusor instability
   b. Detrusor hyperreflexia, e.g. multiple sclerosis, spinal trauma
3. Mixed incontinence
4. Urethral diverticula
5. Congenital abnormalities, e.g. epispadias, ectopic ureter, bladder exstrophy, spina bifida occulta
6. Transient incontinence
   a. Urinary tract infection
   b. Restricted mobility
   c. Constipation
   d. Excessive urine production
      i.   Diuretic therapy
      ii. Diabetes mellitus
      iii. Diabetes inspidus
      iv. Cardiac failure
      v.   Hypercalcemia
   e. Confusion, e.g. dementia, acute illness
   f. Atrophic urethritis and vaginitis
7. Pharmacological causes, e.g. diuretics, tranquilizers, cholinergic agents, prazosin
8. Fistulae, e.g. urethral, vesical, ureteral
9. Overflow incontinence
   a. Hypotonic detrusor
   b. Rarely urethral obstruction
10. Urethral instability
11. Functional.

It is important to determine whether the urine loss is continuous or intermittent.

Continuous urine loss is rare. It is usually seen when there is an ectopic ureter or fistula; the women will often complain of nocturnal incontinence as opposed to nocturnal enuresis. This occurs most often following pelvic surgery or as a result of malignancy, or radiotherapy. Obstetric fistulae are more commonly seen in the Third World. These patients should be separated from another category of women who complain that they are never dry. Patients from this group often suffer from severe intermittent urinary incontinence, rather than a continuous loss of urine. This occurs in women who have had multiple previous operations and have a fixed and fibrosed 'drainpipe' urethra.

The pattern of intermittent urinary incontinence should be linked with associated activity, such as physical exercise, laughing, putting the key in the front door, sexual intercourse or orgasm. The severity of the incontinence can be quantified not only by volume but also by the type and number of pads required in 24 h and the magnitude of the provoking stimulus. Often there is little relation between the findings of urodynamic tests and the symptoms described by the patient in her day-to-day life. This reflects modification in behavior and lifestyle to ameliorate the condition and reduce the impact on the woman's life. It does not, however, reduce the importance of the symptoms described.

Stress incontinence

Stress incontinence is the involuntary loss of urine on an increase in intra-abdominal pressure, such as when coughing, sneezing, running and lifting. There is no associated urgency. The urine is usually lost in small discrete amounts.[11,12] This must be differentiated from urge incontinence.

Urge incontinence

Urge incontinence is a type of urinary incontinence occurring in association with the symptom of urgency (a strong sudden desire to void). Often women will describe getting the sensation of the desire to void and not getting to the toilet in time. The quantity of urine lost can be a few drops on lowering the undergarments prior to voiding or can be quite a large volume and it is not uncommon for the patient to describe at least one occasion where the urine has poured down both legs uncontrollably. The urge incontinence may be triggered by changes in temperature, opening the front door or hearing running water and occasionally takes place during sexual intercourse at orgasm. The main coping strategy for this symptom is increasing voiding frequency, thus pad usage or counting the incontinent episodes are not useful in assessing the severity of the condition. The symptom of urge incontinence has a limited sensitivity of 78% and a specificity of 39% in the diagnosis of detrusor instability.[5] This contrasts with the findings of Farrar et al,[13] where women with urge incontinence were found to have detrusor instability in 80% of cases.

Mixed incontinence

In mixed urinary incontinence, which is very common, where the patient has both symptoms of stress and urge incontinence, it is very important to determine the balance between the two symptoms, and which troubles her the most.

Coital incontinence

Urinary incontinence can occur during sexual intercourse either on penetration or during orgasm. Urinary leakage on penetration is more likely to occur in women with urethral sphincter incompetence and with a cystocele.[14] The urinary incontinence is not associated with urgency. Leakage with orgasm is associated with urgency and is thought to be related to detrusor instability.[15,16]

Nocturnal enuresis

Nocturnal enuresis is urinary loss during sleep. It is important to differentiate between this complaint and waking with urgency and then leaking before arriving at the toilet, which is urge incontinence. Nocturnal enuresis can be primary or secondary. Primary nocturnal enuresis start in childhood and can persist into adulthood, the woman never having consistently been dry at night.[17] Secondary nocturnal enuresis is when the incontinence restarts in adulthood following a period of night-time continence, even if it resolved in childhood. The causes for this can be abnormal circadian secretion of antidiuretic hormone, detrusor instability, abnormal control of the micturition reflex or abnormal sleep pattern. A family history should be sought and the presence of diurnal symptoms noted.

Post-micturition dribble

After voiding is completed, a woman may complain of intermittent urinary loss per urethran. This symptom may be related to a urethral diverticulum, a cystourethrocele or detrusor instability. Where detrusor contractions occur after the completion of voiding, urgency will often accompany the urinary leakage. Post-micturition dribble should be distinguished from terminal dribble, which is continuous after the main flow of urine.

Giggle incontinence

This form of incontinence is found in young women. It has a clear history and is difficult to reproduce during investigation. The problem usually resolves with time and rarely occurs after 25 years of age.

Urgency

Urgency is a strong and sudden desire to void which is inappropriate and if not relieved can result in urge incontinence. If this symptom is recorded more often than once a week it may be considered abnormal.

Hesitancy

Hesitancy is not common in women. It is a delay in initiating a urinary stream when the woman wishes to void. The volume voided on these occasions should be noted as small volumes (<100 ml) are difficult to void in normal women. However, hesitancy when voiding a full bladder may be an indication either that the urethral sphincter is not relaxing when the detrusor contracts (detrusor–sphincter dyssynergia) or that the detrusor muscle is not contracting effectively during voiding, or that there is psychological inhibition of bladder contraction, which occurs in women who can only void when alone. This symptom does not discriminate between any of these problems. Women with detrusor instability may complain of hesitancy and poor stream but this probably relates to the small volumes of urine passed by them in response to urgency.

Straining to void

The intra-abdominal pressure is increased during the valsalva maneuver which increases the intravesical pressure and this can improve bladder emptying. The urinary stream is impaired and may be intermittent, each transient increase in flow being associated with an increase in intra-abdominal pressure.

Incomplete emptying

This symptom is a sensation that urine is left in the bladder after micturition. The sensation can be due to fluid remaining in the bladder or can be secondary to an abnormality of sensation or due to after-contractions in women with detrusor instability: these women do not always have increased post-micturition urinary residual volumes.

Women with prolapse can suffer from functional obstruction and may have increased urinary residual volumes. A cystocele can act as a sump and a rectocele can press anteriorly on the urethra in women who void by straining, preventing complete emptying.

Poor stream

Decreased urinary stream often described as 'decreased force'. As the urine flow rate is dependent on the volume of urine passed this should be assessed with reference to a frequency/volume chart. A reduced urine flow can be due to reduced voided volumes, bladder outflow obstruction (rare in women) and decreased bladder contractility. This can be neuropathic (lower motor neurone lesions) or myopathic.

Urethral pain

Dysuria

This is pain on passing urine and is experienced in the urethra. Dysuria is often described as 'burning on passing urine' and can be aggravated by sexual intercourse. As an isolated symptom it is associated with urinary tract infections or urethritis.

Bladder pain

Suprapubic pain is associated with inflammation of the bladder, bladder stones or tumor. The pain more commonly occurs after micturition as the bladder mucosa closes down. Some women complain of pain after voiding and have detrusor instability. The pain has been found to coincide with contractions. The presence of bladder pain is an indication for cystoscopy and bladder biopsy. Suprapubic pain may also be associated with pathology outside the bladder but within the pelvis. Endometriosis on the bladder may cause dysuria which is present at certain times in the menstrual cycle. Pelvic inflammatory disease may cause dysuria, but the woman will then have symptoms of vaginal discharge and pyrexia.

Loin pain

This pain originates in the flank and radiates to the groin of the ipsilateral side. The pain is referred from the sensory nerves innervating the kidney and ureter; there are many causes and these may be listed as follows:

1. Vesicoureteric reflux
2. Renal trauma
3. Acute ureteric obstruction
   a. Stone
   b. Blood clot
   c. Papillary necrosis
4. Chronic ureteric obstruction
   a. Tumor, e.g. transitional cell carcinoma, renal cell carcinoma, Wilms tumor
   b. Ureteric stricture
   c. Retroperitoneal fibrosis
   d. Stone
   e. Congenital anomaly

5. Renal inflammation
   a. Pyelonephritis
   b. Perinephric abscess
6. Renal infarction.

Acute or chronic obstruction of the urinary tract can cause pain. This becomes more acute as the pressure generated within the urinary tract is higher. Women with detrusor instability may complain of loin pain associated with urgency and this may indicate vesicoureteric reflux.

Hematuria

Blood in the urine should always be investigated and never be ignored.

NEUROLOGICAL HISTORY

Women should be questioned about any alteration in sensation and motor power in the legs or perineum. The latter may be described as altered sensation during sexual intercourse or an inability to feel their urinary stream during micturition. Fecal incontinence is described as diarrhea which causes staining of underwear or urgency to defecate. Worsening symptoms of back pain with urinary and neurological symptoms must be treated rapidly and seriously as these may indicate a worsening central intervertebral disk prolapse. Neurological symptoms can also be a result of peripheral neuropathy associated with diabetes mellitus, cerebrovascular accidents, Parkinson's disease or multiple sclerosis.

GYNECOLOGICAL SYMPTOMS

The lower urinary tract has receptors to estrogen.[18] Thus it is important to ask the patient about changes in urinary symptoms during the menstrual cycle and to note whether she is menopausal. The majority of women complaining of urological symptoms have coexisting gynecological pathology.[19] As vaginal prolapse alters the range of treatments for urinary incontinence, enquiries about symptoms of vaginal prolapse and prolapse affecting micturition and defecation should be made. Over 40% of women with urethral sphincter incompetence will also have significant cystoceles,[6] making this an important symptom affecting the management of a woman's urinary incontinence. A vaginal prolapse can mask urethral sphincter incompetence.[20] It is important to identify the prolapse before a urodynamic test, so that a vaginal ring can be inserted during the provocative phase of urodynamics to expose any underlying urethral sphincter incompetence. Previous continence operations have an important influence on the future success of continence surgery, as the urethral sphincter may be altered by scarring and damage to sphincter innervation by previous vaginal surgery, as well as distorsion and narrowing of the bladder neck. Operations on the uterus may interfere with the innervation of the bladder, particularly after radical hysterectomy for carcinoma.

PAST MEDICAL HISTORY

It is important to record all past major abdominal and pelvic surgery, and urinary complications as a result of the surgery should be noted. The postoperative course can often be revealing, particularly when women have been unable to void spontaneously and required catheterization; this could indicate prolonged overdistension which can lead to voiding difficulties due to detrusor hypotonia.[21] Surgery to the spine and neurological impairment after this must be recorded particularly in relation to any possible nerve damage. Operations on the large bowel, particularly those involving dissection at the side wall of the pelvis such as abdominoperineal resection of the rectum, may result in denervation.

Conditions increasing abdominal pressure such as chronic cough or constipation can produce the symptom of stress incontinence and make a minor problem more severe; they are also implicated in the development of vaginal prolapse.[22] Cardiac and renal failure can produce frequency and nocturia through polyuria. Endocrine disorders such as diabetes mellitus or diabetes insipidus may lead to polyuria and polydipsia. Chronic diabetes mellitus can produce frequency as a result of overflow incontinence secondary to a hypotonic detrusor and impaired bladder sensation. There does appear to be an association between schizophrenia and detrusor instability.[23] Additionally, women suffering from dementia may not empty their bladders frequently and may not be aware of the need to void. The number of proven urinary tract infections during the past 2 years should be recorded. Childhood enuresis is particularly important as often these patients have detrusor instability.

The obstetric history should include parity, length of labor, mode of delivery and weight of largest infant, although such information has not been shown to be very useful as the details of labor are not recalled accurately. Caesarean section or epidural block during labor and the retention of urine post partum are possible precipitators of voiding difficulties.[24,25]

DRUG HISTORY

Many drugs affect the lower urinary tract. Diuretics can produce urgency, frequency and urge incontinence.[26] Benzodiazepines sedate and may cause confusion and secondary incontinence, particularly in elderly patients. Alcohol impairs mobility, produces a diuresis and can impair the woman's perception of bladder filling. Anticholinergic drugs impair detrusor contractility and may cause urinary retention with secondary overflow incontinence. These include antipsychotic drugs, antidepressants, opiates, antispasmodics and anti-Parkinsonian drugs. Drugs improving urine storage are listed below:

1. Anticholinergic drugs
   a. Propantheline bromide
   b. Emepronium bromide/carrageenate

2. Musculotrophic drugs
    a. Oxybutynin chloride
    b. Dicyclomine chloride
    c. Flavoxate hydrochloride
3. Calcium antagonists
    a. Nifedipine
    b. Flunarizine
4. Tricyclic antidepressants
    a. Imipramine
    b. Doxepin
5. β-adrenoceptor agonists
    a. Terbutaline
    b. Salbutamol
    c. Isoprenaline
6. α-Adrenoceptor antagonists
    a. Phenoxybenzamine
    b. Prazosin
7. Prostaglandin synthetase inhibitors
    a. Flurbiprofen
    b. Indomethacin
8. Neurotoxins
    a. Capsaicin
9. Reduce urine production
    a. Desmopressin
10. Increased outlet resistance
    a. α-Adrenergic agonists
        i. Phenylpropanolamine hydrochloride
        ii. Midodrine
    b. β-Adrenergic antagonists
        i. Propranolol
11. Estrogens.

Sympathomimetic drugs, which are often found in cold remedies, can increase the urethral sphincter resistance and produce voiding difficulty. Prazosin is a postsynaptic α-adrenergic blocker used to treat hypertension which has been found to cause urethral relaxation and urinary incontinence.[27] The following drugs improve bladder emptying:

1. Increased detrusor contractility
    a. Cholinergic agents
        i. Carbachol
        ii. Bethanechol
    b. Anticholinesterase
    c. Prostaglandins
        i. E_2
        ii. F_{2a}
2. Decreased outlet resistance
    a. α-sympathetic blocking agents
        i. Phenoxybenzamine
        ii. Phentolamine
        iii. Prazosin

b. Striated muscle relaxants
  i.   Baclofen
  ii. Dantrolene
  iii. Diazepam.

GENERAL EXAMINATION

Before examining the woman it is important to reassure her about the possibility of urinary leakage and explain that she should not be embarrassed as a result of it. The woman's mobility and mental state play a role in her ability to react to her incontinence problem and may influence management. The woman's mental state should as far as possible be assessed as well as her motivation and manual dexterity. This is important in terms of likely patient compliance with possible treatments and follow-up. It is important to perform a screening neurological examination testing the tone, strength and movement of the lower limbs. It is particularly useful to test the abduction and spreading of the toes, as the innervation for the lateral abductors comes from S3. The anal tone should be assessed and gentle tapping of the clitoris will produce a reflex contraction of the anal sphincter (bulbocavernosus reflex). Additionally, a voluntary cough should cause a reflex contraction of the anal sphincter. An intact sacral reflex can be tested by stroking the skin lateral to the anus, which should elicit a contraction of the external anal sphincter.

GYNECOLOGICAL EXAMINATION

The condition of the vulval skin is important as there may be signs of excoriation, edema and erythema, due to exposure of the skin to urine on the vulva for prolonged periods of time, and concomitant candidiasis. Vaginal atrophy may be seen, particularly in women who experienced the menopause more than 10 years previously.

Any cystocele, rectocele or uterine or vaginal vault descent should be assessed, as this can have an important bearing on the urinary symptoms of the patient.[20] Genital prolapse can be best assessed using a Sims' speculum with the patient in the Sims' or (left lateral) position and coughing and straining. Genital prolapse can now be quantified using the methods produced by the International Continence Society committee on the standardization of terminology.

To demonstrate stress incontinence the woman should have a full bladder.[28] Often women will empty their bladder prior to gynecological examination, rendering the demonstration of stress incontinence impossible. Bonney described a test of bladder neck elevation[29] which he claimed indicated the likelihood of curing stress incontinence with a vaginal repair. The patient, whose bladder should not recently have been emptied, is told to cough violently and the escape of urine is noted. The index and middle finger of the examiner's hand should be inserted into the vagina and the anterior vaginal wall pressed against the subpubic angle but without pressing on the urethra. The patient is now told to cough again. If the pressure of the fingers prevents the leak, the operation of anterior colporrhaphy, if properly carried out, will cure her. The Bonney test produces occlusion of the urethra which is not reproduced surgically. Thus Bonney's test is positive irrespective of the urodynamic diagnosis and cause of the urinary leakage and is of no practical use.[30,31]

If the woman is likely to need incontinence surgery, vaginal mobility and scarring should be assessed. The urethra should be examined for any discharge, inflammation or fixation. If a woman is complaining of a discharge or has had a recent onset of symptoms of urgency and frequency it may be useful to obtain swabs to culture for chlamydia and gonococcus. The anterior vaginal wall should be examined for masses which may be a urethral diverticulum or a urethral or vaginal cyst. A bimanual examination should be performed to exclude abnormal pelvic organs, masses and uterine impaction and it can also exclude a large post-micturition urinary residual.[32] Pelvic masses such as ovarian cysts and uterine enlargement greater than that of 12 weeks' gestation can cause pressure symptoms resulting in frequency: often the symptoms resolve once the mass has been removed. Finally, rectal examination is particularly important in the elderly to exclude fecal impaction, which can aggravate urinary incontinence.

Q-TIP TEST

The mobility of the urethra and bladder neck can be evaluated by inserting a sterile, lubricated, Q-tip cotton bud into the urethra to the level of the bladder neck. The patient is then asked to strain. The rotational movement of the bladder neck around the symphysis pubis causes the Q-tip to move, cranially. The angle of the Q-tip is measured relative to the horizontal using an orthopedic goniometer. The resting and straining angles are measured and the difference between the two is calculated. A change of >30° is thought to represent a hypermobile urethra. This test does not establish the diagnosis of stress incontinence[33] and does not add any extra information to history and examination.[34,35,36] However, it is thought by some clinicians to indicate the most appropriate continence procedure when genuine stress incontinence has been diagnosed and may predict the failure of incontinence surgery.[37]

CONCLUSION

History and examination do not allow the diagnosis of female urinary disorders but guide future investigation and management. In some cases a very obvious cause can be found and dealt with, avoiding the need for further investigations which may be embarrassing, expensive and invasive.

REFERENCES

1 Griffiths DJ, McCracken PN, Harrison GM, Gormley EA. Relationship of fluid intake to voluntary micturition and urinary incontinence in geriatric patients. Neurourol Urodynam 1993; 12: 1–7.
2 Carter PG, McConnell AA, Abrams P. The significance of atrial natriuretic peptide in nocturnal urinary symptoms in the elderly. Neurourol Urodynam, 1992; 11: 420–421.
3 Norgaard JP. Pathophysiology of nocturnal enuresis. Scand J Urol Nephrol 1991; Suppl 140: 7–31.
4 Jarvis GJ, Hall S, Stamp S, Millar Dr, Johnson A. An assessment of urodynamic examination in the incontinent woman. Br J Obstet Gynaecol 1990; 87: 893–896.
5 Sand PK, Ostergard DR. Incontinence history as a predictor of detrusor stability. Obstet Gynecol 1988; 71: 257–259.
6 Cardozo LD, Stanton SL. Genuine stress incontinence and detrusor instability – a review of 200 patients. Br J Obstet Gynaecol 1980; 87: 184–188.
7 Wise BG, Cutner A, Cardozo LD, Kelleher CJ, Burton G, Abbott D. Do detailed symptom questionnaires negate the need for urodynamic investigation? Neurourol Urodynam 1992; 11: 353–355.
8 Larsson G, Abrams P, Victor A. The frequency/volume chart in detrusor instability. Neurourol Urodynam 1991; 10: 533–543.
9 Larsson G, Victor A. The frequency/volume chart in genuine stress incontinent women. Neurourol Urodynam 1992; 11: 23–31.
10 Bates P, Bradley WE, Glen E et al. First report on the standardisation of terminology of lower urinary tract function. Urinary incontinence. Procedures related to the evaluation of urine storage – cystometry, urethral closure pressure profile, units of measurement. Br J Urol 1976; 48: 39–42.
11 James ED, Flack FC, Caldwell KPS, Martin MR. Continuous measurement of urine loss and frequency in incontinent patients. Br J Urol 1971; 43: 233–237.
12 James ED. The behaviour of the bladder during physical activity. Br J Urol 1978; 50: 387–394.
13 Farrar DJ, Whiteside CG, Osborne JL, Turner-Warwick RT. A urodynamic analysis of micturition symptoms in the female. Surg Gynecol Obstet 1975; 141: 875–881.
14 Kelleher CJ, Cardozo LD, Wise BG, Cutner A. The impact of urinary incontinence on sexual function. Neurourol Urod 1992; 11: 359–360.
15 Field SM, Hilton P. The prevalence of sexual problems in women attending for urodynamic investigation. Int Urogynecol J 1993; 4: 212–215.
16 Sutherst JR. Sexual dysfunction and urinary incontinence. Br J Obstet Gynaecol 1979; 86: 387–388.
17 Foldspang A, Mommsen S. Adult female urinary incontinence and childhood bedwetting. J Urol 1994; 152: 85–88.
18 Iosif CS, Batra S, Ek A Ashedt B. Estrogen receptors in the human female lower urinary tract. Am J Obstet Gynecol 1981; 141: 817–820.
19 Benson JT. Gynecologic and urodynamic evaluation of women with urinary incontinence. Obstet Gynecol 1985; 66: 691–694.
20 Rosenzweig BA, Pushkin S, Blumenfeld D, Bhatia NN. Prevalence of abnormal urodynamic test results in continent women with severe genitourinary prolapse. Obstet Gynecol 1992; 79: 539–542.
21 Hinman F. Postoperative overdistension of the bladder. Surg Gynecol Obstet 1976; 142: 901–902.
22 Spence-Jones C, Kamm MA, Henry MM, Hudson CN. Bowel dysfunction: a pathogenic factor in uterovaginal prolpase and urinary stress incontinence. Br J Obstet Gynaecol 1994; 101: 147–152.
23 Bonney W, Gupta S, Arndt S, Anderson K, Hunter DR. Neurobiological correlates of bladder dysfunction in schizophrenia. Neurourol Urodynam 1993; 12: 347–349.
24 Kerr-Wilson RHJ Thompson SW, Orr JW, Davis RO, Cloud GA. Effect of labor on the postpartum bladder. Obstet Gynecol 1984; 64: 115–118.
25 Kerr-Wilson RHJ, McNally S. Bladder drainage for Caesarean section under epidural analgesia. Br J Obstet Gynaecol 1986; 93: 28–30.
26 Fantl JA, Wyman JF, Wilson M, Elswick RK, Bump RC, Wein AJ. Diuretics and urinary incontinence in community-dwelling women. Neurourol Urodynam 1990; 9: 25–34.

27 Hoffman BB, Lefkowitz RJ. Adrenergic receptor antagonists. In: Gilman AG, Rall TW, Nies AS, Taylor P (eds.) Goodman and Gilman's the pharmacological basis of therapeutics, 8th edn. New York: Pergamon Press, pp 221–243.

28 Robinson H, Stanton SL. Detection of urinary incontinence. Br J Obstet Gynaecol 1981; 88: 59–61.

29 Berkeley C, Bonney V. A text book of gynaecological surgery, 3rd edn. London: Cassell, 1935.

30 Migliorini GD, Glenning PP. Bonney's test – fact of fiction? Br J Obstet Gynaecol 1987: 94: 157–159.

31 Bhatia NN, Bergman A. Urodynamic appraisal of the Bonney test in women with stress urinary incontinence. Obstet Gynecol 1983; 62: 696–699.

32 Norton PA, Peattie AB, Stanton SL. Estimation of residual urine by palpation. Neurourol Urodynam 1989; 8: 330–331.

33 Bergman A, McCarthy TA, Ballard CA, Yanai J. Role of the Q-tip test in evaluating stress urinary incontinence. J Reprod Med 1987; 32: 273–275.

34 Fantl JA, Hurt WG, Bump RC, Dunn LJ, Choi SC. Urethral axis and sphincteric function. Am J Obstet Gynecol 1986; 155: 554–558.

35 Walters MD, Diaz K. Q-tip test: a study of continent and incontinent women. Obstet Gynecol 1987; 70: 208–211.

36 Walters MD, Shields LE. The diagnostic value of history, physical examination and the Q-tip cotton swab test in women with urinary incontinence. Am J Obstet Gynecol 1988; 159: 145–149.

37 Bergman A, Koonings PP, Ballard CA. Negative Q-tip test as a risk factor for failed incontinence surgery in women. J Reprod Med 1993; 34: 193–197.

7 Frequency/volume charts

History taking plays an integral part in the management of all urinary symptoms and frequency/volume charts are often used in this context as an adjunct to patient questionnaires and visual analog scales.

The frequency/volume chart (also referred to as bladder or voiding record, urinary diary or incontinence chart) is a semi-objective recording used to assess the frequency of micturition and volume of urine output, the volume of fluid intake and the number of incontinent episodes or pad changes over a given period of time. In addition, the voiding pattern can be observed and other symptoms such as urgency of micturition may be evaluated. It also offers the advantage of assessing the severity of urinary symptoms in the patient's home environment.

Many different types of frequency volume chart have been described,[1,2,3] covering a time period of 3–14 days. Information such as the diurnal and nocturnal frequency of micturition, the mean and maximum voided volumes, the total urine output and diuresis over a 24 h period may be extracted from the charts,[4] and these values may be used to assess the severity of symptoms and their etiology as well as the efficacy of treatment. Furthermore, it has been suggested that they help to diagnose genuine stress incontinence, detrusor instability, bad voiding habit, anxiety, chronic infection, acontractile bladder and premenstrual tension.[5]

Controversy exists over the value of this type of record for there is little agreement on the ideal duration of the chart, or the discriminative value of the data obtained, whilst there remains concern over the reproducibility of the data.

Despite these problems frequency/volume charts are still widely used because they yield semi-objective data which may help in diagnosis and management. For example, fluid intake may be found to be excessive (Fig. 7.1) and thus contributing to the presenting complaint, or urinary frequency may be found to be only diurnal and not nocturnal, suggesting a psychosomatic element to the underlying problem (Fig 7.2).

'NORMAL' VALUES

To try and establish 'normal' values for variables such as fluid intake and urine output, daytime frequency, nocturia and maximum and average voided volumes, Larsson & Victor[6] studied 151 asymptomatic women volunteers, aged 19–81 years, using a 48-hr frequency/volume chart. The

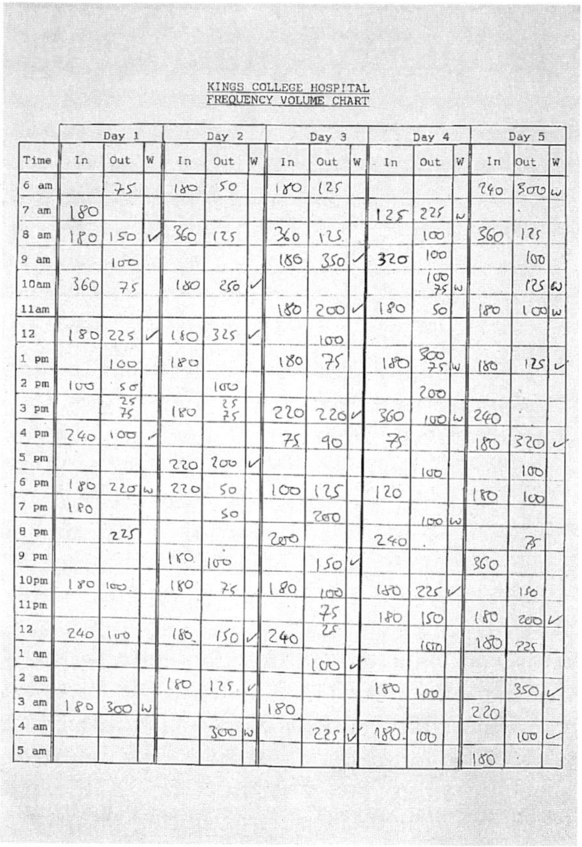

KINGS COLLEGE HOSPITAL
FREQUENCY VOLUME CHART

Fig. 7.1 Frequency/volume chart showing excessive fluid intake

results for the total volume voided and frequency of micturition were reported as means per 24 h. The mean voided volume was calculated by dividing the 48-h total voided volume by the frequency of micturition (Table 7.1).

Table 7.1 Normal frequency/volume chart data

	Mean	SD	Range
Total volume voided dl/24h	14.3	4.87	6.0–31
Frequency/24h	5.8	1.41	3–11
Mean volume voided (ml)	250	79	90–610
Largest single volume voided (ml)	460	174	200–1250

From Larsson and Victor 1988[6]

The diurnal distribution of micturition can be described in different ways. In this study nightly voids when the woman was woken by an urge to void were chosen for presentation. Using these criteria 24 women (15.9%) reported waking up with an urge to void during the night, but none of them more than three times in 48 h. The mean age of these women was slightly greater than, but did not differ significantly from, the rest of the study group.

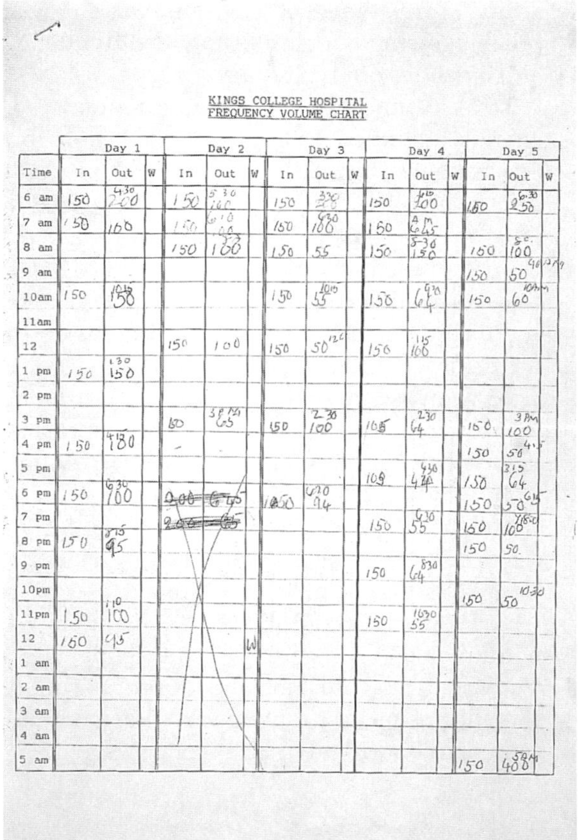

Fig. 7.2 Poorly recorded frequency/volume chart showing marked diurnal frequency but little or no nocturnal frequency of micturition

The data collected in this study were based on recordings of micturition behavior in presumably normal women, and the authors emphasized that it remained to be established in what way micturition patterns might differ in various pathological states.

CHART DURATION

The time period during which charts should be completed is an aspect over which there is a diversity of opinion. Current standard practice is to ask patients to complete a chart for at least 5 days, as this is thought to give more information than a 1-day chart, assuming that the chart will be correctly completed for the length of time requested. However, Abrams et al[1] recommended a 7-day record, Larsson & Victor [6] suggested a 48-h chart, whilst Sommer et al[7] used a 3-day chart and Wyman et al[8] a 2-week chart.

The 1-week record was chosen by Abrams et al[1] as it allows assessment of micturition patterns at home and at work. They found these charts to be well accepted and enthusiastically completed.

Wyman et al[8] compared the results obtained from the first week of a 2-week urinary diary with the results from the second week and found strong correlations between the two, suggesting that a 1 week diary is a reliable method for assessing the frequency of voluntary micturitions and episodes of involuntary urine loss.

To assess the value of a 5-day frequency/volume chart versus a 1-day chart we studied 150 women attending the urodynamic clinic for the assessment of urinary symptoms.[9] The results recorded on the first day of a 5-day chart (Fig. 7.2) were compared with the subsequent results where more than 1 day of the chart was completed. The data for 1 day chart completion were not normally distributed, therefore Spearman's rank correlation coefficients and their probability were calculated. A highly significant correlation was found between the two sets of results for all the recorded and calculated values (p < 0.0001).

To compare these results further, a technique based on the supposition that the longer records (>1 day) are more accurate than the record of the first day alone, was employed. The >1-day data were taken as the standard from which the data obtained on day 1 for each individual patient were subtracted (Fig. 7.2). In Fig. 7.3 two clinically important limits have been set where the value of maximum voided volume on day 1 is over estimated by <50 ml or <100 ml. It can be seen that 26 (39.3%) results were identical, 38 (57.6%) were accurate to within 50 ml and 51 (77.2%) to within 100 ml. Therefore, although the correlation coefficient is statistically significant and there is good agreement using Kappa statistic, using a 1-day record the maximum voided volume is over-estimated by >10 ml in 22.8% of cases.

REPRODUCIBILITY

The reproducibility of a 48 h chart described by Larson & Victor[6] was assessed by comparing the data obtained from the 2 separate days of the same chart and from two charts completed by the same individual. The

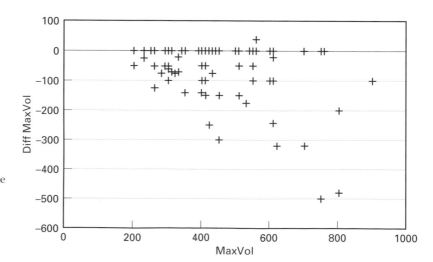

Fig. 7.3 The difference in the maximum voided volume recorded on 1-day and >1–day frequency/volume charts (ml), plotted against the volume recorded on the >1–day chart (ml)

reproducibility of the chart was excellent but they suggested that the observation time of the chart should be lengthened to strengthen the reliability of the recordings, and that social factors such as being at work influence the results obtained.

Wyman et al[8] studied 50 community-dwelling women volunteers using a urinary diary for 2 consecutive weeks. They concluded that test–retest analysis of a 1 week diary showed that the data are highly reproducible and indicated that the charts are a reliable method for assessing the frequency of voluntary micturitions and episodes of involuntary urine loss.

DISCRIMINATIVE VALUE

Various claims as to the discriminative value of frequency/volume charts have been made anecdotally.[5,10] Most of these reports give examples of typical charts in various urological disorders but do not critically analyze the use of such charts in routine clinical practice.

Abrams et al[1] state that voiding patterns suggestive of a particular type of bladder and urethral pathology may be demonstrated at a relatively early stage in the investigation using frequency voiding charts, though no data are supplied to support their value as a diagnostic tool. Wyman et al[8] reported a modest but significant correlation between the patient's history and information obtained using a 'urinary diary' (Table 7.2).

Table 7.2 Relationship between history and urinary diary for weekly diurnal and nocturnal micturition frequency in women with urethral sphincter incompetence alone and women with detrusor instability with or without concomitant sphincter incompetence

		History		Diary		Significance	Correlation	
		Mean	SD	Mean	SD	p value	r	p
Diurnal	SI	70.2+/−33.6		59.6+/−20.9		0.056	0.66	0.0001
Frequency	DI+/−SI	71.2+/−25.3		62.1 +/−16.2		NS	0.25	NS
Nocturnal	SI	8.4+/−6.6		7.9+/−5.6		NS	0.66	0.0001
Frequency	DI+/−SI	8.7+/−7.6		9.5+/−4.4		NS	0.56	0.02

SI = Sphincter incompetence (n = 34); DI +/− SI = detrusor instability with or without sphincter incompetence (n = 16). Data are expressed as mean +/− SD. Modified from Wyman et al 1988[8].

The data show that there is a large range of results in both the diagnostic groups using both techniques. In addition, the authors found that the data obtained were similar in women with sphincter incompetence alone (n = 34) and women with detrusor instability with or without concomitant sphincter incompetence (n = 16), suggesting a poor discriminative value for their frequency/volume chart. Interestingly, there was no significant correlation between the two methods of recording in women with an element of detrusor instability, suggesting that women with detrusor instability are less likely to report their symptoms accurately.

To try and clarify this issue we performed a study in which the results obtained from the 5–day frequency/volume chart of 81 women who had completed at least 1 day of the chart were correlated with the subsequent urodynamic diagnosis made on videocystourethrography. We hoped to ascertain whether data from the frequency/volume chart could help to differentiate between the most common diagnoses, especially genuine stress incontinence and detrusor instability. The Wilcoxon rank test was employed to compare the different diagnostic groups.

Only nocturnal frequency and maximum voided volume showed a statistically significant difference between the two groups; nocturnal frequency was more common and the maximum voided volume was smaller in the patients with detrusor instability.

When all the patients with genuine stress incontinence with or without detrusor instability (n = 46) were compared with all the patients with other diagnoses (n = 32), no statistical difference was found between the two groups. It is therefore not possible to distinguish patients with genuine stress incontinence from those with other diagnoses using frequency/volume data. However, when comparing all patients with detrusor instability with or without genuine stress incontinence (n = 30) with all those with other diagnoses (n = 48), statistical differences were found in average nocturnal frequency, which was significantly increased ($p < 0.025$), and volume at first void ($p < 0.05$); maximum voided volume ($p < 0.01$) and average volume voided ($p < 0.025$), all of which were significantly reduced.

We then studied the correlation between frequency/volume charts and cystometric variables and found that it was possible to relate measured variables on the frequency/volume chart to bladder capacity and maximum detrusor pressure, although all the correlations were weak.

To assess if these are of any predictive value in discriminating between the commonly encountered diagnostic groups, the data obtained from the frequency/volume chart were plotted against the maximum detrusor pressure obtained on provocative subtracted cystometry (Fig 7.4). We found that the frequency/volume chart values were of little if any discriminative value in detecting detrusor instability.

Anecdotal reports of associations between frequency/volume charts and underlying urinary tract pathology are of interest, especially as most practitioners can recall instances where the frequency/volume chart has

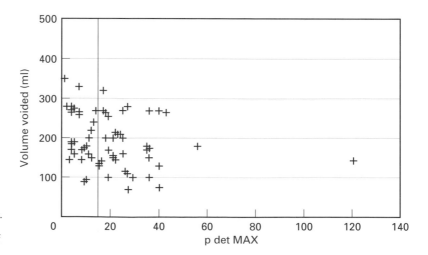

Fig. 7.4 Plot of maximum detrusor pressure at subtracted cystometry and average recorded volume on the frequency /volume chart. The line at 15 cmH$_2$0 represents the normal cut-off

been useful both diagnostically and as an aid to choosing appropriate therapy; however, applied as a routine in clinical practice the data obtained would seem to be of limited discriminative diagnostic value.

CHART COMPLETION

This is an issue that has been poorly addressed as none of the previously reported studies has used frequency/volume charts in a routine clinical setting.

In our study[9] chart completion was assessed in 106 consecutive cases. These women were sent a 5 day frequency volume chart as part of their routine work-up prior to investigation of lower urinary tract symptoms. Fewer than half the patients correctly completed the chart recording values in ml for the full 5 days (40%), although far more women attempted to fill in the chart (86%)

CONCLUSIONS

Frequency/volume charts may yield useful information for individual patient assessment. They may provide information with regard to voiding pattern, frequency of micturition, fluid intake and urine output, as well as the number of incontinent episodes and pad changes. These are particularly useful in the assessment of symptom severity and the effects of treatment.

It is, however, important to remember that when they are used as a routine part of patient assessment they are poorly completed. Moreover, the data that are obtained should be treated with caution as there is a wide range in all the readings and they are of little or no discriminative value.

REFERENCES

1 Abrams P, Feneley R, Torrens M. Urodynamics. New York: Springer-Verlag: 1983; pp 15–17.
2 Autry D, Luazon F, Holiday PJ. The voiding record: an aid in decreasing incontinence. Geriatr Nurs 1984; 5: 22.
3 Ouslander JG, Urman HN, Uman GC. Development and testing of an incontinence monitoring method. Am J Geriat Soc 1986; 34: 83–87.
4 Klevmark B. Miksjonslistens parametre, diagnostiske prototyper og bruk for kontroll av behandling. Nord Med 1987; 102: 340–342.
5 Corcoran M, Brown ADG, Chisholm GD. Urinary symptoms and the value of daily frequency/volume charts at the gynaecological clinic. Proceedings of the 12th World Congress of Gynecology and Obstetrics, 1988 pp: 507–508.
6 Larsson G, Victor A. Micturition patterns in a healthy female population, studied with a frequency/volume chart. Scand J Urol Nephrol 1988; Suppl 114: 53–57.
7 Sommer P, Bauer T, Nielsen KK et al. Voiding patterns and prevalence of incontinence in women. A questionnaire survey. Br J Urol 1990; 66: 12–15.
8 Wyman JF, Choi SC, Harkins SW, Wilson MS, Fantl JA. The urinary diary in evaluation of incontinent women: a test-retest analysis. Obstet Gynecol 1988; 71: 812–817.
9 Barnick C, Cardozo L. Unpublished data, 1993.
10 George NJR, Barnard RJ, Blacklock NJ. Frequency volume charts revealing physiological abnormalities. Proceedings of the 11th Annual Meeting of the International Continence Society, 1981: pp 67–68.

8 Uroflowmetry

INTRODUCTION

Uroflowmetry is an essential part of any urodynamic assessment. It is relatively simple and is non-invasive and gives objective evidence of voiding dysfunction. The first flowmeter was described in 1956 by von Garrelts.[1] The original design utilized a strain gauge weighing transducer placed under a cylindrical receptacle into which the patient voids (Fig. 8.1). The weight of fluid is electronically converted to give a simultaneous flow rate. In addition, the total volume of fluid can be measured. It is important to appreciate that the strain gauge is in fact measuring a change in mass and that for this reason it needs to be calibrated for fluid of the correct density. This method has been shown to be accurate for both clinical and experimental use.[2] Other commonly used devices include an electronic dipstick,[3] a rotating disk[4] ultrasound[5] and the displacement of air from a container.[6] The signal produced by flowmeters is electronically filtered to give a smooth curve. Insufficient filtering would result in too much electronic interference and it would be impossible to read results accurately. Too much filtering of the signal would cause the reading to be unrepresentative of the actual flow rate. Technical aspects of commonly used flowmeters are discussed in a paper produced by the International Continence Society.[7]

RECORDING A FLOW RATE

To obtain a record of flow parameters, the patient is asked to void into the flowmeter when her bladder is comfortably full. Preferably this should be carried out in private. The maximum flow rate and the volume voided are recorded. In addition, the average flow rate, the flow time and the time to maximum flow may be determined (Fig. 8.2).

The normal trace is bell-shaped with a peak flow of at least 15 ml/s for a volume voided of at least 150 ml of urine.[8] A normal recording is shown in Fig. 8.3. A reduced maximum flow rate may be due to an inadequate voided volume or to voiding difficulties (Fig. 8.4). In addition, the shape of the curve may be altered and suggest evidence of abdominal straining on voiding.

Different authors give different values for the lower limit of normal for the maximum flow rate for different volumes voided.[9,10] Backman[11] tried

A

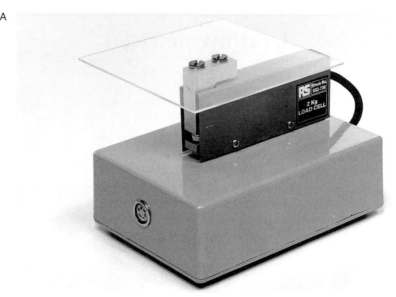

Fig. 8.1 A weighing transducer for measuring flow rates

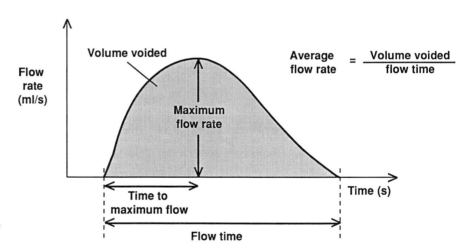

Fig. 8.2 Uroflowmetry curve and derived measurements

to overcome the problem of different voided volumes by constructing nomograms for the maximum flow rate with different volumes in the female. However, the data were insufficient to be reliable.

NOMOGRAMS

More recently, Haylen et al[12] constructed nomograms for maximum flow rates (Fig 8.5) and average flow rates (Fig. 8.6) in both normal females and normal males. Their study consisted of 249 female volunteers who passed between 15 and 600 ml of urine. They found no effect of parity or age on parameters measured. Equations for the nomogram graphs were calculated (Fig 8.7).

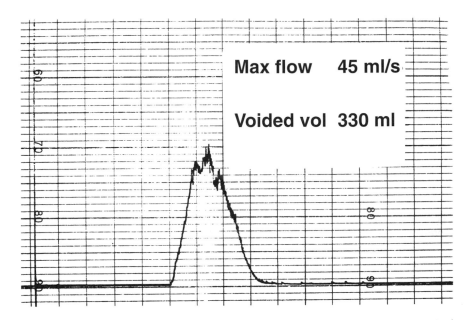

Fig. 8.3   A normal flow rate curve

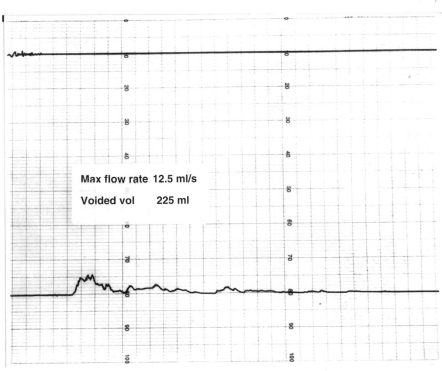

Fig. 8.4   A flow rate curve suggestive of voiding difficulties

These equations give a mean maximum flow rate of 21 ml/s for a voided volume of 150 ml. In addition, a voided volume of 80 ml will result in a mean maximum flow rate of 15 ml/s. This is largely in agreement with the previous studies already discussed, as in these the actual voided volume was not taken into account.

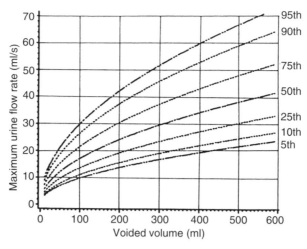

Fig. 8.5 Peak flow rates for women according to Haylen et al 1989b[12] with permission

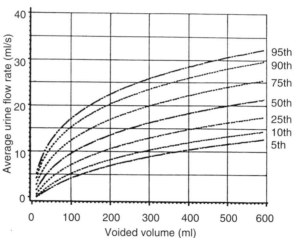

Fig. 8.6 Average flow rate nomograms for women according to Haylen et al 1989[12] with permission

Ln (maximum flow rate) = 0.511 + 0.505 × Ln (voided volume)
[root mean square error = 0.340]

Square root (average flow rate) = –0.921 + 0.869 × Ln (voided volume)
[root mean square error = 0.640]

Fig. 8.7 Liverpool nomogram equations in women

THE SIGNIFICANCE OF THE FLOW RATE

A reduced flow rate will not determine whether the cause is due to an outflow problem or detrusor dysfunction. The position adopted by the patient may alter the recorded flow rate. Moore & Richmond[13] found that a high proportion of women crouch over the toilet rather than sit and that this reduces the average flow rate recorded. It may be that parameters recorded in the urodynamic clinic are unrepresentative. Wijkstra et al[14] described a low-cost portable flowmeter which enabled multiple recordings to be made in the patient's home. Although this may be more reliable, diagnoses are not made on a single flow rate alone but rather in conjunction with cystometry with or without other investigations.

More recently, workers have been concerned with increases in flow rate. Haylen et al[15] compared flow rates in patients referred for urodynamic investigation to their original nomograms.[12] They found evidence of increased maximum flow rates in patients with detrusor instability. In men 86% of results on or above the 75th centile were in those subjects with detrusor instability. In women differences were less marked, with 50% of those on or above the 90th centile having detrusor instability.

Other authors have derived new parameters from the flow curve. Acceleration in flow rate has been used to study voiding in both men and women.[16,17,18] It is defined as the peak flow rate divided by the time to peak and does not vary with the volume voided.[17] This may reflect the velocity of opening of the bladder neck.[18] Cucchi[17] demonstrated that the acceleration in flow rate was significantly greater in women with detrusor instability than in those with genuine stress incontinence and normal controls, and concluded that this may reflect an increased speed of detrusor contraction.

PRESSURE/FLOW MEASUREMENT

Further analysis of flow rates involves pressure/flow studies. There is much controversy in this field and standardized terminology and definitions have not been established. In simple terms, where the maximum voiding pressure is high and the flow rate is low, this will signify outflow obstruction, and where both the maximum voiding pressure and flow rate are low, this will signify poor detrusor function. However, the standard limits for detrusor pressure have not been defined and therefore assessment is subjective. In addition, in cases of outflow obstruction, the detrusor decompensates with time resulting in both low detrusor pressure and a low flow rate.

There have been attempts to derive parameters which signify whether the voiding difficulty is due to detrusor hypotonia or outflow obstruction. The original concept was of a urethral resistance factor for which various equations have been derived. These are all derived from the detrusor pressure and flow rate.[19] They suffer from the fact that the urethra is not a rigid tube but rather distensible, thus making calculated factors unreliable.

The International Continence Society[20] recommends that the peak flow rate and the detrusor pressure at that flow be marked on a graph (Fig 8.8) to separate those women with obstructed flow from those with unobstructed flow. In addition, from the urodynamic recording, certain measurements have been defined but the limits for normality have yet to be established (Fig. 8.9).

The whole pressure/flow plot can also be demonstrated graphically (Fig. 8.10) and various parameters calculated these pressure/flow plots. The exact meaning of these calculated parameters and interpretation of the trace remain uncertain and their use in clinical practice is not established.

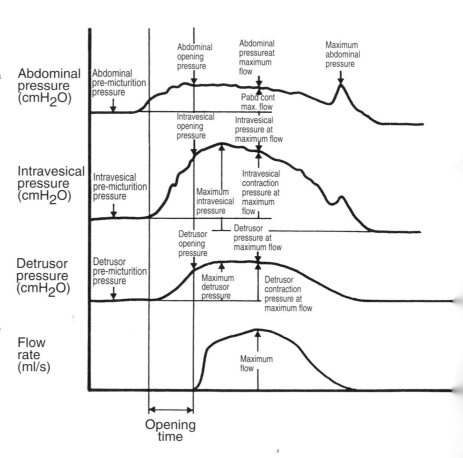

Fig. 8.8 Presentation of pressure/flow data on individual patients in three groups obstructed, equivocal and unobstructed. (From Abrams et al 1990. The standardisation of terminology of lower urinary tract function. Br J Obstet Gynaecol 97 (Suppl 6): 1–16, with permission.)

Fig. 8.9 Pressure/flow recordings of micturition with International Continence Society recommended nomenclature. Opening time: the time elapsed from the initial rise in detrusor pressure to onset of flow. Pre-micturition pressure: the pressure recorded immediately before the initial isovolumetric contraction. Opening pressure: the pressure recorded at the outset of measured flow. Maximum pressure: the maximum value of the measured pressure. Pressure at maximum flow: the pressure recorded at maximum flow rate. Contraction pressure at maximum flow: the difference between pressure at maximum flow and pre-micturition pressure. (From Abrams et al 1990. The standardisation of terminology of lower urinary tract function. Br J Obstet Gynaecol 97 (Suppl 6): 1–16, with permission.)

Further guidance as to whether or not urine flow is obstructed may be gained using urethral pressure profilometry (see Ch. 11). A combination of the micturition urethral pressure and pressure/flow recording performed simultaneously has been described both as a theoretical model[21] and in men with outflow obstruction[22] to calculate the cross-sectional

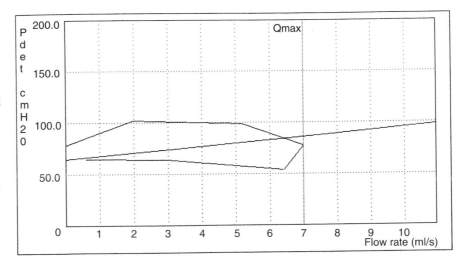

Fig. 8.10 A pressure/flow curve derived from a computerized urodynamic recording. Calculated parameters derived by the computer are as follows. Total volume (V) 28 ml. Max flow rate (Qmax) 7.00 ml/s. Average flow rate (Qave) 4.00 ml/s. Resting pressure (Pres) 65 cmH$_2$O). Average voiding pressure (Pvoid) 12 cmH$_2$O. Passive ura resistance (PURR) 3.00 cmH$_2$O/[ml/s]. Voiding time (T) 0:07 m:s. Flow time (Tflow) 0:07 m:s. Work done in voiding (Wvoid) 71 cmH$_2$Os

area of the urethra at the point of obstruction. Further development of this technique in women may enable more accurate assessment of whether or not voiding difficulties are due to outflow obstruction or detrusor hypotonia. However, as yet the differential diagnosis remains somewhat subjective.

CONCLUSION

In summary, measurement of the peak flow rate is a simple, non-invasive test. It gives much valuable information but further data from the flow curve and in combination with pressure/flow studies will help reveal the whole clinical picture.

REFERENCES

1 von Garrelts B. Analysis of micturition: a new method of recording the voiding of the bladder. Acta Chir Scand 1956; 112: 326–340.
2 Nyman CR, Boman J, Gidlof A. Von Garrelt's uroflowmeter, a technical and clinical evaluation. Proceedings of the 7th Annual Meeting or the International Continence Society, Portoroz, 1977: 88–90.
3 James ED. A novel 'dip-stick' type urine volume and flow rate monitor. Proceedings of the 7th Annual Meeting of the International Continence Society. Portoroz, 1977: 85.
4 Rowan D, Mackenzie AL, McNee S, Glen E. A technical and clinical evaluation of the Disa uroflowmeter. Annual Proceedings of the 6th Meeting of the International Continence Society, Antwerp, 1976.
5 Rollema HJ. An ultrasonic volumeter for uroflowmetry. Annual Proceedings of the 6th Meeting of the International Continence Society, Antwerp, 1976.
6 Gierup J, Ericsson NO, Okmian L. Micturition studies in infants and children. Scand J Urol Nephrol 1969; 3: 1–8.
7 Rowan D, James ED, Kramer AEJL, Sterling AM, Suhel PF. Urodynamic equipment: technical aspects. J Med Engineering and Technology 1987; 11: 57–64.
8 Stanton SL. In: Stanton SL, Tanagho EA (eds)Surgery of female incontinence. Ch. 2: Investigation of incontinence. 2nd edn. Berlin; Springer-Verlag, 1986: pp 23–56.
9 Farrar DJ, Osborne JL, Stephenson TP et al. A urodynamic view of bladder outflow obstruction in the female: factors influencing the results of treatment. Br J Urol 1976; 47: 815–822.

10 Massey JA, Abrams PH. Obstructed voiding in the female. Br J Urol 1988; 61: 36–39.

11 Backman K–A. Urinary flow during micturition in normal women. Acta Chir Scand 1965; 130: 357–370.

12 Haylen BT, Ashby D, Sutherst JR, Frazer MI, West CR. Maximum and average flow rates in normal male and female populations– the Liverpool nomograms. Br J Urol 1989b; 64: 30–38.

13 Morre KH, Richmond D. Crouching over the toilet seat: prevalence, and effect upon micturition. Neurourol Urodyn 1989; 8 (4): 422–424.

14 Wijkstra Hl, Kersten PL, Debruyne FMJ. A low cost digital portable uroflowmeter. Neurourol Urodyn 1991; 10 (4): 423–424.

15 Haylen BT, Parys BT, Anyaegbunam WI, Ashby D, West CR. Urine flow rates in male and female urodynamic patients compared with the Liverpool nomograms. Br J Urol 1990; 65: 483–487.

16 Susset JG. Development of nomograms for application of uroflowmetry. In: Hinman, F Jr (ed) Benign prostatic hypertrophy. Ch. 49. Springer–Verlag, New York:1983 pp 523–538.

17 Cucchi A. Acceleration of flow rate as a screening test for detrusor instability in women with stress incontinence. Br J Urol 1990a; 65: 17–19.

18 Cucchi A. Acceleration of flow rate in obstructed detrusor instability. Br J Urol 1990b; 66: 26–29.

19 Bates CP, Bradley WE, Glen ES et al. Third report on the standardisation of terminology of lower urinary tract function. Br J Urol 1980; 52: 348–350.

20 Abrams P, Blaivas JG, Stanton SL, Andersen JT. The standardisation of terminology of lower urinary tract function. Br J Obstet Gynaecol 1990; 97 (Suppl 6): 1–16.

21 Palmer MA, Desmond AD. Elimination of the influence of intravesical pressure on the micturitional urethral pressure profile by calculation of urethral cross-sectional area: an experimental study. Br J Urol 1994a; 73: 279–283.

22 Palmer MA, Desmond AD. Simultaneous measurement or urethral opening pressure and urethral cross-sectional area during voiding cystometry. Br J Urol 1994b; 73: 275–278.

Cystometry

INTRODUCTION

Cystometry is the central and most important of the urodynamic investigations. It evaluates the pressure–volume relationship of the urinary bladder during both filling and voiding phases. Cystometry is used to assess detrusor activity, sensation, capacity and compliance. It is usually undertaken in conjunction with other urodynamic studies. These include particularly uroflowmetry and imaging studies, but other techniques may also be indicated. Double-channel subtracted cystometry is the technique most often employed and the availability of this investigation is now quite widespread.

The function of the bladder is primarily that of a storage organ. It must also be able to evacuate its contents at appropriate intervals and the intravesical pressure and its relationship to the maximum urethral pressure are vital to both of these functions. The bladder is normally able to store relatively large volumes of urine at low pressure. It then reflexly contracts at a certain volume resulting in complete bladder emptying. Following bladder training in childhood, this voiding reflex is under central inhibition from the higher centers so that voiding only occurs at appropriate times and places. The bladder is unique in that it is a smooth muscle organ which is under partial somatic control. Although cystometry forms the crux of urodynamic studies, its results need to be taken in context with the patient's history, clinical examination and the findings of other urodynamic investigations.

HISTORY

In 1882, Mosso and Pellacani[1] described the first cystometer (Fig. 9.1) and assessed the behavior of the bladder during filling in both animals and humans. Utilizing a water manometer to measure intravesical pressure, which was recorded on a smoked drum, they noted that introduction of additional volumes into the bladder did not result in an increase in pressure. Their technique was modified by Rose[2] in 1927, who introduced cystometry as a clinical test of detrusor function. Several years later, Denny-Brown & Robertson[3] assessed, for the first time, the activity of the urethra and bladder neck, as well as measuring bladder pressure, and introduced the concept of co-ordinated lower urinary tract activity.

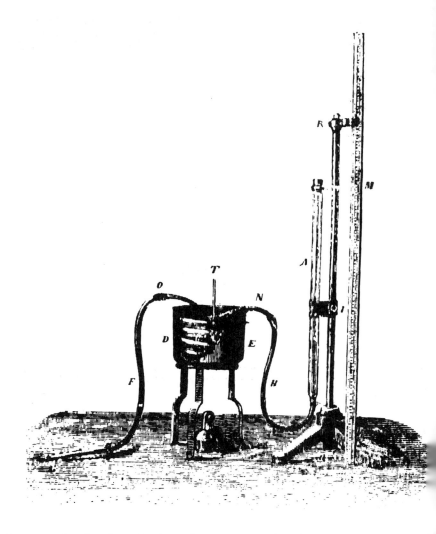

Fig. 9.1   Cystometer used by Mosso and Pellacani in 1882

Improved technology in the 1950s, in particular the advent of pressure transducers, allowed accurate and consistent recordings to be made and Scandinavian workers[4,5] began the description of the normal function of the lower urinary tract. There was a great expansion in the development of urodynamic studies over the subsequent 30 years and a gradual implementation of them into clinical practice. Zinner[6] introduced the term 'urodynamics' in 1963 and Bates et al[7] pioneered the concept of combined filling and voiding cystometry in conjunction with urinary flow studies and radiological assessment of the bladder and urethra. Since then there has been a constant improvement in equipment design including the use of sophisticated computers (Fig. 9.2).

INDICATIONS

Ideally, all women with lower urinary tract dysfunction should undergo cystometry, but in centers where urodynamic investigations are not readily

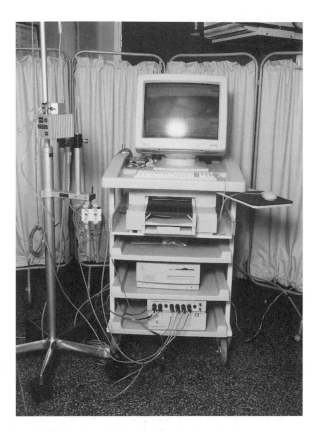

Fig. 9.2 Modern urodynamic equipment, based on a micro processor. For combined urovideo studies (courtesy of Dantec Ltd.)

available, the following indications may be employed:

- mixed stress and urge incontinence
- forthcoming surgery for genuine stress incontinence
- failure to respond to conservative management
- severe unexplained frequency
- recurrent urinary tract infections
- suspected voiding difficulties
- failed incontinence surgery
- neurogenic bladder dysfunction.

TECHNIQUE

Prior to cystometric examination a detailed history should be taken. This is most easily achieved by a standardized questionnaire[8] which avoids the omission of important information. Examination is then performed and should include pelvic assessment and a local neurological examination. A completed frequency/volume chart is helpful and the urine should be demonstrated to be sterile prior to cystometry. This latter point is important as the presence of a urinary tract infection may give artefactual cystometric findings. A current lower urinary tract infection may also be exacerbated by the catheterization and manipulation which occur during urodynamic investigation.

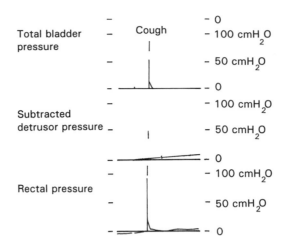

Fig. 9.3   Pressure changes on coughing at the beginning of the study

Artefacts

Accurate interpretation of an incorrectly performed study is extremely difficult. Therefore, it is of the utmost importance to check carefully that the equipment is recording correctly and all transducers and pressure monitoring lines are working appropriately prior to commencing the study and also during the investigation. Imprecise balancing of the monitoring equipment is the most common cause of artefactual recordings and will give rise to incorrect detrusor pressure measurements and possibly subsequent misdiagnoses. This may be due to air in the pressure monitoring lines or incorrect positioning of 3-way taps. Accurate balancing is tested at the beginning of each study by asking the patient to cough once or more. This results in a similar rise in both rectal and intravesical pressure with a 'bounce' on the subtracted detrusor pressure graph (Fig. 9.3). In those patients who are unable to cough, such as women with a high spinal lesion, suprapubic pressure can be employed to check that the lines are balanced. Other possible causes of artefactual results are incorrect placement of pressure lines and poor calibration of monitoring equipment. If the rectal catheter is not placed above the anal sphincter then artefacts due to anal contractions are likely.

Single-channel cystometry

The measurement of bladder pressure during filling is the most useful single test of bladder function. The patient should be awake, unanesthetized, and neither sedated nor taking drugs that affect bladder function. There are a number of methods by which cystometry can be performed and these vary in complexity. The simplest and cheapest technique requires only an intravenous giving set, a 12F catheter and a central venous pressure (CVP) line (Fig. 9.4). With the patient supine, the bladder is filled by gravity, with normal (0.9%) saline. Using the CVP line and 3-way tap, intermittent recordings of bladder pressure can be made. The disadvantages of this technique are that intravesical and not detrusor pressure is measured, the measurement is intermittent rather than continuous and voiding phase measurements are not possible. Some of these problems may be overcome by using a fine (1-mm) fluid-filled catheter

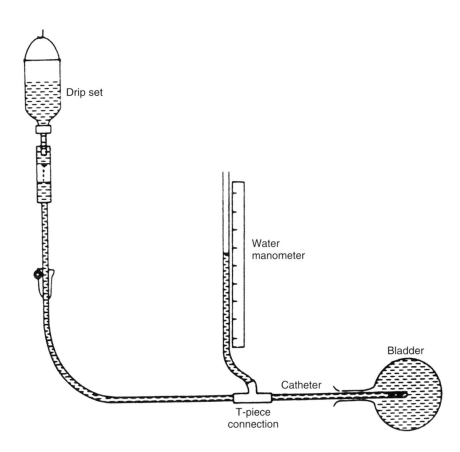

Drip set

Water
manometer

Bladder

Catheter

T-piece
connection

Fig. 9.4 Simple water
manometer cystometer

placed in the bladder, alongside the filling catheter, and connected to a
pressure transducer instead of the CVP line. This will make possible continuous bladder pressure measurement as well as intravesical pressure
measurement during voiding, once the filling catheter has been removed.
However, the major problem with single-channel cystometry is that as
the bladder is an intra-abdominal organ, changes in intra-abdominal
pressure due to movement, coughing or posture change will also be
recorded and make interpretation of the results difficult.

Double-channel cystometry

Double-channel cystometry involves the continuous measurement of
both intravesical and rectal pressure (Fig. 9.5). All systems are zeroed at
atmospheric pressure. For external transducers the reference point is the
level of the superior edge of the symphysis pubis. For catheter-mounted
transducers the reference point is the transducer itself. The rectal pressure
is an indicator of intra-abdominal pressure and the electronic subtraction
of this value from the intravesical pressure will give the detrusor pressure,
which is a true indicator of bladder function. This form of cystometry is
the most commonly performed as it makes accurate diagnosis easier. The
rectal pressure is determined by a 2-mm fluid-filled catheter inserted into
the rectum, beyond the anal canal, and connected to a pressure transducer.
The end of the catheter is protected from fecal blockage by a finger stall

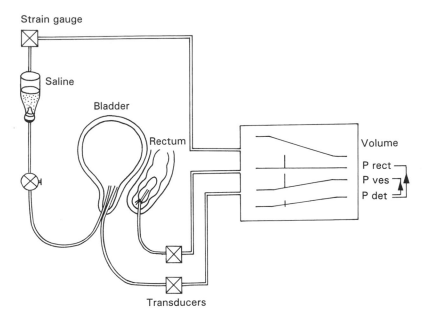

Fig. 9.5 Diagramatic illustration of twin-channel subtracted cystometry

or condom (Fig. 9.6). Bladder volume during filling is determined by a force transducer from which is suspended the filling reservoir. The weight change as the fluid enters the bladder is an accurate indicator of the bladder volume. The increased accuracy of diagnosis with double-channel cystometry generally outweighs the disadvantages of higher cost, greater complexity of equipment and increased invasiveness.

Definitions

At this stage it may be useful to establish some definitions.

Intravesical pressure is the pressure within the bladder.

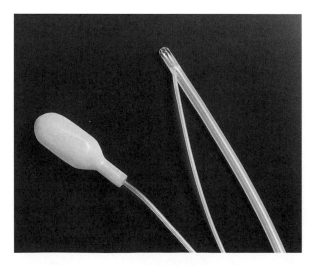

Fig. 9.6 The filling catheter shown with intravesical and rectal pressure measuring lines

Abdominal pressure is taken to be the pressure surrounding the bladder. It is generally estimated from rectal, vaginal or, less commonly, extraperitoneal pressure.

Detrusor pressure is that component of intravesical pressure that is created by forces, both active and passive, in the bladder wall. It is estimated by subtracting abdominal pressure from intravesical pressure.

Bladder sensation is difficult to evaluate because of its subjective nature. It is usually assessed by questioning the patient about her feeling of bladder fullness during cystometry. Commonly used descriptive terms include 'first desire to void', 'normal desire to void', 'strong desire to void' and 'urgency'.

First desire to void is when the woman is aware that the bladder is filling and feels that she could void.

Normal desire to void is defined as the feeling that leads the patient to pass urine at the next convenient moment, but voiding can be delayed if necessary.

Strong desire to void is defined as a persistent desire without the fear of leakage.

Urgency is a strong desire to void accompanied by fear of leakage or fear of pain.

Maximum cystometric capacity is the volume at which the patient (with normal sensation) feels she can no longer delay micturition. In the presence of sphincter incompetence the maximum cystometric capacity may be significantly increased by occlusion of the urethra, e.g. by a Foley catheter. In the absence of sensation the maximum cystometric capacity is the volume at which the clinician decides to terminate filling.

Functional bladder capacity is assessed from a frequency/volume chart (urinary diary).

Maximum (anesthetic) bladder capacity is the volume measured after filling during a deep general or spinal anesthetic. The fluid temperature, filling pressure and filling time should be specified.

Compliance indicates the change in volume for a change in pressure. It is calculated by dividing the volume change by the change in detrusor pressure during that change in bladder volume. Compliance is expressed as ml/cmH_2O.

Filling phase

This phase of the cystometric examination tests the ability of the bladder to accomodate an increase in volume. The filling catheter is usually inserted following a uroflowmetry examination, thus enabling determination of residual urine. Local anesthetic gel can be used to anesthetize the urethra and provide lubrication for insertion of the catheters but is not usually required. Intravesical pressure is measured by a 1-mm fluid-filled catheter which is inserted at the same time as the filling catheter by 'piggy-backing' the distal end into a side hole of the filling catheter (Fig. 9.6). Transducer-tipped catheters are also available for measuring bladder pressure but, although convenient, are generally quite expensive and prone to damage. The rectal pressure line (2 mm diameter) is inserted above the anal sphincter to prevent artefact from rectal contractions. Both pressure measuring lines are attached to pressure transducers and cleared of any air bubbles which would dampen pressure transmission. Accurate balancing is checked by asking the patient to cough. The transducers are aligned to the upper border of the pubic symphysis to give zero pressure.

As filling is commenced, the woman is asked to indicate when she first feels as if she could void and this volume is recorded as 'first desire to void'. She is asked to try to inhibit the urge to void until she can no longer tolerate further fluid in her bladder. Filling is then ceased and the volume of instilled fluid is recorded as the 'maximum cystometric capacity'. The filling catheter is removed at this stage, leaving the pressure monitoring lines in situ. The bladder should not be overstretched as this may interfere with subsequent flow rates.

During the filling phase the patient is asked to cough several times, both as a test for stress incontinence and also as a provocative maneuver to elicit unstable contractions. After removal of the filling catheter, the table on which the patient is lying is tipped to the upright position, or alternatively the patient assumes the erect position. The detrusor pressure response to the change in posture is noted and the transducers are realigned to the level of the pubic symphysis if necessary. Serial coughs are used to elicit the sign of stress incontinence. The grading system of genuine stress incontinence that we use is 'severe' if significant leakage occurs on the first cough, 'moderate' if leakage occurs after several coughs and 'mild' if incontinence only occurs after vigorous and prolonged coughing. Although this method is somewhat subjective, it is easily applied and is helpful in determining subsequent appropriate management options. While the patient is in the erect position, other provocative measures are also employed to generate unstable contractions. These include heel bouncing, the sound of running water and rinsing hands in cool water.

Variable factors

1 Route of filling The bladder is usually filled via a urethral catheter. A 12F urethral catheter is appropriate for adult women. A smaller fluid filled catheter is usually used as well to monitor bladder pressure. This enables the larger filling catheter to be removed when filling is complete in order to allow voiding studies to be performed. Bladder filling may also be achieved by an antegrade method using diuretics and a large fluid load.[9] This method is slow, cystometric capacity cannot be determined and a catheter still has to be introduced into the bladder for pressure measurements. If a suprapubic catheter is in situ then this can be used satisfactorily for bladder filling. It has been suggested that this route may be more physiological and could be used routinely,[10] especially in children. However, insertion may be traumatic to the patient and this technique has not gained favor.

2 Filling medium The bladder can be filled with either gas or liquid. The latter is usually used in the United Kingdom but gas is often used in the United States. Normal (0.9%) saline is most often employed as the filling medium unless radiological screening is also being performed, in which case contrast medium is used. The cystometric findings are not affected by this choice of liquid media.[11]

Carbon dioxide is the gas usually used for gas cystometry. This is popular in the United States as it is quick and easy to perform[12] and the same equipment can be used for cystometry, urethral pressure profilometry and endoscopy.[13] Another advantage is the absence of viscous drag effects. However, carbon dioxide has an irritant effect on the bladder which may give rise to artefactual results. Other disadvantages are its compressibility,[14] leakage and difficulty in measuring urine flow rate and residual volume.

3 Temperature of the filling medium The infusion of cold fluid into the bladder may trigger a detrusor contraction. Therefore, in order not to affect the results of the cystometry artificially, the temperature of the filling medium should be between room and body temperature. However, the instillation of ice-water (Bor's test) is occasionally used as a test for neurological disorders.

4 Rate of filling Bladder filling may be physiological, with or without diuresis, or via a urethral catheter. Physiological filling is generally too slow for routine clinical use although it is appropriately used in ambulatory urodynamic studies. Filling via a catheter may be incremental, as in the early days of cystometry when 50–100 ml was added at regular intervals, or continuous, as is usually the case today. The filling medium may flow under the force of gravity, or for more accurate filling rates with the aid of a peristaltic pump which is a standard option in most modern urodynamic machines. Filling rates are designated as either 'slow' (< 10 ml/min), 'medium' (10–100 ml/min) or 'fast' (> 100 ml/min). Most urodynamic units use continuous filling at between 50 and 100 ml/min.[15] We fill, using gravity, at a rate of approximately 100 ml/min. Fast filling is a provocative test for patients with detrusor instability. However, a stable bladder will not be 'provoked' into instability by fast bladder filling.[11,16] A different situation exists in patients with neurological abnormalities in whom slow fill is essential to reduce artefactual bladder activity.[17]

5 Posture of the patient Cystometry may be performed with the patient either supine, seated or standing. Some consider the seated position to be the most physiological.[18] Change of posture during cystometry is a provocative test for detrusor instability.[19] The standing position should be included at some stage of the cystometric investigation as this results in a better correlation between the patient's symptoms and the urodynamic findings.[20] We perform the filling phase of the examination with the woman supine, and then have her stand for the voiding phase and further assessment for genuine stress incontinence.

6 Who performs the investigation? Nurses, continence advisors and technicians can be taught to perform urodynamic investigations competently. The accurate interpretation of the cystometrogram trace requires detailed knowledge of what actually occurred during the investigation, the patient's subjective responses and the provocative measures used, and how these relate to the pressure recordings. Careful annotation of important events on the graph paper is extremely helpful. However, optimally the investigation should be performed by the person who has subsequently to make the decisions on diagnosis and on the appropriate therapy, or recommendations for it, and this is the doctor.

Voiding phase

Once the filling catheter has been removed, and serial coughs performed, the patient is asked to void. This is preferably performed in conjunction with the measurement of urine flow parameters. Although more comfortable for the patient in the seated position, the voiding phase of the cystometric examination can be performed in the erect position, as may be required when concomitant radiological screening is being performed. However, not all women are able to void while standing. The maximum detrusor pressure during voiding is noted, as is the presence of any abdominal straining used to aid bladder emptying. The 'stop' test may be employed to assess detrusor contractility. For this the patient is asked to inhibit voiding midstream. As the bladder neck contracts prior to detrusor relaxation, there is a rise in detrusor pressure due to this isometric detrusor contraction, termed 'P det iso'.

NORMAL CYSTOMETRIC PARAMETERS

Residual urine should be less than 50 ml. The first sensation to void is usually experienced at 150–250 ml with fast-fill cystometry but may be almost at capacity with slow filling. A strong desire to void is usually present at 400 ml and the normal bladder can hold between 400 and 600 ml. The detrusor pressure rise on filling is < 15 cmH$_2$O to 500 ml and < 10 cmH$_2$O to 300 ml. Provocation of the normal bladder by rapid filling, change of posture, coughing, etc. will not provoke abnormal detrusor activity. There is no loss of urine and only slight descent of the bladder base on coughing in the erect position. Voiding occurs with a detrusor pressure rise of < 60 cmH$_2$O and a peak flow rate of > 15ml/s for a voided volume of at least 150 ml. The normal bladder can cease voiding on command. When this occurs the urinary stream is interrupted at the mid-urethra and the fluid proximal to this point is 'milked back' into the bladder.

HOW SENSITIVE IS CYSTOMETRY?

The diagnosis of detrusor instability can only be made following cystometric examination and this is also the most common 'positive' diagnosis made by cystometry (genuine stress incontinence is diagnosed by demonstrating urethral leakage at times of raised intra-abdominal pressure and in the absence of abnormal detrusor activity). Because this is the only way in which detrusor instability can be diagnosed, it is difficult to determine the sensitivity of the test. It is certainly not 100% sensitive, although the real number of false negative results is unclear. The use of provocative measures such as rapid bladder filling, coughing, posture change, heel bouncing and hand rinsing is important in minimizing the number of false negative findings.

It has been demonstrated that 55% of women who complain of urge incontinence[21] and 70% who complain of urgency[22] have no evidence of detrusor instability. In addition, 55% of women with genuine stress incontinence also complain of urge incontinence.[23] Making an accurate prediction of the cystometric diagnosis from the clinical history and examination is difficult. Jarvis et al[24] found that an experienced clinician was correct only 65% of the time.

We, however, do not feel that the bladder is such an 'unreliable witness' but that many of the discrepancies described above relate to the imperfect sensitivity of cystometry as a diagnostic test for detrusor instability. We re-examined 50 women with symptoms suggestive of detrusor instability in whom initial cystometry showed no abnormality. In over half of this group a cystometric abnormality was found on the second occasion and this was detrusor instability in most cases.[25] This concept is also supported by the findings of studies using ambulatory urodynamics which seem generally to be more sensitive in the diagnosis of detrusor instability.[26] A stable bladder will not be made to contract inappropriately by provocative measures, therefore the problem of false positive diagnoses of detrusor instability should not arise.

AMBULATORY URODYNAMICS

This technique involves the assessment of lower urinary tract function over many hours while the patient undertakes normal daily activities. It is suggested that this will give more realistic results than those obtained in the artificial environment of the urodynamic laboratory. Multichannel urodynamics can be performed using this method and it may be more sensitive for the diagnosis of detrusor instability than standard urodynamic assessment.[27,28] There has been some concern that ambulatory urodynamics may result in a significant number of false positive diagnoses of detrusor instability,[29] but this does not seem to be the case.[30] As yet it has not gained widespread acceptance. It is probably most beneficial in those symptomatic women in whom standard multichannel cystometry did not reveal any abnormality.

CYSTOMETRY INTERPRETATION

Lower urinary tract dysfunction may be caused by an abnormality of bladder structure or detrusor muscle function, or disturbance of the neural or psychological control systems. Any urodynamic diagnosis made should correlate with the woman's symptoms and signs. Abnormalities of bladder function during the filling phase of cystometry may relate to detrusor activity, bladder sensation, bladder capacity or compliance.

The measurement of urinary residual volume following voiding is an integral part of urodynamic assessment. It can be estimated by ultrasound and radiography but is most often determined initially by catheterization after a urine flow study. Normal women are able to void to completion and their urinary residual volume should certainly be < 50 ml. The residual may be increased, in the absence of voiding difficulties, in women with a large cystocele, a bladder diverticulum or vesicoureteric reflux. Voiding in unfamiliar surroundings may lead to unrepresentative results, as may voiding on command with a partially filled or overfilled bladder. An isolated finding of residual urine should therefore be confirmed before being considered significant.

Detrusor activity is interpreted from the measurement of detrusor pressure (obtained by subtracting abdominal pressure from the intravesical pressure). Normal detrusor activity is indicated by minimal rise in detrusor pressure during bladder filling. There is also an absence of involuntary contractions despite provocation. Such a bladder is described as 'stable'.

Overactive detrusor function is characterized by involuntary contractions during the filling phase, which may be spontaneous or provoked and which the patient cannot completely suppress. These involuntary detrusor contractions may be triggered by a number of provocative procedures such as rapid filling, coughing, jumping and change of posture. When the detrusor muscle is shown objectively to contract, spontaneously or on provocation, during the filling phase while the patient is attempting to inhibit micturition, it is described as unstable.[31] Unstable detrusor contractions may be asymptomatic and are usually phasic in type (Fig. 9.7) Detrusor contractions during the filling phase of 15 cmH$_2$O are significant

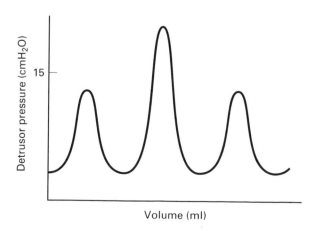

Fig. 9.7 Detrusor instability–phasic type

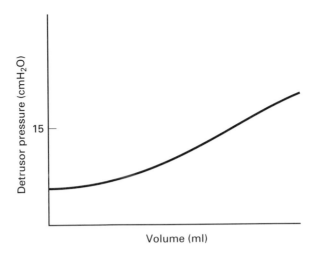

Fig. 9.8 Cystometrogram trace indicating low compliance

So too are contractions of lower amplitude if they are associated with symptoms of urgency or incontinence. The presence of unstable contractions does not necessarily imply a neurological disorder.

Where detrusor overactivity occurs in the presence of objective evidence of a relevant neurological disorder the appropriate term is detrusor hyperreflexia. The use of poorly defined terms such as hypertonic, systolic, uninhibited and spastic should be avoided.[31] A gradual increase in detrusor pressure without subsequent decrease is best regarded as a change of compliance (Fig. 9.8).

There are a number of possible causes of low bladder compliance: interstitial cystitis, radiation cystitis, upper motor neurone lesion, chronic bacterial cystitis and detrusor overactivity. Of these it is probable that a form of detrusor overactivity is one. Excessively rapid bladder filling may give a cystometric appearance suggestive of low bladder compliance. However, this artefact is evident by subsequent 'decay' of the detrusor pressure once bladder filling ceases (Fig. 9.9).

Bladder sensation during filling can be classified by both qualitative and objective measurements. It can be classified as either normal, increased, reduced or absent. Usually sensation is assessed qualitatively by questioning the patient during bladder filling regarding the sensation of

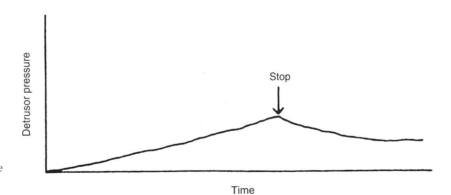

Fig. 9.9 Artefactual appearance of low compliance due to too rapid bladder filling

bladder fullness. Descriptive terms commonly used are 'first desire to void', 'normal desire to void', 'strong desire to void' and urgency. Normal ranges for the bladder volumes at which these sensations occur are difficult to define due to the subjective nature of the experiences. However, patient sensations of first desire to void at < 150 ml and severe urgency at < 400 ml, in the absence of other abnormalities, are indicative of bladder hypersensitivity. Sensory function in the lower urinary tract can also be assessed by semi-objective tests involving the measurement of urethral or bladder sensory thresholds to a standard applied stimulus. The stimulus is most commonly electrical but may be mechanical or chemical. The sensory threshold is defined as the least current which consistently produces a sensation perceived by the patient during stimulation at the site under investigation.

During the voiding phase of a cystometric examination detrusor activity may be normal, underactive or acontractile. Normal detrusor contractility is indicated by a voluntarily initiated detrusor contraction that is sustained and can usually be suppressed voluntarily. In the absence of outflow obstruction, a normal detrusor contraction will result in complete bladder emptying. For a given detrusor contraction, the magnitude of the recorded pressure rise will depend on the degree of outlet resistance. The detrusor pressure at maximum flow is generally between 40 and 65 cmH$_2$O and should result in a maximum flow rate of > 15 ml/s. Some women are able to void satisfactorily without a rise in detrusor pressure. This is particularly so in those with genuine stress incontinence who may be able to void at normal flow rates by relaxing their pelvic floor and urethra alone.

Detrusor underactivity is defined as a detrusor contraction of inadequate magnitude and/or duration to cause bladder emptying within a normal

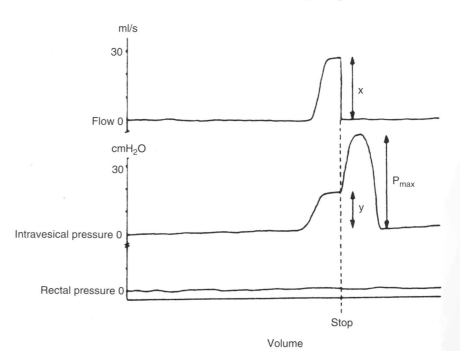

Fig. 9.10 Cystometrogram trace indicating P det iso

timespan.[31] Detrusor underactivity during micturition may coexist with detrusor overactivity during filling. An acontractile detrusor is one that cannot be demonstrated to contract during cystometric examination.[31] Detrusor areflexia refers to acontractility due to an abnormality of nervous control and denotes the complete absence of a centrally co-ordinated contraction.

The 'stop' test may be used to assess detrusor contractility. During micturition the woman is instructed to inhibit voiding. Urine flow should be able to be suddenly interrupted by closing the urethra. As the bladder neck closes more rapidly than the detrusor relaxes, the detrusor contraction becomes isovolumetric and increases to a maximum (P det iso) (Fig. 9.10).

This value is an important indicator of detrusor muscle power and may aid in selecting women at increased risk of voiding problems following incontinence surgery, i.e. those women with a low P det iso may be more likely to have voiding difficulties as incontinence surgery usually increases bladder outflow resistance. In the presence of a normally functioning detrusor the P det iso should exceed 50 cmH$_2$O.[32] This value may be reduced in women with detrusor failure due to long-standing outflow obstruction. Some women with poor urethral sphincter function may only be able to achieve cessation of urine flow by detrusor inhibition which takes several seconds. If the woman is unable to interrupt her own stream, the P det iso may be determined by physically occluding the urethra during voiding by rapidly withdrawing a balloon.[33] The detrusor pressure rise during voiding may be low or even absent in women due simply to relaxation of the urethra; the 'stop test' is of particular importance in these women. Voiding cystometry should preferably be assessed in conjunction with a concomitant flow study (see Fig. 8.9).

Outlet obstruction, which is rare in women, is suggested by a low flow rate in the presence of a high detrusor pressure, particularly if voiding is also incomplete. A low flow rate may also be due to an underactive detrusor resulting in a poor or interrupted flow rate. In this instance abdominal straining may be used to aid bladder emptying.

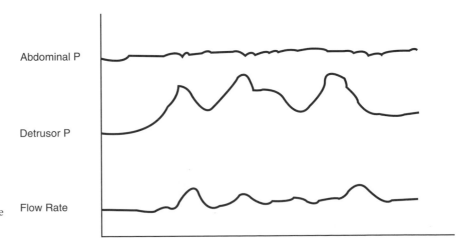

Abdominal P

Detrusor P

Flow Rate

Fig. 9.11 Pressure flow trace in detrusor–sphincter dyssynergia

Detrusor–sphincter dyssynergia occurs when the urethral sphincter mechanism contracts against a detrusor contraction or fails to open at attempted micturition. It is seen in patients with neurological abnormalities such as spinal injury or multiple sclerosis and occasionally after radical pelvic surgery. It may also occur in children. Spasms of urethral over-activity occur with a resultant intermittent flow pattern. The intravesical pressure rises as urine flow stops and falls as the flow recommences (Fig. 9.11). Vesicoureteric reflux may result and incomplete bladder emptying is common.

REFERENCES

1 Mosso A, Pellacani P. Sur les fonctions de la vessie. Arch Ital Biol 1882; 1: 205–212.
2 Rose DK. Cystometric bladder pressure determinations: their clinical importance. J Urol 1927; 17: 487–501.
3 Denny-Brown D, Robertson EG. On the physiology of micturition. Brain 1933; 56: 149–189.
4 Von Garrelts B. Intravesical pressure and urinary flow during micturition in normal subjects. Acta Chir Scand. 1957; 114: 49–66.
5 Enhorning G. Simultaneous recording of intravesical and intraurethral pressure. Acta Chir Scand (Suppl) 1961; 276: 1–68.
6 Zinner NR, Paquin AJ. Clinical urodynamics, 1: studies of intravesical pressure in normal human female subjects. J Urol 1963; 90: 719–730.
7 Bates CP, Whiteside CG, Turner-Warwick R. Synchronous cine/pressure flow/cystourethrography with special reference to stress and urge incontinence. Br J Urol 1970; 42: 714–723.
8 Cardozo LD, Stanton SL, Bennett AE. Design of a urodynamic questionnaire. Br J Urol 1978; 50: 269–274.
9 Hodgkinson CP. Direct urethrocystometry. Am J Obs Gyn 1960; 79: 648–664.
10 Bryndorf J, Sandoe E. The urodynamics of micturition. Danish Medical Bulletin 1960; 7: 65–71.
11 Arnold EP, Brown A. Webster J. Videocystourethrography with synchronous detrusor pressure and flow recording. Annals of the Royal College of Surgeons 1974; 55: 90–98.
12 Bradley WE, Trimm GW, Scott FB. Cystometry III. Cystometers. Urology 1975; 6: 843–848.
13 Robertson JR. Gas urethroscopy with pressure studies. Clinics in obstetrics and gynaecology. Gynaecological urology. London: Saunders, 1979, pp 39–49.
14 Gleason DM, Bottaccini MR, Drach GW. Urodynamics. The Urol 1976; 115: 356–361.
15 Torrens MJ. A comparative evaluation of carbon dioxide and water cystometry and sphincterometry. Proceedings of the 7th International Continence Society Meeting 1979, Portoroz.
16 Ramsden PD, Smith JC, Pierce JM, Ardran GM. The unstable bladder–fact or artefact? Brit J Urol 1977; 49: 633–639.
17 Thomas DG. Clinical urodynamics in neurogenic bladder dysfunction. Urologic Clinics of North America 1979; 6(1): 237–253.
18 Torrens MJ. The control of the hyperactive bladder by selective sacral neurectomy. MD Thesis 1974, Bristol.
19 Turner-Warwick R. Some clinical aspects of detrusor dysfunction. J Urol 1975; 113: 539–544.
20 Mayo ME. Detrusor hyperreflexia: the effect of posture and pelvic floor activity. J Urol 1978; 119: 635–638.
21 Cantor TJ, Bates CP. A comparative study of symptoms and objective urodynamic findings in 214 incontinent women. Brit J Obs & Gynae 1980; 87: 889–892.
22 Abrams PH. The clinical contribution of urodynamics. In: Abrams PH, Fenley RC, Torrens M (eds) Urodynamics, Berlin: Springer-Verlag. 1983; p 142.
23 Cardozo LD, Stanton SL. Genuine stress incontinence and detrusor instability: a review of 200 cases. Brit J Obs & Gynae 1980; 87: 184–190.
24 Jarvis GJ, Hall S, Stamp S, Miller DR, Johnson A. An assessment of urodynamic examination in incontinent women. Brit J Obs & Gynae 1980; 87: 893–896.
25 Benness CJ, Barnick CG, Cutner A, Cardozo LD. Normal urodynamics findings in

symptomatic women–who to believe, the patient or the test? Int Urogyn J 1990; 1(3): 173–174.

26 James ED. Continuous monitoring. Urologic Clinics of North America 1979; 6(1): 125–135.

27 Bhatia NN, Ostergard DR. Urodynamics in women with stress urinary incontinence. Obstet Gynecol 1982; 60: 552.

28 Mulder AF, Vierhout ME. Combined ambulatory urodynamics and pad testing. Neurourol Urodynam 1991; 10(4): 420–421.

29 Van Waalwijk van Doorn ES, Remmers A, Janknegt RA. Extramural ambulatory urodynamic testing of the lower urinary tract in volunteers. Neurourol Urodynam 1990; 9(4): 380–381.

30 Robertson AS, Griffiths CJ, Ramsden PD, Neal PD. Ambulatory monitoring and conventional urodynamic studies in normal volunteers. Neurourol Urodynam 1991; 10(4): 418–419.

31 Abrams P, Blaivas JG, Stanton SL, Andersen JJ. The standardisation of terminology of lower urinary tract function. Scand J Urol Nephrol 1988; Suppl 114: 5–18.

32 Griffiths DJ. The bladder. In: Urodynamics, the mechanics and hydrodynamics of the lower urinary tract, Bristol: Adam Hilger. 1980.

33 Coolsaet BLRA. The stop-flow test and its implications in bladder function. Proceedings of the 76th American Urological Association Meeting, Boston, 1981.

10 Pad weighing test

Pad weighing tests offer the possibility of objectively measuring urine loss. This can be very helpful when assessing individual patient symptoms, as there is considerable evidence that subjective assessment of urine loss is often incorrect.[1,2,3,4,5] Objective measurement is also essential when comparing treatments and results from different centers and is mandatory when the results of research are being reported. Urodynamic evidence of urinary loss remains the 'gold standard' for the diagnosis of incontinence,[6] however, there is still no standardization of the severity of incontinence when the diagnosis is made by urodynamic investigation. For the above reasons several tests have been devised to quantify the amount of urinary loss in incontinent patients.

These tests all have some sort of collecting device ranging from electrical sensors through to perineal pads. The loss is measured over a standard time and in addition bladder capacity and exerise regimens may be standardized. However, although pad testing appears to have good potential objectively to measure urine loss there are some problems.

The first problem is that urine is not the only substance contributing to the pad weight. Sutherst et al[7] noted that up to 1 g/h pad weight increase occurs in 95% of normal women. Versi & Cardozo[6] felt that the upper normal limit was 1.4 g/h, while Jorgensen studied 24-h tests and estimated a maximum normal loss of 8 g/24 h. Menstruation, infection and periovulation can also complicate measurements.

Secondly, pad testing may not be measuring normal conditions. This is particularly true in 1- or 2-h testing where the activities done during the test may be quite different from the normal activities of the patient. In a research setting this is not very important but in a clinical setting it must be taken into account.

The third potential problem with pad testing is that its sensitivity may vary with different medical conditions. Detrusor instability may alter with different outside conditions such as cold weather or running water. The longer tests will assess this better but there is possibly a loss of standardization.

With the introduction of any new investigation it is important to analyze the validity and reproducibility of the test. It is possible to get a good historical overview of pad testing by reviewing papers studying its validation and reproducibility.

URILOS, THE ELECTRIC NAPPY

In 1971[8] Urilos, a specially designed nappy with electrodes within it was described. If a fluid touched the nappy then a change in electrical conductivity occurred. The advantage of this technique is that it can record the time of incontinence and therefore relate it to a specific action or event. However, there is no clear relationship between the amount of loss and the recording signal and there have been technical problems that have led to inaccuracies being reported.[9,10] The equipment was rather specialized so it was only practical in a specialist unit.

PAD-WEIGHING TESTS

In 1974 Caldwell reported a technique of weighing perineal pads to record urine loss.[11] However, no objective work was done on this technique until 1981 when Sutherst et al and Walsh et al reported studies looking at pad weighing tests done at the Royal Liverpool Hospital.[7,12]

Sutherst studied 100 incontinent women and 50 continent women. All the women had a 'comfortably' full bladder and they were given preweighed perineal pads. They were encouraged to do whatever activity made them leak for an hour and the pad was changed every 10 min. They estimated that the normal increase in pad weight because of perspiration and vaginal discharge was up to 1.0 g/h or no greater than 0.5 g per pad. Walsh used a 2–h test to study 56 elderly women who were known to be incontinent and 6 healthy volunteers. They felt they were recording 94% of all urinary loss (the rest leaked around the pads), that the normal mean pad weight gain was 1.2 g/h and that the mean evaporative effect on a wet pad was 1.3 g. Neither group validated the test or checked its reproducibility but the test began to be used in units around the world.

The 1-hour test

In 1983 the International Continence Society attempted to standardize the pad weighing test. Standard conditions were described, the exercise was standardized and the fluid intake was set.[13] Again the test had not been validated or shown to be reproducible and there was no attempt to standardize the bladder volume.

Reproducibility

Since 1983 a number of authors have attempted to document the reproducibility of the 1–h pad weighing test. Mundt-Pettersen et al tested and then retested 20 women and noted that the results could differ by as much as a factor of two.[14] Another Swedish group retested 19 women and found reasonable reproducibility but a persistent skewing of the data.[15,16]

In 1987 Jorgensen et al[17] reported on 81 women. They retested 18 women and found a correlation of 0.68 between the two tests. Importantly, the correlation increased to 0.93 if initial bladder volume and total diuresis during the test were compared with urine loss. Data from a different study from the same institution[18] showed very similar retest correlations if bladder volumes and diuresis during the test were taken into account.

Several authors have attempted to modify the 1-h ICS pad test by standardizing the bladder volume at which the test is done. Kinn & Larsson[16,19] used maximum cystometric capacity and then retested at 75% of that volume with a correlation of 0.74. Fantl et al[20] filled the bladder via a catheter and retested 67 women. Patients with different diagnoses were tested with a correlation of 0.97 for stress incontinence and 0.84 for detrusor instability. However, there were wide individual variations especially in women with stress incontinence. In 1988, Lose et al[21] used a standard volume of 50% of maximum cystometric capacity to fill the bladder. The correlation was 0.97 but there were individual variations of up to 24 g. It is still unclear whether the variations in reproducibility are physiological variations or inherent inaccuracies of the test but it is now accepted that to get the best result from a 1-h test, bladder volume needs to be known.

Validation

There have been very few attempts scientifically to validate the pad test. In the paper by Jorgensen et al,[17] 49 patients underwent 1-h pad testing and videocystourethrography. There was only a 50% correlation between a positive pad test and videocystourethrography. However, it was the pad test that was recording the higher numbers of women leaking so perhaps this is a criticism of videocystourethrography.

Versi & Cardozo[6] compared 1-h pad testing and videocystourethrography in 99 women. Using a normal group of controls they estimated the average pad loss in 'dry' women to be 1.4 g/h. Using this cut-off, 14 of the 99 women who had proven genuine stress incontinence had a false negative pad test. Interestingly, there was no relationship between the severity of the incontinence and the false negative rate.

As these have been the only formal attempts to validate 1-h pad testing it is difficult to gauge the sensitivity and specificity of the test. It does appear that it may not be sensitive enough for research purposes or for complex cases.[16]

Home and long-term testing

Wilson et al[22] postulated that pad testing undertaken at home would be more physiological, although they still used a standardized exercise regimen. The results showed very little difference between the two types of 1-h pad test (home and hospital). They felt the advantage of the home test may be cost savings, although it is difficult to see how the bladder volumes could be standardized.

Twenty-four-hour and 48-h tests have been devised to try and mimic 'normal' conditions and to attempt to increase the specificity but more importantly the sensitivity of the 1-h test. Ali et al[23] first reported a comparison of a 12-h home test and a 1-h test. They showed similar results in both tests.

Victor & Asbrink[24] reported a 48-h test. Patients weighed their own pads and performed normal activities. In 1987 Victor et al published a comparison of a 48-h test and a 1-h test.[25] They were unable to show any correlation between the two tests. The correlation between two 48-h tests was 0.90. The difference in results comparing the 1-h test and the 48-h test was thought to be due to an increased sensitivity in the 48-h test and it was thought that the 48-h test is probably better at demonstrating urge incontinence. The 48-h test was also thought to need less hospital staff and to be independent of the patient's activity.

Lose et al[26] compared two 24-h pad tests and a 1-h ward test in 31 women with proven stress or mixed incontinence. Eighteen (58%) women were classified as incontinent after the 1-h test, whereas 28 (90%) were classed as incontinent after the 24-h test. On retesting with another 24-h test there were variations of over 100%. The authors felt that this was due to variations in patient activity and if the activity could be standardized then the 24-h test could be used in a more quantitative way rather than as a screening test. However, it is difficult to see how the level of activity over 24-h could be standardized.

The authors felt that other advantages of the 24-h test were that it is performed in familiar surroundings, provocative activities that are known to induce leakage can be used, it can be independent of the mobility of the patient and the total number of pads used can be a guide to how many pads may be needed by the patient. In addition, it may be better at demonstrating urge incontinence and it did not involve hospital staff to perform the test.

In 1989 Kralj reported to the International Continence Society the results of a comparison of the standard ICS pad test, the ICS test done at cystometric capacity, the ICS test done at two-thirds bladder volume and a 48-h home test. All the results were compared against patient histories of their symptoms. There are some difficulties comparing the results of objective and subjective tests[16] but the 48-h test had a sensitivity of 0.92 and the ICS standard test had a sensitivity of 0.45. Interestingly, the best test for urge incontinence was the maximum capacity test (0.73) and the best test for stress-type symptoms was the two-thirds capacity test (0.73).

CONCLUSIONS

It is now accepted that short pad testing needs to be done at standard volumes. Therefore the patient needs to be catheterized, which means hospital staff must be involved. Ultrasound estimation of bladder volumes can be used to avoid this problem. A standard bladder volume makes the shorter tests more reproducible than the home tests, but the short tests are not very sensitive. There has been little work looking at measurement of different types of incontinence. Home tests do have a high sensitivity but reproducibility is not very good. Again it is not really known how different types of incontinence affect the test.

Pad tests have a useful role particularly where the symptoms and urodynamic results are at variance. They have not yet been properly validated and the reproducibility is still suspect. However, as further work is done these questions will eventually be answered.

REFERENCES

1 Jarvis GJ, Hall S, Stamp S, Millar DR, Johnson A. An assessment of urodynamic examination in incontinent women. Br J Obstet Gynaecol 1980; 87: 893–896.
2 Frazer MI, Sutherst JR, Holland EFN. Visual analogue scores and urinary incontinence. Br Med J 1987; 295: 582.
3 Versi E, Cardozo LD, Anand D, Cooper D. Symptom analysis for the diagnosis of genuine stress incontinence. Br J Obstet Gynaecol 1991; 98: 815–819.
4 Robinson H, Stanton SL. Detection of urinary incontinence. Br J Obstet Gynaecol 1981; 88: 59–61.
5 Katz GP, Blaivas JG. A diagnostic dilemma: when urodynamic findings differ from the clinical impression. J Urol 1983; 129: 1170–1174.
6 Versi E, Cardozo L. Perineal pad weighing versus videographic analysis in genuine stress incontinence. Br J Obstet Gynaecol 1986; 93: 364–366.
7 Sutherst J, Brown M, Shawer M. Assessing the severity of urinary incontinence, in women by weighing perineal pads. Lancet 1981; 1: 1180–1181.
8 James ED, Flack FC, Caldwell KPS, Martin MR. Continuous measurement of urine loss and frequency in incontinent patients. Br J Urol 1971; 43: 233–237.
9 Stanton SL, Ritchie D. Urilos: the practical detection of urine loss. Am J Obstet Gynecol 1977; 128: 461–463.
10 Wilson PD, Samarrai MT, Brown ADG. Quantifying female incontinence with a particular reference to the Urilos system. Urol Int 1980; 35: 298–302.
11 Caldwell KPS. Clinical use of the recording nappy. Urol Int 1974; 29: 172–73.
12 Walsh JB, Mills GL. Measurement of urinary loss in elderly incontinent patients. A simple and accurate method. Lancet 1981; 1: 1130–1131.
13 Bates P, Bradley W, Glen E et al. Fifth report on the standardisation of terminology of lower urinary tract function. Bristol: International Continence Society Committee on Standardisation of Terminology, 1983.
14 Mundt-Pettersen B, Matthiasson A, Sundin T. Reproducibility of the 1 hour incontinence test proposed by the ICS standardisation committee. Proceedings of the 14th Annual Meeting of the ICS. Boston: International Continence Society. 1986. pp 90–91.
15 Klarskov P, Hald T. Reproducibility and reliability of urinary continence assessment with the 60 minutes test. Scand J Urol Nephrol 1984; 18: 293–298.
16 Victor A. Pad weighing test – a simple method to quantitate urinary incontinence. Ann Med 1990; 22: 443–447.
17 Jorgensen L, Lose G, Thorup Andersen J. One-hour pad weighing test for assessment of female urinary incontinence. Obstet Gynecol 1987; 69: 39–42.
18 Lose G, Gammelgaard J, Juul Jorgensen T. The one-hour pad weighing test: reproducibility and the correlation between the test result, the start volume in the bladder and the diuresis. Neurourol Urodyn 1986; 5: 17–21.
19 Kinn AC, Larsson B. Pad test with fixed bladder volume in urinary stress incontinence. Acta Obstet Gynecol Scand 1987; 66: 369–371.
20 Fantl JA, Harkins SW, Wyman JF, Choi SC, Taylor JR. Fluid loss quantitation test in women with urinary incontinence: a test-retest analysis. Obstet Gynecol 1987; 70: 739–743.
21 Lose G, Rosenkilde P, Gammelgaard J, Schroeder T. Pad weighing tests performed with standardised bladder volume. Urology 1988; 32: 78–80.
22 Wilson PD, Mason MV, Herbison GP, Sutherst JR. Evaluation of the home pad test for quantifying incontinence. Br J Urol 1988; 64: 155–157.
23 Ali K, Murray A, Sutherst J, Brown M. Perineal pad weighing test: comparison of the one hour ward test with twelve hour home pad test. Abstract. Proceedings of the 13th Annual Meeting of the ICS. Aachen: International Continence Society 1983, pp 380–382.
24 Victor A, Asbrink AS. A simple 48 hour test for the quantification of urinary incontinence. Abstract. Proceedings of the 15th Annual Meeting of the ICS, London: International Continence Society 1985; pp 507–508.
25 Victor A, Larsson G, Asbrink AS. A simple patient administered test for objective quantitation of the symptom of urinary incontinence. Scand J Nephrol 1987; 21(4): 277–279.
26 Lose G, Jorgensen L, Thunedborg P. 24 hour home pad weighing test versus 1 hour ward test in the assessment of mild stress incontinence. Acta Obstet Gynecol Scand 1989; 68: 211–215.

Urethral pressure profilometry

INTRODUCTION

The first report of urethral pressure measurements was by Bonney[1] and described a technique known as retrograde sphincterometry. In 1939 Simons[2] described a method of measuring the intraurethral pressure using a balloon catheter, and this was subsequently used by other workers.[3]

Subsequent to this a fluid perfusion device was used to measure the intraurethral pressure.[4,5] This enabled pressure changes along the length of the urethra to be determined together with simultaneous recording of the intravesical pressure.[5]

The advent of solid state microtransducers resulted in a new catheter being used for urethral pressure profilometry (UPP). The catheter is made of soft metal material with two pressure-tip transducers a set distance apart (Fig. 11.1). Due to the expense of solid state microtransducers and the fact that adequate sterilization is required between patients, there has been a move by some workers towards previously used disposable catheters.

DIFFERENT URETHRAL PRESSURE PROFILE CATHETERS

There are three main varieties of disposable catheter systems used for urethral pressure measurements: the open-sided catheter with a variable

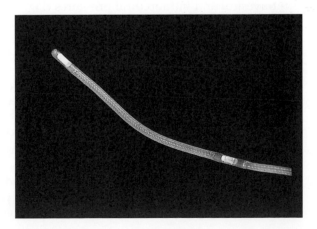

Fig. 11.1 A urethral pressure profile catheter (Gaeltec)

number of side holes, the open-ended catheter and the balloon catheter. These three measuring devices are compared in a paper by Jonas & Klotter.[6] The overall conclusion is that the balloon catheter is superior as it records real wall pressure, but its disadvantage is that it requires exact calibration for each test to obtain good results.

Ask & Hök[7] produced a paper looking at different pressure-measuring devices. They examined water-filled catheters, balloon catheters and microtransducers. The advantages and disadvantages of each system are discussed.

With balloon catheters, the frequency of the response is determined by the properties of the catheter-manometer system. It integrates the pressure over the length and circumference of the whole balloon. This will reduce disturbances due to local variations, but an average is obtained rather than a point measurement. In addition, if the balloon is deformed by pressure variations, this will affect the cross-sectional area of the balloon and hence the measurements will be distorted.

The advantage of the water-filled infused catheter is that the infused fluid will prevent blockage. However, any sudden rise in pressure will result in tissue contact initially blocking the side hole, resulting in a raised pressure until the infusing fluid clears the blockage. Not all fluid systems have an adequate frequency response time to measure stress profiles.

Microtransducers have an adequate response time for all aspects of UPP. The side wall mounting of the transducers provides a more reproducible recording of both mechanical and fluid pressures in a collapsible tube. In addition, some workers have used multiple transducers along the catheter to assess stationary recordings of the urethral pressure profile.[8] Overall it would appear that microtransducers are most applicable to UPP and are the system adopted by most units.

THE URETHRAL PRESSURE PROFILE RECORDING

Simultaneous urethrocystometry was first popularized by Asmussen & Ulmsten.[9] The catheter is gradually withdrawn (Fig. 11.2) at a constant rate along the urethra enabling simultaneous recording of the intravesical and intraurethral pressures (Fig. 11.3). Electronic subtraction of these recordings can be made. Many different parameters of the resultant trace can be analysed. It is important to appreciate that the technique is a measure of urethral function and not detrusor function, as only the intravesical pressure is recorded.

The profile can be assessed both at rest and during stress. During rest, the standard parameters analysed include: maximum urethral pressure (MUP), maximum urethral closure pressure (MUCP), functional urethral length (FUL) and anatomical urethral length (AUL)[10, 11, 12] (Figs. 11.3, 11.4 and 11.5). Other authors have analyzed the length to peak[10] and the area under different sections of the curve.[12,13]

The catheter can then be withdrawn at a standard rate while the patient gives repeated coughs, thus producing a stress pressure profile (Figs. 11.4 and 11.5). The same measurements can then be recorded. In addition, a

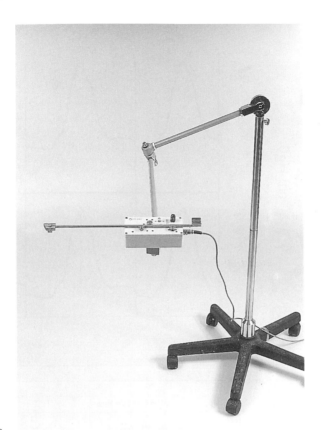

Fig. 11.2   A urethral pressure profile catheter mounted in the withdrawal device (Weist)

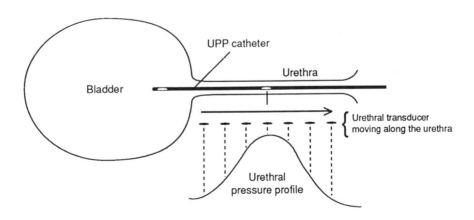

Fig. 11.3   Urethral pressure profilometry technique

loss of urethral closure pressure on raised intra-abdominal pressure can be noted. Also the pressure transmission ratio (PTR) can be determined. This is defined as the increment in urethral pressure on stress as a percentage of the simultaneously recorded increment in intravesical pressure (Fig. 11.4). A convenient method is to divide the urethra into quartiles and calculate the PTR for each quartile.[12,14]

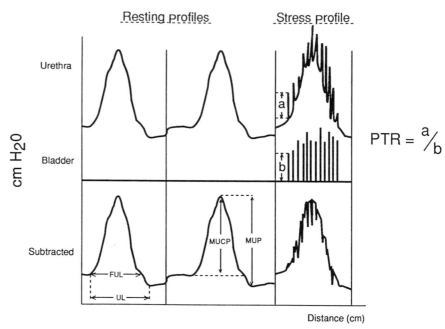

Fig. 11.4 A urethral pressure profilometry trace demonstrating the parameters measured

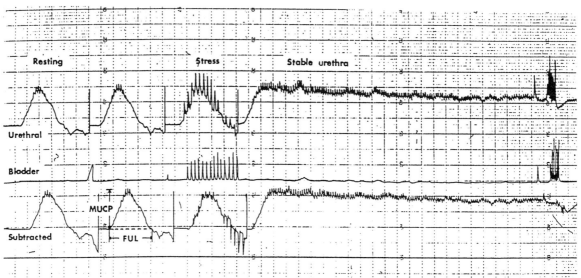

Fig. 11.5 A normal urethral pressure profilometry trace

Finally, while the patient is at rest, with the transducer at the point of MUP for 2 min, a tracing can be obtained. This can be used to measure urethral vascular pulsations[15,16] and to look for evidence of urethral instability and urethral relaxation.[17,18,19,20]

Data on the use of UPP in the determination of lower urinary tract dysfunction are contradictory. Rud[21] studied resting parameters in continent women in different age groups. The mean results in women of fertile ages is shown in Table 11.1. In postmenopausal women he found a decrease in all parameters.

Table 11.1   Urethral pressure profilometry parameters according to Rud 1980[20]

Parameter	Age Group (years)			
	16–20	21–25	26–30	31–35
Number of women	18	24	18	11
MUCP (cmH$_2$O)	85	90	73	84
MUP (cmH$_2$O)	106	110	94	104
FUL (mm)	27	30	30	29
AUL (mm)	34	37	37	36

Table 11.2   Maximum urethral closure pressure and functional urethral length in normal controls

Study	Mean age +s range	Number	MUCP (cmH$_2$O)	FUL (mm)
Henriksson et al 1977[21]	39 (20–64)	14	53	25
Van Geelan et al 1981[13]	25.4 (19–35)	27	84	32
Hilton & Stanton 1983b[10]	46.1 (25–74)	20	68	24
Sorensen et al 1988a[22]	32 (28–43)	10	62	32
Versi 1990[12]	49.7 (SD = 6.8)	102	52	29

Other studies have examined these parameters in women of different ages and the results are not in total agreement (Table 11.2). Differences may be due to a variety of factors: age ranges, parity of women, race, the technique employed and whether or not the women were proven to be urodynamically normal (this was only true in the study by Versi.[12]) A standardized method is proposed by the International Continence Society.[11] They suggest that the position of the patient,[22] the bladder volume, pressure-measuring device and rate of catheter withdrawal be recorded. In addition, Anderson et al[23] suggest that the direction of the pressure transducers should be lateral at the 3 or 9 o'clock position.

It has been suggested that urethral pulsations in the urethral pressure profile may influence the measurement of the MUCP. Urethral pulsations will vary according the estrogen status of the patient and probably indicate the degree of vascularization of the urethra.[10,24] The correlation of the size of pulsations with clinical symptomatology has not been determined.

DIAGNOSIS OF GENUINE STRESS INCONTINENCE

The resting profile has been used to diagnose genuine stress incontinence. Although the MUP and MUCP are significantly reduced in women with genuine stress incontinence compared to normal controls,[10,12] there is considerable overlap between groups[12]. Hilton & Stanton[10] found the same to be true with regard to urethral length and Versi[12] with regard to FUL and AUL. All parameters were significantly lower in women with genuine stress incontinence in the stress pressure profile,[10,12] but again there was considerable overlap. A negative stress pressure profile is recorded when the intravesical pressure exceeds the intraurethral pressure with a cough.[10,25] However, it has been shown that the size of the cough influences the stress curve, thus making its analysis unreliable.[26]

Pressure transmission ratios are a test of the dynamic response of the urethra to raised intra-abdominal pressure. Several authors have suggested its use in differentiating those women with and those without genuine stress incontinence.[10,27,28] Values of less than 90–95% in at least one quartile are suggestive of genuine stress incontinence. However, other studies deny its specificity.[12,29] Thind et al[30] state that the rise in urethral pressure is made up of two components, one being active and the other passive. Furthermore, in continent women the rise in urethral pressure precedes the rise in intravesical pressure. This finding may account for some of the differences in other studies, especially when comparing results of continence operations. Other factors that have been shown to affect transmission ratio results include the bladder volume at which the recording was obtained.[32] Thus, as with the rest of the profile, the method should be standardized to give reproducible results.

Other authors have attempted to use Valsalva leak point pressure as a more sensitive test than UPP in the assessment of women with genuine stress incontinence.[32,33] During this test the patient strains and the degree of straining necessary to cause leakage of urine is measured. Bump et al[3] found this urodynamic parameter to be reproducible but dependent on the size of urethral catheter. Swift & Ostergard,[33] however, found poor correlation of Valsalva leak point pressure and the MUCP and found no satisfactory cut-off point to determine those patients with a low-pressure urethra. It may be that the poor correlation between the two parameters is due to the fact that they are measuring two different entities: Valsalva leak point pressure measures a dynamic response of the urethral sphincter mechanism, whereas the MUP is measuring static components. Van Venrooij et al[34] used a parameter derived from both the above. They determined the ratio of the relative leakage pressure (urethral leakage pressure minus the intravesical resting pressure) to MUCP. They found that the average value was 0.5. The place of this parameter in assessing urodynamic abnormalities has yet to be determined, however.

TREATMENT OF GENUINE STRESS INCONTINENCE

Although UPP will not make possible a diagnosis of genuine stress incontinence, some workers have suggested its use both in planning the type of surgery to be carried out and as an aid during the operation itself. Several authorities have suggested a cut-off of 20 cmH$_2$O of MUCP for predicting poor outcome for incontinence surgery.[35,36,37] It has been suggested that in these patients a sling, or even artificial sphincter should be considered.[35,37,38,39,40] Others, although identifying a low urethral pressure as a risk factor for failure of retropubic surgery, do not consider that the increased complication rate of sling procedures is justified as a reasonable cure rate can still be obtained with a colposuspension.[42]

In addition to UPP predicting a potentially poor outcome, it has been suggested that peroperative profilometry can be of benefit to confirm that adequate resistance has been achieved.[42] These authors suggest that a closure pressure of at least 60 cmH$_2$O and a twofold increase prior to the suspension should be aimed for. There is, however, little corroborative evidence as to the use of per-operative profilometry.

ASSESSMENT OF VOIDING DIFFICULTIES

When a patient has either a low flow rate or an increased post-micturition residual, a diagnosis of voiding difficulty can be made. Voiding cystometry can be used to help determine whether or not the primary pathology is outflow obstruction. In this situation, the detrusor pressure will be raised, indicating that the detrusor is trying to overcome an outlet obstruction. If the pathology is poor detrusor function, then the detrusor pressure will be low and there will be a low flow rate (see Ch. 8). However, with time, the detrusor decompensates if it is working against an outflow obstruction, and therefore the voiding cystometry findings are similar in both situations.

The resting urethral pressure profile trace can help differentiate between the two clinical entities. The MUCP will be raised in cases of outflow obstruction but not in cases of poor detrusor function. There are, however, no data on the upper limit of normal but a markedly raised MUCP in association with a low peak flow rate would indicate obstruction. Thus UPP can help plan the correct treatment of voiding difficulties and prevent inappropriate urethrotomy in cases of poor detrusor function, which will result in a combination of voiding difficulties and genuine stress incontinence.

DIAGNOSIS OF URETHRAL DIVERTICULUM

A further use of UPP is in the diagnosis of urethral diverticulum.[43] On the resting trace, the presence of a biphasic curve indicates the possibility of a diverticulum. However, this configuration may also occur in some cases of genuine stress incontinence, in particular after continence surgery. Although a useful aid, it is probably not superior to video-cystourethrography or cystourethroscopy.

URETHRAL INSTABILITY

More recently, the association between variations in urethral pressure (at the point of MUCP at rest) and abnormal detrusor function has been examined. This phenomenon is known as urethral instability, which has been defined by the International Continence Society[11] as an involuntary fall in intraurethral pressure in the absence of detrusor instability, resulting in the leakage of urine. Other workers have defined it as urethral pressure variations exceeding either 15 cmH$_2$O[17] or 20 cmH$_2$O.[19] Possibly the relative drop in MUP is of paramount importance and other

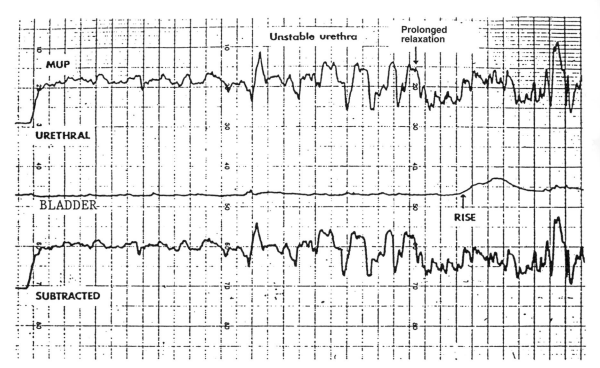

Fig. 11.6   A urethral pressure profilometry trace demonstrating urethral instability associated with detrusor contractions

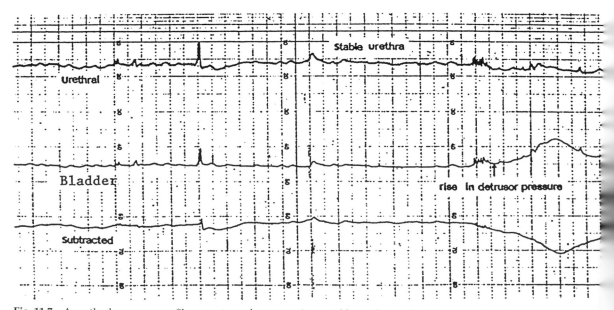

Fig. 11.7   A urethral pressure profilometry trace demonstrating a stable urethra and a detrusor contraction

studies have defined the phenomenon as being due to variations in the MUP at rest of at least one-third of its value[18] (Fig. 11.6).

Several authors have shown a higher incidence of urethral instability in women with detrusor instability[44,45] (Fig. 11.6). The correlation between lower urinary tract symptoms and the presence of instability remains unclear.[17,18]

Further studies have examined the relationship between urethral relaxation and subsequent detrusor contraction. They have suggested that in some cases of detrusor instability, the primary pathology lies in the urethra rather than the bladder itself.[70,44,46] In these patients, unstable detrusor contractions are preceded by urethral relaxation[47] (Fig. 11.6 and 11.7).

SUMMARY

It would thus appear that UPP is a useful tool in the investigation of lower urinary tract dysfunction. It will not make possible a diagnosis of genuine stress incontinence but may help in the preoperative assessment. We have found it an invaluable tool in the assessment of voiding difficulties, but to date normal ranges have not been well documented. Its full potential especially with regard to detrusor instability has only recently been realized, and it may be that in the future it will have a role in targeting specific treatments for this condition.

REFERENCES

1 Bonney V. On diurnal incontinence of urine in women. J Obstet Gynaecol 1923; Br Emp 30: 358–365.
2 Simons I. Studies in bladder function. 2. The sphincterometer. J Urol 1936; 35: 96–102.
3 Enhorning G. Simultaneous recordings of the intravesical and intraurethral pressure. A study on urethral closure in normal and stress incontinent women. Acta Cir Scand 1961; Suppl 276: 1–68.
4 Toews HA. Intraurethral and intravesical pressures in normal and stress-incontinent women. Obstet Gynecol 1967; 29: 613–624.
5 Brown M, Wickham JEA. THe urethral pressure profile. Br J Urol 1969; 41: 211–217.
6 Jonas U, Klotter HJ. Study of three urethral pressure recording devices: theoretical considerations. Urological Research 1978; 6: 119–125.
7 Ask P, Hök B. Pressure measurement techniques in urodynamic investigations. Neurourol Urodynam 1990; 9: 1–15.
8 Ulmsten U, Forman A, Hök B, Lindström K, Gewers G, Olsson CO. A new multitransducer catheter for intraluminal pressure recording in vivo. Electromedica 1980; 1 (80): 9–12.
9 Asmussen M, Ulmsten U. Simultaneous urethrocystometry with a new technique. Scand J Urol Nephrol 1976; 10: 7–11.
10 Hilton P, Stanton SL. Urethral pressure measurement by microtransducer: the results in symptom-free women and in those with genuine stress incontinence. Br J Obstet Gynaecol 1983b; 90: 919–933.
11 Abrams P, Blaivas JG, Stanton SL, Andersen JT. The standardisation of terminology of lower urinary tract function. Br J Obstet Gynaecol 1990; 97 (Suppl 6): 1–16.
12 Versi E. Discriminant analysis of urethral pressure profilometry data for the diagnosis of genuine stress incontinence. Br J Obstet Gynaecol 1990; 97: 251–259.
13 van Geelen JM, Doesburg WH, Thomas CMG, Martin CB. Urodynamic studies in the normal menstrual cycle: the relationship between hormonal changes during the menstrual cycle and the urethral pressure profile. Am J Obstet Gynecol 1981; 141: 384–392.
14 Versi E, Cardozo L, Cooper DJ. Urethral pressures: analysis of transmission pressure ratios. Br J Urol 1991; 68(3): 266–270.

15 Versi E, Cardozo L. Urethral vascular pulsations. Proceedings of the 15th Annual Meeting of the International Continence Society, London. 1985, pp 503–504.

16 Schultze H, Wolansky D. Urethralwandpulsationen bei schwangeren, kontinenten und stressinkontinenten Frauen. (Urethral vascular pulsations in pregnant, continent and urinary stress incontinent women). Zent B1 Gynakol 1990; 112: 19–22.

17 Ulmsten U, Henriksson L, Iosif S. The unstable female urethra. Am J Obstet Gynecol 1982; 144: 93–97.

18 Tapp AJS, Cardozo LD, Versi E, Studd JWW. The prevalence of variation of resting urethral pressure in women and its association with lower urinary tract function. Br. J. Urol 1988a; 61: 314–317.

19 Low JA, Armstrong JB, Mauger GM. The unstable urethra in the female. Obstet Gynecol 1989; 74: 69–74.

20 Bergman A, Koonings PP, Ballard CA. Detrusor instability. Is the bladder the cause or the effect? J Reprod Med 1989; 34: 834–838.

21 Rud T. Urethral pressure profile in continent women from childhood to old age. Acta Obstet Gynecol Scand 59: 331–335.

22 Henriksson L, Ulmsten U, Andersson K–E. The effect of changes of posture on the urethral closure pressure in healthy women. 1977; Scand J Urol Nephrol 11: 201–206.

23 Anderson RS, Shepherd AM, Feneley RCL. Microtransducer urethral pressure profile methodology: variations caused by transducer orientation. 1983; J Urol 130: 727–728.

24 Schreiter F, Fuchs P, Stockamp K. Estrogenic sensitivity of α-receptors in the urethra musculature. Urol Int 1993; 31: 13–19.

25 Beck RP, Maughan GB. Silmultaneous intraurethral and intravesical studies in normal women and those with stress incontinence. Am J Obstet Gynecol 1964; 89: 746–753.

26 Schick E. Objective assessment of resistance of female urethra to stress. A scale to establish degree of urethral incompetence. Urol 1985; 26: 518–526.

27 Farghaly SA, Shah J, Worth P. The value of the intraurethral pressure transmission ratio in the assessment of female stress incontinence. Arch Gynecol 1985; Suppl 237: 366. Abstract.

28 Fantl JA. Genuine stress incontinence: pathophysiology and rationale for its medical management. Obstet Gynecol Clin North Am 1989; 16: 827–840.

29 Rosenzweig BA, Bhatia NN, Nelson AL. Dynamic urethral pressure profilometry pressure transmission ratio. What do the numbers really mean? 1991; Obstet Gynecol 77: 586–590.

30 Thind P, Lose G, Jorgensen L, Colstrup H. Variations in urethral and bladder pressure during stress episodes in healthy women. Br J Urol 1990; 66: 389–392.

31 van Waalwiijk van Doorn ESC, Remmers A, Weil EHJ, Janknegt RA. Transmission ratio related to bladder filling in volunteers. Neurourology Urodynamics 1991; 10(4): 446–447.

32 Bump RC, Elser DM, McClish DK. Valsalva leak point pressures in adult women with genuine stress incontinence: reproducibility, effect of catheter caliber, and correlations with passive urethral pressure profilometry. Neurourol Urodyn 1993; 12(4): 307–308.

33 Swift SE, Ostergard DR. A comparison of stress leak-point pressure and maximal urethral closure pressure in patients with genuine stress incontinence. Obstet Gynecol 1995; 85(5): 704–708.

34 van Venrooij GE, Blok C, van Riel MP, Coolsaet BL. Relative urethral leakage pressure versus maximum urethral closure pressure. The reliability of the measurement of urethral competence with the new tube-foil sleeve catheter in patients. J Urol 1985; 134(3): 592–595.

35 McGuire EJ. Urodynamic findings in patients after failure of stress incontinent operations. Prog Clin Biol Res 1981; 351: 78–82.

36 Weil A, Reyes H, Bischoff P, Rottenburg RD, Krauer F. Modifications of the urethral rest and stress profiles after different types of surgery for urinary stress incontinence. Br J Obstet Gynaecol 1984; 91: 46–55.

37 Sand PK, Bowen LW, Panganiban R, Ostergard DR. The low pressure urethra as a factor in failed retropubic urethropexy. Obstet Gynecol 1987; 69: 399–402.

38 Koonings PP, Bergman A, Ballard CA. Low urethral pressure and stress urinary incontinence in women: risk factor for failed retropubic surgical procedure. Urol 1990; 36: 245–248.

39 Blavis JG, Olsson CA. Stress incontinence: classification and surgical approach. J Urol 1988; 39: 727–731.

40 Meschia M, Bruschi F, Barbacini P, Amicarelli F, Ceosignani PG. Recurrent incontinence after retropubic surgery. J Gynecol Surg 1993; 9: 25–28.

41 Richardson DA, Ramahi A, Chalas E. Surgical management of stress incontinence in patients with low urethral pressure. Gynecol Obstet Invest 1991; 31: 106–109.

42 Gearhart JP, Williams KA, Jeffs RD. Intraoperative urethral pressure profilometry as an adjunct to bladder neck reconstruction. J Urol 1986; 136: 1055–1056.

43 Summitt RL, Stovall TG. Urethral diverticula: evaluation by urethral pressure profilometry, cystourethroscopy, and the voiding cystourethrogram. Obstet Gynecol 1992; 80(4): 695–699.

44 Low JA. Urethral behaviour during the involuntary detrusor contraction. Am J Obstet Gynecol 1977; 128: 32–42.

45 Weil A, Miege B, Rottenberg R, Krauer F. Clinical significance of urethral instability. Obstet Gynecol 1986; 68: 106–110.

46 Hindmarsh JR, Gosling PT, Deane AM. Bladder instability. Is the primary defect in the urethra? Br J Urol 1983; 55: 648–651.

47 Wise BG, Cardozo LD, Cutner A, Benness CJ, Burton G. The prevalence and significance of urethral instabiity In women with detrusor instability. Br J Urol 1993; 72: 26–29.

12 Cystourethroscopy

NTRODUCTION

Cystourethroscopy enables the inside of the bladder and urethra to be visualized. The procedure can be performed for a number of indications, either diagnostic or therapeutic. Local or general anesthesia can be employed. In the United Kingdom it is usual to infuse normal saline into the bladder to facilitate visualization but in North America gas cysto-urethroscopy using carbon dioxide is often employed. This is less messy than conventional fluid-filled cystourethroscopy but has the disadvantage of being unphysiological (carbon dioxide dissolves in urine to produce carbonic acid, which is irritant to the bladder).

Contemporary rigid endoscopes incorporate three essential features–a rod-lens system, a fiber optic bundle for transmission of light from an external source to the bladder and an irrigating channel to flush away blood and dilate the bladder under direct vision. Such a system is shown in Fig 12.1. This type of endoscope can accommodate different telescopes

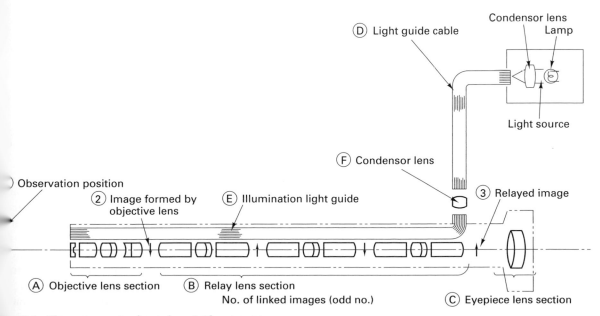

12.1 The components of a modern rigid cystoscope

Field of view & apparent field of view

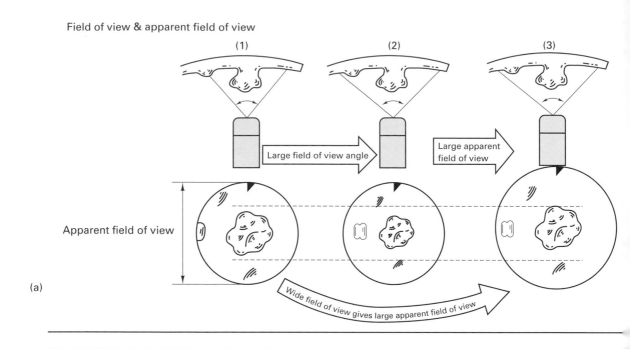

(a)

Direction and field of view angle

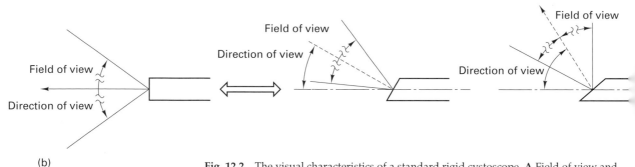

(b)

Fig. 12.2   The visual characteristics of a standard rigid cystoscope. **A** Field of view and apparent field of view. **B** Direction and field of view

which will vary with their field of view and direction of view (Fig 12.2 Both rigid and flexible cystoscopes are used in current urological practic The advantages of the rigid cystoscope are that visualization is mu clearer and more magnified, and difficult manipulative procedures c easily be carried out through the large instrument channel. The disa vantage of a rigid cystoscope is that it usually requires either general spinal anesthesia and this had led to the widespread use of a flexib cystoscope for simple diagnosis. The flexible cystoscope is particula easy to use in the female bladder but one has to contend with the mc limited view and a relative inability to carry out manipulative procedur It is possible to take small mucosal biopsies with ease but more diffic procedures such as ureteric catheterization and tumour fulguration dema a significant amount of experience with a flexible cystoscope. Figure 1 shows a flexible cystoscopy in progress.

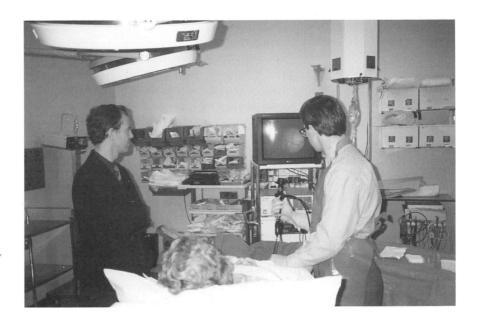

Fig. 12.3 A flexible cystoscopy in progress. Ideally, an endoscopic CCD allows both operator and patient to monitor the procedure. No anesthesia is required. A biopsy can easily be taken and even small tumors can be fulgurated through the cystoscope with minimal discomfort

RIGID CYSTOSCOPY

The rigid cystoscope is the definitive diagnostic and manipulative instrument for the urethra and bladder. It is such a versatile tool that Kelling in 1901 first used it as a laparoscope and it was also the first endoscope used for percutaneous intrarenal surgery by Wickham in 1982. Four commonly used angled view telescopes are used in this system. The 30° angled lens is used for more accurate, direct on-line work such as taking a biopsy, fulguration with diathermy and ureteric intubation with a catheter. The 70° angled lens is less commonly used now by urologists but it has always had the advantage of looking into more restricted corners of the bladder. In fact, a 120° backwards-looking lens was once a standard telescope. Many urologists are now working with a 12° lens for all cystourethroscopic procedures and this is ideal for the female urethra and will supersede the 0° telescope. The application of both the 70° and 120° telescope has been superseded by the advantageous diagnostic facility of the flexible, steerable cystoscope. Various optional add-ons to the cystoscope are available, including bridges, integrated cold cup biopsy forceps and an Albarran lever. The Albarran lever can more accurately guide a ureteric guide wire, catheter or diathermy probe on to a more exact point, but this will become obsolete when manufacturers start making integrated cystoscopes with smooth, straight-working channels.

An estimate of the residual urine can be gauged and a sample sent for culture. Cystoscopic examination of the bladder should take place in a systematic way so that no area is missed and should always include an inspection of the urethra, which is best carried out whilst withdrawing the instrument in a female. Start with the trigone and note the number, position and shape of the ureteric orifices. A chronically refluxing ureter will have a golf hole appearance. Reflux is sometimes seen during video-urodynamics and its relevance quite rightly questioned.

The normal cystoscopic appearance of a ureteric orifice that resembles a winking (a bolus of urine comes down 2–3 times each minute) 'Asian eye implies that no further investigations for reflux are usually required. An edematous trigone is commonly seen in females and whilst this is labelled trigonitis it usually only reflects subclinical concentrations of bacteria and in the absence of other cystoscopic abnormalities is not regarded as pathological. The bladder mucosae are then inspected in a clockwise fashion ending at 12 o'clock, where the normal air bubble is present in every bladder. Depress the dome of the bladder with one hand to move the bubble. A small tumor can sometimes lurk unnoticed behind it. If hematuria has been a presenting symptom then the clockwise inspection should be repeated with a 70° telescope.

During the cystoscopy, the bladder will have been filled with saline or water. Water can safely be used for diagnostic cystoscopy but must be replaced by a non-ionic solution such as glycine if diathermy is to be used. Diathermy will cause polarization within an ionic solution, with the production of numerous bubbles that impair visualization. Some centers do not even use sterile water and have as low morbidity with infections as anyone. However, where cost is not a significant issue, a fresh bag of sterile saline with a new giving set should ideally be used for each patient to maintain the highest levels of sterility when retrograde flow may have occurred. The normal bladder only holds 400–500 ml before over-stretching produces reactions that the anesthetist will identify before the surgeon. Therefore, run the irrigation fluid in slowly and once there is enough to hold the bladder open for close inspection, turn the irrigation off. This is usually at 150–200 ml. The irrigation will only be needed subsequently to wash the lens if a biopsy is taken. At the end of the procedure, re–insert the sheath and trocar to drain the bladder.

When a biopsy of an identified lesion or a randomly selected piece of mucosa is needed, try to stay away from the very sensitive trigone and remember that the dome of the bladder is probably intraperitoneal whilst dilated. The cold cup biopsy will not cause a problem but the subsequent fulguration with diathermy to the site of prevent hemorrhage may cause extravesical damage if not applied accurately and carefully. If a diagnosis of interstitial cystitis is suspected and a cystodilatation is contemplated remember to do this before the biopsy is taken. The bladder is thin and does not take much tension to produce a large tear.

Tears of the bladder with extravesical leaks can always be managed conservatively, when they are extraperitoneal, by prolonged catheterization (5–7 days). However, if an intraperitoneal leak is suspected and sometimes the peritoneal contents can be viewed through an iatrogenic bladder window then open repair is recommended. Rarely a peritoneal leak is missed but this should be suspected postoperatively when there are oliguria, non-obstructed kidneys on ultrasound, normal central venous pressure and a rising serum urea out of proportion to a slightly rising creatinine. In these cases, most of the urine is running into the peritoneal cavity and being reabsorbed. Prompt surgical exploration quickly resolves this but it is a clinical problem that is often allowed to go undiagnosed unsuspected.

Ureteric catheterization is a urogynecological maneuver often under used. In cases of recurrent urinary tract infections, hematuria or positive urine cytology where no bladder cause can be found then being able to identify at least which upper renal tract is the source helps the diagnostic process considerably. In these instances, a 7F ureteric catheter with an end hole should be slid up each ureter for approximately 10cm. They may have to be introduced over a guide wire (and the wire then removed). A diuresis is needed. The anesthetist should be asked to give 20 mg of intravenous frusemide together with an intravenous saline drip. The urine from each ureteric catheter can then be sampled.

FLEXIBLE CYSTOSCOPY

The fundamental principle of a flexible endoscope is the efficient transmission of light in one direction and an optical image in the opposite direction along precisely engineered bundles of optical fibers. Each of these fibers has an outer coating with a different refractory index from its core and so light is efficiently guided through each fiber with almost 100% of the photons bouncing back into the central 'stream'. The multifiber composition gives a cross-sectional appearance similar to an insect's eye and for this reason the visual acuity can never match that of a rigid rod-lens system. However, by increasing the number and quality of fibers, a good image is obtained and easily counterbalanced by the flexibility of the whole telescope. If there is a significant disadvantage to these flexible endoscopes in general it is their susceptibility to mishandling. Careful cleaning and storage is required to prevent fibers breaking. The life of a flexible telescope is probably only 20% of its rigid counterpart. Always have an up-to-date maintenance contract.

The flexible cystoscope has transformed our urological practice. The majority of cystoscopic procedures are diagnostic with perhaps a biopsy and this can now be done without fuss using only a topical anesthetic. Using two flexible cystoscopes, and sterilizing one (7 min) whilst using the other, it is not unreasonable for a surgeon to complete 8–10 procedures in one hour, and these can be done in out-patients.

As with rigid cystoscopy, a complete inspection of the bladder requires a systematic approach. The same clockwise steps are suggested with the added bonus that it is possible to look back on oneself at the bladder neck. In contrast to the case with standard rigid endoscopes, the image is magnified and the biopsies are much smaller. This latter fact, whilst sometimes frustrating the histopathologist, does mean that secondary diathermy fulguration is not usually required but adequate bites of detrusor muscle are not usually obtained. Ureteric catheterization is possible but only by the initial placement of a guidewire under flexible cystoscopic vision, removal of the cystoscope and subsequent railroading of a ureteric catheter over the guidewire. Because of the smaller working channel, irrigation is slower and does not allow drainage of residual urine.

If a flexible cystoscope is passed into a bladder full of urine then the view is a little murky. In these cases, the urine should be drained with a catheter and a washout given before reintroduction of the flexible cystoscope.

CONCLUSION

Although it is unusual to discover cystoscopic abnormalities in women who complain only of incontinence, it is important to undertake cysto urethroscopy in those individuals who present with mixed symptoms including urgency, frequency and dysuria, or those with recurrent urinary tract infections or voiding difficulties. The investigation may not always be helpful but in some cases will reveal the underlying pathology. A bladder biopsy may be useful in differentiating between follicular and interstitial cystitis and will therefore guide the clinician to the appropriate form of treatment.

Cystourethroscopy is an invasive but relatively low risk procedure which can be undertaken on women of any age as a day case. The choice between flexible or rigid instrumentation and local or general anesthesia will depend upon the needs of the individual and the equipment available. Repeat cystoscopies may be required in those patients in whom a bladder lesion has been identified and subsequently treated, in order to assess treatment efficacy.

REFERENCES

1 Bramble FJ. The clam cystoplasty. BJ Urol 1990; 66: 337–341.
2 Mundy AR, Stephenson TP. Clam ileocystoplasty for the treatment of refractory urge incontinence. BJ Urol 1985; 57: 641–646.

13

Electromyography and urethral electric conductance

The normal co-ordinated functions of the bladder and urethra are controlled by a complex set of central and peripheral neurological reflex mechanisms which are as yet not fully understood.[1,2] As a result of efforts to try and understand these mechanisms better a whole range of neurophysiological investigations has evolved, ranging from the very simple, such as quantitative electromyography of the pelvic floor with surface electrodes on the perianal skin or within the vagina, to the highly complex, such as electromagnetic stimulation of cortical centres to measure latencies to the urethral sphincter.

The more complex investigations give more accurate information as to the site of any neurological lesion but they require expensive equipment, tend to be more difficult to perform and are more invasive and unpleasant for the patient; moreover, the results need careful skilled interpretation. They should only be performed in specialist centres and their place in the clinical assessment of patients with lower urinary tract dysfunction remains uncertain.

One major problem in the use of neurophysiological techniques for investigating the lower urinary tract is that current techniques measure conduction in large myelinated nerve fibers and striated muscle, whilst the detrusor muscle of the bladder is a smooth muscle innervated largely by small, unmyelinated autonomic nerves. Consequently, the striated urethral and anal sphincters and the pelvic floor and their nerve supply are usually studied in isolation from the bladder, a fact which may reduce the validity of any conclusions and the clinical relevance of the results.

Electromyography (EMG) is the study of electrical potentials produced by the depolarization of muscle fibers. It is predominantly used to study striated muscle because the potentials produced are sodium-mediated and of relatively high amplitude and are thus relatively easy to record. Smooth muscle fibre activity is dependent on calcium ion exchange, which produces low current density. This can only be properly assessed using techniques involving intracellular microelectrodes.

The electrical activity of individual motor units is recorded as a motor unit action potential (MUAP), where a motor unit consists of the muscle fibers innervated by branches from the motor neurone of a single anterior horn cell. This motor unit activity can be recorded using surface electrodes which record quantitative data on muscle activity or by various types of needle electrode which record smaller areas of activity and may be used for qualitative assessment of innervation. The potentials are of small

Fig. 13.1 Electromyogram recording from urethral sphincter showing continuous activity at rest

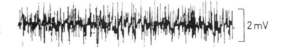

2 mV

amplitude (20–2000 MV) and are of brief duration (3–15 ms). The recorded signals therefore require amplification and filtering before they can be analyzed.

Normally, a stimulus has to be applied to the muscle in order to activate it, but the urethral sphincter shows continuous motor activity in order to maintain urethral pressure and urinary continence and thus does not require any form of stimulation before recordings can be obtained (Fig. 13.1). The muscle fibers responsible for this continuous activity are probably slow twitch Type 1 muscle fibers of which the urethral sphincter is predominantly composed.[3]

As urine collects within the bladder the urethral sphincter contracts with motor units firing at a rate of 2–8 Hz. During coughing or other provocative activity there is a marked increase in the amount of muscle activity, with an increased number of motor units in the firing pattern. This is called 'recruitment' and increases urethral occlusive forces and helps to maintain continence. These 'recruited' muscle fibers are probably the ones that are under voluntary control.

The onset of micturition is marked by inhibition of motor unit activity which results in a reduction in intraurethral pressure. Under normal circumstances this is followed, within a few seconds, by a detrusor contraction and the passage of urine. This co-ordination of urethral relaxation and detrusor contraction is essential for normal voiding and may be affected by upper motor neurone neurological diseases such as multiple sclerosis or spinal cord injury.[4] The resulting asynchronicity causes abnormal voiding and is called 'detrusor–sphincter dyssynergia'.

TECHNIQUES

Surface electrodes

Surface electrodes have the advantage that they are relatively non-invasive and are thus well tolerated. They give quantitative information about muscle activity rather than data for qualitative analysis. They are useful in determining the timing of muscle activity either in relation to voiding or in relation to a stimulus applied at a distant site when measuring sensorimotor nerve latencies.

Bipolar surface electrodes are placed close to the muscle being studied and may thus be placed on the perianal skin or may take the form of anal plug electrodes (Fig. 13.2), sponge-mounted intravaginal electrodes (Fig. 13.3) or catheter-mounted intraurethral electrodes. The depolarizing potentials produced by muscle activity are recorded on EMG recording apparatus, having been amplified and filtered.

Their use has been compared to the use of needle pelvic floor/external sphincter EMG in adults[5] and to a catheter-mounted ring electrode or an anal plug electrode in children.[6] Both these studies show that correlation

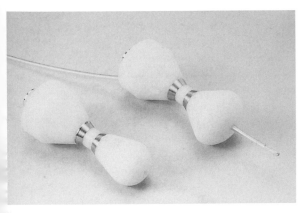

Fig. 13.2   Anal plug electrodes

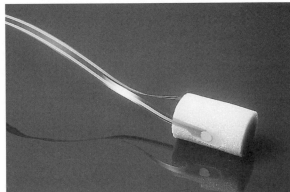

Fig. 13.3   Sponge-mounted intravaginal electrode

between the results of these different recording methods is good. They conclude that skin surface electrodes are painless, easy to use and well tolerated, and that the recordings obtained are reproducible.

Anal plug electrode

The anal plug electrode is an hour-glass shaped device which is inserted into the anus so that the two circumferential recording surfaces which are mounted on it are positioned in the region of the external anal sphincter (Fig. 13.2). It is apparently easy to use and insert but it is rather unpleasant for the patient and may cause artefact by producing a strong urge to defecate which may inhibit the micturition reflex. It has been a favoured test in the past, particularly as it was used in early studies of detrusor–sphincter dyssynergia.[7] One major disadvantage of the test, when used in the investigation of lower urinary tract function or dysfunction, is that the assumption that the anal sphincter and the pelvic floor and urethral sphincter act synchronously is not always correct. In particular, confusion may arise when there is a partial or unilateral neurological lesion or in multiple sclerosis.[8,9]

Vaginal electrodes

The use of disposable vaginal surface electrodes[5] was developed by Lose et al.[10] This technique involves placing into the vagina a box-shaped sponge plate on which are mounted two silver chloride surface electrodes. When positioned correctly, under auditory control, the electrodes are located on the anterior vaginal wall just below the mid-urethra. The slightly compressed sponge ensures good contact between the electrode and the recording surface. The advantage of the technique is that it monitors the urethral sphincter rather than the functionally distinct anal sphincter. The results of this technique have been compared with EMG recordings made using a periurethral coaxial needle electrode and have been found to give qualitatively similar results.[11] The vaginal electrode therefore offers a simple, reliable and well-tolerated technique for evaluating urethral sphincter activity during urodynamic studies in women.

Catheter-mounted electrodes

Experiments with catheter-mounted ring electrodes were performed in order to overcome the problem of possible dissociation of the urethral and anal sphincter in certain disease states. It is particulary useful in recording urethral sphincter activity and may thus be used in the study of motor latencies to this muscle.

The electrode consists of a thin cylinder which fits on to a Foley catheter. Wound on to the cylinder are two lengths of platinum wire separated by a distance of approximately 1 cm. These act as the two recording electrodes. The technique produces good results[12] but has two main disadvantages: first it is relatively invasive, and secondly, simultaneous flow studies cannot be performed while it is in situ.

Needle electrodes

Two main types of needle electrode are used in EMG. These are the concentric needle electrode (CN) and the single-fiber needle electrode (SF). These two techniques are quite different from each other and will be individually discussed.

Concentric needle electrode

Concentric needle electrodes consist of a hollow needle which serves as the reference electrode, and an insulated wire electrode mounted within it which serves as the active electrode.

The use of CN EMG was first reported in 1953 by Franksson & Petersen,[13] who published further data using this technique in 1955.[14] Most of the early studies performed using this technique concentrated on simultaneous CN EMG and cystometric recordings in order to study the timing of urethral sphincter relaxation.[4,15,16] They evaluated EMG of the urethral and anal sphincters during bladder filling, reflex EMG activity during voiding, and voluntary suppression of reflex EMG activity. These 'kinesiological' studies of normal and abnormal subjects showed that at rest minimal electrical activity is observed in the urethral and anal sphincters. With increased bladder filling there was a gradual increase in motor unit activity due to more motor units firing at an increased rate; this was found to be suppressed just before the onset of voiding when there was complete electrical silence. In subjects with upper motor neurone lesions they demonstrated an increase in the activity of the striated sphincter during voiding. Thus CN EMG was used primarily in the diagnosis of detrusor–sphincter dyssynergia and was mostly performed in subjects with a proven diagnosis of upper motor neurone disease.

The constant activity produced by tonic firing of motor units within the urethral sphincter is ideal for individual motor unit analysis and later studies have focused on the qualitative analysis of the recorded potentials with respect to their amplitude, duration and polyphasic pattern.[17] A number of patterns have now been recognized to be associated with different types of neurological lesion.

Complete lower motor neurone lesions such as those seen following radical pelvic surgery or damage to the sacral spinal cord initially cause complete electrical silence. After 12–21 days low-amplitude (50–100 microV) diphasic or triphasic potentials of short duration (0.5–2 ms) are seen. These are called 'fibrillations'. They are difficult to detect and i may be difficult to diagnose them with any certainty because when

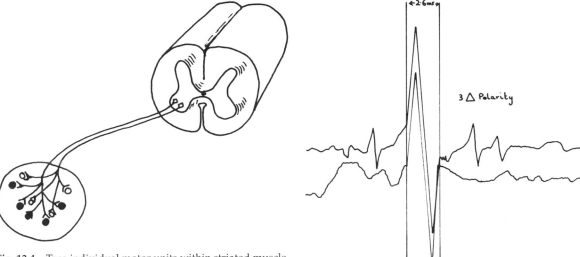

Fig. 13.4 Two individual motor units within striated muscle prior to partial dennervation

Fig. 13.5 Normal motor unit potential of short duration and with few changes in polarity. Two recordings are superimposed to identify the limits of the motor unit more clearly

sphincter activity is being studied the tonic activity of small motor units cannot be suppressed and complete electrical silence is not possible.

Partial lower motor neurone lesions, such as damage to the cauda equina and pelvic nerve, lead initially to a decrease in the number of motor units, which fire at higher frequency in order to maintain muscle strength. Those muscle fibers that have become denervated become reinnervated either by regrowth of the axon from the site of injury or by collateral reinnervation from the axons of adjacent motor units which have survived the partial lesion (Fig. 13.4 and 13.5). When this occurs a single axon comes to supply a greater number of muscle fibers and thus the MUAP becomes more complex, leading to a polyphasic electrical discharge when the motor unit is activated (Figs. 13.6 and 13.7). Initially, the new communicating axonal buds are unmyelinated and conduct slowly, thus prolonging the motor unit potential duration, but in time they become myelinated and their conduction velocity increases so that the motor unit potential duration decreases whilst the amplitude of the potential is increased. In summary, typical findings following partial denervation and reinnervation are a decreased number of rapidly firing, polyphasic, high-amplitude motor units of prolonged duration.[18]

Analysis of motor units from the urethral sphincter reveals a normal duration of less than 6 ms with no more than 5 turns of 100 microV or more amplitude, fewer than 5 phase reversals and an amplitude of between 0.15 and 0.5 mV. The amplitude is proportional to the size of the muscle fiber and is influenced by the distance between it and the recording electrode, and so is less commonly evaluated.

Another pattern that has been reported in women with urinary retention[19] and in women with neurological disease[20] is decelerating bursts and

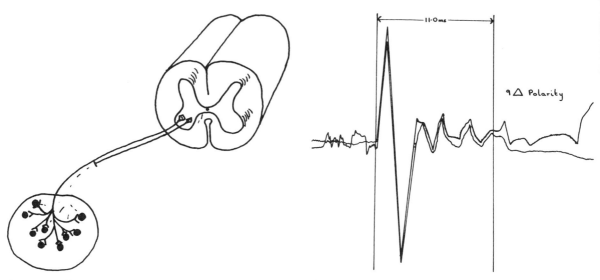

Fig. 13.6 Following partial denervation the remaining axons come to supply more muscle fibers leading to more complex motor units

Fig. 13.7 More complex motor unit potential following partial denervation and reinnervation

complex repetitive discharges, also known as pseudomyotonia. The meaning of these abnormal discharges is not clearly understood but they may be associated with impairment of urethral sphincter relaxation.

Single-fiber EMG

Single-fiber EMG uses a CN electrode with a recording surface of 25 Hm in diameter situated on the side of the electrode 3 mm from the tip. The diameter of the muscle around the SF needle from which recordings are obtained is therefore about one-third of that sampled using a CN electrode at 300 Hm. The electrodes are used to record the fiber density of the muscle under study. In a normally innervated muscle the muscle fibers of each motor unit are widely distributed so that it is unlikely that the SF electrode with its small recording diameter will pick up more than one or two muscle fibers of the same motor unit. This means that recorded potentials are usually monophasic or biphasic in nature. When reinnervation has occurred following nerve injury, the number of muscle fibers near the electrode which are innervated by the same neurone increases, and the potentials become polyphasic. If this sampling technique is carried out at 20 different sites within a given muscle, the fiber density of that muscle may be obtained. Single-fiber EMG is a useful technique for studying the anal sphincter;[21] however, it is difficult to apply this technique to the urethral sphincter because it is small and relatively inaccessible. Thus it is difficult to sample the muscle at different sites, and to date no sufficiently large studies have been reported.

Nerve conduction studies

A large number of different techniques have been employed to study the conduction of central and peripheral nervous pathways to the bladder and urethra. The principle behind these studies is that a neurological lesion in the pathway that is being tested causes a delay in conduction, and thus a prolonged latency between the stimulus and the muscular response. The techniques used vary in the type of stimulation that is used, the site at which this stimulus is given, the site at which the response is measured and the technique and equipment used for detecting it. They include studies of the sacral reflex arc, distal motor latencies of the pudendal and terminal motor nerves, spinal stimulation, cortical evoked responses and transcutaneous electrical or electromagnetic cerebral stimulation, and are listed as follows:

1. Sacral reflex arc
   a. Bulbocavernous reflex
   b. Anal reflex
   c. Urethral reflex
2. Distal motor latencies
   a. Pudendal
   b. Terminal motor
3. Spinal stimulation
4. Cortical evoked responses
5. Cerebral stimulation
   a. Electrical
   b. Electromagnetic

In addition the amplitude of the muscle response and the intensity of the stimulus required to produce it may be recorded to try and assess sensory and motor thresholds, but these values depend too much on the type of stimulation and recording techniques to be of much clinical value.

Sacral reflex arcs

The bulbocavernous reflex is used in the differential diagnosis of bladder problems as it provides a convenient method of assessing the integrity of S2 through to S4 and their afferent and efferent connections.[22,23] Classically the bulbocavernous reflex is evoked by manual compression of the glans penis or the clitoris and the reflex contraction is sought either by placing a finger in the anal canal or by palpation of the skin behind the scrotum in the midline to locate the bulbocavernous muscle.[24]

Alternatives to this technique involve electrical stimulation with recording of the latency of the response by measuring electrical activity of the urethral sphincter and urethral pressure changes.[25] Using this type of technique Bilkey et al,[26] in a large study of 108 normal subjects and 110 with neurological lesions, found that in normal women the mean latencies were 37.4 ± 5.5 s at the striated urethral sphincter and 38.6 ± 4.0 s at the external anal sphincter. The mean reflex latency was significantly shorter in women with upper motor neurone disease and was increased in patients with lower motor neurone disease.

The anal reflex is the dimpling of the anal skin produced by pricking the perianal skin. Latencies are now measured between electrical stimulation of the perianal skin and anal sphincter contraction, using CN electrodes, an anal plug or perianal surface electrodes to record electrical activity.[27,28] The neuronal control of this reflex is not as simple as would be expected. First there is a very early response at 2–8 ms, which is probably due to direct efferent nerve stimulation,[28,29] and secondly the longer normal latency of around 200 ms depends on the stimulus intensity and also tends to habituate, probably indicating that it is polysynaptic.[30]

The urethral reflex was described by Bradley et al.[31] The reflex response of the anal sphincter was recorded following urethral stimulation via a stimulating electrode mounted on an indwelling catheter. Similar work has also been performed by Galloway et al.[32] Although testing this reflex may be useful in the investigation of male impotence, the clinical use of this additional information in the assessment of lower urinary tract dysfunction is uncertain.

Distal motor latencies

Distal motor latencies, pudendal nerve conduction times and spinal stimulation are all used to study different parts of the motor pathway to the pelvic floor, anal sphincter and urethral sphincter. The latency of the motor nerves is studied by applying an electrical stimulus to different parts of the nerve supply, ranging from proximal spinal stimulation to distal pudendal nerve stimulation. In order to do this the electrical stimulus to the nerve is set to an intensity that will stimulate all the nerve fibers. The time taken for distant muscle to respond is recorded as the motor latency. Usually this response is measured using a CN electrode. The conduction time in the different parts of the motor pathway can be assessed and if the conduction distance between stimulation sites is measured then the conduction velocity of the nerve can be calculated:

$$\text{Conduction velocity (m/s)} = \frac{\text{Conduction distance (mm)}}{\text{Conduction time (ms)}}$$

Where: Conduction time = proximal – distal motor latency

A prolonged latency is used as a measure of denervation; however, what is assessed is the conduction of the fastest conducting fibers and not the integrity of the nerve as a whole. The latency is prolonged if all the fast-conducting fibers are damaged or when conduction in these nerves is slowed by a demyelinating process.

The pudendal and pelvic nerves lie deep within the pelvis so their conduction time is difficult to assess. Access can only be gained by insertion of long needles or by a technique devised by Kiff & Swash[33] whereby the pudendal nerve is stimulated using a rubber finger stall, on which are mounted two stimulating electrodes and two recording electrodes. The pudendal nerve is located by feeling for the ischial spine, and two series of five supramaximal stimuli (50 V square wave stimulus 0.1 ms duration) are applied via the stimulating electrode at the tip of the device. Recordings of anal sphincter activity are taken via the two recording electrodes at its base and the terminal motor latency of the pudendal nerve (PNTML) is calculated. Using this device the pudendal nerve may also be stimulated whilst measurements are taken from the urethral sphincter, using a CN electrode, to give the perineal terminal motor latency.[34]

Transcutaneous spinal stimulation

Transcutaneous spinal stimulation may also be applied directly to the spinal cord using a technique pioneered by Merton & Morton[35] and modified by Snooks & Swash.[34] They delivered a single impulse of 800–1000 V, decaying with a time of 50 ms through saline-soaked pads applied to the lumbar spine, whilst the urethral response was measured using an intraurethral surface electrode to give a spinal latency measurement of around 5 ms. By stimulating at different levels of the spine they were able to calculate spinal latency and a spinal latency index. No comment is made in their study as to how well the test was tolerated!

Cerebral stimulation

The integrity of central motor pathways to the urethral sphincter have also been studied using electrical and electromagnetic stimulation. Electrical stimulation involves placing electrodes on the vertex (anode) and just below the hairline (cathode). Thiry & Deltenre[36] studied 40 patients using this technique applying a 750-V discharge and recording the response in the urethral sphincter using a CN electrode. They found that the method could be used to assess the various segmental and suprasegmental influences on the behavior of the external urethral sphincter but that 'unfortunately the poor tolerance of the subjects to the scalp sensations caused by the electrical stimulus was a major limitation to its clinical use'.

More recently the use of electrical stimulation has been obviated by the introduction of facilitated transcranial stimulation of the cerebral cortex using a magnetic stimulator. This technique is easier to use and less painful.[37] The stimulus is applied using a magnetic neural stimulator which provides a maximum output of at least 1000 J. The latency to the urethral sphincter is about 29 ms and the central conduction time calculated by subtracting the spinal latency is around 18 ms.

PELVIC FLOOR AND URETHRAL INNERVATION AND INCONTINENCE

In 1980 Niell & Swash[21] demonstrated evidence of peripheral denervation of the striated anal sphincter in subjects with fecal incontinence. Since then a large number of studies have been performed investigating the role of denervation in fecal and urinary incontinence and prolapse and it is now accepted that it may have a role in the etiology of these conditions.

Koll and Swash[33] showed that the PNTML was increased in women with idiopathic (neurogenic) fecal incontinence and that the delayed conduction occurs distally and not at a spinal level. The outcome of this work was the hypothesis that damaged peripheral innervation might be the mechanism by which vaginal delivery caused incontinence and prolapse.

In order to investigate this Snooks et al[38] studied a group of women immediately following delivery and at 2 months post partum. They showed that PNTML was increased in the first 48–72 h following vaginal delivery (n = 57), but that this was no longer significant at 2 months following delivery when compared with a control group (n = 40). In this study only one woman had urinary incontinence following delivery but her PNTML measurements were normal both at 48 – 72 h and at 2 months, as was her anal sphincter fiber density.

In 1986 Snooks et al[39] concluded that vaginal delivery might cause damage to the pudendal nerves. Using SF EMG they demonstrated an increased fiber density of the anal sphincter when comparing results obtained before and after delivery (n = 51). They did not show any increase in the PNTML when controls were compared to primigravidae who had a normal delivery, but did find a significant increase in those primiparae who had a forceps delivery (n = 9) and those women who had a prolonged second stage (n = 10).

These studies prompted Allen et al[40] to perform a large study of nulliparous women (n = 96) to establish whether childbirth causes damage to the striated muscles and nerve supply of the pelvic floor. They found evidence of damage to the innervation of the pubococcygeus muscle following delivery. Perineal nerve terminal motor latency was not performed antenatally but results obtained in the immediate post partum period were within the normal range and no different from values obtained at 2-month follow-up. Thus they concluded that any damage to the pudendal nerve caused by the first vaginal delivery is too small to be detected by conduction time tests.

Gilpin et al[42] in a histochemical study of the anterior and posterior pubococcygeus muscle, showed significant differences in the structure and histochemistry of the posterior pubococcygeus in women with stress incontinence and prolapse (n = 16) when compared with normal controls (n = 11), but did not find similar differences in the anterior pubococcygeus muscle.

Smith et al,[42] using SF EMG of the pubococcygeus, found that the fiber density was increased in parous compared to nulliparous women and in women with stress incontinence compared to normal parous women. They found no difference in the fiber density of stress incontinent women with prolapse compared to those with prolapse alone. Observations that fiber density of the pelvic floor is increased in women with genuine stress incontinence show that there has been substantial reinnervation, which might be considered to be a favorable rather than an unfavorable outcome with regard to muscle function. In a further study by the same authors,[43] the perineal nerve terminal motor latencies to the urethral sphincter and the PNTML to the anal sphincter were studied. Women with stress incontinence of urine with or without prolapse had a significantly prolonged perineal nerve terminal motor latency compared with women with normal urinary control.

In the only long-term study performed to date, Snooks et al[44] studied 14 of 24 women who had been recruited into a 5-year follow-up study of the effect of childbirth on the pelvic floor. In this study only the innervation to the anal sphincter was assessed using SF EMG and PNTML. They found that both of these were significantly altered and also that there was a reduction in the anal maximum squeeze pressure. They concluded that denervation of the pelvic musculature is the major etiological factor in the pathogenesis of stress incontinence of urine and feces.

From these studies it would seem that peripheral nerve damage may be implicated in the etiology of genuine stress incontinence and that this may be related to childbirth, but in most of the studies urodynamics had not been performed and the diagnosis of genuine stress incontinence was based on symptoms alone. Conclusions about urethral sphincter innervation made on the basis of measurements taken from the functionally and anatomically distinct, but conveniently placed, anal sphincter or pubococcygeus muscle must also be treated with caution, as this may lead to erroneous impressions of urethral innervation.[17] In addition, none of the authors have attempted to correlate innervation and pelvic floor or urethral function, so that whilst innervation as measured is altered, this may not reflect a change in function. For example, nerve conduction studies have certain shortcomings in that what is recorded is the conduction time of the fastest transmitting nerve fibers. Damage to the rest of the innervation of that muscle cannot be assessed. Thus changes in nerve conduction times may not relate to changes in the function of the muscle studied.

Studies of the EMG–force relationship of skeletal muscles show that it is dependent on the firing rate and the recruitment control strategy used by a muscle. Muscles that use motor unit recruitment to obtain the initial 50% of their maximum force and use firing rate increase to complement the remaining 50% have a nearly linear EMG–force relationship. Muscles that use recruitment to obtain 60% and up to 100% of their maximal force demonstrate progressive increase in non-linearity of their EMG–force curves.[45,46] The recruitment control strategy of the urethral sphincter has not been adequately documented.

In two studies where urodynamics have been performed to confirm genuine stress incontinence, the anal sphincter showed evidence of partial denervation in women with genuine stress incontinence, prolapse or both, and there was a significant increase in the conduction time to the urethral sphincter in women with genuine stress incontinence with or without prolapse when compared with controls.[41] Work performed in our own unit[47] showed no statistically significant difference in urethral sphincter EMG parameters when women with urodynamically proven genuine stress incontinence (n = 33) and a continent control group (n = 35) were compared. Our findings suggested that denervation and reinnervation of the striated urethral sphincter is not a major etiological factor in the development of genuine stress incontinence. In a further study[48] we aimed to investigate the relationship between innervation and function of the urethral sphincter. Comparing CN EMG and urethral pressure profile parameters in 36 women, we found a significant correlation between variables indicating denervation and reinnervation and variables indicating improved resting urethral function. No correlation was found between any of the measured EMG variables and urethral function during cough-induced stress.

The theory that pelvic floor function is not grossly affected by changes in innervation is supported by work on patients with hereditary motor sensory neuropathy in whom gross neurophysiological disturbances are recorded in the absence of stress incontinence of urine.[49]

The conclusion that altered innervation produced by the trauma of vaginal delivery is responsible for the later development of genuine stress incontinence may be incorrect, for although denervation has been shown to be caused by childbirth, and many women with genuine stress incontinence are parous, this does not imply a causal relationship between denervation and genuine stress incontinence.

Tapp et al[50] showed that women with genuine stress incontinence (n = 148) are not, as one might expect from the EMG data presented above, of higher parity than age-matched continent controls (n = 89). Using multiple regression analysis controlling for age, menopausal age and ponderal index they also found no difference between the two groups in the number of vaginal deliveries or birthweight of the heaviest baby. These data would seem to contradict the hypothesis that denervation caused by childbirth is a major etiological factor in the pathogenesis of genuine stress incontinence.

CONCLUSION

Clinical neurophysiology involves a complex collection of techniques for stimulating and recording neurological activity. By applying these techniques to different levels of the neurological pathways they can be more clearly understood, and neurological lesions may be accurately identified. It has important applications in the investigation of lower urinary tract dysfunction, the exact etiology of which often remains elusive, and in which co-ordinated reflex neurological activity is vital. The techniques are, however, usually invasive and unpleasant, and whilst they improve our understanding of the etiology of lower urinary tract dysfunction, the results obtained to date have had little effect on clinical management. For despite considerable research into the role of altered innervation of the pelvic floor and urethral sphincter in the etiology of genuine stress incontinence, there is still some controversy over its importance. This is due partly to the difference in techniques used in these various studies and partly to assumptions about urethral innervation based on data obtained from the pubococcygeus muscle or the anal sphincter.

URETHRAL ELECTRIC CONDUCTANCE

In urethral electric conductance (UEC) tests, a 7F flexible silicone probe is inserted into the urethra. Mounted on it are two gold-plated, 1-mm wide brass ring electrodes separated by 1mm. Two lengths of probe are used: a 'short' 50-mm and a 'long' 250-mm probe (Fig. 13.8).

The electric conductance of urothelium is considerably lower than that of urine or saline, therefore the amplitude of a weak current passed between the two electrodes will change as urine enters the urethra.[50] This is recorded as the conductivity of the urethra and can be used to identify bladder neck opening and also entry of fluid into the distal urethra.

By withdrawing the device through the urethra at rest and during coughing, resting and stress, urethral conductance profiles may be obtained.[51] This allows for accurate determination of the region of the bladder neck and can be used to assess bladder neck opening and involuntary urine loss along the whole length of the urethra, and gives similar information to the stress urethral pressure profilometry.[52] It has been used in conjunction with urethral pressure profilometry to compare

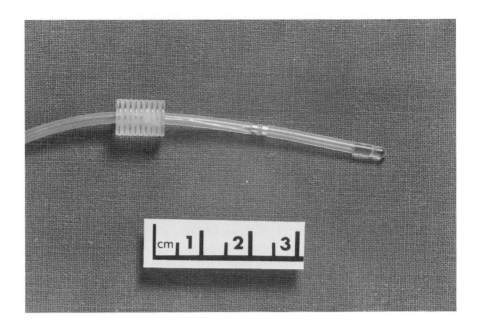

Fig. 13.8 Distal urethral conductance recording electrode

distal urethral electric conductance (DUEC) and urethral pressure profilometry measurements accurately.[53]

More commonly, UEC is combined with provocative cystometry. The 'short' catheter is usually used for this as it is relatively fixed in position external to the urethral sphincter. In the normal young female the detrusor is stable on cystometry; there are negative UEC deflections during coughing, indicating closure of the internal urethral meatus (IUM); and the urethra remains closed during provocation. However, in 55% of normal women aged 30–50 years, coughing increases the conductance at the IUM and the proximal urethra indicating bladder neck opening and fluid entry into these parts of the urethra. The remaining part of the urethra stays closed.[54,55] In women with genuine stress incontinence or detrusor instability, or a mixture of the two, different patterns of UEC and cys-

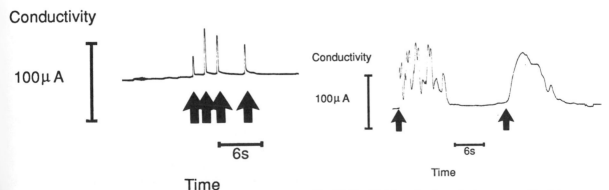

Fig. 13.9 Distal urethral conductance record in genuine stress incontinence. The arrows represent coughs

Fig. 13.10 Distal urethral conductance record in detrusor instability. Note the urine loss between coughs leading to increased conductivity

tometry traces are recorded, which apparently improve diagnostic accuracy over cystometry alone[56] (Figs. 13.9 and 13.10).

In distal urethral electrical conductance (DUEC), the 'short' probe is used. It has a collar on it to fix it in place, which allows for standard placement of the electrodes 15 mm from the external urethral meatus and distal to the zone of maximum urethral pressure. It has been used per se to demonstrate incontinence. Holmes et al,[57] using visual examination and a pad test, compared to DUEC, demonstrated incontinence in 39% and 44% of patients respectively. The sensitivity of the test has been compared with the International Continence Society's 1 h pad test and found to be positive in 96% of those women in whom the pad test was also positive.[58] However, it must be remembered that the reproducibility of the pad test used in this study is poor.

Two main DUEC patterns have been identified which have been used to distinguish between genuine stress incontinence and detrusor instability. Peattie et al[59] found that a reliable diagnosis could be made in this way and also found that the DUEC had a significantly higher pick-up of abnormalities compared with conventional cystometry. They concluded that DUEC diagnosis of genuine stress incontinence or detrusor instability is sufficient if patients are considered for conservative treatment, and it has subsequently been suggested that DUEC is a useful screening test in the investigation of female incontinence.[60]

One further proposed role for this technique is that is may be useful as an intraoperative tool in the surgical management of genuine stress incontinence. Janez & Plevnik,[67] in an uncontrolled study of 50 women with urodynamically proven genuine stress incontinence, found that perioperative use of the UEC during the Stamey procedure allowed for accurate placement of elevating sutures, and restoration of urethral competence at minimum elevation of the sutures, factors which they felt were important in achieving the high (86%) cure rate that was found in their study.

However, despite the fairly extensive research that has been performed using this technique, it has failed to gain widespread popularity as a routine test.

REFERENCES

1 Bradley WE, Rockswold GL, Timm GW, Scott FB. Neurology of micturition. J Urol 1976; 115: 481–486.
2 Mahoney DT, Laferte RO, Blais DJ. Integral storage and voiding reflexes. Urology 9: 95–106.
3 Gosling JA, Dixon JS. Light and electron microscopic observations on the human external urethral sphincter. J Anat 1981; 129: 216 (Abstract).
4 Blaivas JG, Sinha HP, Zayed AH, Labib KB. Detrusor-external sphincter dyssynergia: a detailed electromyographic study. J Urol 1981; 125: 545–548.
5 Maizels M, Firlit C. Paediatric urodynamics: a clinical comparison of surface versus needle pelvic floor/external sphincter electromyography. J Urol 1979; 122: 518–522.
6 Nielsen KK, Kristensen ES, Qvist N et al A comparative study of various electrodes in electromyography of the striated urethral and anal sphincter in children. Br J Urol 1985; 57: 557–559.
7 Anderson JT, Bradley WE. The syndrome of detrusor-sphincter dyssynergia. J Urol 1976; 116: 493–495.

8 Vereecken RL, Verduyn H. The electrical activity of the paraurethral and perineal muscles in normal and pathological conditions. Br J Urol 1970; 42: 457–463.

9 Nordling J, Meyhoff HH. Dissociation of urethral and anal sphincter activity in neurogenic bladder dysfunction. J Urol 1979; 122: 352–356.

10 Lose G, Andersen JT, Kirstensen JK. Disposable vaginal surface electrode for urethral sphincter electromyography. Br J Urol 1987; 59: 408–413.

11 Lose G, Tanko A, Colsturp H, Andersen JT. Urethral sphincter electromyography with surface electrodes: a comparison with sphincter electromyography recorded via periurethral coaxial, anal sphincter needle and perianal surface electrodes. J Urol 1985; 133: 815–818.

12 Nordling J, Meyhoff HH, Walter S, Anderson JT. Urethral EMG using a new ring electrode. J Urol 1978; 120: 571–573.

13 Franksson C, Petersen I. Electromyographic recording from the normal human urinary bladder, internal urethral sphincter and ureter. Acta Physo Scand 1953; 29 (suppl 106): 150–156.

14 Franksson C, Petersen I. Electromyographic investigation of disturbances in the striated urethral sphincter. Br J Urol 1955; 27: 154–161.

15 Blaivas JG, Labib KL, Bauer SB, Retik AB. A new approach to electromyography of the external urethral sphincter. J Urol 1977; 117: 773–777.

16 Mayo ME. The value of sphincter electromyography in urodynamics. J Urol 1979; 122: 357–360.

17 Di Benedetto M, Yalla SV. Electrodiagnosis of striated urethral sphincter dysfunction. J Urol 1979; 122: 361–365.

18 Fowler CJ, Kirby RS, Harrison MJG, Milroy EJG, Turner-Warwick R. Individual motor unit analysis in the diagnosis of disorders of urethral sphincter innervation. J Neurol Neurosurg Psych 1984; 47: 637–641.

19 Fowler CJ, Kirby RS. Electromyography of the urethral sphincter in women with urinary retention. Lancet 1986; 2: 1455–1456.

20 Potenzoni D, Juvarra G, Bettoni L, Stagni G. Pseudomyotonia of the striated urethral sphincter. J Urol 1983; 130: 512–513.

21 Niell ME, Swash M. Increased motor unit fibre density in the external anal sphincter muscle in ano-rectal incontinence: a single fibre EMG study. J Neurol Neurosurg Psychiatry 1980; 43: 343–347.

22 Lapides J, Bobbitt JM. Diagnostic value of bulbocavernosus reflex. JAMA 1986; 162: 971–972.

23 Hart BL. Bulbocavernosus reflex in the paraplegic and intact dog. J Urol 1966; 95: 384–386.

24 Bors EJ. Neurogenic bladder. Urol Surv 1957; 7: 177–185.

25 Yalla SV, Di Benedetto M, Blunt KJ, Sethi JM, Fam BA. Urethral striated sphincter responses to electrobulbocavernosus stimulation. J Urol 1977; 119: 406–409.

26 Bilkey J, Awad EA, Smith AD. Clinical application of sacral reflex latency. J Urol 1983; 129: 1187–1189.

27 Pedersen E, Harving H, Klemar B, Torring B. Human anal reflexes. J Neurol Neurosurg Psych 1978; 41: 813–818.

28 Henry M, Swash M. Assessment of pelvic floor disorders and incontinence by electrophysiological recording of the anal reflex. Lancet 1978; 1: 1290–1291.

29 Pedersen E, Klemar B, Shroder HD, Torring B. Anal sphincter responses after perianal electrical stimulation. J Neurol Neurosurg Psych 1982; 45: 770–773.

30 Voducek DB, Janko M, Lokar J. Direct and reflex responses in perineal muscles on electrical stimulation. J Neurol Neurosurg Psych 1983; 46: 67–71.

31 Bradley WE, Brantley-Scott F, Timm GW. Sphincter electromyelography. Urol Clin North Am 1974; 1(1): 69–80.

32 Galloway NTM, Chisholm GD, McInnes A. Patterns and significance of the sacral evoked response (the neurologist's knee jerk). Br J Urol 1985; 57: 145–147.

33 Kiff ES, Swash M. Slowed conduction in the pudendal nerves in idopathic (neurogenic) faecal incontinence. Br J Surg 1984; 71: 614–616.

34 Snooks SJ, Swash M. Perineal nerve and transcutaneous spinal stimulation: new methods for investigation of the urethral striated sphincter musculature. Br J Urol 1984; 56: 406–409.

35 Merton PA, Morton HB. Stimulation of the cerebral cortex in the intact human subject. Nature 1980; 285: 227–231.

36 Thiry AJ, Deltenre PF. Neurophysiological assessment of the central motor pathway to the external urethral sphincter in man. Br J Urol 1989; 63: 515–519.

37 Eardley I, Nagendran K, Kirby RS, Fowler CJ. A new technique for assessing the efferent innervation of the human striated urethral sphincter. J Urol 1990; 144: 948–951.

38 Snooks SJ, Swash M, Setchell M, Henry MM. Injury to innervation of pelvic floor sphincter musculature in childbirth. Lancet 1984; 2: 546–550.

39 Snooks SJ, Swash M, Henry MM, Setchell M. Risk factors in childbirth causing damage to the pelvic floor innervation. Int J Colorect Dis. 1986; 1: 20–24.

40 Allen RE, Hosker GL, Smith ARB, Warrell DW. Pelvic floor damage and childbirth: a neurophysiological study. Br J Obstet Gynaecol 1990; 97: 770–779.

41 Gilpin SA, Gosling JA, Smith ARB, Warrell DW. The pathogenesis of genitourinary prolapse and stress incontinence of urine. A histological and histochemical study. Br J Obstet Gynaecol 1989; 96: 15–23.

42 Smith ARB, Hosker GL, Warrell DW. The role of partial denervation of the pelvic floor in the aetiology of genitourinary prolapse and stress incontinence of urine. A neurophysiological study. Br J Obstet Gynaecol 1989a; 96: 24–28.

43 Smith ARB, Hosker GL, Warrell DW. The role of pudendal nerve damage in the aetiology of genuine stress incontinence. Br J Obstet Gynaecol 1989b; 96: 29–32.

44 Snooks SJ, Swash M, Mathers SE, Henry MM. Effect of vaginal delivery on the pelvic floor: a five year follow-up. Br J Surg 1990; 77: 1358–1360.

45 Solomonow M, Baratta R, Zhou BH, Shoji H, D'Ambrosia R. Historical update and new developments on the EMG-force relationships of skeletal muscles. Orthopaedics 1986; 9: 1541–1543.

46 Solomonow M, Baratta R, Shoji H, D'Ambrosia R. The EMG-force relationships of skeletal muscle; dependency on contraction rate and motor units control strategy. Electromyogr Clin Neurophysiol 1990; 30: 141–152.

47 Barnick CGW, Cardozo LD. Denervation and reinnervation of the urethral sphincter in the aetiology of genuine stress incontinence: an electromyographic study. Br J Obstet Gynaecol 1993a; 100: 750–753.

48 Barnick CGW, Cardozo LD. A comparison of bioelectrical and mechanical activity of the female urethra. Br J Obstet Gynaecol 1993b; 100: 754–757.

49 Voducek DB, Zidar J. Pudendal nerve involvement in patients with hereditary motor sensory neuropathy. Acta Neurol Scand 1987; 76: 457–460.

50 Tapp A, Cardozo LD, Versi E, Montgomery J, Studd J. The effect of vaginal delivery on the urethral sphincter. Br J Obstet Gynaecol 1988; 95: 142–146.

50 Plevnik S, Vrtacnik P, Janez J. Detection of fluid entry into the urethra by electrical impedence measurement: electric fluid bridge test. Clin Phys Physiol Meas 1983; 4: 309–313.

51 Plevnik S, Holmes DM, Janez J, Mundy AR, Vrtacnik P. Urethral electric conductance (UEC)- a new parameter for evaluation of urethral and bladder function: methodology of the assessment of its clinical potential. Proc Int Cont Soc London, 1985; 15: 90–91.

52 Asmussen M, Ulmsten U. Simultaneous urethrocystometry with a new technique. Scand J Urol Nephrol 10: 7–11.

53 Plevnik S, Janez J, Vrtacnik P. Superimposition of urethral closure pressure profiles using urethral conduction measurements. Neurourol Urodyn 1985; 4: 129–134.

54 Janez J, Plevnik S, Trsinar B, Mihelic M. Bladder neck and urethral behaviour during stress in continent female: an age stratified study. Proc Int Cont Soc Boston, 1986; 16: 433–434.

55 Janez J, Plevnik S, Vrtacnik P. Assessment of bladder neck mechanism during coughing by urethral electric conductance measurement: UEC-metry. Neurourol Urodynam 1987; 3: 179–180.

56 Holmes DM, Plevnik S, Stanton SL. Bladder neck electrical conductance activity in female urinary urgency and urge incontinence. BJ Obstet Gynaecol 1989; 96: 816–820.

57 Holmes DM, Plevnik S, Stanton SL. Distal urethral electric conductance (DUEC) test for the detection of urinary leakage. Proc Int Cont Soc London, 1985; 15: 94–95.

58 Mayne CJ, Hilton P. The distal urethral conductance test: standardisation of method and clinical reliability. Neurourol Urodyn 1988; 7: 55–60.

59 Peattie AB, Plevnik S, Stanton SL. Distal urethral electrical conductance: a screening test for female urinary incontinence? Neurol Urodyn 1988; 7: 173–174.

60 Creighton SM, Plevnik S, Stanton SL. Distal urethral electrical conductance (DUEC) - a preliminary assessment of its role as a quick screening test for incontinent women. BJ Obstet Gynaecol 1991; 98: 69–72.

61 Janez J, Plevnik S. UEC-controlled Stamey proceedure. Neurourol Urodynam 1989; 8: 338–339.

14 Radiology of the lower urinary tract

INTRODUCTION

Imaging of the lower urinary tract can be of great benefit in the management of women with lower urinary tract dysfunction. The modalities that are most useful are radiology and ultrasound, with much lesser roles for computerized tomography and magnetic resonance imaging. This chapter reviews the radiological procedures used for assessing the lower urinary tract. These range from plain films of the pelvis and abdomen to sophisticated realtime screening of the bladder and urethra combined with simultaneous pressure and flow recordings.

HISTORY

Uroradiology began in 1923 when Osborne and associates[1] noted that urine in the bladder was radio-opaque in patients treated with intravenous sodium iodide for syphilis. Two decades later, beadchains were used by Barnes[2] to determine urethral configuration radiographically. In 1949, Muellner[3] described the fluoroscopic assessment of bladder base morphology during coughing and noted the presence of funnelling of the bladder neck in some women. Jeffcoate & Roberts,[4] in 1952, reported the loss of the posterior urethrovesical angle in cystourethrography on women with stress incontinence. This gave rise to a theory on the pathogenesis of genuine stress incontinence which has only been discredited in recent years. Cineradiology of the lower urinary tract was introduced in the 1950s. The combination of this technique with pressure and flow studies was described and popularized by Bates and colleagues[5] in the 1970s and is essentially the same as the technique used in many units today.

PLAIN FILMS

A plain film of the abdomen can be used to screen for urinary calculi or as the first film in an intravenous urogram. It is sometimes referred to as a 'KUB examination' (kidneys, ureters and bladder). Many urinary calculi contain calcium and may be detected on a routine film (Figs. 14.1 and 14.2). Bony abnormalities of the pelvis may accompany developmental anomalies of the lower urinary tract and will be apparent on a plain film. For example, symphyseal separation may occur in association with

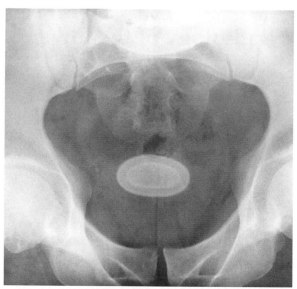

Fig. 14.1 Plain abdominal X-ray indicating a bladder calculus

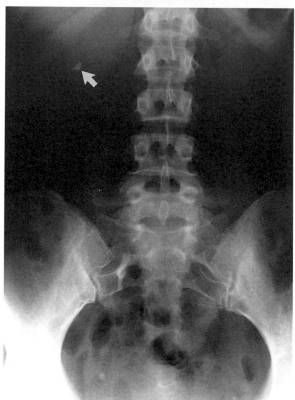

Fig. 14.2 Plain abdominal X-ray indicating a calculus in the (R) renal pelvis

epispadias or bladder exstrophy (Fig. 14.3) or myelomeningocele (Fig. 14.4). Acquired symphyseal separation may follow symphysiotomy or trauma. A plain abdominal X-ray may also reveal a foreign body in the bladder or urethra (Fig. 14.5).

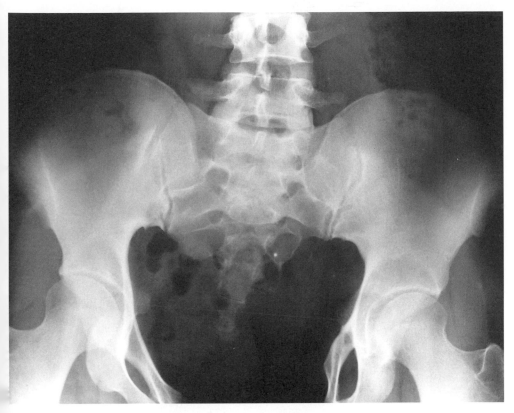

Fig. 14.3   Severe symphyseal separation in a woman with bladder exstrophy

INTRAVENOUS UROGRAPHY

This is one of the most frequently performed contrast-agent-enhanced procedures in diagnostic radiology. The technique has changed little over 40 years, although with newer contrast agents it is now safer and more comfortable for patients. Intravenous urograph (IVU) remains the primary modality for visualizing the kidneys, pelvicalyceal system and ureters and for assessing calculi and renal infection. Common indications are as follows:

- recurrent UTIs
- microscopic hematuria
- diagnosis of congenital abnormalities
- diagnosis of calculi
- diagnosis of bladder diverticula
- suspected urinary fistula
- preoperative assessment of large pelvic masses
- assessment of possible injury to urinary tract
- staging of gynecological malignancy.

It will be seen that these include assessment of women with recurrent urinary tract infections (UTIs) or hematuria, as well as the diagnosis of

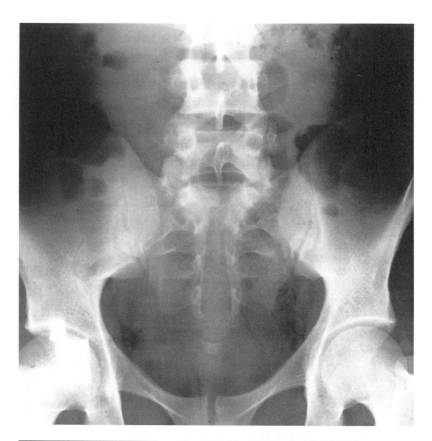

Fig. 14.4 Abnormality of bony pelvis associated with myelomeningocele

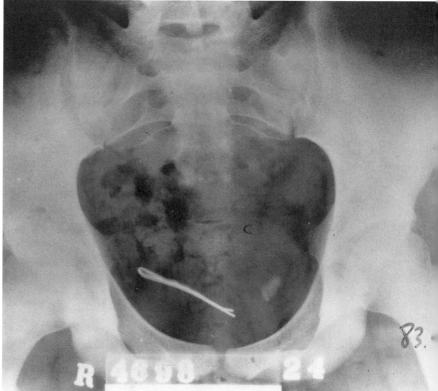

Fig. 14.5 Foreign body in bladder seen on plain X-ray of abdomen

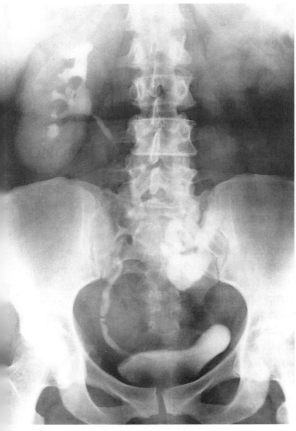

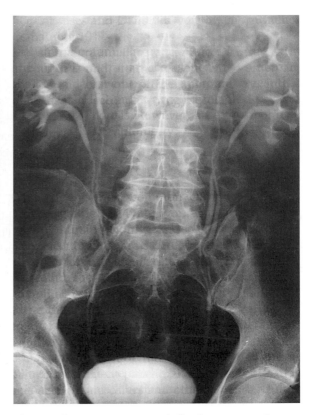

Fig. 14.7 Intravenous urogram indicating two ureteric systems on each side

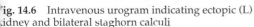

ig. 14.6 Intravenous urogram indicating ectopic (L) .idney and bilateral staghorn calculi

calculi and congenital anomalies of the urinary tract (Figs. 14.6 and 14.7). Operative damage to the urinary tract may present postoperatively with unilateral or bilateral loin tenderness or persistent fever and should be assessed by IVU.

The disadvantages of the IVU are the exposure of the patient to ionizing radiation, the possibility of adverse reaction to contrast agents and the potentially nephrotoxic effect of the contrast agents. The technique involves the rapid intravenous injection of an iodinated contrast agent (typically 300 mg iodine/kg bodyweight). An immediate film of the renal areas is obtained (nephrogram phase). More films of the renal areas are obtained at about 5 min to demonstrate the contrast-filled pelvicalyceal system (pyelogram phase). The ureters may be compressed by a tight band around the lower abdomen to provide better filling of the pelvis and calyces with contrast medium. At 10 min a full-length abdominal film is obtained to demonstrate ureters and bladder. A post-micturition film may be obtained to assess the residual volume of contrast agent in the bladder. Variations include tomograms when appropriate, administration of a diuretic to precipitate flow and demonstrate possible pelviureteric junction obstruction, prone films and delayed films to demonstrate the level of an obstruction.

CYSTOURETHROGRAPHY

This can be a useful study in the assessment of women with urinary symptoms. Cystourethrography will indicate the resting position of the urethrovesical junction in relation to the symphysis pubis as well as its downward and posterior movement with straining (Figs. 14.8 and 14.9). It is helpful in the diagnosis of urethral diverticula and tumors and stones of the lower urinary tract (Fig. 14.10). The selection of an appropriate contrast material is important, as some can irritate the bladder leading to artefactual findings.

Technique Following emptying of the bladder and insertion of a urethral catheter, the bladder is filled to capacity with contrast medium under low pressure. The catheter, filled with contrast medium, can be left in the urethra to indicate the urethrovesical junction. A modification, described by Stanton,[6] describes the introduction of a heavy barium paste into the bladder followed by a lighter radiopaque dye. The barium highlights the bladder base and urethrovesical junction, whereas the dye outlines the remainder of the bladder. Films are obtained in both supine and erect positions with the patient coughing and straining. The occurrence of incontinence is noted once the catheter is removed and films are also taken during and after voiding.

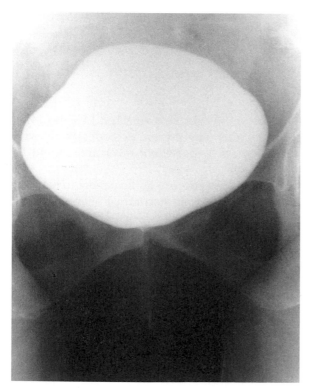

Fig. 14.8   Cystogram indicating position of bladder base at rest (compare with Fig 14.9)

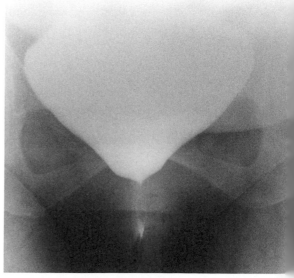

Fig. 14.9   Cystogram indicating descent of bladder base on straining as well as some loss of urine

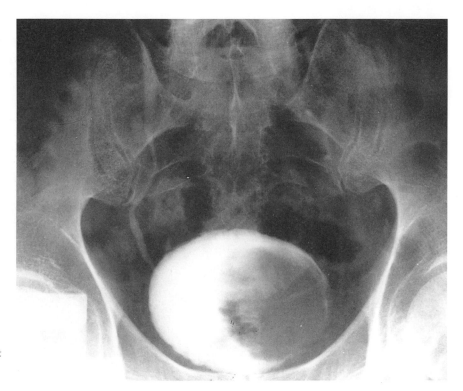

Fig. 14.10 Cystogram phase of an intravenous urogram indicating a large filling defect in the bladder from a transitional cell carcinoma

Normal anatomy of the urethrovesical junction is characterized by a well-supported position opposite the lower border of the symphysis pubis, absence of funneling and minimal descent with stress. The base of the bladder is usually flat in the supine position, but may be conical in appearance on standing. Loss of the posterior urethrovesical angle as described by Green[7] is no longer considered a valid concept in the pathophysiology of genuine stress incontinence. The bladder neck should be inspected at rest. It is open in some women and the incidence of this varies with the urodynamic diagnosis, being greatest in those with genuine stress incontinence.[8]

Cystourethrography can be of assistance in assessing the patient with neurological abnormality. An overactive bladder may appear as a 'pine tree' shape due to bladder wall hypertrophy (Fig. 14.11) or may be associated with urethral funneling. The poorly contracting hypotonic bladder will appear as a large, contrast-filled balloon, possibly containing calculi.

In all patients the voiding cystourethrogram is useful in diagnosing vesicoureteric reflux, which may be present in those women with recurrent urinary tract infections and pyelonephritis. Bladder diverticula are uncommon in women and are most often associated with outlet obstruction. They are best demonstrated in the oblique projection. Trabeculation of the bladder is also a sign of outlet obstruction or may be a result of chronic cystitis. It is manifest radiologically as an increase in internal foldings of the bladder mucosa. Bladder tumors, which are less

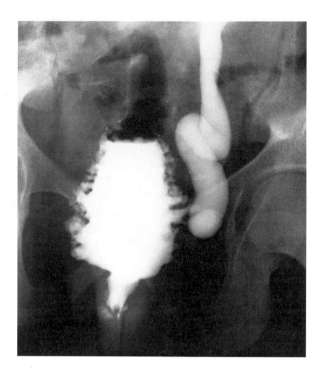

Fig. 14.11 Neurogenic bladder on cystogram indicating 'pine tree' shape of the bladder and (L) ureteric reflux

common in women than men, may appear as a filling defect or cystourethrography.

Vesicovaginal fistulae may be detected by noting passage of contrast agent from the bladder into the vagina (Fig. 14.12), although small fistulae are not easily seen. Urethral disorders, such as diverticulae and urethrovaginal fistulae, may also be detected by voiding cystourethrography.

VIDEOCYSTOURETHROGRAPHY

In this technique the lower urinary tract is screened radiologically while there is synchronous recording of bladder function by urodynamic techniques. Realtime visualization of the bladder and urethra is undertaken and can be stored on videotape for review at a later time. A coexisting image of the pressure tracings can be recorded on the videotape adjacent to that of the bladder morphology. Videocystourethrography (VCU) provides information regarding the morphology of the bladder, bladder neck and urethra. Urine loss can be demonstrated and residual urine estimated. Fistulae of the lower urinary tract and urethral diverticulae will usually be demonstrated by this technique. Videocystourethrography is generally regarded as the 'gold standard' of urodynamic investigations against which other techniques are compared.

Bladder function during VCU is assessed by double-channel cystometry which involves the continuous measurement of both intravesical and rectal pressures. The rectal pressure is an indicator of intra-abdominal pressure and the electronic subtraction of this value from the intravesical

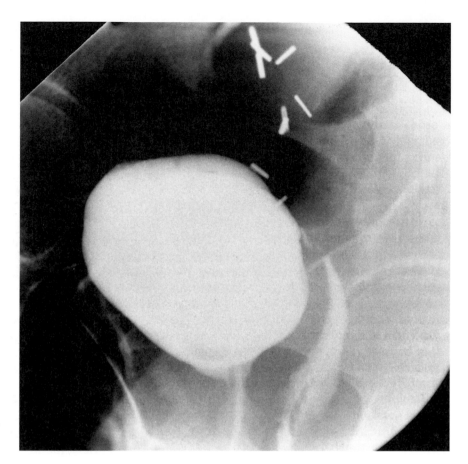

Fig. 14.12 Vesicovaginal fistula seen on cystogram in a woman who had recently had surgery for cervical malignancy

pressure will give the detrusor pressure, which is a true indicator of bladder function. Intravesical pressure is measured by a 1-mm fluid-filled catheter which is inserted at the same time as the filling catheter. Rectal pressure is determined by a 2-mm fluid-filled catheter inserted into the rectum, beyond the anal canal. Both catheters are connected to pressure transducers. Further information regarding this investigation is present in Ch. 9.

There is some controversy regarding the indications for VCU and whether it should be performed routinely or selectively. Some common indications are as follows:

- failed incontinence surgery
- complexity of case in tertiary referral center
- equivocal results after routine urodynamics studies
- neurological disease
- lower urinary tract dysfunction in children.

We have demonstrated that VCU does provide important additional information in a small group of women,[9] compared to cystometry alone, and not all of these additional diagnoses will be made using a selective VCU policy. Therefore, where facilities are available, and particularly in tertiary referral centers, routine VCU is the investigation of choice. Where radiological screening is not available, most women with lower urinary tract dysfunction can be investigated adequately by cystometry alone which will differentiate between genuine stress incontinence and detrusor instability. Some of the additional information gained by radiological screening may also be obtained by ultrasound examination and this may be worthwhile where radiological facilities are not available. The radiation exposure of VCU varies quite widely but is approximately 4 mSv for a typical examination. This is less than the exposure for an intravenous urogram.

ANTEROPOSTERIOR AND LATERAL FILMS

Whereas some information can be gained while screening the patient in the supine position, assessment of bladder base descent and incontinence is best performed in the erect position. Anteroposterior films are used to study mobility and position of the bladder base. In women without significant prolapse the bladder base does not usually descend below the level of the inferior border of the symphysis pubis on coughing and straining. Where a cystocele is present the bladder base usually descends below this level. In the anteroposterior view it is difficult to differentiate between descent of the bladder neck and the bladder base because of superimposition. There is a typical appearance of the bladder neck in the anteroposterior view following suprapubic incontinence surgery.

Lateral and oblique views are more appropriate to assessment of the position of the bladder neck and urethra at rest and on straining. They are also the most appropriate view for inspecting the urethra during voiding to exclude urethral diverticula or fistulae. In women with a large cystocele, it is not uncommon to see residual contrast agent in the 'sump' of the cystocele on the post-void film. This is an important finding as it may be related to symptoms of frequency and urgency or recurrent urinary tract infections.

POSITIVE PRESSURE URETHROGRAPHY

This technique is important in the diagnosis and management of urethral diverticula. The diagnosis of this condition is difficult and is often missed on physical examination and cystourethroscopy. The technique should be used in conjunction with a voiding cystourethrogram. Positive pressure urethrography was described by Davis & Cian[10] in 1956 to assess urethral anatomy. They filled the urethra with contrast agent using a double-balloon catheter. Urethral diverticula have been found much more often since the introduction of this technique.

CONTRAST MEDIA

The essential feature of contrast media is that they have a different coefficient of absorption of X-rays relative to the surrounding tissue

They are generally iodine-containing compounds. In recent years there has been the development of a new generation of 'low osmolality' agents which are significantly less toxic than the traditional ionic agents. In particular, the 'non-ionics' are much better tolerated. They have a reduced incidence and severity of subjective side effects as well as a lower incidence of major adverse reactions.

The incidence of severe reactions to ionic contrast media is approximately 1 in 1000 with a mortality rate, following intravascular injection, of 1 in 40 000.[10] With non-ionic contrast media the incidence of severe reactions is 1 in 25 000.[11,12] The frequency of these reactions is significantly higher in individuals with histories of asthma or hypersensitivity of some kind. Significant reactions may be characterized by the following features: alterations in blood pressure, bronchospasm, laryngospasm, cardiac arrhythmias, angio-edema, pulmonary edema, angina, loss of consciousness and convulsions. Patients with a history of reaction to contrast media in the past have a fourfold increase in risk of reacting to a subsequent injection. The reaction is usually not more severe than the original reaction. Women who have had a previous life-threatening reaction should be examined with caution although often have no reaction on re-examination. Pretreatment with steroids should be considered and substituting non-ionic contrast media for ionic media is probably worth the increased cost if the latter was previously used.[13] The risk of reaction when the contrast medium is instilled into the bladder, as opposed to intravenous injection, is probably considerably lower than the rates indicated above but should not be ignored.

When severe reactions occur the patient's airway should immediately be maintained and oxygen and subcutaneous adrenaline should be administered. Intravenous physiological fluids should be given and blood pressure and heart rate monitored. Appropriate fluid replacement alone has been reported to be an effective treatment for contrast-induced anaphylaxis[14] and is therefore of high priority.

REFERENCES

1 Osborne ED, Sutherland CG, Scholl AJ, Rowntree LG. Roentgenography of urinary tract during excretion of sodium iodide. JAMA 1923; 80: 368–373.
2 Barnes AC. The roentgenologic study of urethral sphincter strength in the female. J Urol 1942; 59: 1252.
3 Muellner SR. The etiology of stress incontinence. Surg Gynecol Obstet 1949; 88: 237.
4 Jeffcoate TN, Roberts H. Observations on stress incontinence of urine. Am J Obstet Gynecol 1952; 64: 721.
5 Bates CP, Whiteside CG, Turner-Warwick R. Synchronous cine/pressure/flow/ cystourethrography with special reference to stress and urge incontinence. Br J Urol 1970; 42: 714.
6 Stanton SL. Radiological techniques for evaluation of bladder and urethra. In: Ostergard DR. Gynecologic urology and urodynamics, 2nd edn. Baltimore: Williams and Wilkins, 1985.
7 Green TH. Development of a plan for the diagnosis and treatment of urinary stress incontinence. Am J Obstet Gynecol 1962; 83: 632.
8 Benness CJ, Cutner A, Cardozo LD. Bladder neck competence in women with lower urinary tract symptoms. Int Urogynecol J 1990; 1(3): 173.
9 Benness CJ, Barnick CG, Cardozo L. Is there a place for routine videocystourethrography in the assessment of lower urinary tract dysfunction? Neurourol Urodynam 1989; 8: 299–300.

10 Davis JH, Cian LG. Positive pressure urethrography: a new diagnostic method. J Urol 1956; 75: 753.
11 Katayama H, Yamaguchi K, Kozuka T, Takashima T, Seez P, Matsuma K. Adverse reactions to ionic and nonionic contrast media. Radiology 1990; 175: 616–618.
12 Ansell G. Adverse reactions to contrast agents: scope of problem. Invest Radiol 1970; 5: 374–384.
13 Benness GT, Fischer HW. Reactions to ionic and non-ionic contrast media. Radiology 1989; 170: 282.
14 Obeid Al, Johnson L, Potts J, Mookherjee S, Eich RH. Fluid therapy in severe systemic reaction to radiopaque dye. Ann Intern Med 1975; 83: 317–321.

15

Ultrasound and magnetic resonance imaging of the lower urinary tract

ULTRASOUND

Ultrasound has many advantages over other imaging techniques in that it is possible to visualize fluid-filled structures without the use of contrast. If pressure studies are not carried out catheterization is not necessary, and this eliminates the risk of urinary tract infection. Ultrasonography allows soft tissues to be seen, including the kidney, bladder wall, urethra and urethral sphincter. The main advantage with ultrasound is that there is no ionizing radiation used and this means that tests may be repeated as frequently as required. There is no risk to the patient or ultrasonographer from ionizing radiation, and urine within the bladder and urethra is clearly visualized. The installation and operating costs of ultrasound are significantly less than those of similar radiological equipment.

The main disadvantage of ultrasound is that the waves do not penetrate air and thus the probe always requires a coupling medium to image any structures. Also, the probe has a limited field of view and therefore only certain parts of the urinary tract can be visualized at one time, and until recently this was only possible in one plane. With the advent of three-dimensional ultrasound it is now possible to image a volume of tissue and review the image without the patient being present.[1,2] Orientations not usually possible and magnifications not used at the time of imaging can be produced. The disadvantage of this method of imaging is that it takes 4–5 s to scan the area of interest, so that for dynamic images a clear picture may not be seen. The ultrasound image itself depends on the echogenicity of the tissues rather than density, so tissues which have a high echogenicity appear white on the ultrasound image and those with a low echogenicity, and this includes structures which are fluid-filled, appear black. This is important when interpreting scans of soft tissues.

Due to the bony enclosure of the pelvic organs, ultrasound imaging is limited to the transabdominal, transvaginal, transrectal and perineal approaches. The images obtained do require experience to interpret and each approach has limitations and advantages. The type of probe and frequency of ultrasound wave (1–10 MHz) emitted determines what is seen and the quality of the ultrasound image obtained. Ideally, the higher the frequency the better the resolution of the imaged soft tissue structures, but unfortunately the increased frequencies have reduced depth of penetration due to attenuation.

The kidney

To image the kidneys the patient should be examined while lying supine. The right kidney is visualized through the liver, which acts as an acoustic window, and the left kidney can be visualized through the spleen if there is splenomegaly. Alternatively, a left posterior lateral approach with the patient being raised to 45° can be used to visualize the left kidney.

Measurements of the longest length can be made by rotating the probe; the accuracy is within 1 cm in 95% of patients[3] and for an accurate measurement of the kidney volume it is assumed to be an ellipsoid. Proper assessment of the entire kidney is done with the probe scanning in a transverse orientation and the probe can be moved from one side to the other to visualize the kidney adequately (Fig. 15.1).

The renal capsule is a well-defined hypoechoic structure. The inner edge of the renal parenchyma is not as well defined, as there are multiple echoes from the pelvicalyceal fat.[5] The parenchyma is relatively hypoechoic and with the medullary pyramids can be differentiated as hypoechoic oval areas adjacent to the pelvicalyceal system.[6] It is important to measure the parenchymal thickness, as a reduction may indicate scarring secondary to childhood pyelonephritis, reflux or infarcts. Sometimes the appearance of scarring may be imitated by fetal lobes which can persist into adulthood. This is easily differentiated as the indentations between the fetal lobes are always in between the renal medullary pyramids.[7] The cortical thickness can be measured, but the distance recorded is dependent on the angle and approach used as well as the size and age of the patient. To measure cortical thickness the distance from the capsule to the outer edge of the medullary pyramids is recorded. The parenchymal thickness is the measurement from the capsule to the outer edge of the pelvicalyceal fat echoes; is reproducible and correlates well with the intravenous urogram.[3]

The renal pelvis is usually filled with hyperechoic fat tissue; however, there is dilatation of the collecting system dark areas of fluid appear within the pelvis. Care must be taken in diagnosing dilatation as this may be seen if the bladder is full or if the patient is undergoing a diuresis.[8] To exclude obstruction a renal scan should be repeated after the patient has voided or when the patient is not having a significant diuresis. Ultrasound is sensitive at detecting dilatation but it cannot diagnose the degree of obstruction, a severe obstruction may only lead to mild pelvicalyceal dilatation.

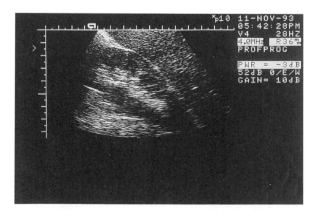

Fig. 15.1 Normal kidney with cortex and bright sinus echoes

Dilatation of the pelvicalyceal system should only be diagnosed when an enlarged rounded renal pelvis communicates with the calyces and these should obviously communicate with each other. In reporting the dilatation may be graded as mild, moderate or severe but this is really a qualitative description.[9,10] If there is marked obstructive dilatation the renal parenchyma may be thinned.[11,12]

During pregnancy the collecting system is often dilated and this can be seen as early as 12 weeks' gestation.[13] With increasing gestation the percentage of women with dilated collecting systems increases such that by 36 weeks over 60% of women have dilated pelvicalyceal systems.[13,14] There is more dilatation of the right kidney than the left and within 2 days of delivery these changes may disappear. Possible reasons why this occurs might be the enlarged uterus pressing on the ureters and the increased blood levels of progesterone, which causes smooth muscle relaxation and increased blood flow.[14]

Ultrasound is also useful for detecting abnormalities of the upper urinary tract such as duplex, ectopic or horseshoe kidneys.

The urethra and surrounding structures

The normal anatomy of the proximal urethra has been imaged transabdominally using small mechanical sector scanners. The initial attempts at viewing the urethral sphincter with ultrasound were transabdominal using 3.5-MHz probes.[15,16] This approach was not useful for imaging the size and dimensions of the sphincter as the distance between the ultrasound probe and the urethral sphincter was large, and there was reduced resolution due to the low ultrasound frequencies used. Without catheterization only 35% of urethral sphincters were visualized with this approach.[15] The introduction of a catheter into the urethra alters the position of the urethra relative to the symphysis pubis as well as the dimensions of the urethra and urethral sphincter. Hennigan & DuBose[17] described the normal anatomy of the female urethra using a 3.5-MHz transducer transabdominally. They described the urethral sphincter as having an anteroposterior diameter just inferior to the bladder of 1–1.5 cm and the transverse diameter was slightly larger. In the transverse plane the urethra and 'surrounding tissues' were described as an ovoid 'bull's-eye'. The sonographic texture was described as less echogenic than the surrounding connective tissue. Unfortunately, the subjects were not questioned about urinary symptoms, the only inclusion criterion being visualization of the urethra. Thus women were selected with a bias to those women with visualized urethral sphincters and as no data were collected about urinary symptomatology these dimensions cannot be considered as a normal reference range.

In a larger study[18] volunteers were scanned as well as women referred for pelvic masses. The urethral sphincter was imaged using the transabdominal approach and a 3.5-MHz transducer. Unfortunately, although the authors comment on urinary symptoms in the study group, they did not specify which women had symptoms. None of these women underwent urodynamics or any objective tests for urinary incontinence. There was no correlation between the urethral sphincter measurements and the degree of bladder filling. Age did not appear to affect the urethral sphincter measurements. The mean values reported by this group were 1.30 (±+0.36) cm longitudinally by 1.33 (±+0.43) cm transversely and 0.96 (±+0.32) cm anteroposteriorly.

The transrectal approach has been used to visualize the urethral sphincter in men and women to enable accurate placement of concentric needles for electromyography.[19,20] This approach was also used to measure the urethral sphincter in women with abnormal myotonic-like electromyographic activity.[21] These women have voiding dysfunction and urinary retention as the urethral sphincter does not relax during micturition.

Measurement of bladder volume

This is useful in the estimation of post-micturition residual urine volumes. There is no need for urethral catheterization and the concomitant risk of infection. It is particularly useful in the assessment of patients with voiding difficulties for whatever cause.

The transabdominal approach has traditionally been the method by which the organs of the pelvis have been visualized ultrasonically. The transonic window of a full bladder is required to visualize the pelvis, and this is the ideal method to measure bladder volume.[22–31] Bladder volume is measured by imaging the maximal cross-sectional area in sagittal and transverse planes of the fluid within the bladder. Measurements are made of the maximal anteroposterior diameter, transverse diameter and caudal–cranial diameter.

Various methods of calculating this volume have been proposed.[26] All of these calculations approximate the bladder to the volume of a sphere, so correction factors need to be applied. This reduces the inaccuracy to ± 20%. At low volumes the bladder approximates to an ovoid structure with the major axis in the transverse plane; at larger volumes the bladder is more spherical in shape as the dome of the bladder distends, the trigone remaining fixed and unchanged. Below 50 ml of volume transvaginal scanning has been proposed as a more accurate method of measurement;[32,33,34,35] however, at larger volumes it is certainly as inaccurate.[36]

In premenopausal women with recurrent urinary tract infections the diagnostic yield of investigations such as intravenous urography is low, altering management in fewer than 2% of cases.[37,38] Transabdominal ultrasound has been found to be more informative by demonstrating uterine and ovarian pathology as well as post-micturition residuals where urography has been unhelpful.[39]

Transabdominal ultrasound is useful for detecting bladder diverticula (Fig. 15.2). These diverticula may result from increased detrusor pressures due to detrusor instability or increased outflow resistance. Dynamic assessment of diverticula is important as expansion may occur with filling of the bladder and this may continue on micturition. This may reduce the efficiency of bladder emptying and result in a post-micturition urinary residual. Common complications of diverticula include calculi due to urinary stasis and transitional cell carcinoma in 5% of cases.[40] These can be excluded using ultrasound but it may not be technically possible

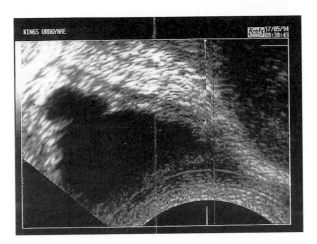

Fig. 15.2 Bladder with diverticulum. The contents of the diverticulum are easily imaged

on cystourethroscopy. Calculi can be differentiated from carcinomas as they produce an acoustic shadow and move if the patient alters position.

The majority of bladder cancers are exophytic and papillary in shape: this enables easy visualization on transabdominal ultrasound with a filled bladder. The major role of transabdominal ultrasound is in the surveillance of selected patients with resected bladder tumors and it has been proven to be successful over long periods of time.[41] Transabdominal and transrectal ultrasound have been used to replace flexible cystoscopy in the detection of recurrent bladder tumors: the majority of tumors were identified by both techniques. In view of the invasive nature of, and the morbidity associated with, flexible cystoscopy,[38,42] ultrasound may have a useful role in the follow-up of recurrent bladder tumors. Ultrasound was preferred by the majority of patients.[41] Ultrasound has been found to be the method of choice for imaging tumors of the trigone in women.[43]

Transvaginal ultrasound

Transvaginal ultrasound images the urethral anatomy and the relationships of the urethra with the urethrovesical junction. Attempts using the abdominal approach have not visualized the bladder neck clearly,[15,44] and markers such as Q-tips or pediatric feeding tubes have been used. Using the transvaginal approach the anatomy can be clearly visualized[45,46,47,48] (Fig. 15.3); the precise position of the urethra is seen as a hyperechoic area. The urethra can only be seen clearly after catheterization if frequencies less than 5 MHz are used. The vaginal probe can easily distort the urethrovesical anatomy by pressing on the urethra,[49] so results from this technique must be interpreted with care. The resting position of the bladder neck has been noted to be more caudal in women with stress incontinence than in continent women and during the valsalva maneuver the bladder neck has been noted to descend more than in healthy women.[46,47,48] Detrusor pressures are not measured during these procedures and detrusor instability cannot be reliably diagnosed. Involuntary opening of the bladder neck in the absence of an increase in abdominal pressure has been suggested to indicate the presence of detrusor instability.[45]

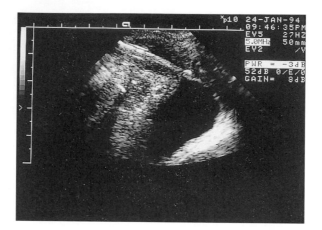

Fig. 15.3 Transvaginal ultrasound image of the urethra and bladder neck

Incontinence procedures for genuine stress incontinence have been assessed postoperatively using vaginal ultrasound. The Burch colposuspension has been found to increase the approximation of the bladder neck to the symphysis pubis and arrest the descent of the bladder neck during the valsalva maneuver.[47,48] The absence of these features was found in recurrent genuine stress incontinence. The Gittes and Stamey suspension procedures were also successful in arresting the descent of the bladder neck during the valsalva maneuver but approximation of the bladder neck with the symphysis pubis did not occur.[48] Failure of the suspension procedure after initial success was associated with a return of mobility of the bladder neck observed on ultrasound. Ultrasound may be useful in the assessment of the bladder neck after continence procedures.

The transvaginal ultrasound approach allows clear visualization of the urethra and urethral diverticula.[50] The position and contents of a diverticulum and ostium can be seen in relation to the urethra and the rhabdosphincter, making this the imaging modality of choice.[50] Bladder wall thickness of an empty bladder (less than 50 ml) can be measured transvaginally.[51] This is a reproducible sensitive method of screening for detrusor instability. A mean bladder wall thickness greater than 5 mm has a positive predictive value of 94% for the diagnosis of detrusor instability[52] (Fig. 15.4).

Three-dimensional transvaginal ultrasound has been used to measure the levator ani hiatus. This hiatus is significantly larger in women with vaginal wall prolapse than in asymptomatic women.[53]

Translabial ultrasound

The ultrasound probe is placed between the labia and the pelvis is imaged parasagittally. A view of the bladder neck, urethra and vagina, is obtained but the symphysis pubis, casts an acoustic shadow over the dome of a full bladder. The ultrasound waves are emitted parallel to the axis of the urethra, so that the longitudinal smooth muscle around the urethra is hypoechoic and appears echo-poor in comparison to the vaginal and transrectal approaches. The rhabdosphincter, however, is perpendicular to the ultrasound waves and appears echogenic (Fig. 15.5).

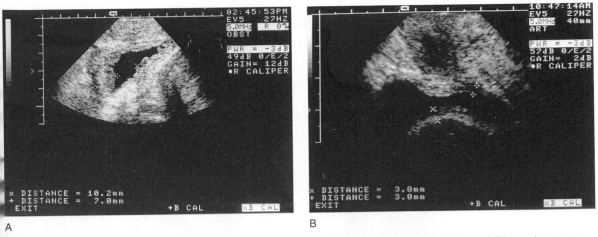

Fig. 15.4 Transvaginal bladder wall thickness of a woman with (**A**) diagnosed detrusor instability and (**B**) genuine stress incontinence

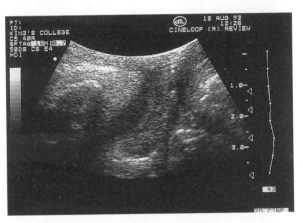

Fig. 15.5 Translabial sagittal section through the urethra and rhabdosphincter

Translabial ultrasound is the method of choice of imaging the rhabdo-sphincter.[1] This method of sonography does not impede movement of the bladder neck or vaginal prolapse.[54] It has been suggested as a replacement for radiological screening[55] and a chair has been designed for scanning during voiding. The probe is fixed in a steerable mount controlled at a distance.[56]

The volume of the urethral sphincter has been measured using the transperineal approach with both two-dimensional and three-dimensional ultrasound. Two-dimensional volume estimation of the urethral sphincter assumes the rhabdosphincter is an ellipsoid structure. The measured volumes do not discriminate between the different causes of urinary incontinence.[57] Three-dimensional ultrasound has been used to estimate the volume of the rhabdosphincter (Fig. 15.6); the volume of the sphincter in women with diagnosed genuine stress incontinence is significantly smaller than in women with detrusor instability. Unfortunately, the two groups are not sufficiently distinct to allow this to be diagnostically useful.[1]

The volume of the rhabdosphincter does correlate significantly with the area under the curve of the resting urethral pressure profile[51] (Fig. 15.7).

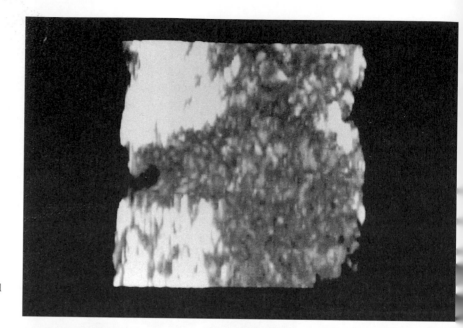

Fig. 15.6 Three-dimensional ultrasound reconstruction of the female urethra

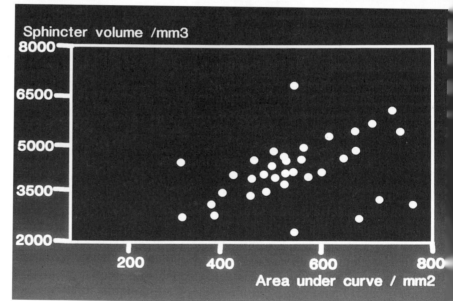

Fig. 15.7 Volume of the rhabdosphincter measured on three-dimensional ultrasound plotted against the area under the urethral pressure profile curve. They represent women who underwent vaginal repairs. These women have low rhabdosphincter volumes for relatively high area under the curves

Three-dimensional ultrasound allows images to be obtained from planes impossible to obtain by any other method (Fig. 15.8). The pelvic floor muscle has been measured using this approach and may have applications in the clinical setting.[58] The transperineal approach cannot be used in voiding or during stress situations as it inhibits micturition.

Transrectal ultrasound

In transrectal ultrasonography the probe is inserted with the woman in the left lateral position. Chairs have been developed such that the subject

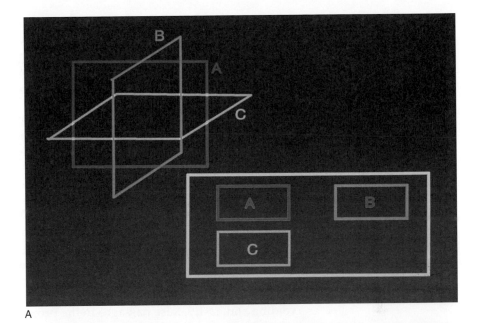

A

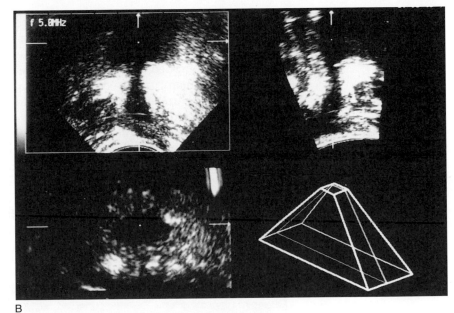

B

Fig. 15.8A Two-dimensional representation of a three-dimensional ultrasound scan. Three planes perpendicular to each other are shown A, B, C. **B** Ultrasound scan of a woman with genuine stress incontinence; plane C is an oblique plane cross-sectional through the urethra, but images the rhabdosphincter as a hyperechoic structure

may sit and void while the bladder neck is being scanned. As with all endosonography, acoustic coupling gel is put inside a condom which is used to protect the subject and the probe. The outside of the condom is also lubricated with gel prior to insertion. With the patient in this position a sagittal view of the bladder neck is obtained anteriorly. The bladder base, neck, urethra and symphysis pubis are visualized clearly. A good image may not be obtained if the rectum is full of flatus or feces. The probe can be used to measure post-void residuals and visualize movement of the bladder neck.[59] Occasionally, dilated ureters may be visualized, but although the ureteric urine jets can be visualized entering the bladder, vesicoureteric reflux cannot be diagnosed.

Transrectal ultrasound has been suggested as an alternative method of imaging during urodynamic studies and this has been compared with radiology.[60,61] The position of the probe in the rectum does not appear to alter the pressures measured during urodynamics; however, the woman may feel inhibited from voiding due to the probe's position.[62] Additionally, the probe may move if the patient has a significant degree of rectal prolapse and anterior vaginal wall prolapse may be moved by the rectal probe. In urological patients who do not have sensation in the anus and rectum, this method of visualization is useful. However, it should be borne in mind that sacral cord reflexes may still be intact and altered by the insertion of the probe. The bladder neck and proximal urethra have been visualized with transrectal ultrasound during voiding and this has been found to be an aid to diagnosis. The images are similar to those obtained during videocystourethrography,[60,63] and have been used to diagnose catheter-induced hyperreflexia, posterior ledge at the bladder neck during voiding and, lastly, false passages in the proximal urethra.[64,65,66]

Color Doppler imaging

Blood flow measurements within the bladder wall are reduced at bladder volumes greater than 30 ml, so it is extremely important to ensure that the bladder is emptied prior to imaging. Most women (90%) empty their bladders to less than 10 ml[33] so that catheterization is not usually necessary.

Color Doppler ureteric jets have been studied and the distance of the ureteric jet origin from the midline has been correlated with vesicoureteric reflux; the velocity and longitudinal angle have not been found to be useful to diagnose this[67] (Fig. 15.9). The velocity and frequency of the ureteric jets correlate with the state of hydration of the subject, both increasing with increased hydration.

The vascular supply to the trigone, bladder neck and terminal part of the ureter is from the inferior vesical artery. The fundus of the bladder is supplied by the superior vesical artery. Intramural bladder blood flow has been measured at the edge of the trigone where the ureters insert.

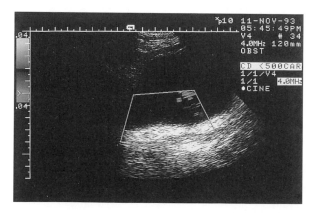

Fig. 15.9 Ureteric jet on color Doppler ultrasound

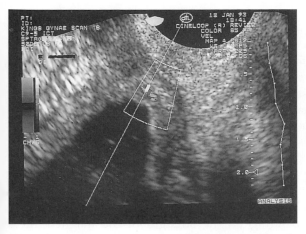

Fig. 15.10   Color Doppler blood flow within the bladder of a woman with detrusor instability

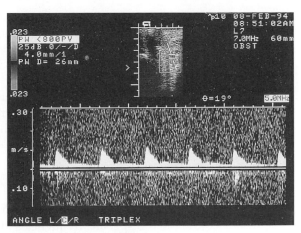

Fig. 15.11   Velocity waveform of the inferior vesical artery; note the notch after the systolic peak

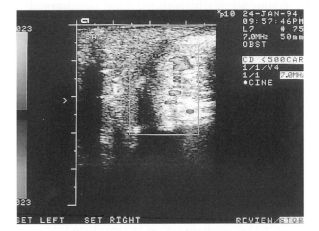

Fig. 15.12   Color Doppler blood flow of the inferior vesical arteries' branches supplying the urethra

This is easily identified by imaging the ureteric jets of urine entering the bladder on color Doppler ultrasound. Transvaginal color Doppler ultrasound can detect blood flow in the fundus of the bladder in women with detrusor instability and in young women (Fig. 15.10). In women with genuine stress incontinence blood flow is rarely seen in the fundus. Intramural blood flow in normal asymptomatic women and women with urodynamically diagnosed genuine stress incontinence and detrusor instability all show little change with age.[68,69] The inferior vesical artery can be visualized using the transperineal approach; the velocity waveform has a characteristic notch[70] (Fig. 15.11). In young women a large periurethral vascular plexus can be seen, which is fed by two lateral vessels[71] (Fig. 15.12). Women with genuine stress incontinence have lower peak and mean velocities and pulsatility indices than women with detrusor instability.[68] The reduced blood flow to the bladder neck in women with genuine stress incontinence falls further with increasing age and there is a negative correlation with age. This has important implications for medical treatment of genuine stress incontinence, as estrogens are thought to act by increasing urethral blood flow. Thus blood flow measurement may predict those likely to benefit from estrogen treatment.

Conclusion

Ultrasound offers a useful method by which the bladder, urethra and surrounding tissues may be studied and measured. This additional information may help clinical assessment and treatment.

MAGNETIC RESONANCE IMAGING

Magnetic resonance imaging (MRI) depends on the protons 'wobbling' at specific frequencies depending on the strength of the magnetic field applied. When a stronger magnetic field is applied on one side of a patient, different parts of the body have protons 'wobbling' at different frequencies, which allows their position to be localized. The proton, once stimulated by a magnetic pulse, emits a radio frequency signal. The time taken to attain the baseline state depends on the tissue around the proton. At different times after a stimulation different tissues can be imaged. The emitted radio frequency is analyzed and an image like a conventional computerized tomogram (CT) is generated. Air and calcium do not contain protons and always appear black on MRI. This method of imaging is non-invasive and non-ionizing and allows tissue density to be determined. Using surface coils which are attached to the patient like a belt[72] increased resolution with slices as thin as 3 mm can be obtained.

Computerized tomography is of no value in imaging the pelvis in urogynecology as the images take a long time to be produced, so that the woman has to stay still for a considerable length of time, and views in only the coronal section are produced. Magnetic resonance imaging does not involve this problem to the same degree and soft tissues can be imaged with greater contrast resolution than is the case with CT. The completed image can be viewed from multiple planes and different views can be generated. There are two main imaging modes: T1 and T2 weighed images. T1 weighed images are useful for determining anatomy, as fat appears white with a high signal and fluid appears black with a low signal. Other tissues appear as intermediate shades of grey. T2 weighed images can produce more artefacts but produce high-contrast images of the internal anatomy of organs. This is useful for tumor visualization.[73,74,7] The fluid within the bladder is white with a high signal and muscle has a low signal. Scans are contraindicated in any patient with metal implants, patients unable to co-operate and those suffering from severe claustrophobia.

The speed of the scan dictates the length of time the patient has to remain still. Each 'slice' can take between 3 and 12s. To image the pelvis up to 45 min is required. The individual pelvic organs are easy to image. Using a surface coil either external or internal high-resolution imaging of a specific area can be carried out.

Prolapse

The movement of prolapse has been studied using fast scan MRI.[76] Using graded Valsalva maneuvers and maximal pelvic contraction, the movement of pelvic organs in women with diagnosed prolapse and in asymptomatic controls was compared. Views in the sagittal plane were used for comparison and descent and elevation of the structures within the pelvis were compared to a line from the inferior border of the symphysis pubis to the last coccygeal joint. Limits of normality were defined on the basis of findings in the 11 asymptomatic women. The bladder base, and cervix should not descend more than 1 cm below the pubococcygeal line. The rectum, as assessed by the lowest point of air in the rectum, should not be lower than 2.5 cm below the pubococcygeal line. A low-signal intensity structure was noted between the inferior border of the symphysis pubis and the vesicourethral junction. This imaging technique clearly delineated enteroceles. However, the use of such technology to image structures which can be assessed clinically is contentious, especially as the cost for each study is between £150 and £450.[77]

Stress incontinence

The image resolution of the urethra, bladder neck and surrounding tissues can be enhanced by using a belt-type surface coil placed at the level of the symphysis pubis. Using T2 weighing the paraurethral fibrous tissue and musculature can be visualized.[78] In asymptomatic women extensions from the levator muscle arcuate line medially to the bladder neck and proximal urethra are seen. These have been referred to as the 'urethropelvic' ligaments and are characterized on MRI as being musculofascial (Fig. 15.13). The features on MRI scanning associated with continence are horizontal urethropelvic ligaments, proximity of the bladder neck to the symphysis pubis, and the vagina having an 'H' shape with the anterior vaginal wall conforming well to the urethra.[79] Women with genuine stress incontinence have urethropelvic ligaments directed in an obliquely

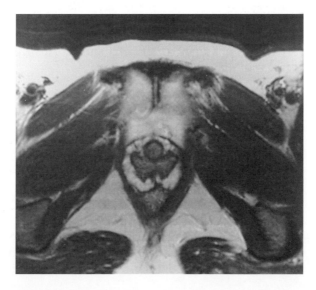

Fig. 15.13 Transverse section through the pelvis showing the attachment between the vagina and the pelvic floor and also the urethra. Image is 4-mm section using a GE Sigma 1.5T, Milwaukee, Wi. Fast-spin echo sequences. T2 weighed. (Illustration kindly provided by Dr M. Quinn)

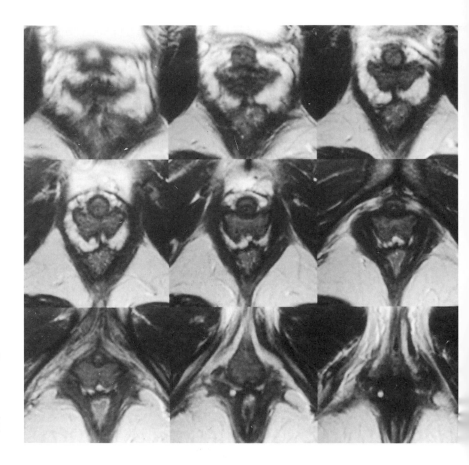

Fig. 15.14 Multiple cross-sectional images through the pelvis. Image is a 4-mm section with 0-mm interslice gap using a GE Sigma 1.5T, Milwaukee, Wi. Fast-spin echo sequences. T2 weighed. (Illustration kindly provided by Dr M. Quinn)

downward course and anterior vaginal wall prolapse is imaged as a change in shape of the vagina (it becomes an inverted 'U' shape) (Fig. 15.14). The urethra appears as a white structure reflecting the vascular plexus and the smooth muscle bundles in between loosely woven connective tissue. The surrounding circular muscle appears black on the image. After repeated failed continence surgery some women have intrinsic damage to the sphincter mechanism. This can be visualized as deficient areas of tissue.

Bladder carcinoma

The preoperative staging of patients with extensive disease is important in planning therapy. This method of imaging has been found to be accurate at determining the depth of invasion of tumor and sensitive at detecting perivesical fat.[80] The detection of macroscopic lymph node involvement was accurate in 60% of patients.

Conclusion

Magnetic resonance imaging gives clear anatomical images of the lower urinary tract. In the future these may be useful in planning treatment of women in whom continence surgery has previously failed.

REFERENCES

1 Khullar V, Salvatore S, Cardozo LD, Hill S, Kelleher CJ. Three dimensional ultrasound of the urethra and urethral sphincter–a new diagnostic technique. Neurourol Urodynam 1994; 13: 352–354.

2 Nerstrom H, Holm HH, Christensen NEH, Movild AF, Nolsoe C. 3-dimensional ultrasound based demonstration of the posterior urethra during voiding combined with urodynamics. Scand J Urol Nephrol 1991; 137S: 125–127.

3 Hederstrom E, Forsberg L. Accuracy of repeated kidney size estimation by ultrasonography and urography in children. Acta Radiol Diag 1985; 26: 603–607.

4 Hricak H, Lieto RP. Sonographic determination of renal volume. Radiology 1983; 148: 311–312.

5 Rosenfield AT, Siegel NJ. Renal parenchymal disease. Histopathological-sonographic correlation. AJR 1981; 137: 793–798.

6 Rosenfield AT, Taylor KJW, Grade M, DeGraaf CS. Anatomy and pathology of the kidney by grey-scale ultrasound. Radiology 1978; 128: 737–744.

7 Marchal G, Verbeken E, Ogen R, Moerman F, Baert AL, Lanweryns J. Ultrasound of the normal kidney: a sonographic, anatomic and histologic correlation. Ultrasound Med Biol 1986; 12: 999–1009.

8 Morin ME, Baker DA. The influence of hydration and bladder distension on the sonographic diagnosis of hydronephrosis. J Clin Ultrasound 1979; 7: 192–194.

9 Malave SR, Neiman HL, Spies SM, Cisternino SJ, Adamo G. Diagnosis of hydronephrosis: comparison of radionuclide scanning and sonography. AJR 1980; 135: 1179–1185.

10 Dalla-Palma L, Bazzochi M, Pozzi-Mucelli RS, Stacul F, Rossi M, Agostini R. Ultrasonography in the diagnosis of hydronephrosis in patients with normal renal function. Urol Radiol 1983; 5: 221–226.

11 Sanders RC, Bearman S. B-scan ultrasound in the diagnosis of hydronephrosis. Radiology 1973; 108: 375–382.

12 Ellenbogen PH, Scheible FW, Talner LB, Leopold GR. Sensitivity of grey scale ultrasound in detecting urinary tract obstruction. AJR 1978; 130: 731–733.

13 Cietak KA, Newton JR. Serial qualitative maternal nephrosonography in pregnancy. Br J Radiol 1985; 58: 399–404.

14 Peake SC, Roxburgh HB, Langlois SlP. Ultrasonic assessment of the hydronephrosis of pregnancy. Radiology 1983; 146: 167–170.

15 White RD, McQuown D, McCarthy TA, Ostergard DR. Real-time ultrasonography in the evaluation of urinary stress incontinence. Am J Obstet Gynecol 1980; 138: 235–237.

16 Wexler JD, McGovern TP. Ultrasonography of female urethral diverticula. AJR 1980; 134: 737–740.

17 Hennigan HW, DuBose TJ. Sonography of the normal female urethra. AJR 1985; 145: 839–841.

18 de Gonzalez EL, Cosgrove DO, Joseph AE, Murch C, Naik K. The appearances on ultrasound of the female urethral sphincter. Br J Radiol 1988; 61: 687–690.

19 Hill S, Khullar V, Cardozo LD, Athanasiou S. Ultrasound electromyography–a new technique. Int Urogynaecol J 1995; 6: 243 (Abstract).

20 Hasan ST, Hamdy FC, Schofield IS, Neal DE. Transrectal ultrasound guided needle electromyography of the urethral sphincter in males. Neurourol Urodynam 1995; 14: 359–364.

21 Rickards D, Noble JG, Milroy EJG, Fowler CJ. Ultrasound evaluation of the urethral sphincter in women with obstructed voiding dysfunction. J Urol 1992; 147: 221A.

22 Poston J, Joseph AEA, Riddle PR. The accuracy of ultrasound in the measurement of changes in bladder volume. Br J Urol 1983; 55: 361–363.

23 McLean GK, Edell SL. Determination of bladder volumes by gray scale ultrasonography. Radiology 1978; 128: 181–182.

24 Mainprize TC, Drutz HP. Accuracy of total bladder volume and residual urine measurements: comparison between real-time ultrasonography and catheterization. Am J Obstet Gynecol 1989; 160: 1013–1016.

25 Griffiths CJ, Murray A, Ramsden PD. Accuracy of and repeatability of bladder volume by means of ultrasonic B-mode scanning. J Urol 1986; 136: 808–812.

26 Hartnell CG, Kiely EA, Williams G, Gibson RN. Real-time ultrasound measurement of bladder volume: a comparative study of three methods. Br J Radiol 1987; 60: 1063–1065.

27 Beacock CJ, Roberts EE, Rees RWM, Buck AC. Ultrasound assessment of residual urine. A quantitive method. Br J Urol 1985; 57: 410–413.

28 Rageth JC, Langer K. Ultrasonic assessment of residual urine volume. Urol Res 1982; 10: 57–60.

29 Hakenberg OW, Ryall RL, Langlois SL, Marshal VR. The estimation of bladder volume by sonocystography. J Urol 1983; 130: 249–251.

30 Roehrborn CG, Peters PC. Can transabdominal ultrasound estimation of postvoiding residual (PVR) replace catheterisation? Urology 1988; 31: 445–449.

31 Pedersen JF, Bartrum RJ, Grytter C. Residual urine determination by ultrasonic scanning. AJR 1975; 125: 474–478.

32 Haylen BT, Frazer MI, Sutherst JR, West CR. Transvaginal ultrasound in the measurement of bladder volumes in women. Br J Urol 1989; 63: 149–151.

33 Haylen BT. Residual urine volumes in a normal female population: application of transvaginal ultrasound. Br J Urol 1989; 64: 347–349.

34 Haylen BT. Verification of the accuracy and range of transvaginal ultrasound in measuring bladder volumes in women. Br J Urol 1989; 64: 350–352.

35 Haylen BT, Frazer MI, Sutherst JR, West CR. Transvaginal ultrasound in the assessment of bladder volumes in women–preliminary report. Br J Urol 1989; 63: 149–151.

36 Baker KR, Drutz HP, Lemieux M-C. Limited accuracy of vaginal probe ultrasound in measuring residual urine volumes. Int Urogynaecol J 1993; 4: 138–140.

37 Spencer J, Lindsell D, Mastorakou I. Ultrasonography compared with intravenous urography in the investigation of adults with haematuria. BMJ 1990; 301: 1074–1076.

38 Fowler JE, Pulaski ET. Excretory urography cystography and cystoscopy in the evaluation of women with urinary tract infection. N Engl J Med 1981; 304: 462–465.

39 McNicholas MMJ, Grifin JF, Cantwell DF. Ultrasound of the pelvis and renal tract combined with a plain film of the abdomen in young women with urinary tract infections: can it replace intravenous urography? Br J Radiol 1991; 64: 221–224.

40 Fox M, Power RF, Bruce AW. Diverticulum of the bladder–presentation and evaluation in 115 cases. Br J Urol 1962; 34: 286–289.

41 Davies AH, Mastorakou I, Dickinson AJ et al. Flexible cystoscopy compared with ultrasound in the detection of recurrent bladder tumours. Br J Urol 1991; 67: 491–492.

42 Flannigan GM, Gelister JSK, Noble JG et al. Rigid versus flexible cystoscopy. A controlled trial of patient tolerance. Br J Urol 1988; 62: 537–540.

43 Fernandez A, Mayayo Dehesa T. Leiomyoma of the urinary bladder floor: diagnosis by transvaginal ultrasound. Urol Int 1992; 48: 99–101.

44 Bhatia NN, Ostergard DR, McQuown D. Ultrasonography in urinary incontinence. Urology 1987; 29: 90–94.

45 Quinn MJ, Beynon J, McC. Mortensen, Smith PJB. Transvaginal endosonography: a new method to study the anatomy of the lower urinary tract in urinary stress incontinence. Br J Urol 1988; 62: 414–418.

46 Quinn MJ, Beynon J, McC. Mortensen, Smith PJB. Vaginal endosonography in the post-operative assessment of colposuspension. Br J Urol 1989; 63: 295–300.

47 Weil EHJ, van Waalwijk van Doorn ESC, Heesakkers JPFA, Meguid T, Janknegt RA. Transvaginal ultasonography: a study with healthy volunteers and women with genuine stress incontinence. Eur Urol 1993; 24: 226–230.

48 Kil PJM, Hoekstra JW, van der Meijden APM, Smans AJ, Theeuwes AGM, Schreinemachers LMH. Transvaginal ultrasonography and urodynamic evaluation after suspension operations: comparison among the Gittes, Stamey and Burch suspensions. J Urol 1991; 146: 132–136.

49 Wise BG, Burton G, Cutner A, Cardozo LD. Effect of vaginal ultrasound probe on lower urinary tract function. Br J Urol 1992; 70: 12–16.

50 Keefe B, Warshauer DM, Tucker MS, Mittelstaedt CA. Diverticula of the female urethra: diagnosis by endovaginal and transperineal sonography. AJR 1991; 156: 1195–1197.

51 Khullar V, Salvatore S, Cardozo LD, Kelleher CJ, Bourne TH. A novel technique for measuring bladder wall thickness in women using transvaginal ultrasound. Ultra Obstet Gynecol 1994; 4: 220–223.

52 Khullar V, Salvatore S, Cardozo LD, Hill S, Kelleher CJ. Ultrasound bladder wall measurement–a non-invasive sensitive screening test for detrusor instability. Neurouro Urodynam 1994; 13: 461–462.

53 Athanasiou S, Hill S, Cardozo LD, Khullar V, Anders K. Three dimensional ultrasound of the urethra, periurethral tissues and pelvic floor. Int Urogynaecol J 1995; 6: 239 (Abstract).

54 Wise BG, Khullar V, Cardozo LD. Bladder neck movement during pelvic floor contraction and intravaginal electrical stimulation in women with and without genuine stress incontinence. Neurourol Urodynam 1992; 11: 309–311.

55 Koelbl H, Bernaschek G. A new method for sonographic urethrocystography and simultaneous pressure-flow measurements. Obstet Gynecol 1989; 74: 417–422.

56 Yamashita T, Ogawa A. Transperineal ultrasonic voiding cystourethrography using a newly devised chair. J Urol 1991; 146: 819–823.

57 Khullar V, Abbott D, Cardozo LD, Kelleher CJ, Salvatore S, Bourne TH. Perineal ultrasound measurement of the urethral sphincter in women with urinary incontinence: an aid to diagnosis? Br J Radiol 1994; 67: 713.

58 Bernstein I, Juul N, Gronvall S, Bonde B, Klarskov P. Pelvic floor muscle thickness measured by perineal ultrasonography. Scand J Urol Nephrol 1991; 137S: 131–133.

59 Richmond DH, Sutherst JR, Brown MC. Screening of the bladder base and urethra using linear array transrectal ultrasound scanning. J Clin Ultrasound 1986; 14: 647–651.

60 Brown MC, Sutherst JR, Murray A, Richmond DH. Potential use of ultrasound in place of X-ray fluoroscopy in urodynamics. Br J Urol 1985; 57: 88–90.

61 Bergman A, McKenzie CJ, Richmond J, Ballard CA, Platt LD. Transrectal ultrasound versus cystography in the evaluation of anatomical stress urinary incontinence. Br J Urol 1988; 62: 228–234.

62 Richmond DH, Sutherst J. Transrectal ultrasound scanning in urinary incontinence: the effect of the probe on urodynamic parameters. Br J Urol 1989; 64: 582–585.

63 Shabsigh R, Fishman IJ, Krebs M. Combined transrectal ultrasonography and urodynamics in the evaluation of detrusor-sphincter dyssynergia. Br J Urol 1988; 62: 326–330.

64 Shapeero LG, Friedland GW, Perkash I. Transrectal sonographic voiding cystourethrography: studies in neuromuscular bladder dysfunction. AJR 1983; 141: 83–90.

65 Perkash I, Friedland GW. Catheter induced hyperreflexia in spinal cord injury patients: diagnosis by sonographic voiding cystourethrography. Radiology 1986; 159: 453–88.

66 Perkash I, Friedland GW. Posterior ledge at the bladder neck: crucial diagnostic role of ultrasonography. Urol Radiol 1986; 8: 175–88.

67 Marshall JL, Johnson ND, De Campo MP. Vesicoureteric reflux in children: prediction with colour Doppler imaging. Radiology 1990; 175: 355–358.

68 Khullar V, Cardozo LD, Kelleher CJ, Abbott D, Bourne TH. Blood flow in the lower urinary tract in women with genuine stress incontinence and detrusor instability. Ultra Obstet Gynecol 1993; 3 (Supp 2): 105 (Abstract).

69 Khullar V, Cardozo LD, Kelleher CJ, Abbott D, Bourne TH. Blood flow in the lower urinary tract in normal women. Ultra Obstet Gynecol 1993; 3 (Supp 2): 106 (Abstract).

70 Khullar V, Cardozo LD, Bourne TH, Kelleher CJ. Description and validation of the inferior vesical artery. Ultra Obstet Gynecol 1993; 3 (Supp 1): 35.

71 Mattox TF, Sinow R, Renslo R, Bhatia NN. The physiology of periurethral vasculature using colour flow doppler. Proceedings of the 22nd Meeting of the International Continence Society, Halifax 1992; 161 (Abstract).

72 Barentsz JO, Lemmens JAM, Ruijs SHJ et al. Carcinoma of the urinary bladder: MR imaging with a double surface coil. AJR 1988; 151: 107–112.

73 Fischer MR, Hricak H, Crooks LE. Urinary bladder MR imaging. I. Normal and benign conditions. Radiology 1985; 157: 467–470.

74 Fischer MR, Hricak H, Tanagho EA. Urinary bladder MR imaging. II. Neoplasm. Radiology 1985; 157: 471–477.

75 Doorns GC, Hricak H. Magnetic resonance imaging of the pelvis: prostate and urinary bladder. Urol Radiol 1986; 8: 156–165.

76 Yang A, Mostwin JL, Rosenshein NB, Zerhouni EA. Pelvic floor descent in women: dynamic evaluation with fast MR imaging and cinematic display. Radiology 1991; 179: 25–33.

77 Ghoniem GM, Shoukry MS, Yang A, Mostwin J. Imaging for urogynaecology, including new modalities. Int Urogynaecol J 1992; 3: 212–221.

78 Klutke C, Golomb J, Barbaric Z, Raz S. The anatomy of stress incontinence: magnetic resonance imaging of the female bladder neck and urethra. J Urol 1990; 143: 563–566.

79 Klutke CG, Raz S. Magnetic resonance imaging in female stress incontinence. Int Urogynaecol J 1991; 2: 115–118.

80 Buy J, Moss AA, Guinet C et al. MR staging of bladder carcinoma: correlation with pathologic findings. Radiology 1988; 169: 695–700.

16 Ambulatory urodynamics

INTRODUCTION

Laboratory urodynamics is unphysiological as it uses retrograde bladder filling and is necessarily provocative, in the filling rate and the actions the women are asked to perform. It is not surprising that on occasions the clinical history and the test result do not concur. Ambulatory urodynamics has been developed in an attempt to measure lower urinary tract function under more physiological conditions. A physiological environment is important, as there is a strong link between incontinence and the women's activities in daily life, and this facilitates the study of the incontinence. This cannot be studied during routine urodynamics, as the woman is asked not to void during bladder filling and this may lead to cortical suppression of detrusor activity. Ambulatory urodynamics facilitates the observation of bladder function under more 'normal' conditions and this may lead to a better understanding of bladder pathophysiology.

To allow a woman to be ambulant either telemetry, long cables or portable recording units have been used. Initial attempts involved the use of a pressure-sensitive radio pill.[1] The pressure information was transmitted by telemetry from a radio pill within the bladder; this method allowed the measurement of intravesical pressure without a foreign body within the urethra, but the cost of the radio pill, the limited range of transmission (30 cm) and occasional difficulty in retrieval prevented its wider use.

The use of fluid-filled lines for ambulatory urodynamics is not recommended as they are prone to movement artefact and the pressures measured are dependent on the position of the pressure transducer relative to the tip of the fluid-filled line, altering the baseline measurements as the woman changes posture. In spite of these problems Tsuji et al[2] used natural filling and described increased phasic activity in spinal injury patients.

James[3] described air probes where a small-diameter air-filled tube was inserted into the bladder. The end of the tube was sealed by a meniscus of urine. Air is not prone to movement artefacts but if fluid traveled down the tube then artefacts appeared. This was prevented by covering the tube end with a compliant balloon. The position of the catheter relative to the transducer was unimportant, but changes occurred with temperature which caused drift in the pressure measurement. This type of catheter is also difficult to calibrate.

Initially radio telemetry[4,5] was used but at distances greater than 50 m interference was marked. Thuroff et al[6] used telemetry to perform urodynamic measurements, but the woman was kept in a room under closed-circuit television, allowing her to void and exercise without disturbance. This method was thorough but prohibitively expensive and time-consuming. Thus a tape recording system[7] using the analog output of microtip pressure transducers was tried. As the recorders had a limited capacity, the pressures were only recorded if they went above a threshold value. Unfortunately, if a patient was symptomatic during the test but without recorded pressure at the time, this left a diagnostic quandary about interpretation; also the level of the threshold was difficult to set.

Griffiths et al[8] developed an ambulatory system which employed microtip pressure transducers with a recorder using a digital solid state memory. This meant that pressures would be recorded digitally and then transferred and reviewed at the end of the test. This allowed the trace to be expanded or compressed easily without loss of information.

EQUIPMENT

Ambulatory systems have three main components: the transducers, the recording unit (including patient markers) and the analysing system. Solid state transducers (Fig. 16.1) measure the pressure impinging on them and are less likely to have movement artefact. There are problems of drift during the test but in most systems this is less than 3 cmH$_2$O over 5 hrs.[9] As most transducers have the pressure-sensitive membrane inset a few millimeters from the catheter exterior, artefactual pressure rises may be recorded by the intravesical transducer touching the bladder wall. To detect this we routinely insert two pressure transducers within

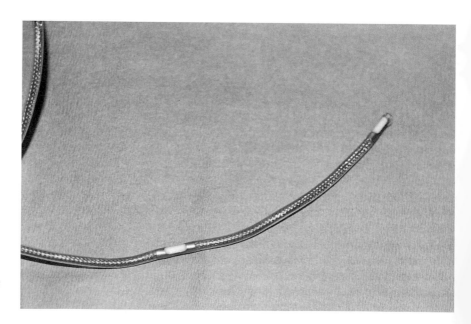

Fig. 16.1 Microtip transducer (Gaeltec): note the recessed transducer sensing plate

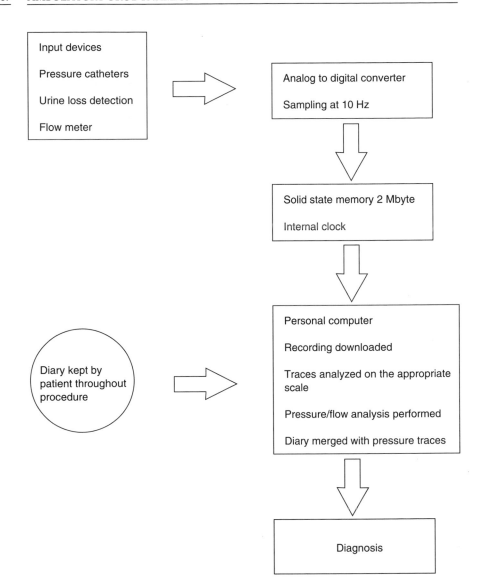

Input devices

Pressure catheters

Urine loss detection

Flow meter

Analog to digital converter

Sampling at 10 Hz

Solid state memory 2 Mbyte

Internal clock

Diary kept by patient throughout procedure

Personal computer

Recording downloaded

Traces analyzed on the appropriate scale

Pressure/flow analysis performed

Diary merged with pressure traces

Diagnosis

Fig. 16.2   An ambulatory urodynamic system and reviewing system

the bladder. An intravesical pressure change is considered significant only if it is recorded on both transducers.

The recording system (Fig. 16.2) should be portable and ideally battery-powered. Sampling of the pressures should be greater than 4 Hz and the memory should be digital as this enables the trace to be compressed. Some recorders only register pressures if the detrusor pressure is above a threshold value,[10] but this produces the problems already outlined.

The patient's own symptoms are important in the interpretation of the trace, and a diary should therefore be used to record them. The recording system should have a method of marking events on to the trace. This allows accurate interpretation of traces in conjunction with the diary. The diary used in our unit is shown in Fig. 16.3. Many systems have multiple

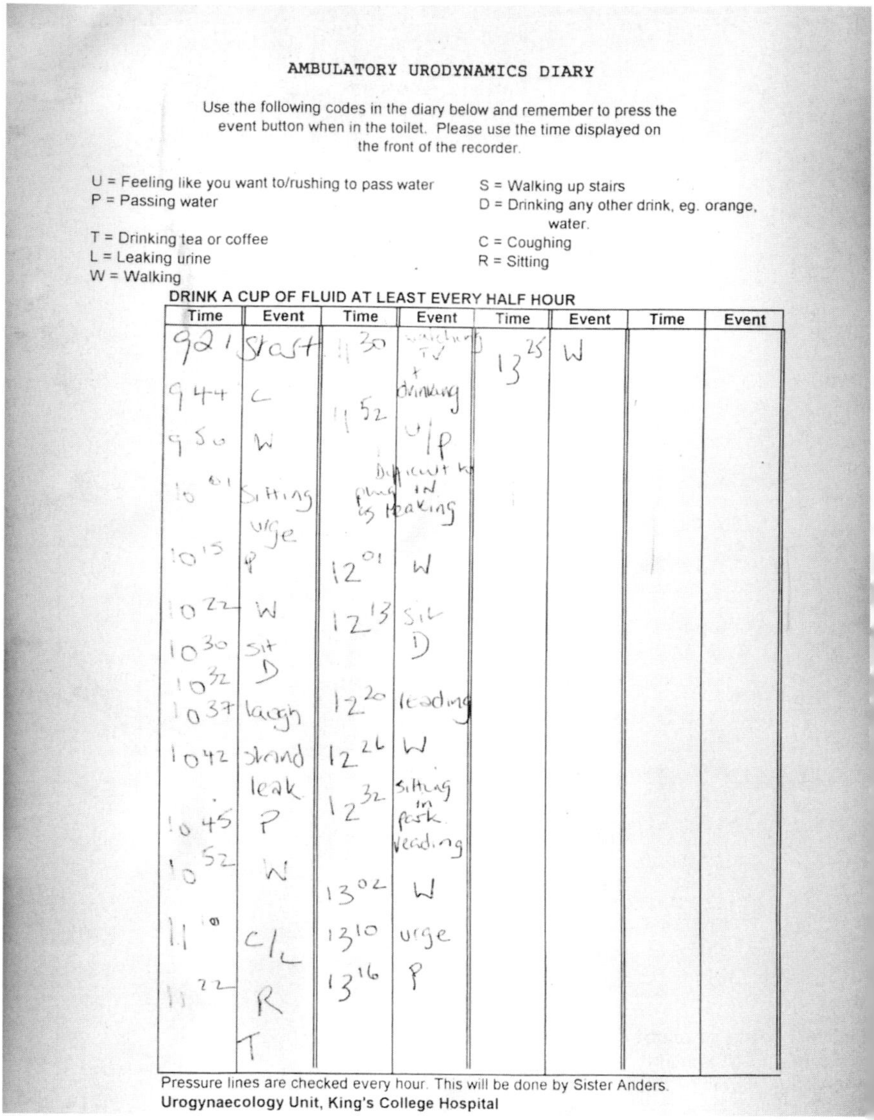

AMBULATORY URODYNAMICS DIARY

Use the following codes in the diary below and remember to press the event button when in the toilet. Please use the time displayed on the front of the recorder.

U = Feeling like you want to/rushing to pass water
P = Passing water
T = Drinking tea or coffee
L = Leaking urine
W = Walking
S = Walking up stairs
D = Drinking any other drink, eg. orange, water.
C = Coughing
R = Sitting

DRINK A CUP OF FLUID AT LEAST EVERY HALF HOUR

Time	Event	Time	Event	Time	Event	Time	Event
9 21	Start	11 30	watching TV + drinking	13 25	W		
9 44	C	11 52	U/P Difficult [illegible] leaking				
9 50	W	12 01	W				
10 01	Sitting urge	12 13	Sit D				
10 15	P	12 20	reading				
10 22	W	12 26	W				
10 30	sit	12 32	sitting in park reading				
10 32	D	13 02	W				
10 37	laugh	13 10	urge				
10 42	stand leak	13 16	P				
10 45	P						
10 52	W						
11 00	C/L						
11 22	R T						

Pressure lines are checked every hour. This will be done by Sister Anders.
Urogynaecology Unit, King's College Hospital

Fig. 16.3 Ambulatory urodynamic diary filled in by a woman. The commonly used comments have been abbreviated. The diary can also have comments not listed at the top of the diary written in. The timing must relate to the ambulatory unit's internal clock

marker buttons on the recorder (Fig. 16.4). Unfortunately, a substantial minority of patients have difficulty in pressing two buttons correctly thus the use of multiple buttons may be more confusing for the woman as well as the physician. If the wrong button is pressed this does not allow easy interpretation of the trace without a diary. For the diary to be meaningful times should also be noted. The recorder may display the time (Fig. 16.5), or the woman's own watch can be synchronized with the recorder. The recorder should have the facility to connect an electronic nappy: this is important to gain information on urine loss. The recorder used in our unit can connect to a gravimetric flowmeter (Fig. 16.6). This is useful in calculating pressure/flow curves and checking when detrusor

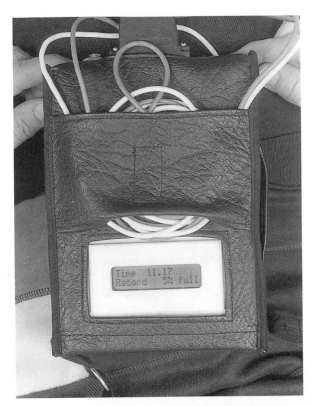

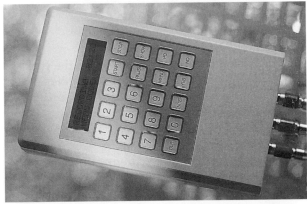

Fig. 16.4 Single marker button ambulatory system (**A**) (Gaeltec) and multiple marker button (**B**) (MMS) ambulatory system

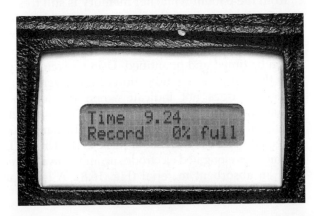

Fig. 16.5 Clock on the ambulatory recording unit (MPR2, Gaeltec)

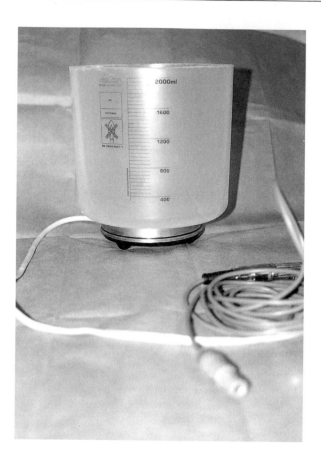

Fig. 16.6 Gravimetric flowmeter used with ambulatory urodynamics

instability has occurred and when the patient was voiding; often detrusor instability is seen before a patient voids.

The pressure traces are downloaded on to a computer, and there are various formats. It is important that diary events are displayed once entered with the pressure recordings, and that in analyzing the recording the appropriate scales are chosen for pressure measurement and time (Fig. 16.7). When interpreting the trace it is important that the patient should be present, as often information may not be written on the diary at a crucial event on the trace, and further information may be obtained from the patient while her memory is still fresh.

To evaluate incontinence it is essential to detect urine loss during the urodynamic test; this allows the interpretation of manometric changes leading to incontinence and is the only method by which incontinence can be timed and quantified. Using a weighed perineal pad for the length of the test gives an indication of the severity of the incontinence, but this method does not indicate when the loss occurred. The timing and quantification of urinary loss and pressure change in the bladder are helpful in determining the cause of urinary leakage. Three methods have been described. The first of these is the Urilos (Exeter) electronic nappy.[11] This uses elongated electrodes arranged in an interleaved fashion embedded in an absorbent material (Fig. 16.8). A low-voltage (50-mV) alternating

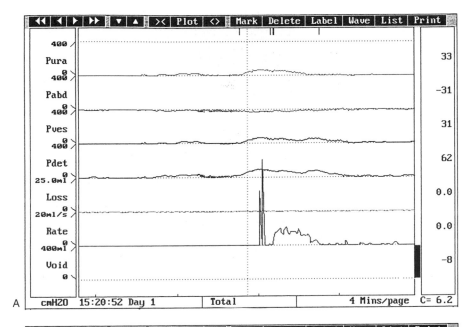

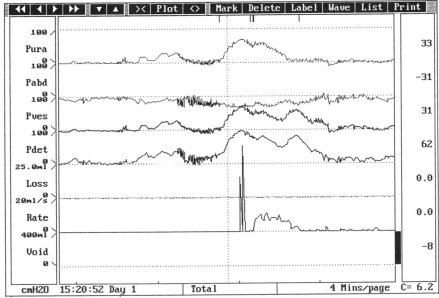

Fig. 16.7 A Y-axis scale too large to allow meaningful examination of the ambulatory urodynamic trace. **B** Same trace as **A** appropriately scaled, showing the detrusor contraction which could not be seen on **A**.

current is passed between the two electrodes. The current crossing between the electrodes increases as the urine loss increases. Unfortunately, this method depends on the electrolytes within the urine, and as this is not constant the pad has to be preloaded with a measured volume of a known electrolyte solution. This method is useful for volumes between 1 ml and 100 ml and is reproducible within 20%. The nappy is bulky but can be cut to a smaller size for ambulatory use and has been found to be adequate in detecting incontinence during ambulatory urodynamic tests.[12] This method is quantitative but losses of

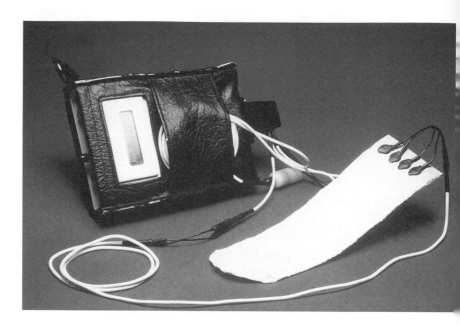

Fig. 16.8 'Urilos' (Exeter) nappy modified for use with an ambulatory system

less than 1 ml may not be detected and once the pad is soaked it does not register further loss.

An alternative method has been to measure the perineal temperature. The temperature of urine (37°C) is warmer than the perineum (30–34°C). When urine leaks the temperature rises transiently. The detection of loss is effective as the urine cools rapidly once it has leaked, allowing detection of further leakage. Using a single temperature detector is not effective in women as the position of the detector in relation to the leaked urine changes, therefore a parallel array of diodes has been used with a separate reference diode.[13] The rate of rise in temperature has been shown to correlate well with the quantity of leaked urine. Problems of interpretation may occur if the patient has her legs together while sitting as this may cause a rise in the perineal temperature.

The catheter within the urethra makes ambulatory urodynamics an ideal method for distal urethral electrical conductivity to be used to detect urinary leakage.[14,15] Two electrodes are mounted on a catheter and an electric current is passed between them. Leakage or voiding of urine causes increased conductance and a larger current passes across the electrodes. The positioning of the electrodes is crucial, in the proximal urethra changes in electrical current would indicate the presence of urine there but not necessarily urinary leakage. This can occur with urethral instability where urethral relaxation allows urine to enter the proximal urethra, which would be interpreted incorrectly as leakage. If the electrodes were not within the urethra then urinary leakage would not be detected. Distal urethral electrical conductance is not used clinically in ambulatory urodynamics and is mainly a research tool.

METHOD OF PERFORMING AMBULATORY URODYNAMICS

At present the regimen we employ is as follows:

1. The urine should be infection-free on urinalysis.
2. The woman is requested to wear clothing with a separate top and bottom prior to the test (Fig. 16.9).
3. If she wishes to evacuate her bowels, she should do this before the pressure transducers are inserted.
4. A urethral Silastic-covered 6F catheter with two pressure transducers (Gaeltec) is inserted with *both* transducers within the bladder. The rectal transducer is on a 6-cm silicone rubber cylinder which is 7 mm in diameter (Fig. 16.10); this is covered with a condom. This allows for comfortable insertion and better retention. Both catheters are strapped firmly with tape to the skin close to the site of insertion; this determines how often the lines will need to be resited (Fig. 16.11). The lines are then looped up and fixed on to the abdomen.
5. The woman is then asked to void and the lines are rechecked.
6. She is told to drink 180 ml/h on the basis of a total daily fluid intake of 2 l. Those women who do not drink this amount of fluid during the test often have normal urodynamic findings.

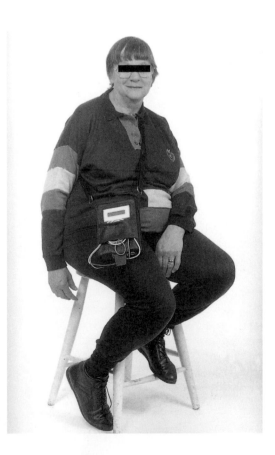

Fig. 16.9 Patient appropriately dressed with ambulatory urodynamic equipment

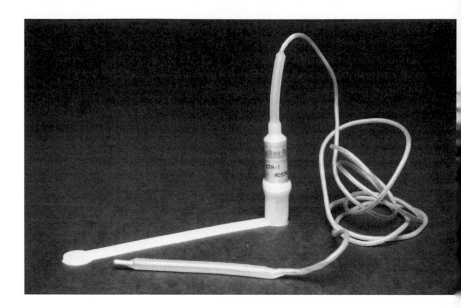

Fig. 16.10   Rectal pressure catheter

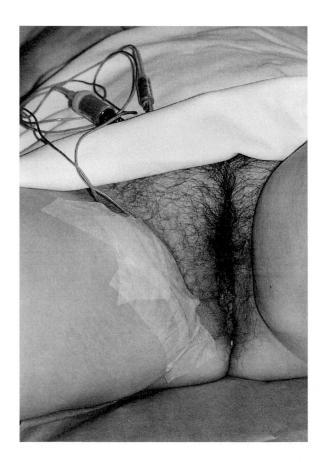

Fig. 16.11   Urethral and rectal pressure lines taped into position

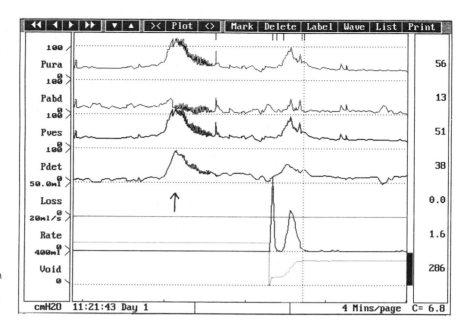

Fig. 16.12 Ambulatory urodynamic trace of a woman with detrusor instability detrusor contractions marked by arrow

7. When she wishes to void, she must press the event marker button *prior* to entering the room and void on the flowmeter. Where a urodynamic system does not have a flowmeter the event marker should be pushed at the initiation of the void.
8. Any other events are noted in the diary and the event marker is also depressed.
9. After each void the lines are checked for their position and if necessary replaced.
10. Provocative maneuvers are carried out with a 'full' bladder for the last half-hour of the test. These are:
    a. Coughing ten times
    b. Ten star jumps
    c. Listening to running water
    d. Anything which causes urinary incontinence.
11. The trace and diary are analyzed with the woman present.

The test length is usually 4 hrs. It must be emphasized that the subject requires close supervision and good patient compliance is essential for a successful test. The diagnosis of detrusor instability is made where the symptom of urgency coincides with a detrusor pressure rise (Fig. 16.12). It is important that this symptom is usually felt by the woman normally, otherwise the presence of the symptom during the test may be due to the catheters.

CLINICAL APPLICATIONS

At present in our unit ambulatory urodynamics is carried out and found to be useful in the following groups of women:

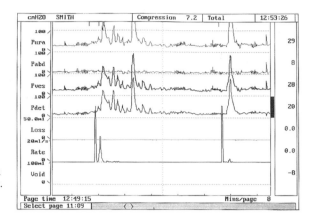

Fig. 16.13 Ambulatory urodynamic trace of a woman suprapubic pain after voiding. Note detrusor contractions after voids

1. Symptomatic women in whom no abnormality was detected during laboratory urodynamics.
2. Women in whom genuine stress incontinence was diagnosed on laboratory urodynamics but who do not complain of stress incontinence as a symptom.
3. Women with mixed urinary incontinence in whom the balance between detrusor instability and urethral sphincter incompetence needs to be clarified.
4. Women with voiding difficulties who are unable to void with pressure lines during laboratory urodynamics. Ambulatory urodynamics allows pressure flow studies to be carried out, thus determining the cause of voiding difficulties.
5. Women with sensory urgency on laboratory urodynamics but normal findings on cystourethroscopy and bladder histology.
6. Women with suprapubic pain after voiding; this has been found to be associated with detrusor contractions once the bladder is empty (Fig. 16.13). This can be treated as detrusor instability but the women will also require cystourethroscopy and bladder biopsy.

CLINICAL STUDIES

Unexplained urinary incontinence

Ambulatory urodynamic studies were undertaken in 100 symptomatic patients (89 male and 14 female)[16] who had undergone standard urodynamic investigations and had a urodynamic result which did not correlate with their symptoms, or in whom previous incontinence surgery had failed. The results of the ambulatory urodynamics were compared with their symptoms as well as the laboratory urodynamic results. Ambulatory urodynamics diagnosed detrusor instability twice as frequently as laboratory urodynamics. Interestingly, 32 patients were diagnosed as normal on laboratory urodynamics but on ambulatory testing only 5 patients were considered normal. This result rather begs the question 'What is normal?' The test could either be very sensitive or alternatively have a high false positive rate for diagnosing detrusor instability. Ambulatory urodynamics only diagnosed 8 patients having urethral sphincter incompetence compared with 13 patients on laboratory urodynamics. Webb et al[11] studied 52 patients who underwent laboratory urodynamics and then ambulatory urodynamics. Laboratory urodynamics had not provided diagnoses which correlated well with the patients' symptoms. Detrusor instability was found on ambulatory monitoring in 31 patients who had not received this diagnosis on the basis of laboratory urodynamics; 11 of these patients were found to have detrusor instability on provocation only, emphasizing the importance of this part of the ambulatory test. Urinary incontinence was detected using the Urilos nappy in 23 women, 13 of whom had detrusor instability and 3 of whom had coexisting urethral sphincter incompetence. In this study detrusor instability and urinary incontinence were detected more frequently on ambulatory monitoring than with laboratory urodynamics.

Normal volunteers

Ambulatory urodynamics performed on 36 female volunteers[17] without lower urinary tract symptoms found 25 to have 'detrusor instability'. Unfortunately, only 17 women also underwent standard cystometry and 3 had detrusor instability. In both the above studies the women were asked to drink more than normal; some drank up to 530 ml/h. This alters the rate of orthograde bladder filling and changes the behavior of the detrusor muscle. The urinary symptoms the volunteers felt during the ambulatory urodynamic test were not felt during their normal daily activities and would therefore be discounted as artefact when analyzed in our unit. The authors suggested the use of the detrusor activity index (DAI) to determine 'normal' limits of bladder activity. This incorporates the number of contractions per hour multiplied by ten added to the mean amplitude and mean duration of uninhibited detrusor contractions. Unfortunately, this index does not take account of leakage or voiding associated with detrusor instability, which may curtail the pressure rise during the detrusor contraction. The investigation of bladder function in women without urinary symptoms needs to be taken further.

Low compliance and detrusor instability

During laboratory urodynamics in the filling phase a tonic detrusor pressure rise (low compliance) may be seen. There are questions about the significance of low compliance and some authorities assert that the pressure rise is a passive phenomenon related to the reduced elasticity of the bladder wall, in which case the pressure rise should not decrease at the end of filling. The other theory is that the increase in pressure is associated with a tonic detrusor contraction. If this is the case the detrusor pressure should decay exponentially at the end of filling as the contracting detrusor relaxes. Webb et al[8] studied patients with neuropathic bladders who developed a detrusor pressure rise greater than 25 cmH$_2$O at a filling rate of 100 ml/min. When these patients underwent cystometry at faster filling rates there was a greater tonic detrusor pressure rise. During the ambulatory test there was a much smaller detrusor pressure rise on orthograde filling, but the frequency of phasic detrusor instability during the test correlated with the size of the pressure rise during the conventional cystometry. The greater number of phasic detrusor contractions during ambulatory monitoring did correlate with dilated upper urinary tracts. Unfortunately, the low compliance on filling during laboratory urodynamics did not correlate with the development of upper tract dilatation. Phasic detrusor contractions during ambulatory urodynamics quantified as the area under the detrusor pressure curve 20 min prior to voiding has been found to correlate with upper tract dilatation.[18] Ambulatory urodynamic studies have also been used to investigate detrusor activity after 'clam' ileocystoplasty,[19] showing reduced pressure rises with detrusor instability after the procedure.

Predicting failure of continence surgery in women

Detrusor instability has to be distinguished from genuine stress incontinence prior to selecting a woman for continence surgery. Detrusor instability is a major risk factor for failure of colposuspension.[20,21] The appearance of detrusor instability after continence surgery in spite of being excluded preoperatively with laboratory urodynamics is also associated with failure.[22,23] No specific cause has been found but it may either be a result of the operation due to excessive dissection or be because detrusor instability was not diagnosed prior to surgery. Ambulatory urodynamics is more sensitive at detecting detrusor instability, but can it predict the development of detrusor instability after surgery? Khullar et al[24] studied 35 women, all of whom were diagnosed as having moderate to severe genuine stress incontinence on laboratory urodynamics. All these women underwent ambulatory urodynamics, and 11 were found to have detrusor instability. Six weeks postoperatively, 6 of these women had developed the irritative symptoms of urgency and urge incontinence; all the other women were asymptomatic. Nine months postoperatively 13 women had irritative symptoms, and these included all the women diagnosed as having detrusor instability on ambulatory urodynamics. On videocystourethrography 9 months after surgery, women were diagnosed as having detrusor instability; these were all women diagnosed as having detrusor instability on ambulatory urodynamics preoperatively. The use of the DAI[17] or the area under the detrusor curve for 20 min prior to voiding[18] may enable more accurate identification of those women who will develop detrusor instability postoperatively.

CONCLUSION

Ambulatory urodynamics is an extremely sensitive method of detecting abnormal detrusor activity. This enables greater understanding of detrusor instability and its relationship with patient symptoms. The detection of detrusor instability in asymptomatic women leads to questions about the relevance of the results obtained in symptomatic women. This needs to be resolved before ambulatory urodynamics can become a standard clinical investigation.

APPENDIX: AMBULATORY URODYNAMIC SYSTEMS

These systems provide a more sensitive method of detecting detrusor instability and may predict the development of detrusor instability after continence surgery. Ambulatory urodynamic systems are more flexible than standard urodynamic systems for the study of bladder function at physiological filling rates and for longer periods with the woman mobile, carrying out activities which provoke urinary problems. All systems should be bought with solid state transducers as with fluid-filled lines the recorded trace will have movement artefacts. Additional to the cost of the basic system, a personal computer is required to review the traces and store the downloaded traces.

DANTEC

This system is based on the original recorder used by van Waalwijk van Doorn. The graphics are monochrome and the system shows events from the diary at the same time as the traces, which is very helpful for review. The system will record for up to 12 h, which is long enough for most purposes. The recorder unit has two event marker buttons and downloads to a personal computer.

GAELTEC (DISTRIBUTED BY LECTROMED LTD)

The Gaeltec MPR2 has the ability to record seven channels for over 24 h. There is one event marker and the machine has a built-in clock display. There is a gravimetric flowmeter attachment and Urilos pad attachment for detecting urinary leakage. Data are transfered through a serial link and the computer to which the traces are downloaded needs at least 2 MB of random access memory. Analysis software is provided in the package.

MMS (DISTRIBUTED BY LEWIS MEDICAL LTD)

The UPS-2020 is a multipurpose ambulatory system which can record for up to 24 h. There are multiple recording buttons which can record up to five user-defined events. Leakage detection and electromyography can also be recorded on the system. The computer to which the traces are downloaded needs at least 2 MB of random access memory to work with this system. The software allows colour graphics with a zoom facility.

SYNETICS

This system records up to six channels at once. The system has a memory capacity of 4 MB and can store recordings over 24 h. The system downloads to a standard personal computer.

WIEST

Camsys 6300 records three pressure channels and one electromyographic channel. The system allows recording over 24 h. The system downloads through a personal computer and can use a Windows environment.

REFERENCES

1 Tsuji I, Kuroda K, Nakajima F. Excretory cystometry in paraplegic patients. J Urol 1960; 83: 839–844.
2 James ED. The behaviour of the bladder during physical activity. Br J Urol 1978; 50: 387–394.
3 Miyagawa I, Nakamura I, Ueda M, Nishida H, Nakashita E, Goto H. Telemetric cystometry. Urol Int 1993; 41: 263–265.
4 Vereecken RL, Puers B, Das J. Continuous telemetric monitoring of bladder function. Urol Res 1983; 11: 15–18.
5 Thuroff JW, Jonas V, Frohneberg D, Petri E, Hohenfellner R. Telemetric urodynamic investigations in normal males. Urol Int 1980; 35: 427–434.
6 Bhatia NN, Bradley WE, Haldeman S, Johnson BK. Continuous monitoring of bladder and urethral pressures: new technique. Urology 1981; 18: 207–210.
7 Griffiths CJ, Assi MS, Styles RA, Ramsden PD, Neal DE. Ambulatory monitoring of bladder and detrusor pressure during natural filling. J Urol 1989; 142: 780–784.
8 Webb RJ, Styles RA, Griffiths CJ, Ramsden PD, Neal DE. Ambulatory monitoring of bladder pressures in patients with low compliance as a result of neurogenic bladder dysfunction. Br J Urol 1989; 64: 150–154.
9 McInerney PD, Harris AB, Pritchard A, Stephenson TP. Night studies for primary diurnal and nocturnal enuresis and preliminary results of the 'clam' ileocystoplasty. Br Urol 1991; 67: 42–43.
10 James ED, Flack FC, Caldwell KPS, Martin MR. Continuous measurement of urine loss and frequency in incontinent patients. Br J Urol 1971; 43: 233–237.
11 Webb RJ, Ramsden PD, Neal DE. Ambulatory monitoring and electronic measurement of urinary leakage in the diagnosis of detrusor instability and incontinence. Br J Urol 1991; 68: 148–152.
12 Eckford SC, Abrams PH. A new temperature sensitive device to detect incontinent episodes during ambulatory monitoring. Neurourol Urodynam 1992; 11: 448–450.
13 Janez J, Rodi Z, Mihelic M, Vrtacnik P, Vodusek DB, Plevnik S. Ambulatory distal urethral electric conductance testing coupled to a modified pad test. Neurourol Urodynam 1993; 12: 324–326.
14 Plevnik S, Vrtacnik P, Janez P. Detection of fluid entry into the urethra by electrical impedance measurement: fluid bridge test. Clin Phys Physiol., Meas 1983; 4: 309–313.
15 van Waalwijk van Doorn ESC, Remmers A, Janknegt RA. Extramural ambulatory urodynamic monitoring during natural filling and normal daily activities: evaluation 100 patients. J Urol 1991; 146: 124–131.
16 van Waalwijk van Doorn ESC, Remmers A, Janknegt RA. Conventional and extramural ambulatory urodynamic testing of the lower urinary tract in female volunteers. J Urol 1992; 47: 1319–1326.
17 Webb RJ, Griffiths CJ, Ramsden PD, Neal DE. Ambulatory monitoring in low compliance neuropathic bladder function. J Urol 1992; 148: 1477–1481.
18 Sethia KK, Webb RJ, Neal DE. Urodynamic study of ileocystoplasty in the treatment of idiopathic detrusor instability. Br J Urol 1991; 67: 286–290.
19 Arnold EP, Webster JR, Loose H et al. Urodynamics of female incontinence factors influencing the results of surgery. Am J Obstet Gynecol 1973; 117: 805–813.
20 Stanton SL, Cardozo LD. Results of the colposuspension operation for incontinence and prolapse. Br J Obstet Gynaecol 1979; 86: 693–697.
21 Cardozo LD, Stanton SL, Williams JE. Detrusor instability following surgery for genuine stress incontinence. Br J Urol 1979; 51: 204–207.
22 Steel SA, Cox C, Stanton SL. Long-term follow-up of detrusor instability following the colposuspension operation. Br J Urol 1985; 58: 138–142.
23 Khullar V, Salvatore S, Cardozo LD, Abbott D, Hill S, Kelleher CJ. Ambulatory urodynamics: a predictor of de-novo detrusor instability after colposuspension. Neurourol Urodynam 1994; 13: 443–444.

17 Computerization

Computers enable large amounts of information to be stored, processed and accessed easily (Fig. 17.1). The rapid improvements in processing capacity and memory of computers have made their introduction into urodynamics useful and increasingly user-friendly. Many companies offer urodynamic equipment which encorporates a computer and urodynamic software. The application of computers in urodynamics is best based on the method and structure of investigation; this enables the collection of data with the minimum disruption to routine investigation. The aim of this chapter is to outline the techniques and individual applications for which computers can be used in clinical practice and research.

PATIENT ADMINISTRATION

Many hospitals have a single system serving all departments.[1,2,3,4,5] These computers are efficient for the general purpose of file management, patient appointments and accounting. Most cannot transfer information to another computer system in a urodynamic clinic. The hospital system is often based on software at least 10 years old and these general computers are often incompatible with the newer urodynamic systems even if networked to smaller personal computers. Programs designed specifically for use in urodynamic clinics are available.[6,7,8] Patient administration programs do not fundamentally alter the care given in urodynamic clinics, but improve the administrative efficiency.

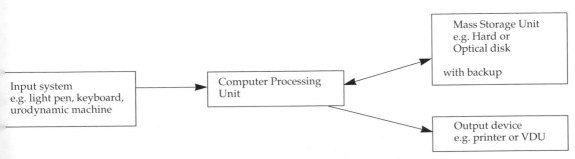

Fig. 17.1 Basic computer system. Note that 'garbage in, garbage out': a computer cannot improve the quality of data.

HISTORY AND EXAMINATION

Information about and from the patient history has traditionally been recorded on paper. In urogynecology there is a standard set of questions which should be asked. There are various paths which may need to be pursued if a woman answers positively to a question relating to another area: these questions are called 'flags.' Thus the standard questionnaire can usefully be recorded on a computer database.[9,10,11,12] The initial method of recording involves the transfer of information from a standard history sheet taken at the time of urodynamics to a computer database at a later point.[13] This enables data from a large number of women to be examined but creates an additional step in the process of clinical assessment and urodynamic investigation. The most important element to remember when information is transferred from a uniform history form on to a computer database is that the registration and format of the data collected should be standardized. The interpretation of massed data is made easy if this has occurred.

The entry of data directly on to a computer database by patients has to be carefully developed.[14] If the women are asked to type information directly on to the database without structured answers, the great variability between answers leads to difficulties in classification and interpretation. The choice of patient replies is structured so that only clear, unambiguous answers are given. The method of reply can be made with a light pen[1] (Fig. 17.3) or using a keyboard. History taking using computer interrogation leads to high patient compliance[16,17] and has been found to elicit symptoms and other factors missed by the clinician.[15] As patients may not understand the questions asked, a nurse or technician must be present throughout the computer interrogation to help the patient if necessary.

The use of computer interrogation in an out-patient setting has been found to result in many correct diagnoses but many unnecessary investigations were suggested.[15] These systems in practice are time-consuming as the patient has to learn how to answer questions and this is often difficult, especially for the elderly. A computer-based record system, when

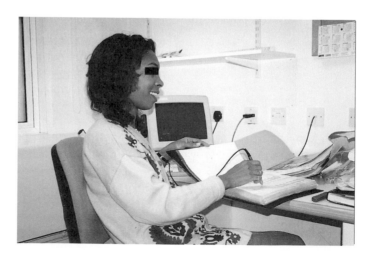

Fig. 17.2 Video display unit and light pen

monitored by a clinician in an open access incontinence clinic, has been found to be useful in cutting down waiting times.[18] A computer which is an expert system gives results which directly affect treatment,[19] but the efficacy of this method of management has not been evaluated.

URODYNAMIC INVESTIGATION

The traditional method of recording urodynamic pressure information is on an analog paper trace for permanent storage. This has the advantage of being cheap, and all pressure information is recorded and can be reviewed without other equipment. Unfortunately, the traces take up a considerable amount of space and require filing, the data have to be digitized to be analyzed for pressure/flow plots,[20,21] accurate copies are difficult to make and the scales for pressures and time cannot be changed for viewing areas of specific interest. If the urodynamic information goes directly into a computer then automated analysis is facilitated and large quantities of data can be stored easily. This method of storage inevitably leads to increased cost, however, as a computer and printer are required.

The analysis of urodynamic pressure information may either be translated online into a digital output (Fig. 17.3) which can be interpreted by a computer in an expert system, or the trace can be photoscanned into the computer, which traces the resulting image with an adjacent scale.[22] The latter method is useful for the development of an expert system by providing a large database of previously obtained values. The sampling rate for an online digital urodynamic machine is 10 samples per second. This can adequately collect information from even a stress urethral pressure profile. The recording of electromyographic activity requires a higher sampling rate of 2000 samples per second.[23] The other parameter

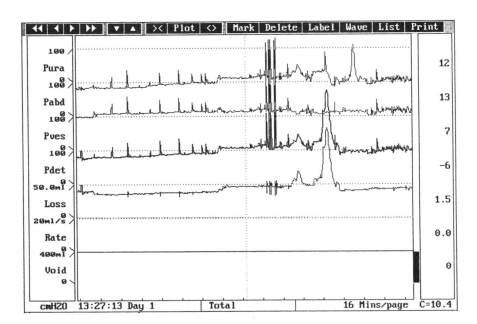

Fig. 17.3 Computerized trace with videocystourethrogram

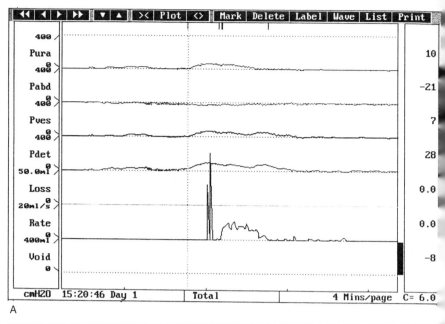

A

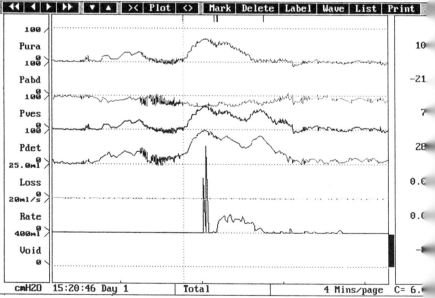

Fig. 17.4 A) Trace on a very large Y-axis scale of detrusor instability. B) Same trace on a corrected Y-axis scale

B

involved in analog to digital conversion is the signal resolution; this determines the smallest change in the pressure measured, which is detected by a digital system. On a channel where the pressures measured vary in the range of 0–250 cmH$_2$O which is converted to a 12 bit (2^{12}) 'word', allows 4096 different levels to be recorded. Thus the signal change which is recorded by this digital system is 0.06 cmH$_2$O, which is more than adequate for most applications. Video images can also be digitized and recorded, together with the pressure trace. These images can be ultrasonographic or radiological. It is important when viewing

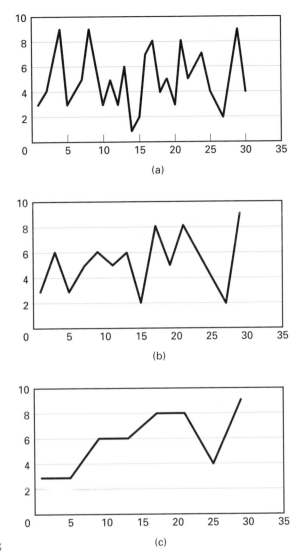

Fig. 17.5A–C Traces with differing degrees of sampling

such traces that care be taken to adjust the speed of the trace and the pressure amplitude on the Y-axis. Significant variations in pressure may be missed with the incorrect setting of scales on a computerized system (Fig. 17.4). The memory used in the storage of traces can be reduced by sampling the finished trace. Unfortunately, if the sampling becomes too infrequent then the trace loses its diagnostic value (Fig. 17.5).

The retention of such a vast amount of information requires a considerable memory size, but this should not pose a problem in the future as memory costs are rapidly decreasing; moreover, with the advent of optical disks a reliable large volume (2000 MB) is now available which could store up to 4000 patient urodynamic traces and records. To reduce the quantity of data stored, periods in a urodynamic record can be skipped and not recorded if certain criteria are met; for example, a flow rate with a zero value is not recorded.

An experimental addition to urodynamic systems for automatic recognition of artefacts and system malfunctions is being developed,[24] but is at a very early stage of development.

The introduction of digital computerized urodynamics has enabled the application of ambulatory urodynamics as a clinical service.[25] The digital sampling and storage of the urodynamic traces has allowed long traces to be recorded and easily reviewed. This is important as reviewing ambulatory urodynamic traces can only be done retrospectively because questioning the patient during the test can affect the results obtained. The review of a trace is focused by the patient's diary kept during the test. The digitized recording allows certain parts of the trace to be magnified and carefully reviewed. Previous techniques for ambulatory recording involved telemetry and paper traces, which were not easy!

DATABASES

The database itself should be 'relational'; this means that files can be linked. This is not only important for processing but it enables different files on the same patient to be associated. In urodynamics this is essential, as for each patient there is demographic information, history and examination and the urodynamic investigation. This feature allows a report about a patient to be produced directly from the database with information drawn from various files and databases. This flexibility is mandatory as a database evolves with time when additional parameters are recorded. It is also important that a database should be easily imported to presentation or statistical packages. All databases should always be backed up on to alternative storage media. This can be backup onto floppy disks, a process which can be time-consuming once a database has attained a certain size, or using magnetic tape drives.

REPORTS

Computer systems have been used to produce a print-out report of relevant data[15] and a range of possible urological management strategies and diagnoses with a probability over 0.1. These expert systems have been found to be correct in over 80% of cases studied.[22] The final output of an expert system should be a letter outlining diagnosis and future treatment.[2] At present all 'expert' systems require a medical expert to screen them as they have a significant false positive rate for diagnoses.[22,26] It is important that the urodynamic trace be reviewed, as a computerized urodynamic machine may record pressures which are either artefactually high or low. The trace should be reviewed on a pressure scale which is not compressed; for female urodynamics this should be no greater than 0–50 cmH$_2$O.

FUTURE DEVELOPMENTS

With the increasing power of computers the digital storage of urodynamic investigations will probably lead to computer-controlled urodynamics, with the computer monitoring the quality and validity of measurements as they are taken. This will mean that the investigator is warned when an investigation is suboptimal and is advised by the computer how to correct the situation. The storage of digital images enables these to be enhanced digitally allowing improved quality. This will probably be the fastest-changing area in urodynamics in the near future.

REFERENCES

1 Bekey BA, Schwartz MD. Hospital information systems. Basle: Marcel Dekker, 1972.
2 Collen MF. Hospital computer systems. New York: Wiley, 1974.
3 Bakker AR. Hospital information systems: scope, design, architecture. Amsterdam: North-Holland, 1992.
4 Leguit FA. The case: Leiden University Hospital information system. In: Bakker AR, Ball MH, Scherrer JR, Willems JL (eds). Towards new hospital information systems (Proceedings of a private IFIP IMIA working conference). Amsterdam: Elsevier, 1988: pp 59–64.
5 Melnick I, Biggs JD. The computer and your practice. Urol Clin North Am 1986; 13: 47–58.
6 Morrison LM, Small DR, Glen ES. Computer applications in a urology department. Br J Urol 1991; 67: 257–262.
7 Engelmann U, van Wallenberg H, Kohl U, Geesken E. Management of clinical data in urology. Br J Urol 1988; 61: 527–530.
8 Harrison GSM. The Winchester experience with the TDS hospital information system. Br J Urol 1991; 67: 532–0.
9 Wickham JEA, Charlton CAC, Richards B et al. A computer-based record and organisation system for a department of urology. Br J Urol 1975; 47: 345–357.
10 Chapple CR, Malone-Lee JG. A microcomputer software package for videocystometry. Neurourol Urod 1987; 6: 209.
11 Cardozo LD, Stanton SL, Bennett AE. Design of a urodynamic questionnaire. Br J Urol 1978; 50: 269–274.
12 Rose MB, Georghiades PA, Dowsland WB. A computer program for urology. Br J Urol 1985; 57: 257–260.
13 Abrams P, Stott M, Lewis P, Roskar E. A computerised urodynamic proforma with teaching facility and automatic report generation. Neurourol Urodynam 1987; 6: 201–202.
14 Quaak MJ, Westerman RF, van Bemmel JH. Comparisons between written and computerised patient histories. BMJ 1987; 295: 184–190.
15 Glen E, Small DR, Morrison LM, Pollock K. Urological history-taking and management recommendations by microcomputer. Br J Urol 1989; 63: 117–121.
16 Pringle M. Using computers to take patient histories. BMJ 1988; 297: 697–698.
17 Lucas RW, Card WI, Knill-Jones RP et al. Computer interrogation of patients. BMJ 1976; 2: 623–625.
18 Glen E, Small DR, Morrison LM, Dawes HA, Cherry L. Computerised urological history taking: its development and application in an open access incontinence resource centre. Int Urogynecol J 1991; 2: 73–76.
19 Kelleher CJ, Cardozo LD. An expert system for the diagnosis of detrusor instability. Int Urogynecol J 1993; 4: 23.
20 Hatano T, Osawa A, Kramer AEJL, Jonas U. Development of a PC-based expert system for lower urinary tract pressure–flow studies. World J Urol 1990; 8: 163–166.
21 Hatano T, Osawa A, Kramer AEJL, Jonas U. Development of a computer-based expert system for lower urinary tract pressure–flow studies. Neurourol Urodynam 1989; 8: 409–410.
22 Hatano T, Osawa A, Kramer AEJL, Jonas U. Entering data into an expert system for lower urinary tract pressure–flow studies. Urol Int 1991; 47(Suppl 1): 48–51.
23 Jonas U, Kramer AEJL. Trends in future urodynamics: computer support–data

base–digitised imaging. Urol Int 1991; 47(Suppl 1): 9–15.

24 Modur PN, Griffiths DJ. Automatic pattern recognition of cystometrogram. Proceedings of the 22nd Annual Meeting of the International Continence Society, Canada. 1992. Abstract.

25 Cardozo LD, Khullar V, Anders K, Hill S. Ambulatory urodynamics: a useful urogynaecological service? Proceedings of the 27th British Congress of Obstetrics and Gynaecology, Ireland, 1995. Abstract.

26 Glen E. Microcomputers and microprocessors in urology: present and future. Br J Urol 1983; 55: 588–590.

Section 4 Clinical Disorders

18 Genuine stress incontinence

INTRODUCTION

Genuine stress incontinence is defined as the involuntary loss of urine when the intravesical pressure exceeds the maximum urethral closure pressure in the absence of detrusor activity.[1] It is a urodynamic diagnosis and is thus not synonymous with the symptom or sign of stress incontinence.

To understand the aetiology and pathophysiology of the condition, it is necessary to have a comprehension of both lower urinary tract anatomy (see Ch. 3) and physiology (see Ch. 3). Armed with this knowledge, it is possible to comprehend the dysfunction which results in genuine stress incontinence and to speculate on the mechanisms via which treatments may effect a cure.

PREVALENCE OF GENUINE STRESS INCONTINENCE

Genuine stress incontinence is the commonest cause of incontinence in women, demonstrable in 40–60% of those investigated. Thomas et al.[2] reported that the symptom of stress incontinence was more common between the ages of 45 and 54, while urge incontinence increased with age between 35 and 64. Kondo et al[3] examined the prevalence of stress incontinence in different age groups and found a maximum prevalence of 43% in the 50-year-old age group. Although the prevalence was less in both younger and older women, in all ages it was more common than the symptom of urge incontinence.

Since genuine stress incontinence is a urodynamic diagnosis, it is more useful to consider the incidence relative to other causes of incontinence. Table 18.1 is a comparison of data from the Leeds Urodynamic Clinic and the Department of Urogynaecology at King's College Hospital.[4]

PATHOPHYSIOLOGY

For continence to be maintained, the urethral and pelvic anatomy must be intrinsically intact, and there should be co-ordinated central and peripheral neurological control. Genuine stress incontinence may occur as a result of an incompetent urethral closure mechanism, anatomical

Table 18.1   A comparison of urodynamic diagnosis between the Leeds Urodynamic Clinic and the Department of Urogynaecology at King's College Hospital

Diagnosis	King's College Hospital (%)	Leeds (after Jarvis) (%)
Genuine stress incontinence (GSI)	44.8	47.5
Detrusor instability (DI)	39.1	37.7
Mixed GSI and DI	8.3	5.2
Sensory urgency	2.9	3.7
Normal urodynamics	5.1	4.4
Chronic retention	–	1.2
Fistula	–	0.3

disturbance of a competent urethral closure mechanism or indeed a combination of both. A defect may be solely responsible or part of a multifactorial cause for the development of genuine stress incontinence.

Neurological factors

Nerve damage may occur by compression or stretching. Partial damage and axonal loss leads to reinnervation from remaining axons such that each axon ultimately supplies a greater number of muscle fibers. The motor units (axon and motor fibers) are therefore larger. Electrophysiological studies have been used to document damage to striated muscle motor innervation.[5] Using single-fiber electromyography (EMG) a quantitative estimate of the number of muscle fibers in a single motor unit (the fiber density) can be obtained. An increased fiber density indicates reinnervation following denervation.[6] Pudendal nerve terminal motor nerve latency has also been used to ascertain damage.[7] An increased latency indicates a denervation injury to the pelvic floor.[7]

In women with stress incontinence, neurophysiological studies have demonstrated partial denervation of the anal sphincter,[8] pubococcygeus[6] and urethral striated sphincter.[9]

Anderson[8] measured fiber density in the external anal sphincter in 35 women with genuine stress incontinence and 14 continent women. The mean fiber density in incontinent women was 1.96 and in normal women 1.5 (p <0.002). These findings were supported by Snooks et al,[10] who showed that incontinence was not found when the single-fiber EMG density was less than 1.9 or when the pudendal terminal motor latency (PTML) was less than 2.5.

Smith et al[6] performed single-fiber EMG of the pubococcygeal muscle in 69 asymptomatic women and 105 women with stress incontinence or genitourinary prolapse or both. Continent women who had borne children demonstrated an increasing fiber density with age when compared with age-matched nulliparous women. Asymptomatic women who were parous had increased pelvic floor denervation but generally not as great as those with stress incontinence. They concluded that the pelvic floor is partially denervated in women with stress incontinence. Furthermore, it was suggested that partial denervation and reinnervation might be part of the normal aging process.

Smith et al[7] demonstrated that PTMLs to the external anal and urethra sphincters were similar in continent nulliparous and multiparous women but latency to the anal sphincter was prolonged in women with genuine stress incontinence. Prolonged PTML was found to correlate well in women with genuine stress incontinence.

Histological evidence supporting the concept of denervation and reinnervation is reported by Gilpin et al,[11] who obtained biopsies from the pubococcygeal muscle of two groups of women, one group with incontinence, the other continent. In the symptomatic women there was a significant increase in the number of muscle fibers showing pathological damage.

In summary, since denervation leads to inefficient muscle function, this may result in weakness of the pelvic floor. Pressure transmission to the proximal urethra is essential for the maintenance of continence. The levator muscle contracts to support the proximal urethra and bladder base and should the levator fail to contract efficiently pressure transmission will be reduced and leakage of urine will occur.

Fascial factors

It has been shown that the vaginal wall forms a supportive sling beneath the urethra.[12] The musculofascial elements of the paraurethral tissue attach to the levator ani and arcus tendineus fasciae pelvis providing further urethral support. Disruption of these tissues may lead to fascial defects and anterior vaginal wall prolapse. Richardson et al[13] described four fascial defects, one of which, the lateral fascial defect, was associated with cystourethrocele and genuine stress incontinence. Anatomically, this consisted of a division of the pubocervical fascia between the vagina and the pelvic wall.

Furthermore, Landon & Smith[14] demonstrated that abdominal wall collagen was less elastic in women with stress incontinence than in continent controls. Sayer et al[15] found that in women with stress incontinence there was abnormal cross-linking in the collagen fibrils of the pubocervical fascia.

Microscopically, type I collagen forms thick strong fiber units, whereas type III collagen forms thin weak and isolated fibers[16]. A reduction in type I collagen compared to type III collagen has been found in women with urodynamically proven genuine stress incontinence. Norton et al[17] reported similar findings in parous women with genuine prolapse and genuine stress incontinence.

Connective tissue elements have also been implicated in the functional properties of the urethra[18] and it has been suggested that the improvement in urethral pressure following estrogen therapy is mediated by a direct effect on fibroblasts.[19]

Muscular factors

Anthropologically, adaptation to the upright position has altered the function of the pelvic floor in humans such that its contractile ability has been substituted for tensile strength. Fascial tissue has replaced muscle and the pelvic floor now acts to support the pelvic organs. Damage and atrophy can occur, leading to incontinence and prolapse.[11,20] However, partial restoration of function is possible with pelvic muscle exercise.

The levator ani muscle is composed of two types of muscle fiber.[21] Type I are small diameter slow twitch fibers suited to prolonged tonic activity and are responsible for normal pelvic floor tone and support of the pelvic organs. The type II fibers are large-diameter fast twitch fibers which are able to contract rapidly and strongly to maintain pelvic support during raised intra-abdominal pressure. Gosling et al[22] showed that type I fibers account for 95% of the muscle mass of the pelvic floor whilst the striated urethral sphincter was found to contain only type II fibers.

In a histological and histochemical study of pelvic floor biopsies obtained from 16 women with genuine stress incontinence and 11 normal controls, Gilpin[11] found that incontinent women had an increased proportion of type I fibers, hypertrophy of the type II fibers and increased abnormality of microscopic muscle characteristics including fiber splitting and cell necrosis. It is postulated that these findings are attributable to partial denervation and indeed the EMG findings corroborate this.

Thus denervation, fascial defects and muscular damage can all lead to the development of genuine stress incontinence.

ETIOLOGY

The etiology of genuine stress incontinence is multifactorial. Those factors that may result in its development are shown below:

1. Increased abdominal pressure
   a. Chronic constipation
   b. Heavy exercise
   c. Abdominopelvic tumors
   d. Chronic pulmonary disease
   e. (Obesity)
2. Urethral incompetence
   a. Urethral hypermobility
   b. Damaged intrinsic sphincteric mechanism
   c. Periurethral fibrosis
   d. Denervation
      i. α-adrenergic blockade
      ii. β-adrenergic stimulation
   e. Hypo-estrogenism
   f. Trauma
      i. Childbirth
      ii. Surgery
   g. Decreased or absent pressure transmission
   h. Decreased or absent reflex striated muscle contraction
3. Bladder overdistension
   a. Neuropathic (overflow incontinence)
   b. Infrequent voiding
4. Congenital abnormalities
   a. Short urethra
   b. Epispadias.

Age

The prevalence of urinary incontinence increases with age. Thomas[2] found that the symptom of stress incontinence was more common before the age of 65, and that the complaints of mixed stress and urge incontinence were more frequent thereafter.

Surgical failure is more likely in the elderly patient[23] due to poor tissues, inefficient healing and loss of urethral closure pressure, the latter a part of the normal aging process.[24]

Racial origin

There is little epidemiological information regarding the racial differences in stress incontinence; however, genital prolapse, enterocele and stress incontinence are less frequent in Negro, Eskimo and Oriental women. Indeed, anatomical differences between Western and Chinese women have been described in a cadaveric study by Zacharrin.[25] The general anatomic relationship of the levator ani muscle and the urethra was similar in both races, but the muscle bundles of the Chinese women were thicker and extended more laterally on the arcus tendineus than those of the Western women. Additionally, the fascia of the pelvic diaphragm extending from the levator ani muscles to the posterior pubourethral ligaments was particularly dense.

Pregnancy and childbirth

The effect of pregnancy and childbirth on the development of genuine stress incontinence is fully explained in Ch. 28.

The menopause

Estrogen receptors have been identified in the female urethra, pubococcygeal muscle and trigone.[26] Urethral closure pressure is dependent upon epithelial, vascular and smooth muscle elements all of which may be adversely affected by estrogen deficiency. However, there is conflicting evidence concerning the therapeutic benefit of estrogen therapy in genuine stress incontinence. This will be further discussed in Ch. 29.

Obesity

It is widely believed that obesity is an etiological factor in genuine stress incontinence although little scientific evidence exists to justify this impression. Dwyer et al[27] reported that obesity was significantly more common in women with stress incontinence than in the normal population. There was, however, no difference in the urodynamic evaluation between obese and non-obese women. This finding has been confirmed by Burton et al.[28]

Surgery is technically more difficult in the obese patient and this may account for the reported reduction in long-term cure rates for incontinence surgery.[29] However, Stanton[23] did not conclude obesity to be a significant factor in failure of surgery.

Often, obese women with a diagnosis of genuine stress incontinence are encouraged to lose weight to help their symptoms, and this view has been reinforced amongst morbidly obese incontinent women. Bump[30] found subjective and objective improvement in 12 incontinent women who had surgically induced weight loss (gastric bypass). The mean weight was 131.5 kg before operation and 88.1 kg after. One year after the operation only 3 women suffered from incontinence and only one required surgery for persistent symptoms. The mechanism for improved continence has been shown urodynamically, including superior pressure transmission and reduced urethral mobility. This is an encouraging report, but without the drastic intervention of surgery, obese women often find it difficult to lose weight with exercise because of their incontinence.

Chronic constipation

Straining at stool and an increased frequency of bowel habit is significantly more common amongst women with stress incontinence and prolapse than in normal controls. It has been suggested that repetitive straining due to constipation may damage pelvic innervation through repeated stretch injury to the nerves. However, constipation, straining at defecation and pelvic floor descent may themselves result from pelvic floor damage at childbirth. The clinical significance of straining at stool therefore remains unclear.

Summary

The etiology of genuine stress incontinence is multifactorial. Pregnancy, vaginal delivery, the menopause and congenital weakness contribute much to its causation. In simple terms, mechanical injury leads to descent of the proximal urethra and bladder base, impairing pressure transmission and allowing leakage of urine. Damage to the nerve supply of the pelvic floor and urethral rhabdosphincter following childbirth predispose to and compound pelvic floor descent. Predisposing factors may include abnormal collagen composition. Constipation, obesity and a chronic cough may exacerbate fascial and nerve damage.

CLINICAL FEATURES IN GENUINE STRESS INCONTINENCE

A detailed history should be taken and a full examination performed as outlined in Ch. 6. The physical examination of patients prior to surgery should also include the assessment of vaginal mobility and establish whether an enterocele is present as this may well influence the type of surgery. The presence of an enterocele should be noted since colposuspension may exacerbate this and a Moschowitz procedure at the time of colposuspension should be considered.

If the patient has undergone previous continence surgery, particular attention should be paid to evaluation of the anterior vaginal wall. The position and degree of elevation of the bladder neck should be noted along with comment on the mobility of the urethra, which should be palpated along its length to assess the degree of scarring not infrequently found after previous operations to cure stress incontinence. Additionally, assessment of the capacity, mobility and fixation of the vagina are of importance when considering surgery.

Stress incontinence as a symptom is the patient's description of involuntary loss of urine associated with coughing, sneezing or physical exercise. As a sign, it is the demonstrable involuntary urine loss with increased intra-abdominal pressure (ICS). However, genuine stress incontinence is a urodynamic diagnosis and can therefore only be made after full investigation.

INVESTIGATION

Methods of investigation are described fully elsewhere in the book. If a woman complains solely of the symptom of stress incontinence, without any symptoms of bladder irritability, there is only a 90% chance that she will have urodynamically confirmed genuine stress incontinence.[31] Such women who prefer to avoid surgery may be allowed a trial of conservative treatment prior to formal investigation. Failure to respond to pelvic floor exercises is an indication for urodynamic studies.

When considering surgery it is unwise to operate without at least excluding voiding difficulties, as the results may be disastrous. A peak urinary flow rate and estimation of post-micturition residual are the minimum investigations required prior to surgery. If urine loss is not demonstrated on examination, a pad test should be performed to verify and quantify the degree of incontinence.[32]

Videocystourethrography is the current investigation of choice for stress incontinence[33] and is mandatory in cases of failed previous surgery. However, subtracted cystometry without fluoroscopy is adequate for most women with stress incontinence. Urodynamic investigation is undertaken not only to diagnose genuine stress incontinence, but also to exclude detrusor instability and voiding difficulties.

Intensive investigation is not required in all cases; indeed, the observation that nearly all women in whom stress incontinence is seen on clinical examination have genuine stress incontinence has led some investigators[34,35] to question whether such women require urodynamic assessment prior to surgery. Nevertheless, treatment without a definitive diagnosis can lead to despondency in patient and physician alike. The majority of patients present with mixed symptoms, and in the knowledge that clinical diagnostic accuracy is poor, treatment without investigation should not be encouraged.

CONSERVATIVE MANAGEMENT OF STRESS INCONTINENCE

Conservative treatment has few complications, does not compromise future surgery and should be available as an option to all incontinent women. The indications for conservative treatment are outlined below:

- extremes of age
- pregnancy or intention to become pregnant
- portpartum condition
- unfitness for surgery
- unwillingness to undergo surgery

- limitation of incontinence to occasional occurrence (e.g. during sport)
- failure to regard incontinence as a major subjective problem
- long waiting lists for surgery
- complicating urodynamic factors, e.g. major voiding difficulty, mixed incontinence.

Conservative treatment is relatively inexpensive and readily available and can be implemented and performed on an out-patient basis prior to specialist consultation. The different types of conservative therapy are shown below:

1. Physiotherapy
   a. Pelvic floor exercises
   b. Vaginal cones
   c. Positive feedback (perineometer)
   d. Faradism
   e. Interferential therapy
   f. Maximal electrical stimulation
2. Drugs
   a. Estrogen
   b. α-Adrenergic agents
3. Mechanical devices
   a. Bladder neck support prosthesis
   b. Contraceptive diaphragm
   c. Hodge pessary
   d. Vaginal tampon.

Physiotherapy

Since physiotherapy is resource-consuming for the service and time-consuming for the patient, application of selection criteria would seem appropriate. Additionally, since good results depend upon patient motivation, properly trained staff are required and appropriate patient follow-up is essential to make this form of treatment effective.

Wilson et al[36] identified predictive factors for successful treatment. Age, degree of incontinence and previous continence surgery were of positive predictive value. However, parity, weight and initial perineometry readings were not predictive of success or failure. Tapp et al[37] suggested that premenopausal patients with a short history of incontinence were more likely to be cured. Subsequently, this group developed criteria for selection of patients for physiotherapy based on a visual analog symptom score and parameters of the stress urethral pressure profile. The different forms of physiotherapy are fully evaluated in Ch. 37.

Mechanical devices

Mechanical devices are particularly useful for patients who have occasional incontinence associated with certain activities (e.g. sport),[38] or who have not responded to other forms of treatment and are unsuitable for surgery.

Nygaard[39] compared the use of a Hodge pessary or a support tampon for reducing the amount of incontinence during aerobic-style exercise. Eighteen women were randomly allocated either to a Hodge pessary, a tampon, or a control group. All women completed all three phases of the study. Objective assessment consisted of pad weight gain during a 40-min exercise regimen. However, genuine stress incontinence was not confirmed on urodynamic testing. The authors used 4 g as the cut-off for incontinence, as assessment of a continent group of women demonstrated this to be the amount of pad weight gain due to sweat and vaginal secretions. Patients were blinded to what form of treatment they had. The control group had a pessary inserted and then removed to try and blind them to the type of device being used. The results demonstrate that overall 36% of women became continent with the use of a pessary and 58% with the use of a tampon. However, in women who lost less than 15 g of urine in the control group, 57% became continent with the pessary and 86% with a tampon. The paper clearly demonstrates the use of a tampon to reduce urine loss during exercise in women with incontinence. It should be noted that the tampon was inserted into the lower third of the vagina to give better urethral support.

Suarez et al[40] assessed the effectiveness of a contraceptive diaphragm in the treatment of urodynamically proven genuine stress incontinence in 12 patients. Eleven patients claimed complete resolution of their genuine stress incontinence. However, two withdrew from the study as they found the device uncomfortable. The authors performed urethral pressure profilometry with and without the device in situ. They confirmed that the diaphragm works by causing relative outflow obstruction.

A bladder neck support prosthesis consisting of a ring with two prongs placed in the vagina to support the bladder neck during exertional activities has also been assessed.[41] It is a device that is inserted and removed by the patient during these specific activities. Thirty-two patients were entered into the study and 25 subjects were dry and 5 were improved but had mild incontinence.

A further device that has been studied but which is not available in this country is the urethral plug.[42] This consists of a urethral plate and a soft stalk with one or two spheres along it. The plug is inserted into the end of the urethra preventing leakage of urine. It is removed to enable voiding. Urethral plugs have not gained much popularity and at the moment are not used in clinical practice.

Another device that is not yet available on the market is the foam barrier.[43] It consists of a small triangular foam pad with a layer of hydrophilic adhesive on one side. It is placed within the vulva and the adhesive covers the urethral meatus preventing leakage of urine. Preliminary data suggest that it may have a use in clinical practice.

Recently, Staskin et al[44] have reported the results of an expandable occlusion device for maintenance of continence in women with stress incontinence. The silicone device is inserted into the urethra with the aid of an attached syringe and a small balloon is inflated to maintain it in place. The device is removed for voiding and when not needed by pulling a short string which deflates the balloon. The data suggest a high degree of satisfaction and continence by users of the device.

Complex devices designed to compress the urethra (Edwards spring) or elevate and compress the urethra (Bonnars device) are now only of historical interest.

Pharmacological therapy

The bladder and proximal urethra contain α-adrenergic receptors. Stimulation results in smooth muscle contraction and an increase in the maximum urethral closure pressure. Phenylpropanolamine (PPA) is a major component of many common cold remedies (Night Nurse, Ornade) and has peripheral α-adrenergic agonist properties similar to those of ephedrine without causing significant central sedation. Stewart et al[45] in an uncontrolled trial found a 59% objective reduction in urine loss in 77 stress incontinent women, and an increase in mean urethral closure pressure of 20%, using PPA. Awad et al[46] found that 11 of 13 women with stress incontinence were significantly improved after 4 weeks of PPA, but Obrink & Brunne[47] found only a 10% subjective improvement in women with severe genuine stress incontinence following PPA therapy.

The number of α-adrenergic receptors in the urethra has been found to increase two-to threefold in animal experiments following estrogen therapy. Beisland et al[48] performed a controlled crossover study of PPA (50 mg twice daily) and estriol (1 mg pv daily), separately and in combination, in 20 stress incontinent women. They found that combined treatment was superior, with 8 patients becoming dry and 9 being improved following combined therapy. The advantage of combination therapy is confirmed in the study by Hilton et al.[49]

SURGERY FOR GENUINE STRESS INCONTINENCE

Since the description of suprapubic cystotomy by Baker-Brown in 1864[50] more than 150 different surgical procedures have been designed for the treatment of genuine stress incontinence. Many of the techniques are similar, variations often consisting of no more than a minor alteration. More importantly, the substantial number of operations described reflects the continuing uncertainty over the precise mechanism of continence, the pathophysiology of incontinence and the ideal surgical cure. Classification of the majority of incontinence operations is shown below:

1. Vaginal procedures
   a. Anterior colporrhaphy
   b. Urethrocleisis
   c. implant
2. Abdominal procedures
   a. Marshall-Marchetti-Krantz operation
   b. Burch colposuspension
   c. Vagino-deturator shelf
3. Needle suspension procedures
   a. Stamey
   b. Pererya
   c. Gittes
4. Operations for intrinsic sphincteric weakness
   a. Sling operations
      i. Organic slings (rectus sheath, fascia lata)
      ii. Synthetic slings (Mersilene, Silastic, Vicryl, Gore-Tex)

       b. Periurethral bulk-enhancing agents
         i. GAX collagen
         ii. Macroplastique
   5. Laparoscopic procedures
       a. Laparoscopic Stamey procedure
       b. Laparoscopic Burch colposuspension
   6. Salvage operations
       a. Artificial urinary sphincter
       b. Neourethra
       c. Urinary diversion (ileal conduit)
       d. Mitroffanoff procedure.

Choice of operative procedure

When the results of different procedures are compared, the patients should ideally be randomized to the different treatment arms. However, with surgery for genuine stress incontinence, the picture is more complicated. In certain situations one procedure may be superior to another, whereas in a different situation the converse may be true. In addition, the surgeon may perform one procedure better than another, which would further influence results. Superimposed on the success rate of the operation is the complication rate. It may be that an operation with a slightly lower success rate is justified due to a markedly reduced complication rate.

There are numerous reports in the literature of different operations with their success rates. Some reports give subjective success rates whereas others concentrate on objective cure rates. Also the length of follow-up is variable. Some studies examine an individual operation whereas others are comparisons of two or more. Where a patient is subjectively cured but objectively not, the question remains whether this is a success or failure. Finally, where an operation is adopted and its success rate reported, it is imperative that the exact method be described, as the operator may have modified the procedure slightly and therefore influenced the results. Ideally, each patient should be selected for the most appropriate operation on an individual basis, and the long-term success of such a policy scrutinized.

Jarvis[51] has recently reported the results of a meta-analysis of the reported success rates of operations where the diagnosis of genuine stress incontinence was made preoperatively. This is a good attempt to compare different procedures, but there are several flaws that may have influenced the results. The subjective results from different centres may be affected by the enthusiasm of the clinicians, length of follow-up is not standardized, the procedures may have been modified by different surgeons, the skill of each surgeon is not known and the appropriateness of patient selection for each operation is also unknown. In addition, objective cure rate criteria included a pad test, a cystometrogram and ultrasonography. The sensitivity of the different outcome variables may have influenced the reported cure rates. The objective cure rates for the different operations[51] reported for first-time procedure and recurrent operations are shown in Tables 18.2 and 18.3. Examination of the confidence intervals would suggest that bladder buttress operations and

Table 18.2   Objective cure rates for first procedure

	Mean (%)	95% confidence intervals
Bladder buttress	67.8	62.85–72.75
Marshall-Marchetti-Krantz	89.5	75.72–100
Colposuspension	89.8	87.55–92.05
Non-endoscopic bladder neck suspension	70.2	64.09–76.31
Endoscopic bladder neck suspension	86.7	75.46–97.94
Sling	93.9	89.18–98.62
Injectables	45.5	28.51–62.49

From Jarvis 1994[4]

Table 18.3   Objective cure rates for recurrent incontinence

	Mean (%)	95% confidence intervals
Bladder buttress	ND	
Marshall-Marchetti-Krantz	ND	
Colposuspension	82.5	76.27–88.73
Non-endoscopic bladder neck suspension	75	45–100
Endoscopic bladder neck suspension	86.4	72.38–100
Sling	86.1	82.41–89.79
Injectables	57.8	43.21–72.39

From Jarvis 1994[51]

injectables are unsuitable for first-time procedures. Those procedures with tight confidence intervals probably result in more reliable cure rates. Interestingly, the mean cure rates for recurrent procedures are not much different from those for first procedures. This may reflect the fact that recurrent operations tend to be performed in centers of excellence where the most appropriate procedure is chosen. In addition, the lower limits of the confidence intervals are less, suggesting a less reliable cure. Thus it would appear that the best operation likely to give a cure should be chosen first time round.

It would appear that a Burch colposuspension should be the first-line procedure as it gives consistently high cure rates and has a lower complication rate than sling procedures. Where previous continence surgery has resulted in a scarred vagina a colposuspension may not be possible. A suburethral sling or needle suspension procedure would be more appropriate. Nulliparous patients with severe urogenital atrophy and those who have received pelvic irradiation will also have restricted vaginal mobility and capacity and should be considered for these procedures.

In some women multiple attempts at continence surgery will result in severe urethral scarring and an artificial sphincter or urinary diversion is the only hope for continence. New techniques using injection of microparticulate silicone at the bladder neck may provide an alternative to major surgical intervention in such patients.

Similarly, if the bladder neck is already well elevated and supported, further elevation procedures are unlikely to provide continence. An artificial sphincter, sling procedure or periurethral injection should be considered.

Anterior colporrhaphy is an excellent operation for repair of a cystocele but is less likely to cure genuine stress incontinence and should be avoided. The procedure may have a place in the elderly or infirm due to its relatively low morbidity, although a needle suspension procedure may be more appropriate in combination with an anterior repair.

For many surgeons the choice of primary operative procedure is based on personal preference; however, Green[52] developed a 'plan for the diagnosis and treatment of urinary stress incontinence'. Although now probably less applicable to the contemporary management of incontinence, this was the first attempt to provide a rational scientific basis for surgical treatment grounded on symptoms, signs and extensive investigation including cystourethrograms. The key assumption of the classification was that the anatomical defect involved in genuine stress incontinence was the loss of the posterior urethrovesical angle and that this could be restored by one of three operative approaches – anterior colporraphy, Marshall-Marchetti–Krantz operation or suburethral sling.

The initial classification divided subjects into type 1 and type II, depending on the degree of loss of posterior urethrovesical angle. Later a further type III group was added, describing a specific urethral defect. The green classification is listed below:

Type I Complete or nearly complete loss of the posterior urethrovesical angle, but with the angle of inclination to the vertical of the urethral axis either normal (range 10–30°) or at least less than 45° as shown on the lateral urethrocystogram.

Type II Loss of the posterior urethrovesical angle and an abnormal angle of inclination to the vertical of the urethral axis, greater than 45° or even reversed (greater than 90°).

Type III Normal posterior urethrovesical angle but with an intrinsic defect in urethral closure either secondary to previous continence surgery or as a primary feature, either idiopathic or as part of a neuropathy.

Anterior colporrhaphy

Introduction

The place of anterior repair as a primary continence procedure is contentious. The operation was first described by Shultz;[53] however, it was Howard Kelly[54] who proposed its use as a continence operation, having identified relaxation of tissue at the bladder neck as a potential etiology of urinary leakage. Via a midline incision, the bladder was dissected free and two silk mattress sutures were inserted to plicate the paraurethral tissue at this level. Redundant vaginal skin was excised and the incision closed. This transvaginal approach for the correction of genuine stress incontinence was the predominant continence procedure for some 40 years.

A more extensive repair was advocated by Pacey,[55] who approximated the pubocervical and cardinal ligaments along with the pubococcygeal muscles and pubocervical fascia. A technique to provide a tissue buttress for the bladder neck and distal urethra using the pubococcygeal and bulbocarvernous muscles was described by Ingelman-Sundberg.[56]

Indications

Anterior colporrhaphy has been used to treat primary genuine stress incontinence in the presence of a cystocele. Although this procedure is probably the best operation for anterior vaginal wall prolapse, it is not the best operation for genuine stress incontinence.

In spite of good evidence that anterior colporraphy gives inferior overall results to those of suprapubic procedures,[57,58] a considerable number of gynecological surgeons continue to perform anterior repair as a primary continence procedure.[59]

Many would now advocate that anterior colporrhaphy be reserved for anterior vaginal wall prolapse without stress incontinence, although it may still have a place in the management of the elderly or infirm in view of its low morbidity and the relatively mild degree of postoperative pain.

The advantages of an anterior repair are that it is quick and easy to perform with few complications and a short hospital stay. It enables a large cystourethrocele to be repaired at the same time, but with regard to incontinence the long-term cure rate is poor. However, the operation may be combined with a needle suspension procedure in those patients with a large cystocele and genuine stress incontinence.

Operative technique

The patient is placed in the lithotomy position and a Foley catheter inserted to delineate the urethrovesical junction. A triangular or diamond-shaped incision is made in the anterior vaginal wall. The vaginal skin is excised, care being taken not to make the initial incision too deep and subsequently remove supportive tissue from beneath the bladder neck and proximal urethra. The bladder is dissected free and mobilized upwards. A Kelly or Pacey suture is then inserted to buttress the bladder neck and thereafter the pubocervical fascia may be coapted (Fig. 18.1). The anterior vaginal wall is repaired with continuous or interrupted mattress sutures.

Complications

Anterior colporrhaphy is relatively easy to perform and complications are rare. They include injury to bladder, urethra and ureter, and hematoma formation. Severe hemorrhage is uncommon. Urinary retention may occur postoperatively. Long-term complications include recurrence of incontinence, narrowing of the vagina (which may lead to dyspareunia and urethral stricture.

Mechanism of continence

Suggested mechanisms include support of the urethra and bladder neck,[52] elevation of the bladder neck above the lowest bladder level,[2] and increased resting intraurethral pressure.[60] It is known that continence depends on adequate resistance of a proximal urethra positioned sufficiently high within the pelvis for pressure transmission to occur. In many patients it is not possible to achieve adequate sustained elevation of the bladder neck and upper urethra with an anterior repair and this accounts for the lower primary success rate and greater relapse rate of the procedure.

Results

Subjective cure rates reported in the literature are variable. Low[61] reports a 48% cure rate and Green[62] a 90% cure rate. Objective cure rates of between 30 and 70% have been reported.[57,58,63,64,65,66] Careful selection of patients increases cure rates to between 80 and 90% [67,68] In an extensive

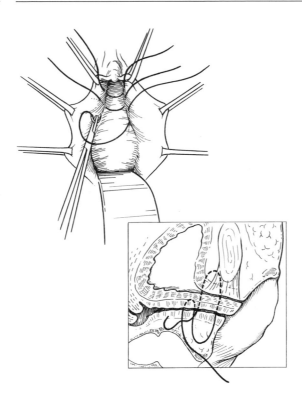

Fig. 18.1 Technique of anterior colporrhaphy for genuine stress incontinence (From Thompson JD, Rock JA (eds) 1992. TeLinde's Operative Gynaecology, 7th edn. JB Lippincott, with permission.)

study of 105 patients, all of whom underwent urodynamic follow-up at 6 weeks, 6 months and 1 and 2 years postoperatively, Beck & McCormack[69] reported an overall 80% cure rate. However, after the technique was modified such that polyglycolic acid (Dexon) sutures were used along with suprapubic rather than urethral catheterization, a 90.9% success rate was achieved.

Urethrocleisis

Introduction

The urethrocleisis operation for stress incontinence was first described by Frewen in 1976.[73] Since his initial report there has been only one further description published in the literature.[74] The procedure is easy to perform, rapid and carries a low morbidity; however, it has not found favor amongst urogynecologists as a primary continence operation.

Operative technique

The original description was of a method of narrowing the urethra, combined with a free urethral graft obtained from the external oblique aponeurosis and secured to the length of the urethra.

A triangular or vertical incision is made in the anterior vaginal wall as for a standard anterior repair. Two vaginal flaps are then elevated and the dissection continues to mobilize the urethra and bladder neck until approximately half the circumference of the urethra is free. Two rows of continuous horizontal Lembert invaginating sutures are placed along the length of the urethra commencing at the bladder neck. A rectangular section of external oblique aponeurosis is then obtained, measuring approximately 3 × 2 cm. This is sutured to the exposed urethra with interrupted non-absorbable sutures. Sufficient narrowing of the urethra is gauged so that it should just admit a 12F Foley catheter. Payne[74] modified the original operation after the first 13 of his series of 62 patients, excluding the urethral graft and performing a urethrocleisis only.

Results

No objective studies exist reporting short- or long-term cure rates for urethrocleisis. The subjective results from Payne's study suggest a 75% subjective cure rate with a further 22% of patients considering themselves improved. Interestingly, 9 out of 10 patients who underwent urethrocleisis plus graft were 'cured', compared with 14 of 23 patients who underwent urethrocleisis alone. It would seem reasonable to suggest that further studies with objective follow-up are indicated to evaluate this simple operation.

Fibrin injection

A new simple procedure has recently been described which can be performed as an out-patient procedure.[75] A Foley catheter is placed in the bladder and the balloon used to identify the bladder neck. A needle is then passed vaginally into the retropubic area to instill local anesthetic. Fibrin sealant is injected either side of the urethra and the urethrovesical area compressed against the back of the symphysis pubis for 15 min. The Foley catheter is then removed and the patient discharged 1 h later. The 24 patients initially reported on had a 63% cure rate (not proven urodynamically). Although the success rate appears poor compared to other procedures, further evaluation is necessary and in addition this procedure is truly a minor one.

Retropubic urethrovesicopexy

Introduction

The limitations of anterior colporrhaphy as a primary continence operation were recognized as early as 1954 by Bailey.[76] Prior to this date a retropubic procedure had been described by Williams, and this involved extraperitoneal dissection of the urethra and bladder neck and the insertion of four pairs of catgut sutures on each side tied to the periosteum of the pubis.

Subsequently, Marshall-Marchetti & Krantz[77] reported surgical elevation of the bladder neck in incontinent males following prostatectomy, with good results; however, the rational application of retropubic procedures to women is credited to Bailey[75] Green[51] and Hodgkinson.[78]

Burch[79] in describing his colposuspension operation recognized that support of the urethra could be achieved by elevation of the vaginal fascia lateral to the urethra, and to avoid the technical difficulty of retaining sutures in the periosteum, inserted the sutures into the ipsilateral iliopectineal ligament (Cooper's ligament), which is better defined and provides greater support. This procedure has since been modified by many surgeons.

Indications

Abdominal operative procedures in appropriately selected patients have a 70–100% cure rate and the long-term results are superior to those of anterior colporrhaphy. The Burch colposuspension and Marshall-Marchetti-Krantz operation (MMK) are now the most widely performed primary procedures for genuine stress incontinence. In the United Kingdom the colposuspension is performed by twice as many gynaecologists as the MMK.[59]

Ideally, urodynamic assessment should be performed prior to consideration of continence surgery; however, not all departments have this facility and therefore clinical evidence of voiding difficulty should be sought, since there is a recognized obstructive effect with the Burch colposuspension.[80] Those patients with symptoms of voiding dysfunction or urodynamic evidence of outflow obstruction should be considered for alternative surgical intervention.

The Marshall-Marchetti-Krantz operation

This procedure, first described by the authors in 1949,[77] has been widely used as a primary continence procedure although in the United Kingdom the Burch colposuspension is performed considerably more frequently.

Operative technique

The patient is placed in the modified lithotomy position and a Foley catheter inserted. A low transverse suprapubic incision is made and the retropubic space entered. The bladder neck and proximal urethra are mobilized from the vagina with the assistance of the index and middle fingers of the surgeon's left hand placed within the vagina. Between one and three sutures are inserted on either side. Each suture should include the paraurethral tissue, the lateral wall of the urethra and a large bite of vaginal wall. A double bite of tissue should be taken if possible. The sutures are then fixed to the periosteum of the superior pubic ramus or the perichondrium of the symphysis pubis (Fig. 18.2). Further sutures may be placed between the anterior surface of the bladder and rectus abdominis to provide additional elevation and support. Care should be taken to avoid overzealous traction on the bladder neck. A Redivac drain should be placed in the retropubic space and a suprapubic catheter used for postoperative urinary drainage.

Complications

The major complication is osteitis pubis (2.5–7%)[51] and abscess formation, requiring antibiotic therapy and possibly incision and drainage. Additionally, problems with retention of the sutures in the periosteum or perichondrium may be experienced.

Results

Many reported series lack objective follow-up. Subjective cure rates of 89%[77] and 90%[81] have been reported. However, studies with objective assessment suggest a far lower cure rate. (Tables 18.4 and 18.5)

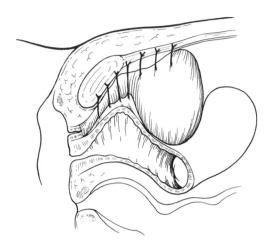

Fig. 18.2 Marshall–Marchetti–Krantz procedure. Sagittal section demonstrating the location of the paraurethral sutures

Table 18.4 Subjective cure rates for anterior colporrhaphy

Reference	No. of patients	% continent	Follow-up (months)
Park & Miller 1988[65]	336	70	60% >60
Pacey 1955[70]	60	65	12–36
Jeffcoate 1961[71]	114	60	24
Jarvis meta-analysis 1994[51]	1481	80.9	>12

Table 18.5 Objective cure rates for anterior colporrhaphy

Reference	No. of patients	% continent	Follow-up (months)
Beck & McCormick 1982[69]	105	80	24
Stanton & Cardozo 1979[57]	25	36	6
Weil et al 1984[63]	30	57	6
Stanton 1985[64]	26	65	3–24
Beck et al 1991[72]	519	64–84	>6
Jarvis meta-analysis 1994[51]	490	72	>12

The Burch colposuspension

Operative technique

The patient is placed in the modified lithotomy position using Lloyd Davies stirrups. The abdomen and vagina are prepared as a sterile operating field to allow manipulation of the vaginal fornices and bladder neck by the surgeon. A Foley catheter is inserted into the bladder and the balloon inflated with 6–10 cm water to enable identification of the bladder neck.

A very low transverse incision is used and the rectus fascia mobilized. Access may be improved by a muscle-cutting incision or division of the recti from their insertion on the symphysis pubis. A self-retaining retractor (Turner-Warwick or Dennis-Brown) is inserted. The abdominal fascia the retropubic space (cave of Retzius) is dissected by blunt and sharp dissection until the paravaginal tissue lateral to the urethra is identified

Table 18.6 Subjective results of Marshall-Marchetti–Krantz procedure

Reference	No. of patients	% continent	Follow-up (months)
Marshall-Marchetti & Krantz 1949[77]	38	74	1–35
Giesen 1962[81]	60	90	>12
Riggs 1986[82]	411	85	6–204
Park 1988[65]	229	72	60–120
Jarvis meta-analysis 1994[51]	6827	92.7	>12

Table 18.7 Objective results of Marshall-Marchetti–Krantz procedure

Reference	No. of patients	% continent	Follow-up (months)
Milani 1985[83]	42	71	>12
Colombo 1993[84]	61	88	24
Jarvis meta-analysis 1994[51]	443	89.2	>12

as a conspicuous white area. Vaginal manipulation assists dissection by elevation of each lateral fornix. The bladder and urethra are further dissected medially off the vaginal fascia to allow good elevation of the fornices (Fig. 18.3).

Two to four sutures of no 1 polyglycolic acid, PDS or Ethibond are inserted into the paravaginal fascia, (Fig. 18.4) ensuring that a good bite of tissue is obtained to secure hemostasis and prevent 'see-sawing'. Some surgeons tie the suture at this point. The needle is then inserted into the ipsilateral iliopectineal ligament. The initial suture is placed at the level of the bladder neck and subsequent sutures more proximally about 1 cm apart. Occasionally, a vertical incision in the vaginal wall may allow elevation of a poorly mobile vaginal fornix secondary to previous surgery or radiotherapy.

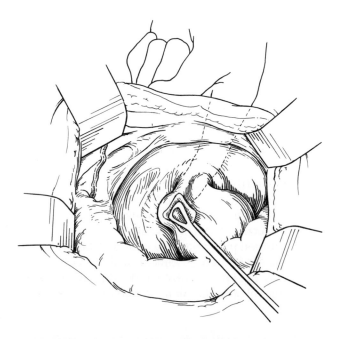

Fig. 18.3 Burch colposuspension. Dissection of the periurethral and paravaginal fascia. The vaginal finger is pushed upward and laterally, with the sponge-holding forceps held firmly

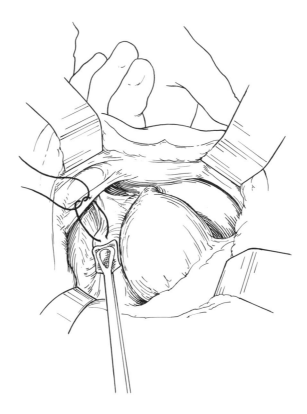

Fig. 18.4 Burch colposuspension. Insertion of the vaginal sutures. The correct point of fixation is determined by pushing the vaginal finger toward the junction of the superior ramus and the body of the symphysis pubis and the suture passed through all layers of the vagina except the mucosa

Once all the sutures are positioned, each lateral fornix is elevated by a\ assistant, allowing the sutures to be tied easily without tension. Normally the vaginal fornices are approximated to the ileopectineal ligament (Figs 18.5 and 18.6), but if the vagina is of restricted capacity, some 'bow stringing' may occur. This does not appear to affect the results. It is th\ practice of some surgeons to inspect the bladder endoscopically c\ initially to instil dye into the bladder to ensure that no sutures hav\ perforated the wall.

The retropubic space is drained using a Redivac suction drain. Depe\ dent upon haemostasis, each side may be drained separately. Suprapubi\ catheterization is advised.[85] Continuous bladder drainage is maintaine\ for 2–6 days, after which the catheter is clamped and the patient e\ couraged to void. Residual urine volumes are measured after each vo\ initially and subsequently at 12-h intervals. When urinary residuals a\ consistently less than 100 ml the suprapubic catheter is removed.

Perioperative complications

Hemorrhage from paravesical veins can be controlled with diathermy\ undersewing. However, most bleeding will be arrested by tying th\ suspension sutures. Bladder or urethral trauma may occur during the\ dissection from the vaginal fascia. Instillation of dilute Bonneys bl\ solution preoperatively allows easier recognition of perforation. The uret\ can be injured or kinked at the level of the most cephalad suture. Th\ may not be recognized at the time of operation and the diagnosis of upp\ tract obstruction will be made late. Perforation of the vaginal epitheliu\

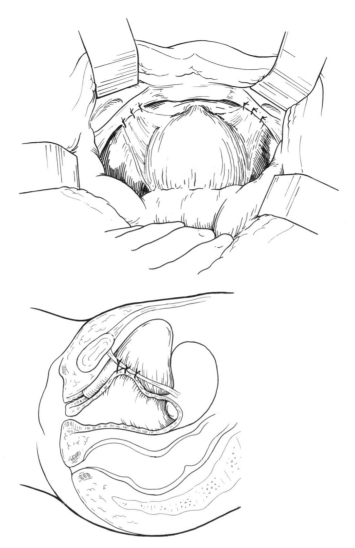

Fig. 18.5 Burch colposuspension. The completed procedure. Three pairs of sutures have been inserted, 1 cm lateral and cephalad of the previous

Fig. 18.6 Burch colposuspension. A sagittal section showing the final position of the bladder neck after elevation. It is useful to compare this figure with Fig. 8.2 (Marshall–Marchetti–Krantz procedure). From Stanton L, Tanagho EA (eds) 1986. Surgery of Female Incontinence, 2nd edn. Springer-Verlag, with permission.)

Postoperative
complications

carries a theoretical risk of retropubic infection but in practice this does not appear to be a problem when prophylactic antibiotics are employed.

Voiding difficulties Voiding difficulty can occur in the early or late post-operative period, perhaps with different etiologies. Late voiding difficulty may represent detrusor decompensation secondary to outflow obstruction.

Voiding difficulties are not uncommon and may be predicted if pre-operative urodynamic assessment shows a reduced peak urinary flow rate of less than 15 ml/s or a maximum voiding pressure of less than 15 cmH$_2$O. Between 12 and 25% of patients who undergo colposuspension are reported to suffer delayed voiding postoperatively and 11–20% have increased residual volumes and reduced flow rates at 3-month follow-up.[23,79] However, Alcalay et al[86] found preoperative factors to be of poor predictive value for postoperative voiding difficulties.

Table 18.8   Voiding difficulties as a result of colposuspension

	Objective voiding difficulties (%)	
	All cases	First operatior
Residual > 100 ml	12	11
Peak flow rate < 15 ml/s	28	26
Residual > 100 ml + PFR < 15 ml/s	2	3

From Cardozo & Cutner 1992[89]

Hilton & Stanton[87] performed postoperative urodynamic studies on 2 women 3 months following Burch colposuspension and found highl significant reduced urinary flow rates and increased voiding pressure. has been shown that in those patients with postoperative voiding di ficulty, the bladder neck is overelevated and relatively fixed.[88] This ha been postulated as the mechanism for postoperative voiding difficulties.

Clinically, many women report concern that their urinary flow rate reduced postoperatively but do not have objective evidence of voidin difficulty (i.e. peak flow rate <15 ml/s and urinary residual >100 ml).

The incidence of voiding difficulties of 100 patients followed up King's College Hospital for between 6 and 12 months is shown Table 18.8.

Enterocele Irectocele formation   This may occur as a result of elevation of th anterior vaginal wall which creates a posterior deficit. If diagnosed pr operatively or recognized at the time of simultaneous hysterectomy Moschcowitz operation can be performed, approximating the uterosacr ligaments and obliterating the pouch of Douglas. The incidence postoperative rectoenterocele is reported to be between 7.6 and 17%.[85,9]

Detrusor instability   It has been shown that detrusor instability arises novo in between 12 and 18.5% of patients postoperatively.[63,86,91,92] occurs more commonly in patients who have undergone previous inco tinence surgery. The incidence of detrusor instability in 100 patier followed up at King's College Hospital for between 6 and 12 months shown in Table 18.9.

Table 18.9   Prevalence of detrusor instability resulting from colposuspension

	Detrusor instability (%)	
	All cases	First operatic
All postoperative cases	14	11
New cases postoperatively	9	5

From Cardozo & Cutner 1992[89]

The cause is not thought to be obstruction and the mechanism remai unknown; however, it seems likely that a proportion of these patie had preoperative detrusor instability that was undetected at cystomet Cardozo et al[91] suggest that damage to the autonomic innervation occ following medial displacement of the bladder base.

Sexual dysfunction It is important to appreciate that incontinence surgery may have deleterious affects on sexual life.[93,94] Elevation of the anterior vagina pulls the posterior vagina upward and forward causing a palpable ridge at the midsection of the posterior vaginal wall. This can lead to dyspareunia, although the tissue relaxes with time. Alteration of the vaginal axis, which allows enterocele formation, also causes positional dyspareunia.

Results

The original subjective report by Burch[79] describes a 100% cure rate in 53 patients, 4 of whom had undergone a previous continence procedure. In a subsequent report by Burch of an extended series of 143 patients, the overall failure rate was 7%. Objective cure rates determined on the basis of postoperative urodynamic studies are usually lower, Hilton & Stanton[87] report a 90% cure rate and Stanton & Cardozo[57] and Galloway[95] 84% cure rates. A comparison of published results with subjective (Table 18.10) and objective (Table 18.11) data are shown below.

The results of Burch colposuspension in patients having undergone previous attempts at continence surgery are uniformly worse. Table 18.12 shows comparative data for patients undergoing subsequent colposuspension.

Table 18.10 Subjective results of Burch colposuspension

Reference	No. of patients	% continent	Follow-up (months)
Burch 1961[79]	53	100	Unstated
Burch 1968[81]	143	93	10–60
Cardozo & Cutner 1992[89]	100	91	6–12
Jarvis meta-analysis 1994[51]	1726	89.6	>12

Table 18.11 Objective results of colposuspension

Reference	No. of patients	% continent	Follow-up (months)
Stanton & Cardozo 1979[57]	25	84	4
Mundy 1983[96]	26	73	12
Stanton 1984[97]	60	83	12
Galloway 1987[95]	50	84	6
Stanton 1976[85]	32	80	6–30
Milani 1985[83]	44	79	>12
Cardozo & Cutner 1992[89]	100	80	6–12
Herbertsson 1993[98]	72	90.3	84–144
Jarvis meta-analysis 1994[51]	2300	84.3	>12

Table 18.12 The results of colposuspension in patients having undergone previous unsuccessful surgery

Reference	% continent	Follow-up (months)
Stanton 1984[97]	65	60
Galloway 1987[95]	63	54
Stanton & Cardozo 1979[57]	77	12
Jarvis meta-analysis 1994[51]	82.5	>12

The vagino-obturator shelf operation and paravaginal repair

Introduction

The vagino-obturator shelf (VOS) procedure and paravaginal repair are relatively similar retropubic procedures. In the United Kingdom they are not widely performed but remain popular in the United States.

The basis for this procedure is that bladder neck support is provided by the anterior vagina and endopelvic fascia which attach to the arcus tendineus fasciae pelvis at the lateral pelvic wall, providing a supportive shelf beneath bladder neck and proximal urethra which resists increases in intra-abdominal pressure and allows urethral compression with straining. Lateral detachment of the vagina and endopelvic fascia from the arcus tendineus fasciae pelvis leads to increased mobility of the bladder neck, reduced urethral compression with straining and hence stress incontinence. Richardson et al[99] identified defects in the endopelvic fasciae and devised the paravaginal repair described below. Turner-Warwick[33] described a similar procedure which is also outlined. The aim of these procedures is to restore the bladder neck to its normal anatomical position without excessive elevation, which may lead to voiding difficulty.

The paravaginal repair

Through a low transverse suprapubic incision, the retropubic space is entered. The loose areolar tissue is broken down digitally and the bladder and vagina reflected medially exposing the lateral pelvic fascia at the level of the bladder neck. The bladder is separated from the pelvic sidewall down to the level of the ischial spine. The arcus tendineus fasciae pelvis is identified as a white band of tissue which runs from the posteroinferior part of the symphysis pubis to the ischial spine. Blunt dissection is continued to this point and the lateral paravaginal defect may be seen either as an avulsion of the vagina from the arcus tendineus fasciae pelvis or as a defect between the latter and the obturator internus.

The repair is performed using non-absorbable sutures and the defect is closed commencing at the level of the bladder neck. The suture is placed through a thick bite of vagina (excluding vaginal epithelium) and then inserted into the arcus tendineus fasciae pelvis and underlying obturator internus. The placement of this suture is of paramount importance since it must lift the urethra back into the pelvis. Subsequent sutures are placed at 1-cm intervals until the defect is closed. Usually three sutures are placed anterior to the first and a further three posterior to it. Insertion of the sutures may be facilitated by insertion of the surgeons hand into the vagina to elevate the appropriate vaginal fornix.

The vagino-obturator shelf procedure differs in that the lateral pelvic fascia is incised at the level of the bladder neck, and the vagina sutured to the obturator internus muscle throughout the length of the incision from the bladder neck to the base.

Complications

The dissection required for a paravaginal repair is less extensive than that required for a Burch colposuspension and therefore perioperative hemorrhage from the paravesical veins is infrequent. However, damage to the obturator vessels can prove troublesome. Injury to the ureters and obturator nerve, both of which are close to the suspensory sutures, may also occur.

Postoperative enterocele and rectocele are considered to be less frequent than with other retropubic procedures because overelevation of the vagina which compromises the support of the peritoneum of the pouch of Douglas, does not occur.

Results

There are no objective studies evaluating long-term cure rates from these procedures. However, Richardson et al[13] report subjective cure in 58 of 60 patients followed up for an average of 20 months. In a later series of 233 patients a 95% subjective cure was observed.[99] Shull[100] also reports high subjective cure rates of 97%.

Endoscopically guided bladder neck suspension

Introduction

Needle bladder neck suspension was first described in 1959 by Pereyra. Numerous modifications of the technique have subsequently been described,[101,102,103,104,105] although the principles of surgical cure are the same.

Indications

Needle bladder neck suspension procedures are indicated for either primary or recurrent genuine stress incontinence. Their use has been advocated in the old or frail in whom formal retropubic procedures may lead to higher morbidity or mortality. Those patients in whom colposuspension may be technically difficult because of poor vaginal mobility or narrowing, or where recurrent surgery has led to scarring, would also be more suited to a needle suspension.

The procedures for the most part are relatively quick and easy to perform. A general anesthetic is not mandatory since regional anesthesia is quite adequate. Hospital stay may be reduced in comparison to that following open retropubic procedures if the primary care team are willing to manage the suprapubic catheter.

The Pereyra procedure

Operative technique The patient is placed in the lithotomy position and a Foley catheter inserted into the urethra. A short transverse incision is made in the midline of the anterior abdominal wall just above the symphysis pubis. The Pereyra needle is passed through the abdominal incision advancing posteriorly guided by a finger in the vagina, emerging through the vaginal wall 2 cm posterior and 1 cm lateral to the urethra. A nylon or Prolene suture is threaded on to the needle (no. 30 stainless steel wire was used originally), which is then withdrawn about 1 cm and rotated so that the eye of the needle may be threaded with the opposite end of the suture. The needle is then withdrawn back through the abdominal wound carrying the suture with it. A loop of suture remains under the anterior vaginal wall. The procedure is repeated on the opposite side after which the abdominal ends are tied together, fixing bladder neck and urethra in a high retropubic position.

1967 modification Pereyra reported his first modification because of a frequent 'cheesewire' effect of the wire suture material cutting through the anterior vaginal wall. This was replaced with catgut. Additionally, he described a technique for plication of the bladder neck, thereby creating a suburethral shelf with concomitant greater support.

1978 modification A further modification (Fig. 18.7A) was described by Pereyra & Lebherz in 1978.[106] The use of catgut as a suspensory suture also resulted in a cheesewire effect, and it was replaced by Prolene. However, a more major alteration was the exploration of the cave of Retzius per vaginam allowing direct observation of each step of the operation.

The lateral attachments of the urethra to the inferior pubic ramus are divided by blunt dissection from the bladder neck to a point proximal to the external meatus. A suture is then passed several times through the endopelvic fascia to include the posterior pubourethral ligaments, plicating the tissue and preventing pull-through. The Pereyra needle is then passed, guided by a finger inserted into the retropubic space per vaginam. The suspensory sutures are then tied to the anterior rectus fascia. This procedure is known as the modified Pereyra operation.

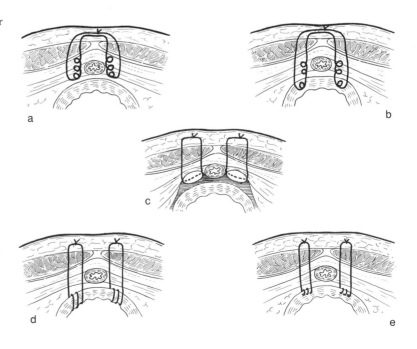

Fig. 18.7 Endoscopic bladder neck suspensions. A cross-section showing the alternative anchoring sutures used for the procedures described in the text. **A** Modified Pereyra: helical stitch through paraurethral ligament and detached endopelvic fascia. **B** Raz operation: helical suture through the endopelvic fascia anchored within the vaginal wall. **C** Stamey procedure, with buttresses placed in fascia adjacent to bladder neck. These are intended to prevent suture pull-through. **D** Gittes procedure (no-incision urethropexy). Sutures are placed through the full thickness of the vaginal wall. (From Karram MM. In: Hurt WG (ed) 1992. Clinical Urogynaecology. Aspen, with permission.)

a b c d e

Postoperative complications Perforation of the bladder occurred in 2 patients in Pereyra's 1967 series and a suture was placed through the bladder in 1 further patient. Cellulitis and retropubic hematoma were also described. Over 30% of patients complained of postoperative urgency lasting up to 3 months. The risk of hemorrhage is greater in those modifications where the retropubic space is explored; however, venous bleeding may be controlled by tamponade from a Foley catheter inserted retropubically. Similar complications have been reported in other series.

Results Pereyra & Lebherz[102] reported a 94.8% subjective cure rate in a series of 172 patients followed up for between 1 and 7 years. Kursch[107] reported the results in 25 patients; 64% described initial cure but this fell to 50% after 1 year. It should be noted that in this series catgut was used as the suspensory suture. Litvak & McRoberts[108] had greater success, with a 91% cure in 35 patients after 3 years, and Backer & Probst[109] reported similar results in 188 patients, 82% of whom still had symptomatic cure between 1 and 9 years after operation.

In an objective comparative study of the Pereyra procedure and Burch colposuspension, Bhatia & Bergman[110] reported an 85% cure rate at 1 year, and in a similar study by Bergman et al,[66] which included anterior colporrhaphy, a 70% success is reported. Leach et al[111] obtained a 90% primary cure rate at 14 months, which betters all objective studies.

The Pereyra procedure is quick and relatively simple but has remained unpopular because it is performed blind, which can lead to perforation of the bladder or urethra. Additionally, misplacement of suspensory sutures has led to outflow obstruction and chronic retention, because of angulation of the proximal or mid-urethra.

The Stamey modification revived interest in needle suspension procedures and resulted in their widespread use as primary continence operations.

The Stamey operation

Introduction The major modification of the Stamey procedure over that of Pereyra was the use of the cystoscope to check that the needle had not passed through the bladder and was located exactly alongside the bladder neck. He designed three blunt-ended needles, one straight, one with an angulation of 15°, the other with an angulation of 30°. Additionally, to prevent the suspensory sutures cutting through the pubocervical fascia, he used a Dacron vaginal buffer on the suspensory nylon suture.

Table 18.13   Subjective results for the Pereyra needle suspension

Reference	No. of patients	% continent	Follow-up (months)
Pereyra 1959[101]	31	90	14
Pereyra & Lebherz 1967[102]	172	95.8	12–84
Litvak & McRoberts 1974[108]	35	88.6	36–60
Backer & Probst 1976[109]	200	82	6–108
Pereyra & Lebherz 1982[112]	162	88.3	6–60
Riggs 1986[81]	225	84	6–184
Jarvis meta-analysis 1994[51]	1886	77.6	

Table 18.14   Objective results for the Pereyra needle suspension procedure

Reference	No. of patients	% continent	Follow-up (months)	Comments
Weil et al 1984[62]		50	6	
Bhatia & Bergman 1985[110]		85	12	
Leach et al 1987[111]	20	90	14	
Bergman et al 1989[66]		65	12	Comparative study with Burch, Pereyra and anterior repair
Karram & Bhatial 1993[113]	93	63	12	
Jarvis meta-analysis 1994[51]	446	70	>12	

Operative technique (Fig. 18.7B) The patient is placed in the lithotomy position and two short incisions (3-cm) made in the abdomen above the pubic symphysis either side of the midline. A Foley catheter is inserted into the bladder and a transverse or inverted T-incision made in the anterior vaginal wall. Using a combination of blunt and sharp dissection the trigone of the bladder is exposed. The Stamey needle is then advanced through the anterior rectus fascia into the vaginal incision lateral to the bladder neck, which is identified by the balloon of the Foley catheter. A 90° cystoscope is inserted into the urethra to observe that the needle has not perforated the bladder and is located properly in the periurethral tissue at the bladder neck.

A no. 2 monofilament nylon suture is threaded through the eye of the needle, which is then withdrawn through the abdominal incision. The needle is then advanced a second time, 1–2 cm lateral to the previous insertion, and guided into the vaginal incision, distal to the first site again using the cystoscope to ensure safe and appropriate placement. The vaginal end of the suture is then threaded through a 1-cm section of Dacron arterial graft into the eye of the needle and withdrawn once more. The suspensory loop is now complete. The procedure is repeated on the opposite side.

Prior to tying the sutures, closure of the bladder neck can be observed via the cystoscope by elevating them. Some idea of the degree of tension required when tying the sutures can thus be gained, and if adequate closure is not obtained the sutures can be removed and repositioned.

Finally, the anterior vaginal incision is closed and the suspensory sutures tied individually over the rectus fascia. The abdominal incision is closed and a suprapubic catheter inserted.

Postoperative complications Infection is probably more common following the Stamey procedure by virtue of the Dacron graft used to buttress the suspensory sutures. Pain in the abdominal incision is not uncommon and may be related to excessive suture tension. Entrapment of the ilioinguinal nerve will lead to pain in the inner thigh, groin or perineum and may be severe. If suspected, the diagnosis may be confirmed by injection of local anesthetic into the inguinal canal. This complication may be obviated if sutures are inserted medial to the pubic tubercle, hence avoiding the superficial inguinal ring where the nerve exits from the inguinal canal.

Voiding difficulties are more common than with retropubic colposuspension, probably because needle procedures are more obstructive

However, it has been suggested that endoscopy of the bladder neck with a forward viewing cystoscope by an assistant at the time the suspensory sutures are tied may help to achieve the optimum position of the bladder neck and avoid excessive tension.[114]

Injury to the structures of the lower urinary tract should theoretically not go unnoticed with appropriate use of the cystoscope. Nevertheless, it may be argued that injury is less likely with the Pereyra procedure since insertion of the needle into the retropubic space is under fingertip control, although migration of the sutures into the bladder may occur at a later date.

Mechanism of continence Mundy[96] suggested that the mechanism by which the Stamey procedure reestablishes continence is by inducing obstruction at the bladder neck. Postoperative voiding dysfunction has been cited as the evidence for this. Hilton & Mayne[115] have shown a significantly reduced peak urine flow rate in those patients cured by the procedure, although similar findings were not found by Leach et al[111] or Wujanto & O'Reilly.[116] In those studies where postoperative video-urodynamics have been performed, lateral views have confirmed the bladder neck to be placed behind the symphysis pubis but without significant angulation of the proximal urethra.

The mechanism of continence is more likely to be simply bladder neck elevation with improved pressure transmission and compression against the posterior aspect of the symphysis pubis.

Results Stamey has reported three studies with subjective cure rates[103,117,118] describing 69%, 93% and 91% success respectively. Hilton & Mayne[115] report an objective 83% cure rate at 3 months, falling to 68% at 4 years. This compares favorably with other studies in which pre- and postoperative urodynamic studies have been performed.[96,119,120]

The Raz needle suspension   The Raz (1981)[104] modification (Fig. 18.7C) differs from Pereyra's 1978 procedure in that an inverted 'U' vaginal incision is made to allow dissection lateral to the urethra and bladder neck. As with the modified Pereyra the retropubic space is entered to allow greater mobilization of urethra and bladder neck and so that the needle may be passed with fingertip control, reducing the chance of injury to either urethra or bladder. Additionally, the suspensory sutures are placed in the endopelvic fascia and include the full thickness of the vaginal wall lateral to the bladder neck. This theoretically obviates the possibility of outflow obstruction since the sutures do not interfere with normal changes that occur in the

Table 18.15   Subjective results of the Stamey endoscopic bladder neck suspension

Reference	No. of patients	% continent	Follow-up (months)	Comments
Stamey 1973[103]	16	69		
Stamey et al 1975[117]	44	93		
Stamey 1980[118]	203	91	6–48	
Kirby & Whiteway 1989[120]	48	75	6–36	
Jones 1989[121]	76	68	7–30	

Table 18.16   Objective results of the Stamey endoscopic bladder neck suspension

Reference	No. of patients	% continent	Follow-up (months)	Comments
Mundy 1983[96]	51	40	12	
English & Fowler 1988[119]	45	58	6	
Peattie & Stanton 1989[122]	44	40	6	Age > 65 years
Hilton 1989[123]	10	80	24	
Hilton & Mayne 1991[115]	100	83	3	Subjective cure rate at years = 65%

urethra during voiding. Cystoscopy is performed to ensure adequate bladder neck elevation and to inspect for any injury to the urethra, bladder or ureters.

The Gittes procedure

The patient is placed in the modified lithotomy position and a Foley catheter inserted. Two short abdominal suprapubic incisions are made 5 cm lateral to the midline. A 30° Stamey needle is passed through the rectus fascia and advanced posteriorly behind the pubis. The anterior vaginal wall is elevated digitally, lateral to the bladder neck as identified by the balloon of the Foley catheter. The needle is then passed through the vaginal wall. A no. 2 nylon suture is threaded into the eyelet and the needle withdrawn into the abdominal incision. The procedure is repeated such that the second pass emerges in the vagina 1–2 cm distal to the first. An unmounted Mayo needle is then used to take a full-thickness bite of the vaginal wall between the two vaginal perforations and the mattress suture threaded and brought forward. The needle is then passed on the contralateral side and the method repeated. Cystoscopy is performed to examine for injury to the bladder, after which the suspensory sutures may be tied and the abdominal incision closed.

Urethrovesical sling procedures

Introduction

Suburethral slings are not widely used as primary surgical procedures for genuine stress incontinence, probably due to the high complication rate. They are sometimes regarded as a 'last ditch' attempt to offer surgical cure when all else has failed; however, this may be an unjust use of the procedure, for which specific indications exist. Usually using a combined abdominovaginal approach, (Figs. 18.8 and 18.9) organic or synthetic material is used both to provide an incompressible suburethral buttress and elevate the bladder neck and proximal urethra.

The procedure was first described in 1907 by Giordano using a vascular gracilis muscle flap which was brought through the rectus fascia beneath the urethra and attached to the pubis. In 1910 Goebell used the pyramidal muscles, detached from the pubis and tied together beneath the urethra. Numerous other organic slings have been described but all suffered the physiological disadvantage of maintaining an adequate vascular supply and the mechanical problem of placing cumbersome tissue suburethrally.

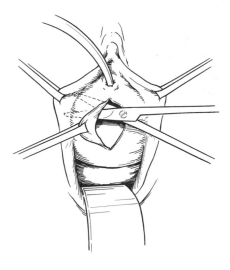

Fig. 18.8 Sling procedure. The anterior vaginal wall is opened at the level of the bladder neck and the retropubic space entered from below. If the combined approach is used, dissection of the retropubic space may be completed abdominally. (From Hurt WG (ed) 1992 Urogynecologic Surgery. Aspen, with permission.)

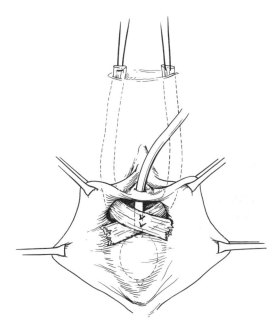

Fig. 18.9 Suburethral sling in which autologous fascia or synthetic material is passed into the retropubic space and tied above the fascia of the rectus abdominis muscle.

In the 1950s Bracht first described the use of a synthetic nylon sling, subsequently Moir[124] used polyethylene gauze (Mercilene) and since then Marlex, Vicryl, Silastic and Gore-Tex have all been used. Only one comparative study between autologous and synthetic slings has been reported[125] and this did not demonstrate a significant difference between the two materials.

Indications

A sling procedure may be considered in patients who have undergone one or more failed attempts at continence surgery and who have developed a functionless, 'drainpipe' urethra because of fibrosis and distortion with reduced urethral mobility. Replacing the proximal urethra intra-abdominally will not restore continence because abdominal pressure transmission cannot occur. Continence in such patients can only be achieved by outflow obstruction.

Several workers have suggested a cut-off of 20 cmH$_2$O of maximum urethral closure pressure for predicting poor outcome for incontinence surgery.[63,126,127] It has been suggested that in these patients a sling, or even artificial sphincter, should be considered.[126,127,128,129,130]

Autologous sling procedures

The Aldridge sling (1942)[174] A triangular incision is made in the anterior vaginal wall and the bladder neck and proximal urethra mobilized. The dissection continues anterosuperiorly to expose the cave of Retzius. A low transverse incision is then made in the abdomen and two strips of external oblique aponeurosis mobilized, leaving the medial end of each attached to the sheath. Each is drawn down through the inner margin of the rectus muscles and sutured beneath the bladder neck, elevating the urethra. Care should be taken to avoid excessive tension, which may lead to retention of urine or avascular necrosis of the urethra. The vaginal and abdominal incisions are then closed.

The Studdiford sling (1944)[175] The Studdiford modification was simply to use several catgut mattress sutures to unite the free ends of the external oblique aponeurotic strips when they were too short to meet in the midline. A more complicated version involved extensive dissection of a strip of rectus sheath passed blindly beneath the bladder neck.

The Millin sling (1947)[176] In this variation the combined abdominovaginal approach is dispensed with and only an abdominal incision is used. The external oblique aponeurotic strips are passed blindly under the urethra following the creation of a suburethral passage using blunt dissection with curved forceps. They are then brought anteriorly through the medial border of the contralateral rectus muscle and sutured together. Not surprisingly, there is an increased risk of urethral damage using this approach.

The operations described above were devised nearly 50 years ago and are now no longer widely used.

Needle suspension fascial slings

The advantage of these procedures is that a smaller length of autologous tissue is required with a concomitant reduction in the degree of abdominal dissection. Rectus abdominis, external oblique or fascia lata can be used as may synthetic material.

A short suprapubic midline incision is made and a fascial patch excised from the rectus fascia. If fascia lata is the preferred material, a 4-cm transverse incision is made 8 cm above the patella and a suitably sized piece of fascia excised, the size depending on individual requirements. The patient is then placed in the modified lithotomy position and an inverted 'U' incision made in the anterior vaginal wall to expose the urethra and bladder neck. Dissection continues anterosuperiorly to enter the cave of Retzius. Adequate mobilization of the urethra and bladder neck should be ensured or elevation will be impeded. The fascial patch is then fixed to the posterior urethra using Vicryl sutures and a Prolene suture inserted into each corner of the patch to include a bite of periurethral fascia.

Under direct fingertip guidance a needle ligature carrier of the Stamey type is passed through the rectus fascia into the vaginal incision and the two free ends of each Prolene suture on the left withdrawn into the left side of the abdominal wound. This is repeated for the sutures on the right. Cystoscopy is now performed to ensure that no damage has occurred to bladder or urethra.

The sutures are secured above the rectus fascia. The use of Silastic mesh has been advocated to anchor the sutures in their anterior attachment; alternatively, if sufficient sling material is available this may be fixed directly.

Synthetic slings

Since Moir[124] first described the use of a Mersilene sling many materials have been used: Marlex (C.R. Bard Incorporated, Massachusetts, USA), Gore-Tex (W.L. Gore and Associates Incorporated) and Silastic (Dow Corning, Reading, UK). The infection rate is no greater than with autologous slings and there is little excess risk of suburethral erosion. The disadvantages of fascial slings, namely dissection and excision of fascia, variable tensile strength, necrosis of vascularized pedicles and difficulty of obtaining adequate length, are all overcome with synthetic materials. However, erosion and voiding difficulty are more common with the latter.

Operative technique The technique for insertion of a synthetic sling is essentially the same as for an autologous one. The procedure may be performed via a combined abdominovaginal approach or suprapubically with blind suburethral dissection. The urethra and bladder neck are mobilized with dissection continuing into the retropubic space and the patch (usually measuring 1.5 × 3.0 cm) fixed beneath the urethra and bladder neck with 4–0 Dexon or Vicryl. A figure of eight Prolene suture is attached to each corner of the patch and passed to the suprapubic incision using a Stamey or Pereyra needle. Cystoscopy is then performed and the vaginal incision closed. The sutures are tied above the rectus fascia, and usually require minimal tension. A Q-tip has been used to evaluate the urethrovesical angle as the suspensory sutures are tied.

Mechanism of continence

Hilton[123] has shown that suburethral sling procedures increase outflow resistance; however, the sling also provides support for the proximal urethra, which is compressed against the sling with increases in intra-abdominal pressure. Beck & McCormack[69] suggested that the greater support given to the proximal urethra as opposed to the bladder neck caused an obstructive effect with raised intra-abdominal pressure.

Complications

Injury to urethra or bladder is not uncommon and should be recognized perioperatively. Wound infection, sinus formation and urinary fistulae (secondary to erosion of the sling) have also been reported. However, the commonest postoperative complication is voiding difficulty, since sling procedures cause significant outlet obstruction. This occurs more frequently with synthetic than autologous slings. Complete retention may necessitate a further operation to loosen the sling or require the patient to perform on-going clean intermittent self-catheterization.

Results

The results of sling procedures have been assessed in many studies, but in most the groups are not homogeneous and reports are based on subjective data with variation in the definition of 'cure' with follow-up for only a short period.

Overall, success rates are good for both autologous and synthetic slings with little difference between the two in terms of cure rates, which are consistently above 75–80%.

Jeffcoate[131] and McClaren[132] reported 76% and 71% cure rates for the Aldridge procedure, whilst Kennedy[133] describes an 87.5% cure for the Millin variation. Results from fascia lata slings vary between 76% and 95%.[125,134,135,136]

Results from synthetic sling procedures are similarly good. Moir[124] reported an 83% success rate with his original 'gauze hammock sling' and Spencer et al[137] in an objective study achieved an 80% cure rate. Using Silastic, Stanton[138] reports an 83% success rate; with Gore-Tex, Horbach et al[139] an 85% cure; and with Marlex, Morgan et al[140] a 77.4% response. Chin & Stanton[141] in a 5-year follow-up of 88 Silastic sling procedures report a 71.4% overall objective cure rate. However, when the number of previous continence operations is considered, in those women who had undergone three or more operations the cure rate falls to 33%. Results (subjective and objective) are summarized in Table 18.17.

Table 18.17   Results of suburethral sling procedures

Reference	Type	% continent
Jeffcoate 1956[131]	Aldridge	76
McClaren 1968[132]	Aldridge	71
Kennedy 1960[133]	Millin	87
Low 1969[134]	Facsia lata	95
Parker et al 1979[136]	Facsia lata	84
Moir 1968[124]	Gauze hammock	83
Spencer et al 1972[137]	Gauze hammock	80
Stanton 1975[138]	Silastic	83
Horbach et al 1988[139]	Gore-Tex	85
Morgan et al 1985[140]	Marlex	77
Chin & Stanton 1995[141]	Silastic	71
Jarvis 1994[51]	All	85

The artificial urinary sphincter

Introduction

Scott et al[142] first described the use of an artificial urinary sphincter in women. The device has several theoretical advantages. First, complete continence can be assured through mechanical occlusion of the urethra (with correct choice of cuff size). Also voluntary relief of sphincteric occlusion allows voiding at an appropriate time for the patient.

Although artificial sphincters are now in regular use, the procedure is performed at few, specialized centers. The technique of implantation is difficult and mechanical failure may still occur even with todays' sophisticated devices. Additionally, they remain expensive.

The AMS series

The original sphincter (AMS 721) consisted of an inflating pump and deflating pump connected to a reservoir with controlling flow valves in the connecting tubes. Poor reliability with this device led to the development of the AMS 742, which was smaller and had fewer components and fewer mechanical failures. This model had a resistor placed between the urethral cuff and the balloon which nullified excesses of detrusor pressure, a potential cause of incontinence if greater than the cuff pressure. Miniaturization of the resistor and its incorporation with the valves into a single control unit led to the AMS 942. This featured automatic reapplication of cuff pressure after voluntary deactivation and voiding. The latest device (AMS 800, Fig. 18.10) incorporates a suspend or resume feature which allows on–off control in the immediate postoperative period. The rationale of this development was to reduce the possibility of cuff erosion, which is assumed to be caused by ischemia secondary to compression of the vascular supply to the tissues beneath the cuff. Advances in silicone technology have provided this device with considerable durability.

The AMS 800 consists of a urethral cuff, a pressure-regulating reservoir, a control pump assembly and connecting tubing. The control pump is placed in the labia majora. To facilitate voiding the pump is squeezed and released, drawing fluid from the cuff into the pump. This is repeated until sufficient fluid has been withdrawn from the cuff to allow voiding. Full repressurization of the cuff occurs automatically in about 3 min.

Indications

Blavias & Olsson[129] recommend the use of the artificial sphincter as the first option in females with sphincter incompetence, believing that tissue that has not been surgically compromised gives the patient the best chance to avoid cuff erosion. Most surgeons would, however, reserve the artificial sphincter for those in whom one or more continence procedures have failed.

Other indications include spinal cord injury, multiple sclerosis, sacral agenesis and severe degrees of spina bifida.

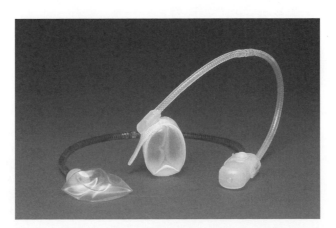

Fig. 18.10 The AMS 800 artificial urinary sphincter

Suboptimal results are likely if detrusor instability or outflow tract obstruction are not excluded prior to surgery. Vesicoureteric reflux must be excluded. The patient should have an adequate bladder capacity and be able void to completion with no residual, although the latter is not imperative if the patient can learn intermittent self-catheterization.

Surgical technique

Meticulous pre- and postoperative attention to the avoidance of infection is of paramount importance. Antibiotic prophylaxis should be given.

A low transverse suprapubic muscle-cutting incision is used. The cave of Retzius is exposed and dissection continued to the level of the bladder neck. A Foley catheter will allow easy identification. In patients who have undergone multiple continence procedures dissection will be difficult. Scott suggests preparing the patient so that perioperative vaginal manipulation can be used to identify the level and extent of the dissection. The endopelvic fascia is incised on each side of the bladder neck and dissection continued until the vaginal wall is reached.

Dissection between the urethra and vagina is hazardous since the urethrovaginal septum is not an anatomical plane. Excessive trauma predisposes to erosion of the cuff. A cutter clamp has been developed to assist in this step. This instrument holds the tissue secure before an integral cutting blade incises the urethrovaginal septum.

The size of cuff required is then determined by measuring the circumference of the bladder neck. With the cuff in place a tubing needle is used to bring the tubing of the cuff through the abdominal fascia into a subcutaneous position lateral to the symphysis. Space is created in the labia majora using blunt dissection from above and the pump assembly placed so that it may be manipulated externally with ease. A balloon reservoir of a size appropriate to that of the cuff is then chosen and the tubing connected after filling.

Since the AS 800 is designed to provide for externally controlled on–off capability, it is routine to perform primary deactivation in all patients in whom the sphincter is implanted. The device should be activated 6–8 weeks postoperatively.

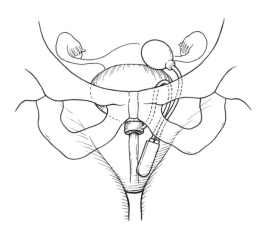

Fig. 18.11 The implanted artificial urinary sphincter. The balloon reservoir lies within the abdomen, with the control pump assembly sited within the labia majora. (Courtesy of American Medical Systems, Minnetonka, MN.)

Complications

Whilst perioperative injury to proximal urethra or bladder may occur, the most severe complication is erosion of the cuff either through the urethra or bladder, although erosion of the pump through the skin of the labia has also been reported. It is likely that many of the cases of cuff erosion are due to chronic infection of the device.

Erosion necessitates removal of the cuff to allow healing of the tissue defect and reimplantation may be attempted at an interval of no less than 3 months.[143]

Mechanical complications continue to occur, Diokno et al[144] reporting a 21% complication rate in a series of 32 patients.

Results

The results from published studies from artificial urinary sphincters are shown in Table 18.18.

Table 18.18   Results of artificial sphincter implantations

Reference	No. of patients	% continent	Follow-up (months)
Scott 1985[145]	39	92	3–72
Donovan et al 1985[146]	31	68	2–59
Diokno 1987[144]	32	91	30
Appel 1988[147]	34	100	24–65
Bhalchandra 1990[148]	24	17	8–66

Periurethral injections

Introduction

The use of periurethral injections of polytetrafluoroethylene (Polytef, Teflon) was first suggested by Berg.[149] He obtained complete cure in three women with several failed continence procedures, all of whom had good urethral support and a normal urethrovesical angle. He postulated that whilst the previous surgery had restored normal anatomy, fixation and scarring of the urethra had prevented continence because the urethra had become 'locked in an open position' – the 'drainpipe urethra' of Jeffcoate.

Politano et al[150] reported a larger series of 15 women and 17 men with encouraging results. However, problems with migration of Teflon to the lung and brain[151] led to concern relating to granuloma formation with fibrosis and scarring. Additionally, Teflon has been shown to be carcinogenic in rats, although no human cases are reported. Such concerns have resulted in the use of bovine glutaraldehyde cross-linked collagen (GAX, Contigen), which is derived from beef dermis and latterly textured polydimethylsiloxane (silicone rubber) particles suspended in a non-silicone carrier gel (Macroplastique – Bioplasty Inc). Autologous fat has also been used as a periurethral bulk-enhancing agent, harvested from the anterior abdominal wall by liposuction. This is certainly a cheaper alternative to GAX collagen and Macroplastique, both of which remain expensive.

The use of injectables as a primary continence procedure is questionable; however, since it may be performed under local anesthetic those patients who are elderly or frail could be considered suitable in addition to the group with urethral fixity.

Operative technique

The procedure can be performed under local, regional or general anesthesia. The patient is placed in the lithotomy position and prepared as for cystoscopy. A 0°, 30° or 70° cystoscope is inserted into the urethra and the delivery needle (Bruning or proprietary Contigen) inserted lateral to the urethral meatus and advanced to the level of the bladder neck (Fig. 18.12). The position of the needle is checked via the cystoscope to ensure that it does not traverse the urethral mucosa. Macroplastique is considerably more viscous than GAX collagen and is best injected through the proprietary needle via the operating port of the cystoscope (Fig. 18.13), directly through the urethral mucosa.

The original description of the procedure involved injection of the material in four quadrants at the proximal and distal third of the urethra; however, the modern technique involves injection at the bladder neck in two opposing lateral planes. The collagen or silicone 'bump' can be visualized through the cystoscope and injection continues until at least 50% of the urethral lumen is occluded, after which the procedure is repeated on the opposite side (Figs. 18.14 and 18.15).

The volume required per injection varies between patients and also according to the periurethral bulking agent used. Frequent reinjections are not uncommon.

Injection can be performed under ultrasound control and this allows accurate insertion of the needle tip to the urethrovesical junction and the 'bumps' to be visualized. This ensures injection at the appropriate site and may improve cure rates (and reduce the need for reinjection).

If the procedure is performed under local or regional anesthetic, the patient can be asked to perform provocative maneuvers immediately afterwards and a further volume injected as appropriate.

Complications

There are **relatively few** complications from injectables for the treatment of genuine stress incontinence. Immediate postoperative retention of urine is relatively frequent and mild urethral discomfort is reported.[152] In some cases the urethral pain may be severe, lasting up to 1 month. Several authors have reported the passage of Teflon plugs per urethram

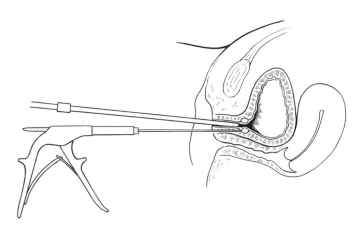

Fig. 18.12 Periurethral bulk-enhancing agents. This diagram demonstrates the paraurethral technique under cystoscopic control

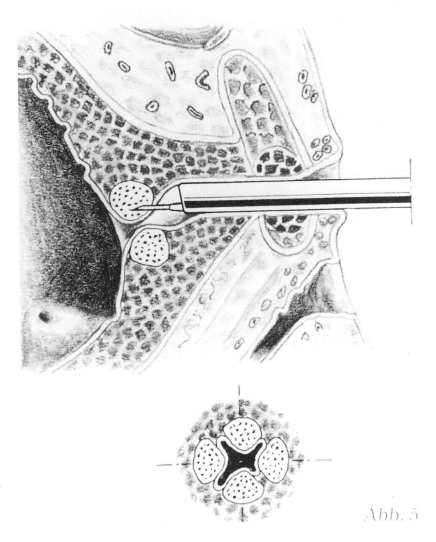

Abb. 5

Fig. 18.13 Periurethral bulk-enhancing agents. An alternative transurethral technique is shown

following intense urethral burning pain. Loss of continence will occur afterwards.

Reports of Teflon migration combined with the significant inflammatory response that it provokes have resulted in relatively little, if any, contemporary use.

Complications

Politano et al[150] reported a success rate of 56% in their mixed group of men and women. A further study by Politano[153] reported a 71% improvement in 51 women. However, Beckingham et al[152] report an initial 80% subjective improvement, falling to 27% at follow-up 3 years later. The authors subsequently abandoned this procedure for the treatment of stress incontinence. A summary of published results for periurethral Teflon injections is shown in Table 18.19.

Recent reports of the results of GAX collagen are similarly diappointing, with poor long-term cure rates (Table 18.20).

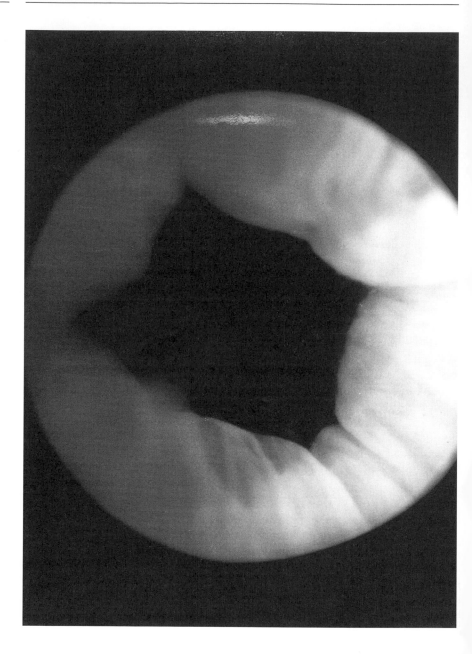

Fig. 18.14 The urethral lumen before injection of periurethral bulk-enhancing agent

Studies using Macroplastique are currently less numerous. However, Buckley et al[161] and Iacovoa et al[162] report 70% and 40% success rates respectively.

The initial optimism that periurethral injections would provide a safe, effective and, in the case of Teflon, cheap treatment of stress incontinence has given way to guarded skepticism. The mechanism of continence with this procedure remains unknown and further evaluation and modification of the technique may improve cure rates.

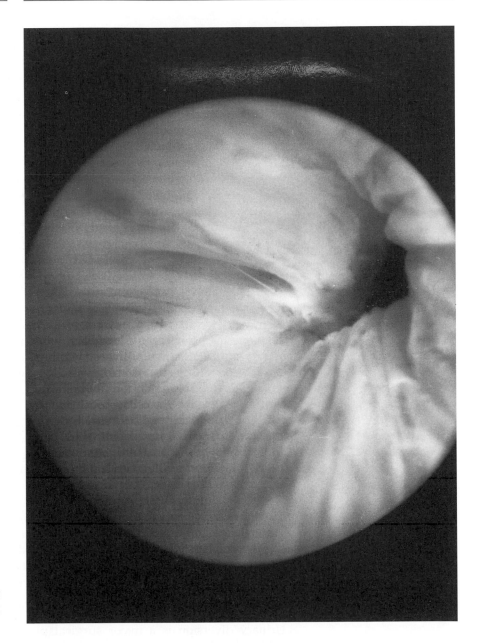

Fig. 18.15 The urethral lumen following injection of periurethral bulk-enhancing agent

Neourethra

Operative Technique

This procedure, described by Tanagho,[163] is useful in women who have had multiple failed continence procedures, who have congenital abnormality or in whom there has been severe trauma.

Via a low transverse suprapubic incision an anterior bladder flap (3 × 3 cm in size) is cut and formed into a tube, using a Foley catheter as a 'mould'. The distal portion remains of the flap should remain contiguous with the urethra. The bladder defect is then closed. The abdomen is then opened and the neourethra enveloped in an omental sheath. The abdominal incision is then closed after placing a

Table 18.19   Results of periurethral Teflon injections for genuine stress incontinence

Reference	No. of patients	% improved	Follow-up (months)
Politano 1982[153]	51	71	6
Lim et al 1983[154]	28	54	9
Schulman et al 1984[155]	56	86	9
Fischer 1986[156]	20	45	12
Beckingham et al 1992[152]	26	27	36

Table 18.20   Results of periurethral GAX collagen injection for genuine stress incontinence

Reference	No. of patients	% continent	Mean volume injected (no. of attempts)	Follow-up (months)
Goldenberg 1994[157]	190	58	NA	6–36
Monga 1995[158]	60	48	10.8 (1.6)	24
Swami et al 1991[159]	66	65%	NA	12
Appell 1989[160]	68	81	NA	12

perivesical drain. Postoperative urinary drainage is by suprapubic catheter.

The anterior bladder wall superior to the internal urethral meatus is required since the detrusor fibers in this area run transversely, so that when the neourethra is formed they are able to exert a compressive force, mimicking a true sphincter.

Complications and results

The complication rate of the procedure is high, with fistula, stricture and failure occurring, although Tanagho[163] reports a 75% subjective improvement. In a small objective study, Gallagher et al[164] report a 63% cure rate.

Urinary diversion

For women in whom all else has failed or in those with neuropathic disease, urinary diversion should be considered. Until recently, an ileal conduit was commonly employed. Continent diversions are now undergoing evaluation and may hold a hope for the future.[165] The complications of such procedures are related to the type of diversion employed, and it is not possible to compare the results with those of other types of continence surgery.

Urinary diversion is a major surgical procedure and although it is considered to be provide a 'final solution' to intractable urinary incontinence, revisional surgery is not uncommon. Cox[166] reports a retrospective review of 18 patients, 7 of whom required further surgery to their ileal loops. The indications included obstruction and stomal or peristomal problems. Urinary diversions are described further in Ch. 36.

Laparoscopic colposuspension

Laparoscopic colposuspension is a new technique (Fig. 18.16)[177] which retains the principle of bladder neck and bladder base elevation but without the need for a traditional low transverse suprapubic incision. Initial reports of the technique[167] described the creation of a pneumo-

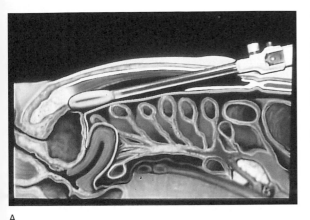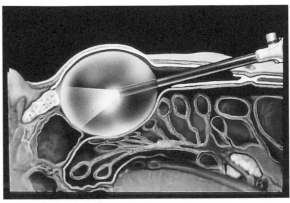

A   B

Fig. 18.16   Laparoscopic colposuspension: balloon dissection of the retropubic space

peritoneum with subsequent incision of the peritoneum above the bladder and dissection of the cave of Retzius. However, it has been shown that retropubic extraperitoneal insufflation is quicker and associated with less trauma.[168]

There are four techniques described. The transperitoneal and retroperitoneal colposuspensions are laparoscopic versions of the open operation described by Burch. The laparoscopic 'Stamey procedure' has been reported by Chapple & Osbourne[168] and a further technique cases Prolene mesh stapled to the paravaginal fascia and Cooper's ligament.[169]

For this procedure to be accepted as an alternative to traditional continence procedures it must be as minimally invasive as the Stamey operation and have the same long-term effectiveness as an open Burch colposuspension.

Equipment

The following equipment will be required:

- high-flow carbon dioxide insufflator
- CCD camera and video monitor
- Veres needle (safety type)
- 0° 10-mm laparoscope
- one 10-mm port and two 5-mm ports with grips and convertors/downsizers
- laparoscopic scissors (diathermy connection)
- laparoscopic dissecting forceps
- Stamey bladder neck suspension needle.
- laparoscopic knot pusher
- laparoscopic needle holder
- suction irrigation

Operative technique

The patient is placed in the lithotomy position with a 25° head-down tilt (Fig. 18.17) and prepared and draped to allow a synchronous pelvic laparoscopy and vaginal procedure to be performed. A urethral Foley catheter is inserted. The video monitor is placed at the foot of the table opposite the surgeon, who will usually stand on the patient's left; alternatively two monitors may be used if available, one each for the surgeon and assistant.

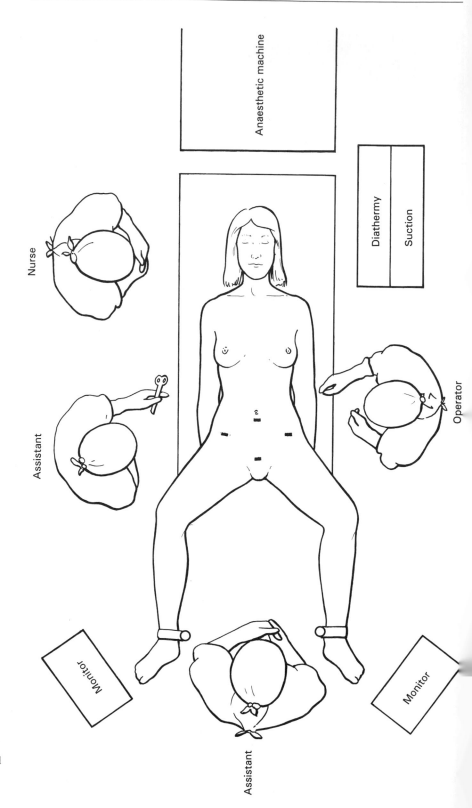

Fig. 18.17 Layout of the operating theatre of staff and equipment for laparoscopic colosuspension

Two different surgical approaches have employed: transperitoneal and retroperitoneal.

Retroperitoneal approach A small incision is made immediately above the symphysis pubis and the Veres needle inserted into the retropubic space. It is important to feel the symphysis with the tip of the needle to prevent inadvertent entry of the peritoneum. The extraperitoneal space is insufflated with 1–1.5 l carbon dioxide. Whilst the pressures will initially be high (in contrast to the case with insufflation of the peritoneal cavity), as the peritoneal lining is stripped caudally, the tension and therefore the inflation pressure fall to the normal range.

A 10-mm port (for the laparoscope) is inserted at the site of the Veres needle, again keeping close to the symphysis pubis. Visual confirmation of entry to the retropubic space is obtained with the laparoscope. Two secondary 5-mm ports are placed proximal and lateral to the laparoscope port as close to the edge of the rectus sheath as possible so as to avoid the inferior epigastric artery. These ports are used for manipulative instruments.

The fatty tissue anterior to the bladder neck is swept medially; care should be taken to avoid hemorrhage from the numerous veins in this area. It is preferable to use soft dissecting instruments and dissection is aided by a finger inserted in the vagina beneath the area of dissection. The paravaginal tissues adjacent to the bladder neck are cleared.

Transperitoneal approach A transverse incision is made 3 cm above the symphysis pubis on the anterior peritoneum between the two obliterated bladder folds. The anterior peritoneum is dissected from the anterior abdominal wall and the retropubic space entered. The bladder is mobilized and paravaginal fatty tissue dissected free. For both techniques the colposuspension is performed using up to three non-absorbable sutures on either side. The knots may be tied intra- or extracorporeally. Occasionally, reduced vaginal capacity and mobility does not allow adequate placement of the suspensory sutures and in this case a modified Stamey procedure is recommended. This involves the passage of a nylon suture by means of a Stamey needle passed through the vagina, guided under direct vision through the retropubic space and out on to the abdominal wall. A minimum of two sutures can then be placed on either side and tied above the rectus sheath. Correct placement of all sutures should be checked with a cystoscope at the end of the procedure. The ports should then be removed under direct vision and the carbon dioxide gas evacuated. A suction drain is not usually required. The 10-mm port will require a fascial suture and the skin can be approximated with either Steristrips or a 3–0 Prolene suture. A urethral catheter may be left in situ for 5 days, although some surgeons have found that this may be removed without complication on the first postoperative day prior to the patient's discharge (Neale, personal communication).

omplications

The recourse to laparotomy for completion of the procedure is not uncommon during the early part of the 'learning curve'. Careful selection of patients who are slim, have had no previous continence surgery and who have adequate vaginal capacity and mobility may reduce the necessity for laparotomy. Profuse hemorrhage from peri-vesical veins may be avoided by careful dissection. However, if severe hemorrhage does occur vision may be impaired, requiring laparotomy to obtain hemostasis. Injury to the bladder may occur and the abdomen opened to effect repair. Postoperative voiding difficulty does not appear to be a significant problem, perhaps due to the lack of postoperative pain, although it may be suggested that this is because elevation of the bladder neck is not as great with a laparoscopic procedure as with an open procedure.

Results

No large series has yet been reported with long-term objective follow-up; however, in a series of nearly 50 laparoscopic colposuspensions a 90% primary cure rate is possible (Neale personal communication). Chapple & Osbourne[168] report a series of 40 patients with a significant number of failures in the first 15 cases. Early failures can be expected as the surgeon progresses along the 'learning curve'. Burton,[170] in a randomized comparison of laparoscopic and open colposuspension with 6- and 12-month objective follow-up, reports a significantly greater failure rate in the laparoscopic group (27%) compared with that in women randomized to the open procedure (3%).

Surgical failure

No continence procedure has yet obtained a long-term cure rate of 100%; therefore surgical failure remains a fact of life. Nevertheless, the surgeon should strive for increased long-term cure rates and investigate fully those patients who return with symptoms of incontinence.

Causes of surgical failure

The causes of surgical failure can be divided into four groups: (1) predisposing factors; (2) de novo causes of incontinence; (3) technical failure; and (4) selection of inappropriate procedure.

Predisposing factors

Age Hilton[123] reported a higher failure rate in older patients for both the Stamey procedure and suburethral sling (mean 67.3 vs 53.4 years) and for the Burch colposuspension[87] (mean 54.8 vs 45.8 years). It is likely that the reduced success rate is due to atrophic tissue changes with poor healing capability, along with 'normal' loss of urethral closure pressure that occurs with age. Some of these changes may be reversible with preoperative administration of estrogen.

Previous continence surgery The association between reduced operative success and previous bladder neck surgery is well established.[23,1?] Multiple attempts at surgical correction may lead to a fixed, immobile urethra surrounded by dense fibrous tissue, the 'drainpipe urethra'. Urethroscopy may reveal a completely patent urethra.

Detrusor instability Detrusor instability coexists in a proportion of patients with stress incontinence and if undiagnosed will reduce the chances of surgical cure. It is widely believed that surgery is relatively contraindicated in the presence of detrusor instability and Stanton et al[23] reported a significantly lower cure rate in such patients compared to those with genuine stress incontinence (43% vs 85%). More recently,[113] further attention has been paid to the management of patients with mixed urinary incontinence, which is discussed further below.

Incorrect diagnosis Stress incontinence is only one of the presenting symptoms of genuine stress incontinence (urethral sphincter incompetence). However, it can occur in other conditions, especially detrusor instability and overflow incontinence. Therefore urodynamic investigation is desirable before embarking upon surgery.

Reduced maximal urethral closure pressure It has been suggested that a maximal urethral closure pressure of less than 20 cmH$_2$O is a predictor of surgical failure.[171] However, considerable overlap exists between the cured and incontinent groups with respect to maximal urethral closure pressure and the relevance of this finding has yet to be established.

De novo causes of incontinence

Detrusor instability Detrusor instability may arise postoperatively in a proportion of women,[86,91,172,173] but it is not judged to be a result of the obstructive nature of some continence procedures. Steel et al[172] report the occurrence of postoperative detrusor instability in 16% of a group of 148 patients following colposuspension. The response to anticholinergic and β-adrenergic drugs was uniformly poor, with only 16% of patients describing any improvement. In this study all patients had a stable detrusor preoperatively, and whilst no specific preoperative or urodynamic variable was identified to predict the development of postoperative detrusor instability, those patients who had undergone previous bladder neck surgery seemed more susceptible. Cardozo et al[91] suggest that repeated dissection at the bladder neck may in some way compromise detrusor function. Future technology might allow prediction of those women who are likely to develop postoperative detrusor instability.

Other causes Chronic retention with overflow may be precipitated in patients with preoperative voiding difficulty. This may develop days or weeks after postoperative catheter removal, even with normal residual urinary volumes prior to discharge.

In the elderly, urinary tract infection, neurogenic and psychogenic factors should be considered.

Technical failure

Suture breakage This may be avoided with the use of non-absorbable suture material of appropriate tensile strength. Nylon or Prolene is recommended. Commonly, the patient complains of a recurrence of incontinence following a fall or a severe bout of coughing.

Suture pull-through Postoperatively, coughing, straining at stool or straining to void may all result in disruption of the sutures from the periurethral tissue, particularly if an inadequate amount of tissue is incorporated in the suture. Similarly, the anterior sutures of retropubic procedures may pull through if poorly secured.

Suture placement Elevation of the bladder neck is crucial to success in the majority of continence procedures. Sutures inserted directly above the bladder neck may lead to total urinary incontinence by holding the proximal urethra open. Sutures placed too distally will fail to achieve adequate elevation and the patient is unlikely to be cured. Careful identification of the bladder neck using a Foley catheter will minimize incorrect placement, and intraoperative endoscopy (an integral part of the Stamey procedure) allows direct visualization of the bladder neck to ensure accurate insertion of sutures.

Incorrect choice of procedure The first operation for stress incontinence is the one most likely to work. Primary surgery is intended to restore the proximal urethra and bladder neck to their normal anatomical location however, when damage to other components of the continence mechanism exists, retropubic repairs may be inadequate. Consideration must be given to all clinical and urodynamic features prior to selection of the surgical procedure.

Improving the results of surgery

While surgery is the appropriate treatment for genuine stress incontinence, detrusor instability is rarely cured by an operation and indeed the symptoms of urgency and frequency may be exacerbated. It is therefore essential to obtain an accurate diagnosis before surgery is contemplated.

Preoperatively the patient should be encouraged to stop smoking and therefore improve any chronic chest disease. Other medical conditions should be treated appropriately. Estrogen therapy may improve the quality of urogenital tissue in postmenopausal women and pelvic floor physiotherapy may be useful both pre- and postoperatively.

Obesity may adversely affect the results of surgery, but there is no conclusive evidence to support this notion. Morbidity is certainly greater and technical difficulty increased in the obese patient. Although obese women should be encouraged to lose weight, this should not be a prerequisite to surgery.

During the course of the procedure it is important to pay particular attention to the number of sutures used and the suture material. Preoperative antibiotic therapy will reduce the incidence of infection and hematoma formation can be prevented with a suction drain. Postoperative urinary drainage using a suprapubic catheter is associated with a lower incidence of urinary tract infection and a shorter time to spontaneous voiding.

It should be remembered that all surgery carries a mortality and morbidity rate whereas urinary incontinence does not. Therefore the indications for surgical intervention must be well established in each case and should be undertaken only at the request of the patient.

Finally, as the first operation is the most likely to cure the patient, the best operation for a given clinical situation should be chosen for the first attempt.

REFERENCES

1 Abrams P, Blavias JG, Stanton SL, Andersen JT. The standardisation of terminology of lower urinary tract function. British Journal of Obstetrics and Gynaecology 1990; 97 (Suppl 6): 1–16.

2 Thomas TM, Plymat KR, Blannin J, Meade TW. Prevalence of urinary incontinence. British Medical Journal 1980; 281: 1243–1245.

3 Kondo A, Kato K, Saito M, Otani T. Prevalence of hand-washing urinary incontinence in females in comparison with stress and urge incontinence. Neurorology and Urodynamics 1990; 9: 330–331.

4 The place of urodynamic investigations. In: Jarvis GJ (ed) Female urinary incontinence. London: Royal College of Obstetricians and Gynaecologists, 1990: pp 15–20.

5 Chantraine A, DeLeval J, Depirieux P. Adult female intra- and periurethral sphincter electromyographic study. Neurourol and Urodynam 1990; 9: 139–144.

6 Smith ARB, Hosker GL, Warrell DW. The role of partial denervation of the pelvic floor in the aetiology of genitourinary prolapse and stress incontinence of urine. A neurophysiological study. British Journal of Obstetrics and Gynaecology 1989; 96: 667–676.

7 Smith ARB, Hosker GL, Warrell DW. The role of pudendal nerve damage in the aetiology of genuine stress incontinence in women. British Journal of Obstetrics and Gynaecology 1989; 96: 29–32.

8 Anderson RS. A neurogenic element to urinary stress incontinence. British Journal of Obstetrics and Gynaecology 1984; 91: 41–45.

9 Snooks SJ, Swash M. Abnormalities of the innervation of the urethral striated sphincter musculature in incontinence. British Journal of Urology 1984; 56: 401–405.

10 Snooks SJ, Badenoch DF, Tiptaft RC, Swash M. Perineal nerve damage in genuine stress incontinence. British Journal of Urology 1985; 57: 422–426.

11 Gilpin SA, Gosling JA, Smith ARB, Warrell DA. The pathogenesis of genitourinary prolapse and stress incontinence of urine. British Journal of Obstetrics and Gynaecology 1989; 96: 15–23.

12 Delancey JOL. Structural support of the urethra as it relates to stress urinary incontinence: the hammock hypothesis. American Journal of Obstetrics and Gynecology 1994; 170: 1713–1723.

13 Richardson AC, Lyon JB, Williams NL. A new look at pelvic relaxation. American Journal of Obstetrics and Gynecology 1976; 126: 568–573.

14 Landon CR, Smith ARB. Biomechanical properties of connective tissue in women with stress incontinence of urine. Neurourol and Urodynam 1989; 8: 369–370.

15 Sayer TR, Dixon JS, Hosker GL, Warrell DW. A study of paraurethral connective tissue in women with stress incontinence of urine. Neurourol and Urodynam 1990; 9: 319–320.

16 Prockap D, Kivirikko K, Tuderman L et al. The biosynthesis of collagen and its disorders. New England Journal of Medicine 1979; 301(1): 13–24.

17 Norton P, Baxter J, Sharp H, Warenski H. Genitourinary prolapse: relationship with joint mobility. Neurourol and Urodynam 1992; 9: 321–322.

18 Gosling JA. The structure of the bladder and urethra in relation to function. Urology Clinics of North America 1979; 6: 31–38.

19 Versi E, Cardozo L, Brincat M, Cooper D, Montgomery J, Studd J. Correlation of urethral physiology and skin collagen in postmenopausal women. British Journal of Obstetrics and Gynaecology 1988; 95: 147–152.

20 Dellee JB. The prophylactic forceps operation. American Journal of Obstetrics and Gynecology 1920; 1–34.

21 Parks AG, Swash M, Urich H. Sphincter denervation in anorectal incontinence and rectal prolapse. Gut 1977; 18: 656–665.

22 Gosling JA, Dixon J, Critchley HOD, Thompson SA. A comparative study of the human external sphincter and perurethral levator ani muscles. British Journal of Urology 1981; 53: 35–41.

23 Stanton SL, Cardozo L, Williams JE, Ritchie D, Allan V. Clinical and urodynamic features of failed incontinence surgery in the female. Obstetrics and Gynaecology 1978; 51: 515–520.

24 Rud T. Urethral pressure profiles in continent women from childhood to old age. Acta Obstet Gynecol Scand 1980; 59: 331–335.

25 Zacharin RF. 'A Chinese anatomy' – the pelvic supporting tissues of the Chinese and occidental female compared and contrasted. Australia New Zealand Journal of Obstetrics and Gynaecology 1977; 17: 1–11.

26 Iosif CS. Stress incontinence during pregnancy and the puerperium. International Journal of Obstetrics and Gynaecology 1981; 19: 13–20.

27 Dywer P, Lee ETC, Hay DM. Obesity and urinary incontinence in women. British Journal of Obstetrics and Gynaecology 1988; 95: 91–96.

28 Burton G, Cardozo LD, Benness B, Wise B, Cutner A. Is obesity a cause of G.S.I? International Journal of Obstetrics and Gynaecology 1991; 4: 356.

29 Hodgekinson CP. Stress urinary incontinence. American Journal of Obstetrics and Gynaecology 1970; 108: 1141–1168.

30 Bump RC. Racial comparisons and contrasts in urinary incontinence and pelvic organ prolapse. Obstetrics and Gynaecology 81(3) 421–425. 1993.

31 Jarvis GJ, Hall S, Stamp S, Miller DR, Johnson A. An assessment of urodynamic examination in incontinent women. British Journal of Obstetrics and Gynaecology 1980; 87: 893–896.

32 Sutherst JL, Brown M, Shawer M. Assessing the severity of urine incontinence in women by weighing perineal pads. Lancet 1981; 1: 1128–1130.

33 Turner-Warwick R. The treatment of female urinary incontinence. Proceedings of the 60 International Continence Society Meeting, Antwerp, 1976.

34 Haylen BT, Sutherst JR, Fraser MI. Is the investigation of most stress incontinence really necessary? British Journal of Urology 1989; 64: 147–149.

35 Hastie KJ, Moisey CU. Are urodynamic investigations necessary in patients presenting with stress incontinence? British Journal of Urology 1989; 63: 155–156.

36 Wilson PD, Al Sammarrai T, Daekin M. An objective assessment of physiotherapy for female genuine stress incontinence. British Journal of Obstetrics and Gynaecology 1987; 94: 575–582.

37 Tapp AJS, Cardozo LD, Hills B, Barnick C. Who benefits from physiotherapy. Proceedings of the 18th Annual Meeting of the International Continence Society, Oslo, Norway. Neurourol and Urodynam 1988; 7: 264–265. Abstract.

38 Nygaard IE. Treatment of exercise incontinence with mechanical devices. Neurourol and Urodynam 1992; 11: 367–368.

39 Nygaard I. Prevention of exercise incontinence with mechanical devices. Journal of Reproductive Medicine 1995; 40(2): 89–94.

40 Suarez GM, Baum NH, Jacobs J. Use of standard contraceptive diaphragm in management of stress urinary incontinence. Urology 1991; 37: 119–122.

41 Davila GW, Osterman KV. The bladder neck support prosthesis: a nonsurgical approach to stress incontinence in adult women. American Journal of Obstetrics and Gynaecology 1994; 171: 206–112.

42 Neilson KK, Kromann-Andersen B, Jacobsen H et al. The urethral plug: a new treatment for genuine stress incontinence in women. Journal of Urology 1990; 144: 1199–1202.

43 Newman DK, Smith DA, Harris T, Diokno A. An external female barrier device in the management of urinary incontinence. Neurourol and Urodynam 1992; 11: 368–369.

44 Staskin D, Bevendam T, Davila G et al. A multicentre experience using an expendable urethral occlusion device for the management of urinary stress incontinence. Neurourol and Urodynam 1994; 13: 380–381.

45 Stewart BH, Banowsky LH, Montague DK. Stress incontinence: conservative therapy with sympathomimetic drugs. Journal of Urology 1976; 115: 559–569.

46 Awad S, Downie J, Kiriluta H. Alpha adrenergic agents in urinary disorders of the proximal urethra. British Journal of Urology 1978; 129: 418.

47 Obrink A, Brunne G. The effect of alpha adrenergic stimulation in stress incontinence. Scandinavian Journal of Urology and Nephrology 1978; 12: 205.

48 Beisland HO, Fossberg E, Moer A. Urethral sphincteric insufficiency in postmenopausal females: treatment with phenlypropanolamine and estriol separately and in combination. Urology International 1984; 39: 211.

49 Hilton P, Tweddell AL, Mayne C. Oral and intravaginal estrogens alone and in combination with alpha-adrenergic stimulation in genuine stress incontinence. International Urogynaecology Journal 1990; 1: 80–86.

50 Baker-Brown I. On diseases of women remedial by operation. Lancet 1864; 1: 263–266

51 Jarvis GJ. Surgery for stress incontinence. British Journal of Obstetrics and Gynaecology 1994; 101: 371–374.

52 Green T. The problem of stress incontinence in the female: appraisal of its current status. Obstetrical and Gynecological Survey 1962; 23: 603–634.

53 Schultze BS. Operative Heilung der urethralen Incontinenz beim Weibe. Cor Bl d allg ärtzl Ver v Thüringen Weimar. 1888; 17: 289.

54 Kelly HA. Incontinence of urine in women. Urologic and Cutaneous Review 1913; 17: 291–293.

55 Pacey K. Pathology and repair of genital prolapse. Journal of Obstetrics and Gynaecology of the British Empire 1949; 56: 1–15.

56 Ingel-Sundberg A. Plastic repair of the pelvic floor. Acta Gynaecologica Scandinavica 1950; 30 (Suppl 7): 318–328.

57 Stanton SL, Cardozo LD. A comparison of vaginal and suprapubic surgery in the correction of incontinence due to urethral sphincter incompetence. British Journal of Urology 1979; 51: 497–499.

58 Stanton SL, Hilton P, Norton C, Cardozo LD. Clinical and urodynamic effects of anterior colporrhaphy and vaginal hysterectomy for prolapse with and without incontinence. British Journal of Obstetrics and Gynaecology 1982; 89: 459–463.

59 Hilton P. Bladder drainage: a survey of practices among gynaecologists in Britain (with unpublished observations regarding surgical practices). British Journal of Obstetrics and Gynaecology 1988; 95: 1178–1189.

60 Beck 1982 Beck RP, The sling operation. In Buchsbaum H and Schmidt J. *Gynaecologic and Obstetric Urology*, 2nd edition, Philadelphia: WB Saunders. pp 199–233.

61 Low JA. The management of severe anatomic urinary incontinence by vaginal repair. American Journal of Obstetrics and Gynecology 1967; 97: 308–315.

62 Green T. Urinary stress incontinence; differential diagnosis, pathophysiology and management. American Journal of Obstetrics and Gynaecology 1975; 122: 368–400.

63 Weil A, Reyes H, Bischoff P, Rottenburg RD, Krauer F. Modifications of urethral rest and stress profiles after three different types of surgery for urinary stress incontinence. British Journal of Obstetrics and Gynaecology 1984; 91: 46–55.

64 Stanton SL, Chamberlein GVP, Holmes DM. Randomised study of the anterior repair and colposuspension operation for the control of genuine stress incontinence. Proceedings of the 75th Annual Meeting of the International Continence Society, London. 1985; 236–237.

65 Park GS, Miller EJ. Surgical treatment of stress urinary incontinence: comparison of Kelly plication, Marshall-Marchetti-Krantz and Pereyra procedures. Obstetrics and Gynaecology 1988; 71: 575–579.

66 Bergman A, Koonings P, Ballard CA. Primary stress urinary incontinence and pelvic relaxation: a prospective randomized comparison of three different operations. American Journal of Obstetrics and Gynecology 1989; 161: 97–101.

67 Warrell D. Anterior repair. In: Stanton SL, Tanagho EJ (eds) Surgery for female incontinence, 2nd edn. Berlin: Springer-Verlag, 1986; 77–86.

68 Walter S, Pleson KP, Hald T, Jensen HK, Pedersen PH.Urodynamic evaluation after vaginal repair and colposuspension. British Journal of Urology 1982; 54: 377–380.

69 Beck RP, McCormack RN. Treatment of urinary stress incontinence with anterior colporrhaphy. Obstetrics and Gynaecology. 1982; 59: 269–274.

70 Pacey HK. Stress incontinence of urine. New Zealand Medical Journal, 1955; 54: 322–324.

71 Jeffcoate TNA. Functional disturbances of the female urethra and bladder. Journal of the Royal College of Surgeons of Edinburgh 1961; 7: 28–47.

72 Beck RP, McCormick RN, Nordstrom L. A 25 year experience with 519 anterior colporrhaphy procedures. Obstetrics and Gynaecology 1991; 78: 1011–1018.

73 Frewen WK. Urethral graft in stress incontinence. In: Communications to the Sixth Annual Congress, International Continence Society. 1976.

74 Payne PR. Urethrocleisis: a simple cure for stress incontinence. British Journal of Obstetrics and Gynaecology 1983; 90: 662–664.

75 Falconer C, Larsson B. New and simplified vaginal approach for correction of urinary stress incontinence in women. Neurourol and Urodynam 1995; 14: 365–370.

76 Bailey KV. A clinical investigation into uterine prolapse with stress incontinence. Treatment by modified Manchester colporrhaphy. Journal of Obstetrics and Gynaecology of the British Empire 1954; 61: 291–298.

77 Marshall-Marchetti AA, Krantz KE. The correction of stress incontinence by simple vesico-urethral suspension. Surgery, Gynecology and Obstetrics 1949; 88: 509–518.

78 Hodgekinson CP. Urinary stress incontinence in the female: a program for preoperative investigation. Clinical Obstetrics and Gynaecology 1963; 6: 154.

79 Burch JC. Urethrovesical fixation to Cooper's ligament for correction of stress incontinence, cystocele and prolapse. American Journal of Obstetrics and Gynecology 1961; 81: 281–290.

80 Lose G, Jorgensen L, Moetrnsen SO, Molsted-Pedersen L, Kristensen JK. Voiding difficulties after colposuspension. Obstetrics and Gynaecology. 1987; 69: 33–38.

81 Giesen JE. A review of 60 Marshall-Marchetti operations. Journal of Obstetrics and Gynaecology of the British Empire 1962; 69: 397–402.

82 Riggs JA. Retropubic cystourethropexy: a review of two operative procedures with long term follow-up. Obstetrics and Gynaecology 1986; 68: 98–105.

83 Milani R, Scalambrino S, Quadri G, Algeri M, Marchesin R. Marshall-Marchetti-Krantz procedure and Burch colposuspension in the surgical treatment of female urinary incontinence. British Journal of Obstetrics and Gynaecology 1985; 92: 1050–1053.

84 Colombo M, Scalambrino S, Marchesin R, Milani R. Way of working of modified Marshall-Marchetti-Krantz urethropexy. Proceedings of the 23rd Annual Meeting of the International Continence Society, Rome. 1993; pp 181–182. Abstract.

85 Stanton SL, Williams JE, Ritchie B. The colposuspension operation for urinary incontinence. British Journal of Obstetrics and Gynaecology 1976; 83: 890–895.

86 Alcalay M, Monga A, Stanton SL. Burch colposuspension: a 10–20 year follow up. British Journal of Obstetrics and Gynaecology 1995; 102: 740–45.

87 Hilton P, Stanton SL. A clinical and urodynamic assessment of the Burch colposuspension for genuine stress incontinence. British Journal of Obstetrics and Gynaecology 1983; 90: 934–939.

88 Dundas D, Hilton P, Williams JE, Stanton SL. Aetiology of voiding difficulty following colposuspension. Proceedings of the 12th Meeting of the International Continence Society, Leiden, Netherlands. 1982; p 132.

89 Cardozo LD, Cutner A. Surgical management of incontinence. Contemporary Reviews in Obstetrics and Gynaecology. 1992; 4: 36–41.

90 Burch JC. Cooper's ligament urethrovesical suspension for urinary stress incontinence. American Journal of Obstetrics and Gynecology 1968; 100: 764–772.

91 Cardozo L, Stanton SL, Williams JE. Detrusor instability following surgery for genuine stress incontinence. British Journal of Urology 1979; 58: 138–142.

92 McGuire EJ, Lyttton B, Kohorn GI, Pepe V. The value of urodynamic testing in stress urinary incontinence. Journal of Urology 1979; 124: 256–258.

93 Haase & Stribsted 1988

94 Poad D, Arnold EP. Sexual function after pelvic surgery in women. Australia New Zealand Journal of Obstetrics and Gynaecology 1994; 34(4): 471–474.

95 Galloway NTM, Davies N, Stephenson TP. The complications of colposuspension. British Journal of Urology 1987; 60: 122–124.

96 Mundy AR. A trial comparing the Stamey bladder neck suspension procedure with colposuspension for stress incontinence. British Journal of Urology 1983; 55: 687–0.

97 Stanton SL. Urethral sphincter incompetence. In Clinical gynecologic urology (ed S.L. Stanton), pp 169–192. C.V Mosby, St Louis. 1984.

98 Herbetsson G, Iosif CS. Surgical results and urodynamic studies 10 years after retropubic colpourethrocystopexy. Acta Obstet Gynecol Scand 1993; 72: 298–301.

99 Richardson AC, Edmonds PB, Williams NL. Treatment of stress incontinence due to paravaginal fascial defect. Obstetrics and Gynaecology 1981; 57: 357–362.

100 Shull BL, Baden WF. A six year experience with paravaginal defect repairs for stress urinary incontinence. American Journal of Obstetrics and Gynecology 1989; 160: 1432–1440.

101 Pereyra AJ. A simplified surgical procedure for the correction of stress incontinence in women. Western Journal of Surgery 1959; 67: 223.

102 Pereyra AJ, Lebherz TB. Combined urethro-vesical suspension and vaginourethroplasty for correction of urinary stress incontinence. Obstetrics and Gynaecology 1967; 30: 537–546.

103 Stamey TA. Cystoscopic suspension of the vesical neck for urinary incontinence in females. Surgery, Gynecology and Obstetrics 1973; 135: 547.

104 Raz S. Modified bladder neck suspension for female stress incontinence. Urology 198_ 18: 82.

105 Gittes RF, Loughlin KR. No-incision pubovesical suspension for stress incontinence. Journal of Urology 1987; 128: 568.

106 Pereyra AJ, Lebherz TB. The revised Pereyra procedure. In: In Buchsbaum H and Schmidt J. Gynaecologic and Obstetric Urology, 2nd edition, Philadelphia: WB Saunders 1978 pp 208–222.

107 Kursch ED, Wainsteim M, Persky L. The Pereyra procedure and urinary stress incontinence. Journal of Urology 1972; 108: 591–593.

108 Litvak AS, McRoberts JW. A modified Pereyra procedure for urinary stress incontinence. Journal of Urology 1974; 12: 89–91.

109 Backer MH, Probst RE. The Pereyra operation. Favourable experience with 200 operations. American Journal of Obstetrics and Gynaecology 1976; 125: 346–352.

110 Bhatia NN, Bergman A. Modified Burch versus Pereyra retropubic urethropexy for stress urinary incontinence. Obstetrics and Gynaecology 1985; 66: 255.

111 Leach GE, Yip CM, Donovan BJ. Mechanism of continence after modified Pereyra bladder neck suspension. Urology 1987; 29: 328.

112 Pereyra AJ, Lebherz TB. Pubourethral supports in perspective: modified Pereyra procedure for urinary incontinence. Obstetrics and Gynaecology 1982; 59: 643.

113 Karram M, Angel O, Koonings P, Tabor B, Bergman A, Bhatia N. The modified Pereyra procedure: a clinical and urodynamic review. British Journal of Obstetrics and Gynaecology 1993; 99: 655–658.

114 Biggers RD. Intraoperative endoscopic evaluation of suprapubic urethropexy. Urology 1987; 29: 268–270.

115 Hilton P, Mayne C. The Stamey endoscopic bladder neck suspension: a clinical and urodynamic investigation, including actuarial follow-up over four years. British Journal of Obstetrics and Gynaecology 1991; 98: 1141–1149.

116 Wujanto R, O'Reilly PH. Stamey needle suspension for stress urinary incontinence. British Journal of Urology 1989; 63: 162–164.

117 Stamey T, Schaeffer AJ, Condy M. Clinical and roentgenographic evaluation of endoscopic suspension of the vesical neck for urinary incontinence. Surgery, Gynecology and Obstetrics 1975; 140: 355–360.

118 Stamey TA. Endoscopic suspension of the bladder neck for urinary incontinence in females: report of 203 consecutive cases. Annals of Surgery 1980; 192: 465–471.

119 English PJ, Fowler JW. Videourodynamic assessment of the Stamey procedure for stress incontinence. British Journal of Urology 1988; 65: 550.

120 Kirby RS, Whiteway JE. Assessment of the results of the Stamey bladder neck suspension. British Journal of Urology 1989; 63: 21–23.

121 Jones DJ, Shah PJ, Worth PH. Modified Stamey procedure for bladder neck suspension. British Journal of Urology 63(2) 153–161. 1989.

122 Peattie AB, Stanton SL. The Stamey operation for the correction of genuine stress incontinence in elderly women. British Journal of Obstetrics and Gynaecology 1989; 96: 983–986.

123 Hilton P. A clinical and urodynamic study comparing the Stamey bladder neck suspension and suburethral sling procedures in the treatment of genuine stress incontinence. British Journal of Obstetrics and Gynaecology 1989; 96: 213–220.

124 Moir JC. The gauze hammock operation. Journal of Obstetrics and Gynaecology of the British Empire 1968; 75: 1–9.

125 Ogundipe A, Rosenzweig BA, Karram MM. Modified suburethral sling procedures for the treatment of recurrent or severe stress incontinence. Surgery, Gynecology and Obstetrics 1992; 175: 173.

126 McGuire EJ. Urodynamic findings in patients after failure of stress incontinent operations. Progress Clinical Biological Research 1981; 351: 78–82.

127 Sand P, Bowen L, Panganiba R, Ostergard D. The low pressure urethra as a factor in failed retropubic urethropexy. Obstetrics and Gynaecology 1987; 69: 399–402.

128 Koonings PP, Bergman A, Ballard CA. Low urethral pressure and stress urinary incontinence in women: risk factors for failed retropubic surgical procedure. Urology 1990; 36: 245–248.

129 Blavias JG, Olsson CA. Stress incontinence: classification and surgical approach. Journal of Urology 1988; 39: 727–731.

130 Meschia M, Bruschi F, Barbacini P, Amicarelli F, Ceosignani PG. Recurrent incontinence after retropubic surgery. Journal of Gynaecological Surgery 1993; 9: 25–28.

131 Jeffcoate TNA. Results of the Aldridge sling operation for stress incontinence. Journal of Obstetrics and Gynaecology of the British Empire 1956; 63: 36–39.

132 McClaren HC. Late results from sling operations. Journal of Obstetrics and Gynaecology of the British Empire 1968; 75: 10–13.

133 Kennedy C. Stress incontinence of urine: a survey of 34 cases treated by the Millin Sling operation. British Medical Journal, 2, 263–267, 1960.

134 Low JA. Management of severe anatomic deficiencies of urethral sphincter function by a combined procedure with a fascia lata sling. American Journal of Obstetrics and Gynaecology 1969; 105: 149.

135 Beck RP, Grove B, Arnusch D, Harvey J. Current urinary stress incontinence treated by the fascia lata sling procedure. American Journal of Obstetrics and Gynaecology 1974;

120: 613–624.

136 Parker RT, Addison WA, Wilson CJ. Fascia lata urethrovesical suspension for recurrent stress urinary incontinence. American Journal of Obstetrics and Gynecology 1979; 135: 843.

137 Spencer TS, Jequier AM, Kersey HJG. The gauze hammock operation in the treatment of persistent stress incontinence. Journal of Obstetrics and Gynaecology of the British Empire 1972; 79: 666–669.

138 Stanton SL, Brindley GS, Holmes DM. Silastic sling for urethral incompetence in women. British Journal of Obstetrics and Gynaecology 1985; 92: 747–750.

139 Horbach NS, Blanco JS, Ostergard JR. A suburethral sling procedure with polytetrafluoroethylene for the treatment of genuine stress incontinence. Obstetrics and Gynaecology 1988; 72: 302–306.

140 Morgan JE, Farrow MD, Stewart RN. The Marlex sling operation for the treatment of recurrent stress urinary incontinence: a 16 year review. Obstetrics and Gynaecology 1985; 151: 224–226.

141 Chin YK, Stanton SL. A follow-up of silastic sling for genuine stress incontinence. British Journal of Obstetrics and Gynaecology 1995; 102: 143–147.

142 Scott FB, Bradley WE, Timm GW. Treatment of urinary incontinence by an implantable urinary sphincter. Urology 1973; 1: 252.

143 Goldwasser B, Furlow WL, Barret M. The model AS 800 artificial sphincter: Mayo Clinic experience. Journal of Urology 1987; 137: 668–671.

144 Diokno RC, Hollander JB, Alderson TP. Artificial urinary sphincter for recurrent urinary incontinence: indications and results. Journal of Urology 1987; 137: 778.

145 Scott FB. The use of the artificial sphincter in the treatment of urinary incontinence in the female patient. Urological Clinics of North America 1985; 12: 305.

146 Donovan MG, Barrett DM, Furlow WL. Use of the artificial urinary sphincter for recurrent female urinary incontinence: indications and results. Surgery, Gynecology and Obstetrics 1985; 161: 17.

147 Appell RA. Techniques and results in the implantation of the artificial urinary sphincter in women with type III stress urinary incontinence by vaginal approach. Neurourol and Urodynam 1988; 7: 613.

148 Parulkar BG, Barrat DM. Application of the AS-800 artificial Sphincter for intractable urinary incontinence in females. *Surgery, Obstetrics and Gynaecology* 171; 131–138.

149 Berg S. Polytef augmentation urethroplasty. Archives of Surgery 1973; 107: 379–381.

150 Politano VA, Small MP, Harper JM, Lynne CM. Periurethral Teflon for urinary incontinence. Journal of Urology 1974; 111: 180–183.

151 Claes H, Stroobants D, Van Meerbeck J, Verbecken E, Knockert D, Baert L. Pulmonary migration following periurethral polytetrafluoroethylene injection for urinary incontinence. Journal of Urology 1989; 142: 821–822.

152 Beckingham IJ, Wemyss-Holden G, Lawrence WT. Long term follow-up of women treated with periurethral teflon injections for stress incontinence. British Journal of Urology 1992; 69: 580–583.

153 Politano VA. Periurethral polytetraflouroethylene injection for urinary incontinence. Journal of Urology 1982; 127: 439–442.

154 Lim KB, Ball AJ, Feneley RCL. Periurethral Teflon injection: a simple treatment for urinary incontinence. British Journal of Urology 1983; 55: 208.

155 Schulman CC, Simon J, Vespes E, Germeau F. Endoscopic injections of Teflon to treat urinary incontinence in women. British Medical Journal 1984; 288: 192.

156 Fischer W, Hegenscheid F, Jende W, Vogler H, Abet L. Is Teflon treatment of female urinary incontinence still justified? Zentrable Gynakol 1986; 108: 833–840.

157 Goldenberg LS. Periurethral collagen injection for patients with stress urinary incontinence. In: Proceedings of the AUA 89th Annual Meeting, San Fransisco J Urol 1994; 151: 479. Abstract.

158 Monga AK, Robinson D, Stanton SL. Periurethral collagen injections for genuine stress incontinence: a 2 year follow-up. British Journal of Urology 76: 156–160. 1995.

159 Swami K, Eckford SD, Abrams P. Collagen injections for female stress incontinence: conclusions of a multistage analysis and results. In: Proceedings of the AUA 89th Annual Meeting, San Fransisco. J Urol 194: 151: 479.

160 Appel RA, Goodman JR, McGuire EJ, et al. Multicenter study of periurethral and transurethral Gax-Collagen injection for urinary incontinence. Neurourol and urodynam 1989; 8: 339–340.

161 Buckley JF, Lingam K, Lloyd SN, et al. Injectable silicone macroparticles for female urinary incontinence. Journal of Urology 1993; 149: 402A Abstract.

162 Iacovou J, Lesberger J, Jones M, Kockelburgh R. Periurethral silicone implants for the treatment of simple stress incontinence. Journal of Urology 1993; 149: 402A.

163 Tanagho EA. Urethrosphincteric reconstruction for congenitally absent urethra. Journal of Urology 1976; 116: 237–242.

164 Gallagher PV, Mellon JK, Ramsden PD, Neal DE. Tanagho bladder neck reconstruction in the treatment of adult incontinence. Journal of Urology 1995; 153: 1451–1454.

165 Kuang-Kuo C, Chang LS, Ming-Tsen C. Urodynamic and clinical outcome of Koch pouch continent urinary diversion. Journal of Urology 1989; 141: 94–97.

166 Cox 1982

167 Albala DN, Scheussler WW, Vancaillie TG. Laparoscopic bladder neck suspension. Journal of Endourology 1992; 6: 137–141.

168 Chapple CR, Osbourne JL. Laparoscopic colposuspension– a new procedure. Minimally Invasive Therapy 1993; 2: 59–62.

169 Ou C, Prestus J, Beadle E. Laparoscopic bladder neck suspension using hernia mesh and surgical staples. Journal of Laparendoscopic Surgery 1993; 3: 563–566.

170 Burton G. A randomised comparison of laparoscopic and open colposuspension. Neurourology and Urodynamics. 1994; 13: 497–498.

171 Sand PK, Bowen LW, Panganiban R, Ostergard DR. The low pressure urethra as a factor in failed retropubic surgery. Obstetrics and Gynaecology 1987; 69: 399–402.

172 Steele SA, Cox C, Stanton SL. Long term follow-up of detrusor instability following colposuspension. British Journal of Urology 1986; 58: 138–142.

173 Jarvis GJ. Detrusor muscle instability – a complication of surgery? American Journal of Obstetrics and Gynaecology 1981; 139: 219.

174 Aldridge AH. Transplantation of fascia for the relief of urinary stress incontinence. American Journal of Obstetrics and Gynecology 1942; 44: 398–411.

175 Studdiford. Transplantation of abdominal fascia for relief of urinary stress incontinence. American Journal of Obstetrics and Gynecology 1944; 47: 764–774.

176 Millin T. Discussion on stress incontinence in micturition. Proceedings of the Royal Society of Medicine 1947; 40: 361–370.

177 Lavin JM, Smith ARB. Laparoscopic colposuspension. In: Smith ARB (ed) The investigation and management of urinary incontinence in women. London: RCOG Press, 1995: pp 96–106.

19

Detrusor instability and hyperreflexia

DETRUSOR INSTABILITY

Introduction

The normal human bladder is a compliant reservoir which only contracts during micturition under voluntary control. Conversely, an unstable bladder is one which contracts involuntarily, or can be provoked to do so.

The motor nerve supply to the bladder is via the parasympathetic nervous system, (S2,3,4), specifically by the pelvic nerve. Its effects are mediated by acetylcholine acting on muscarinic receptors.[1] Sympathetic innervation is derived from the hypogastric nerve and acts predominantly on β-receptors causing relaxation of the detrusor (see Fig. 3.1). Other putative neurotransmitters including adenosine triphosphate and vasoactive intestinal polypeptide may also play a minor role.[2,3] A detrusor contraction is initiated in the rostral pons. Efferent pathways emerge from the sacral spinal cord as the pelvic parasympathetic nerves and run forwards to the bladder. Acetylcholine is released at the neuromuscular junction and results in a co-ordinated contraction. A balance between sympathetic and parasympathetic stimulation is required for normal detrusor function.

Detrusor instability is defined by the International Continence Society as a condition in which the detrusor is shown objectively to contract, either spontaneously or on provocation, during bladder filling, whilst the subject is attempting to inhibit micturition.[4] It is a common condition, and may occur to some degree in up to 10% of the population. It is the second most common cause of urinary incontinence in women, and is demonstrated in about 40% of women who present for urodynamic investigation. The incidence increases with age such that detrusor instability is the most common cause of incontinence in the elderly.[5,6]

In the presence of demonstrable neurological disease, the term 'detrusor hyperreflexia' is used. This distressing condition causes the sufferer much embarrassment and may severely affect her daily life. Although incontinence is often the most unpleasant symptom, urgency, frequency and nocturia and nocturnal enuresis may all occur, and in fact detrusor instability is usually manifested by multiple symptoms.

Our understanding of the pathophysiology of detrusor instability is imperfect and therefore treatment is often empirical and sadly ineffective. Few women are ever completely cured, but many derive considerable symptomatic relief from the treatment regimens currently available.

In women with detrusor instability, there is rarely an obvious cause. It may arise as a result of poorly learnt bladder control as an infant, and indeed bladder retraining together with other behavioral interventions produces good clinical results.

Zoubek et al[7] have studied 46 children with isolated urinary frequency. All were previously toilet trained. In 40% of cases a 'trigger' was identified prior to the onset of symptoms. This often involved problems at school. All cases were self-limiting or resolved following counseling or removal of the trigger. There is a strong association between childhood nocturnal enuresis and detrusor instability presenting in adult life.[8]

The psychoneurotic status of women with detrusor instability has been assessed by several authors with conflicting results. Walters et al evaluated 63 women with incontinence and 27 continent controls using formal psychometric testing.[9] They reported no difference in the test results between women with genuine stress incontinence and those with detrusor instability. Women with detrusor instability scored significantly higher than controls on the hypochondriasis, depression and hysteria scales. They concluded that these abnormalities may be related to incontinence in general and not to the specific diagnosis.

Norton et al[10] psychiatrically assessed 117 women attending the urodynamic clinic prior to urodynamic investigation. There was no increased psychiatric morbidity in women with detrusor instability compared to women with genuine stress incontinence. Interestingly, women in whom no urodynamic abnormality could be detected had the highest scores for anxiety and neuroticism. These levels were comparable to those of psychiatric out-patients.

Moore & Sutherst[11] have evaluated the response to treatment of detrusor instability, using oxybutynin, in relation to psychoneurotic status. Poor responders had a higher mean psychoneurotic score than responders although one-third of poor responders were normal. Patients who responded well to therapy had scores similar to normal urban females. Many women with detrusor instability therefore show little evidence of psychoneuroticism. These last two studies emphasize the need for further research into the physical, and in particular the neurological aspects of detrusor instability.

In the male there is an association between outflow obstruction due to benign prostatic hypertrophy and detrusor instability. In a large study by Webster, however, only one of 3000 women with detrusor instability had bladder neck obstruction on meticulous urodynamic testing.[12] Following incontinence surgery, there is an increased incidence of detrusor instability[13] which may relate to the development of relative outflow obstruction or more likely to the extensive bladder neck dissection performed at operation. The prevalence of detrusor instability in women following multiple incontinence procedures is correspondingly high.

The pathophysiology of the unstable bladder is not fully understood. Increased sensitivity of nerve endings in the bladder to local stimuli may result in abnormal reflex responses resulting in frequency and urgency.[] Low electrical sensitivity thresholds in the posterior urethra of women with urgency syndromes have been demonstrated by Kieswetter.[]

Whether this is responsible for the generation of uninhibited detrusor motor activity has yet to be determined.

Relaxation of the urethra is known to precede contraction of the detrusor in a proportion of women with detrusor instability.[16] This may represent primary pathology in the urethra which triggers a detrusor contraction, or may merely be part of a complex sequence of events which originate elsewhere. It has been postulated that incompetence of the bladder neck, allowing passage of urine into the proximal urethra, may result in an uninhibited contraction of the detrusor. Sutherst & Brown, however, were unable to provoke a detrusor contraction in 50 women by rapidly infusing saline into the posterior urethra using modified urodynamic equipment.[17]

Brading and Turner suggest that the common feature in all cases of detrusor instability is a change in the properties of the smooth muscle of the detrusor which predisposes it to unstable contractions. This change is caused by a long-term reduction in the functional innervation of the bladder wall.[18] They dispute the concept of 'hyperreflexia', i.e. increased motor activity to the detrusor, as the underlying mechanism in detrusor instability.

Clinical presentation

Detrusor instability may present with any or all of the symptoms listed below:

- frequency
- nocturia
- urgency
- urge incontinence
- stress incontinence
- nocturnal enuresis
- coital incontinence.

The most common symptoms are urgency and frequency of micturition, which occur in approximately 80% of patients.[19] Most incontinent women, regardless of the etiology, develop frequency in a conscious effort to leak less. There are, however, many other causes of urgency and frequency (Table 19.1).

Nocturia occurs in almost 70% of cases of detrusor instability. It should be remembered, however, that the prevalence of nocturia is an age-related phenomenon. It is normal over the age of 70 years to void twice, and over the age of 80 to void three times, during the night. Urge incontinence is usually preceded by urgency (a sudden, strong desire to void) and is due to an involuntary detrusor contraction. Some women, however, are unaware of any sensation associated with the detrusor contraction and just notice that they are wet. The symptom of nocturnal enuresis is strongly correlated with the presence of detrusor instability.[8] Incontinence during intercourse is a distressing symptom found both in women with urethral sphincter incompetence and women with detrusor instability. In the former condition, leakage usually occurs on penetration, whereas in the latter it occurs at orgasm.[20]

Table 19.1   Symptoms of 'the urge syndrome' and their causes

Symptom	Causes
Frequency	*Gynecological/urological*
(>7 voids per day)	Detrusor instability
	Sensory urgency
Nocturia	Urinary tract infection
(>1 void per night)	Intravesical lesion
	Interstitial cystitis
Urgency	Small capacity bladder
	Radiation
	Menopause
	Genuine stress incontinence
	Cystocele
	Urinary residual
	Pregnancy
	Abdominal/pelvic mass
	Urethral syndrome
	Urethral obstruction
	Urethral diverticulum
	Psychological
	Excessive fluid intake
	Habit
	Anxiety
	Medical
	Diuretics
	Diabetes mellitus
	Diabetes insipidus
	Congestive cardiac failure
	Neurological (detrusor hyperreflexia)
	Renal failure
Urge incontinence	Detrusor instability
	Sensory urgency
	Urinary tract infection
	Intravesical lesion

Clinical examination is often unhelpful, although general examination will enable mood, mental state and mobility to be assessed. Vulval excoriation and atrophy and the presence of stress incontinence should be assessed. A neurological examination with reference to S2, 3 and 4 outflow may reveal a neuropathic cause for the symptoms.

Routine investigations must exclude local pathology such as infection, calculi and neoplasia, all of which may produce similar symptoms. Sterile urine is mandatory prior to instrumentation of the lower urinary tract, including catheterization at the time of cystometry. Urinary infection may invalidate the results of urodynamic investigations.

A frequency/volume chart will enable excessive fluid intake to be detected, functional bladder capacity to be evaluated and the nature and severity of incontinence episodes to be assessed. The diagnosis of detrusor instability, however, can only be made by subtracted, provocative cystometry. The presence of systolic or provoked detrusor contractions during the filling phase, whilst the subject is attempting to inhibit micturition, is diagnostic of detrusor instability (Fig. 19.1). Figure 19.2 shows the cystometric trace of a patient with detrusor hyperreflexia secondary to a complete T4 spinal cord transection. In the absence of subtracted cystometry, single-channel cystometry provides a useful

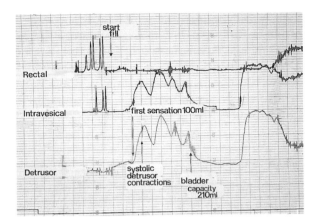

Fig. 19.1 A cystometrogram showing detrusor instability

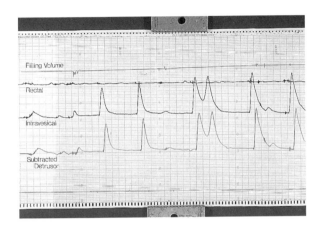

Fig. 19.2 Detrusor hyperreflexia in a spinal injury patient

screening test with fairly high levels of sensitivity, although fairly poor specificity.[21]

Ambulatory monitoring is becoming popular and is believed to be more physiological and therefore more accurate in diagnosing detrusor instability.[22] The test has a greater sensitivity than conventional cystometry in the detection of detrusor instability in women with irritative bladder symptoms. In a large study of women with symptoms of urinary incontinence in whom the findings of conventional urodynamic investigations were normal, detrusor instability was detected in 65% of cases on ambulatory testing.[23] The presence of uninhibited detrusor activity has been detected in asymptomatic 'normal' controls during ambulatory monitoring, and therefore a consensus needs to be reached with regard to normal values.

This technique has recently been used to evaluate the efficacy of oxybutynin (5 mg three times a day) in 50 patients with detrusor instability.[24] The frequency and amplitude of uninhibited detrusor contractions were significantly reduced during the treatment period. Holmes et al[25] have suggested, however, that measurement of bladder neck electrical conductivity may be a more sensitive test in detecting abnormalities in women with urgency and urge incontinence. This technique remains a research investigation and has not been applied to clinical practice.

Other investigations which may provide useful additional information include pad tests, videocystourethrography and distal urethral electric conductance.

Treatment

Women with mild or intermittent symptoms may only require reassurance and simple measures such as decreased fluid intake, avoidance of tea, coffee and alcohol, or a change in voiding habits. Others with more incapacitating symptoms will require further treatment. The methods used attempt either to improve central control, as in behavioral intervention, or to alter detrusor innervation using drugs or surgical techniques. Only when these measures fail are procedures employed which do not treat the instability, but act to increase the size of the reservoir. Conventional bladder neck surgery rarely cures women with detrusor instability, and may make the symptoms of urgency and frequency worse.

The therapeutic options currently employed include:

- drug therapy
- behavioral therapy
- maximal electrical stimulation
- acupuncture
- phenol injections
- augmentation cystoplasty
- urinary diversion.

Many other surgical forms of treatment have been tried in the past, including vaginal denervation,[26] selective sacral neurectomy,[27] cysto-distension[28,29,30,31] and bladder transection.[32] All have been reported to be efficacious initially, but due to high complication rates or long-term relapse have been superseded.

Drug therapy

Still the mainstay of treatment, drugs may be subdivided into groups according to their pharmacological mode of action.

The pharmacological agents commonly used to treat detrusor instability are shown in tables.

Anticholinergic agents The detrusor is innervated by the parasympathetic nervous system (pelvic nerve), the sympathetic nervous system (hypogastric nerve) and by non-cholinergic non-adrenergic neurones. The motor supply arises from S2,3 and 4 and is conveyed by the pelvic nerve. The neurotransmitter at the neuromuscular junction is acetylcholine, which acts upon muscarinic receptors, Anti-muscarinic drugs would seem likely to be of use in the treatment of detrusor instability. Atropine is the classic anticholinergic drug with antimuscarinic activity. Its non-specific mode of action, however, makes it unacceptable for use, due to the high

Table 19.2   Drugs used in the treatment of detrusor instability

Drug	Mechanism of action	Dose
Oxybutynin	Anticholinergic/ direct muscle relaxant	2.5–10 mg two to three times a day
Propantheline	Anticholinergic	15–90 mg four times a day
Imipramine	Anticholinergic/ central action	50 mg twice a day (up to 150 mg in a single dose)
DDAVP (nasal spray)	Reduces urine production	20–40 mg at night
Estrogens	Raise sensory threshold of bladder	

incidence of side effects. Dry mouth, blurred vision, tachycardia, drowsiness and constipation are associated with its use.

Propantheline (Pro-Banthine) is a related drug with fewer side effects. It is a quaternary ammonium analog of atropine with both anti-muscarinic and anti-nicotinic properties, which acts at both the ganglionic level and at the neuromuscular junction. Blaivas et al[33] have shown that intramuscular injection of propantheline abolishes involuntary detrusor contractions in 70% of cases of detrusor instability. However, 50% of patients required short-term intermittent self-catheterization for resulting urinary retention. When given orally in a dose of 15 mg four times a day it is often ineffective. The dose may therefore be increased to as much as 90 mg four times a day, but should be introduced slowly to minimize side effects. Gastrointestinal absorption is aided by taking the drug before meals.[34] Propantheline is a cheap drug with few side effects, and is particularly useful when frequency of micturition is a major problem.

Cornella et al[35] have treated 10 patients with detrusor instability using transdermal scopolamine. Only 3 patients reported symptomatic improvement whilst 9 found the side effects intolerable, requiring discontinuation of treatment in 8 cases. Side effects included ataxia, blurred vision, dizziness, vertigo and severe dry mouth.

Emepromium carageanate is an anticholinergic agent derived from seaweed which, although not available in the United Kingdom, is widely used in Europe and Ireland.

Musculotropic relaxants Oxybutynin (Cystrin, Ditropan) is one of the most effective drugs available. It has a direct spasmolytic effect as well as anticholinergic properties. In the first reported study in 1980, 30 patients were treated in a double-blind placebo-controlled trial.[36] Of the patients treated with oxybutynin, 60% were symptomatically improved compared to 8% of those on placebo. Seventeen patients experienced side effects and 9 of these withdrew from the study because of them.

Oxybutynin has been compared to propantheline in a variable dose crossover trial.[37] It was found to be superior in terms of both symptomatic and cystometric improvement. In a large randomized, double-blind multicenter study conducted by Thuroff et al, the degree of symptomatic improvement and objective improvement in urodynamic parameters was significantly greater for those treated with oxybutynin than for those given either propantheline or placebo.[38] It reduced the degree of urgency experienced by postmenopausal women with detrusor instability, but side effects were frequent.[39] In one study 76% of participants complained of side effects, whilst only 57% derived symptomatic relief.[40]

This is a drug of doubtless benefit, but the dose must be balanced with the patient's ability to tolerate the dry mouth and throat and lingering bad taste which accompany its therapeutic effect. It is contraindicated in patients with glaucoma. It is a drug with a short half-life, and therefore it is rapidly effective following ingestion. A dose may be taken as prophylaxis to control symptoms for short periods, e.g. whilst shopping or at the cinema. The standard dosage is 5 mg orally twice daily but this may be increased up to 10 mg three times a day. Side effects are common at the standard dose and treatment compliance is often poor in the longer term.

In a double-blind, placebo-controlled, crossover study by Moore et al,[41] an alternative dose regimen of 3 mg three times a day has been advocated. Symptomatic cure, or marked improvement, was found in 60% of 53 patients with detrusor instability using this lower dose of oxybutynin, whilst the incidence of side effects resulting in discontinuation of therapy was only 7.5%. Intravesical administration of oxybutynin is effective and a useful alternative for patients with detrusor hyperreflexia who need to self-catheterize or have an indwelling catheter.

Flavoxate (Urispas) is a tertiary amine with a papaverine-like effect on smooth muscle. It inhibits phosphodiesterase, resulting in raised levels of cyclic adenosine monophosphate, which leads to muscle relaxation. It also has analgesic and local anesthetic properties. Commonly prescribed in a dose of 200 mg three times a day, it is poorly absorbed from the gut, and doubt has been cast as to its true efficacy in the treatment of detrusor instability after either oral or parenteral administration. Its effects may be no superior to those of placebo.[42,43] Terflavoxate is a derivative of flavoxate, the efficacy of which has not yet been established.

Calcium channel blockers Any drug which limits the availability of calcium ions will result in smooth muscle relaxation.

Until October 1991, terodiline (Micturin) was the most commonly prescribed drug for the treatment of detrusor instability. It was well absorbed from the gastrointestinal tract, and caused decreased urinary frequency and fewer episodes of incontinence in women with detrusor instability when compared to placebo.[44] It was voluntarily withdrawn by its manufacturer following cardiac adverse events mainly in elderly patients taking the drug.

Verapamil has been used by Bodner et al,[45] alone and in combination with oxybutynin in 14 patients with detrusor hyperreflexia. No clinical improvement was found when using verapamil alone. Thirteen patients showed greater improvement on treatment with combined verapamil and oxybutynin than on treatment with oxybutynin alone. The dose of oxybutynin may be reduced to minimize unwanted side effects, which are common and often lead to discontinuation of therapy.

Other drugs which decrease contractility Imipramine was initially tested as an antipsychotic agent, as it is an analog of chlorpromazine, and was found to have antidepressant properties. It acts by inhibiting reuptake of noradrenaline and 5-hydroxytryptamine into the presynaptic membrane, and thus potentiating their action. This may result in bladder relaxation and increase outlet resistance. It also has anticholinergic and local anesthetic properties. Imipramine sometimes causes the common anticholinergic side effects as well as tremor, sedation and convulsions. If treatment is stopped abruptly, withdrawal reactions may occur involving nausea, vomiting, malaise and depression. ECG changes have been reported, including tachycardia, atrial flutter, atrial fibrillation, ventricular flutter and both atrioventricular and interventricular block.

Imipramine is, however, a most useful drug for the treatment of nocturia and nocturnal enuresis. In a study by Castleden et al,[46] 6 out of 10 elderly patients with detrusor instability became continent at night following treatment with imipramine. A dose of up to 150 mg may be given safely, but the standard dosage is 50 mg twice daily. Other tricyclic anti-depressants such as amitriptyline may be substituted for imiprimine. Imipramine given prophylactically before sexual intercourse may be of benefit to patients with coital incontinence at orgasm.[47]

Antidiuretic drugs 1-Desamino-8-D arginine vasopressin (DDAVP) is a long-acting, synthetic analog of vasopressin, which is a peptide hormone containing eight amino acids. DDAVP can be administered intranasally, or more recently in tablet form, and is effective for 12–24 h, having a half-life of 75 min due to slow metabolic clearance. Whilst it has full anti-diuretic potency and increases permeability in the distal convoluted tubules and collecting ducts of the kidney, unlike vasopressin it has no significant effect on blood pressure. It has a lesser effect on smooth muscle contraction and therefore pallor, colic, bronchospasm, coronary artery or uterine spasm do not occur.

Studies have shown a 50% reduction in urine production following an intranasal dose of 20–40 µg.[48] DDAVP is a useful drug in the treatment of nocturia and nocturnal enuresis. Because the bladder fills more slowly, and the total volume of urine is reduced, the number of uninhibited contractions is diminished. In a double-blind placebo-controlled crossover study involving 21 patients, DDAVP significantly reduced the number of wet nights.[49] Only 6 of the 21 patients, however, had proven detrusor instability. DDAVP causes a significantly greater reduction in night-time voids when compared to placebo.[50] It has been shown to be safe for long-term use,[51] but caution must be used when treating patients with coronary artery disease, hypertension, heart failure or epilepsy.

Hormone replacement therapy Estrogen deficiency following the meno-pause causes changes in all layers of the urethra, which has abundant estrogen receptors.[52] The bladder itself possesses fewer receptors. Of the abundant literature regarding estrogens and the lower urinary tract, there have been few placebo-controlled trials using objective as well as subjective outcome measures.

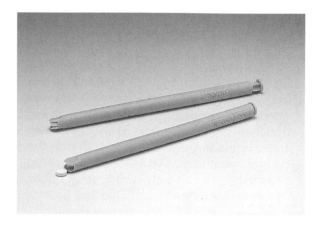

Fig. 19.3 Intravaginal estradiol tablet (Vagifem, Novo)

No studies have shown that estrogen therapy improves incontinence due to detrusor instability. Sensory urgency is, however, improved by estrogen therapy, which is thought to raise the sensory threshold of the bladder.[53] Daily use of a low-dose intravaginal estradiol tablet (Vagifem) in a placebo-controlled trial resulted in significant reduction in the symptom of urgency in a subgroup of postmenopausal women with urodynamically proven sensory urgency (Fig 19.3). No improvement in irritative bladder symptoms was found for women with detrusor instability.[54]

Drugs may be used alone or in combination. Propantheline and imipramine can be used together for the treatment of diurnal and nocturnal frequency. In a similar way, DDAVP may be used in combination with oxybutynin. Drugs may be used in conjunction with other forms of treatment, e.g. bladder retraining.

The choice of drug for each patient depends on the predominant symptoms and the tolerance of side effects (Table 19.3).

Behavioral therapy

This type of treatment is based on the premise that learning is the most important determinant of behavior, and that behavior can be altered as a

Table 19.3 Management of patients with detrusor instability

General	
Decrease excessive fluid intake to 1500 ml/day	
Avoid caffeine-containing drinks and alcohol	
Supply with effective protective pads and pants	
Specific	
First-line treatment is usually with drug therapy	
Symptom	*Drug of choice*
Frequency	Propantheline
	Oxybutynin
	Hormone replacement therapy
Urgency/urge incontinence	Oxybutynin
Nocturia/nocturnal enuresis	Imipramine
	DDAVP
Second-line treatments	Bladder retraining (alone or in combination with drug therapy)
	Maximal electric stimulation
Refractory cases	Augmentation cystoplasty

result of experience. Thus man's behavior is seen as a collection of responses to specific situations. Detrusor instability, in some instances, is viewed as a result of maladaptive learned behavior. Treatment is aimed at either 'unlearning' maladaptive behavior or relearning a more appropriate one.

Bladder drill This was first described as 'bladder discipline' in 1966 by Jeffcoate & Francis.[55] They treated 246 women with urgency incontinence, a condition which we now know as detrusor instability, using a regimen of timed voiding. The interval between voids was gradually increased over a period of days to weeks.

In a study by Frewen in 1978 an 82.5% symptomatic cure rate was found in 40 patients treated with bladder drill for 3 months.[56] He stated that there was a psychogenic or emotive origin for the patients' symptoms. Further studies have produced similar success rates. Of 150 patients with frequency and urgency, 86% were symptomatically cured following 3 months of bladder drill.[57] This was irrespective of the presence or absence of detrusor instability. Frewen suggests that the initial maladaptive pattern of frequency leads to urgency with or without incontinence. Eventually detrusor instability results. If the pattern of frequency can be broken using bladder drill, then the detrusor may reconvert to stability. This may take months to occur.

In 1981 Jarvis compared the efficacy of bladder drill to that of drug therapy and found the former to be superior.[58] These studies suggest that bladder drill is the most effective treatment of idiopathic detrusor instability. In 1983, however, Holmes et al[59] reviewed patients 3 years following bladder drill. Forty-three per cent of patients had relapsed, regardless of initial conversion to a stable bladder following treatment. Bladder drill may be conducted on an out-patient basis but often the patient requires hospital admission for the treatment to be effective. The regimen suggested by Jarvis is commonly employed and is described as follows:

1. Exclude pathology and admit to hospital.
2. Explain rationale to patient.
3. Instruct to void every one and a half hours during the day. She must not void between these times; she must wait or be incontinent.
4. Increase voiding interval by half an hour when initial goal achieved, and continue with two-hourly voiding etc.
5. Give normal volume of fluids.
6. Keep fluid balance chart.
7. Give encouragement.

Biofeedback This involves the use of electronic equipment to monitor a normally unconscious physiological process and relay this information to the individual so that a change in a particular direction may be brought about. The information is fed back as an audible, tactile or visual signal.

In a study of 27 patients with detrusor instability, 81% were improved following four to six 1-h sessions of biofeedback using both audible and visual signals of detrusor activity.[60] The relapse rate at 5 years is unfortunately very high. This type of treatment also requires a great deal of input from motivated doctors or nurses. A pilot study of biofeedback using bladder neck electric conductance has been reported with successful results in females with idiopathic detrusor instability.[61]

Hypnotherapy Freeman & Baxby[62] have treated 50 patients with detrusor instability using this method. Women received 12 sessions of hypnosis during 1 month. Following this 29 were symptom-free and a further 14 were improved. Forty-four underwent repeat urodynamics with 22 converting to a stable bladder. The results of this study have not been substantiated by further studies and hypnotherapy cannot be regarded as a routine treatment option.

All methods of behavioral therapy are complex and time-consuming for both the operator and the patient. For these reasons they are often overlooked in favour of simpler drug regimens.

Acupuncture

The original work was carried out by Philp and colleagues[63] who treated 20 patients with detrusor instability using Chinese acupuncture. Seventy-seven per cent of patients were improved, but only one was converted to a stable bladder on cystometry. Acupuncture is thought to act by increasing levels of endorphins and enkephalins in the cerebro-spinal fluid. Enkephalins are known to inhibit detrusor contractility in vitro.[64] Naloxone, an opiate antagonist, conversely causes decreased bladder capacity and increased detrusor pressures.[65] In 1985 Pigne et al,[66] treated 16 patients with detrusor instability using acupuncture. Fifteen of them were improved in terms of decreased frequency and amount of leakage.

Recently, infrared low-power laser has been used on acupuncture points by Gibson et al.[67] Twenty-eight patients were treated twice a week for 5 weeks. Following this 50% showed a complete symptomatic cure and a further 25% were improved. At follow-up 6 months later 16 had relapsed.

Maximal electrical stimulation

For many years, different forms of electrical stimulation have been utilized in the treatment of detrusor instability and genuine stress incontinence. Stimulation of the proximal end of a transected pudendal nerve was shown to induce bladder relaxation as long ago as 1895.[68] Inhibition of the detrusor following vaginal or anal electrical stimulation using external electrodes is believed to occur via pudendal to pelvic nerve and pudendal to hypogastric nerve reflexes. Long-term, low-amplitude stimulation of pudendal afferents[69] and, more recently, acute maximal electrical stimulation (MES) have proved efficacious in the treatment of detrusor instability.[70]

Ohlsson et al treated 29 patients using MES, administered from a laboratory device.[71] Intravaginal and intra-anal electrodes were used and an alternating rectangular, constant voltage at a frequency of 10 Hz was employed. Four stimulation sessions at weekly intervals were carried out. Transperineal direct stimulation of the pudendal nerve was carried out in patients who showed limited response to external stimulation. The patients were divided into those with an uninhibited overactive bladder and those with idiopathic detrusor instability, on the basis of cystometric findings and the Bor's ice water test. Both groups showed significant reduction in urinary frequency following treatment. The uninhibited overactive bladder group showed a significant increase in functional bladder capacity. Direct stimulation was advantageous in 2 cases where external stimulation was unsuccessful.

Jonasson et al[72] have used short-term home MES to treat 20 women with detrusor instability and 17 with genuine stress incontinence. A vaginal electrode only was employed, using a frequency of 20 Hz and a variable current of 0–90 mA. Stimulation was carried out at home for 20 min a day for 12 weeks. Fourteen of the 20 women with detrusor instability showed subjective improvement and there was a significant reduction in leakage, as judged by pad testing, in 19 cases. In the genuine stress incontinence group, 8 out of 17 were subjectively improved and in 12 cases there was significantly reduced leakage.

We have employed a similar device (Fig 19.4) in a comparative trial of MES and oxybutynin.[73] Both treatments were associated with a significant reduction in reporting of symptoms on visual analog scales, and a reduction in diurnal frequency as measured in a voiding diary. While 20% of the patients who received oxybutynin withdrew due to treatment side effects, MES was universally acceptable, and we feel should be considered as an alternative to current pharmacological agents. A management plan for patients with detrusor instability is shown in Table 19.3.

Surgical techniques

Historically, many different surgical procedures have been utilized but few have stood the test of time.

In 1959, Ingelman-Sundberg described vaginal denervation,[26] which was later employed by Warrell in 1977 with moderate success.[74] Bladder transection was introduced by Turner-Warwick & Ashken in 1967,[32] with good initial results reported by Mundy in 1983.[27] More recent studies, however, have found it to be of little benefit.[75] Torrens & Griffith reported the use of selective sacral neurectomy in 1974 but this technique has

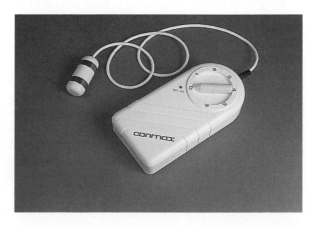

Fig. 19.4 A maximal electrical stimulator with intravaginal electrode

never been employed widely.[28] Bladder distension, introduced by Helmstein as a treatment for carcinoma of the bladder in 1966,[29] was popularized by Dunn et al in 1974.[30] Several subsequent studies have shown it to be of limited efficacy, with a high rate of complications, notably bladder rupture.[31,76] The following operative procedures, however, are of value in selected cases of detrusor instability.

Transvesical phenol injections Transvesical blockade of nerve plexuses adjacent to the bladder has been described using a 25-cm-long needle passed down the side channel of a cystoscope. The tip is introduced midway between the ureteric orifice and the bladder neck and is advanced 2–3 cm. Ten millilitres of 6% aqueous phenol is then injected. The procedure is performed bilaterally.

This was first described by Ewing et al in 1982.[77] In their original work, 76% of patients were dry, with increased bladder capacity and an increase in the volume at which detrusor instability occurred. The majority of their patients had neuropathic bladders, 20 of which were due to multiple sclerosis.

Blackford et al[78] treated 116 women using this method. They reported an 82% success rate in detrusor hyperreflexia, compared to 40% in those with idiopathic detrusor instability. Better results were found in women over the age of 55. They suggested a role for phenol injections in patients with an indwelling catheter and detrusor hyperreflexia who have problems with bypassing due to detrusor contractions. One set of injections may give relief of symptoms and avoid a lifetime of drug therapy. Other studies have also highlighted the possible benefits in the hyperreflexic patient.[79] There is an incidence of retention, requiring intermittent self-catheterization of about 8%. Other complications include sciatic nerve palsy, ureteric sloughing and vesicovaginal fistula.

Subsequent studies, however, have not confirmed these good results. Rosenbaum et al[80] quoted a maximal benefit of 50% in neuropathic bladders after follow-up for 3 months. For idiopathic detrusor instability this figure was only 25%. Very little benefit is maintained beyond 1 year following treatment. They concluded that the temporary nature of any improvement did not warrant the risk of anesthesia in patients with idiopathic detrusor instability. They may be better treated by augmentation cystoplasty. Wall & Stanton[81] found that only 29% of 28 patients responded after one set of injections. Of 11 who underwent a second course, only 3 derived any benefit and there was one case of vesicovaginal fistula.

Augmentation cystoplasty Some patients will not respond to any medical intervention, or find their side effects too incapacitating. They may then have been subjected to cystodistension or phenol injections, as these are still relatively commonly performed procedures. If symptoms are still really severe, augmentation cystoplasty should be considered.

This operation was first described by Bramble[82] for the treatment of 15 patients with enuresis, 87% of whom were cured by the procedure. The operation involves bisecting the bladder in a coronal plane anterior to the ureteric orifices to within 1 cm of the bladder neck. The distance i measured and a corresponding length of ileum is isolated, opened along its antimesenteric border, and sutured as a patch into the defect. This segment is thought to act by absorbing, and thereby reducing, the effect of unstable detrusor contractions. In 1985 Mundy & Stephenson[83] reported a 90% cure rate in 40 patients treated by this method, and in 1987 McRae et al[84] reported cure rates of 90–100% in 59 patients with neuropathic bladders.

There is a significant risk of postoperative voiding difficulties, possibly as a result of diminished voiding pressures, caused by the presence of the ileal segment. This may be overcome by performing a sphincterotomy or by teaching the patient clean intermittent self-catheterization. Less common complications such as urine leakage from the anastomosis, requiring revision, and small bowel obstruction have been described.

Mucus production by the bowel segment occasionally causes distress to the patient, who may have to strain to pass mucus plugs. Ingestion of 200 ml of cranberry juice a day helps to reduce mucus viscidity.[85]

The chronic exposure of the ileal mucosa to urine has given cause for concern with regard to possible malignant change. There is a 5% risk of adenocarcinoma arising in ureterosigmoidostomies, where colonic mucosa is exposed to the N-nitrosamines found in both urine and feces, and a similar risk may pertain to enterocystoplasty. Biopsies of the ileal segment taken from patients with 'clam' cystoplasties show evidence of chronic inflammation and villous atrophy.[86] Chronic inflammation may predispose to adenocarcinoma as in cases of Gilharzia.

There have been reports of cases of adenocarcinoma arising in the ileal segment. Three cases, occurring in patients 7, 22 and 24 years following surgery were reported by Stone et al.[87] All three initially had tuberculosis as a cause of their symptoms: all had been troubled with recurrent urinary tract infections and had high residual urine volumes postoperatively. It is clear, therefore, that patients undergoing augmentation cystoplasty require long-term follow-up.

DETRUSOR HYPERREFLEXIA

The treatment of detrusor hyperreflexia is in general similar to that of idiopathic detrusor instability. Management of patients with neurological disorders is complicated by the clinical features of the underlying condition. Voiding difficulty with residual urine, immobility and lack of manual dexterity, loss of bladder sensation and impaired cognitive function are complicating factors which may alter the basic management of a patient with detrusor hyperreflexia. The particular features of the more common causes of detrusor hyperreflexia are discussed below.

Spinal cord injury

Spinal cord injury (SCI) is a common cause of detrusor hyperreflexia. Motorcycle, car and diving accidents are the major causes of fracture dislocation of the spine and spinal cord injury. Disc prolapse, epidural hematoma or abscess, acute myelitis and surgery for thoracic aortic aneurysm are less common causes of SCI.

All cord injuries which are complete and spare the S2, S3 and S4 segments eventually produce upper motor neurone lesions with resultant detrusor hyperreflexia. However, during the initial phase of spinal shock following suprasacral spinal cord injury, the bladder is areflexic. Urinary retention and overflow incontinence may occur. Effective bladder drainage is essential at this time to avoid overdistension of the bladder, urinary tract infection and upper tract damage with concomitant deterioration in renal function. This may be achieved by suprapubic catheterization or clean intermittent catheterization.

Within 6 to 8 weeks of the injury, reflexic detrusor activity is established. Voiding may be achieved by manual suprapubic compression or stimulation of the genital area. In almost all cases of suprasacral cord injury, the detrusor and urethral sphincter are dysfunctional. Detrusor–sphincter inco-ordination or dyssynergia is present in many cases.

High intravesical pressures may be generated, with subsequent development of trabeculation, bladder diverticula and upper tract dilatation, despite complete bladder emptying. The hyperreflexia must be treated aggressively using anticholinergic agents, even at the expense of increased urinary residuals. Clean intermittent self-catheterization is usually the method of choice to achieve bladder emptying in patients with detrusor–sphincter dyssynergia and those with iatrogenic urinary residuals.

Urinary diversion is rarely indicated in SCI patients, except in cases of extensive pelvic or urethral trauma, urinary fistula, a small fibrotic bladder or severe vesicoureteric reflux.

Intracranial lesions

Cerebrovascular accidents (CVA) commonly give rise to lower urinary tract symptoms. In general, suprapontine lesions result in loss of inhibition of the micturition center and hyperreflexia of the detrusor develops. Management is complicated by loss of sensation and the awareness of the need to void, loss of motor co-ordination and behavioral changes in voiding habits.

Detrusor hyperreflexia may also arise in other intracranial diseases, e.g. Huntington's chorea, cerebellar ataxia, cerebral palsy, Shy-Drager's syndrome, hereditary ataxias and cerebral aneurysms.

Parkinson's disease

Detrusor hyperreflexia is a common finding in patients with Parkinson's disease, occurring in 75% of those with lower urinary tract symptoms.[88] The extrapyramidal system is believed to have an inhibitory effect on the micturition centre and so loss of dopaminergic activity in the substantia nigra, caudate, putamen and globus pallidus results in loss of detrusor inhibition. This theory was challenged by Malone-Lee et al,[89] who found no evidence of a disease-specific Parkinsonian bladder following evaluation of the urodynamic studies of 2526 patients, of whom 76 had Parkinson's disease. He suggested that the urodynamic changes seen in such patients were age-related phenomena. Anticholinergic medication alone or in combination with intermittent self-catheterization are the treatments of choice.

Multiple sclerosis

Urinary symptoms are common in patients with multiple sclerosis (MS) and may occur at some time in up to 80% of cases.[90] Bladder dysfunction may be a feature of the presenting symptom complex, but more commonly lower urinary tract symptoms develop later in the course of the disease.

Detrusor hyperreflexia is the commonest urodynamic abnormality in MS patients, with a reported prevalence of 50–90%. Less frequently detrusor areflexia is present. Detrusor–sphincter dyssynergia commonly coexists with detrusor hyperreflexia with a reported prevalence of 12–88%.

Management is aimed at reducing the high intravesical pressures associated with hyperreflexia and dyssynergia to prevent vesicoureteric reflux and subsequent renal damage. Treatment with oxybutynin, propantheline or imipramine may reduce the degree of incontinence and the severity of irritative bladder symptoms at the expense of increased urinary residuals. In such cases, clean intermittent self-catheterization is employed. Although antispasmodic agents such as baclofen, dantrolene and diazepam may be used to reduce dyssynergia, clean intermittent self-catheterization is usually required.

Regular review is essential as the severity of the neurourological impairment may alter with remission or progression of the disease process.

CONCLUSIONS

Detrusor instability is a common and unpleasant condition which severely affects the lifestyle of many women. The diversity of treatments outlined above emphasizes the lack of understanding of the etiology of this condition. It is vital to make an accurate diagnosis in all women presenting with urinary symptoms, so that appropriate treatment may be initiated.

Urodynamics should be performed in all women, especially if bladder neck surgery is considered, as this is of limited benefit to those with detrusor instability. The role of ambulatory urodynamics in detecting detrusor instability in women with irritative symptoms but normal findings on conventional cystometry is controversial and requires further evaluation.

Treatment should be aimed at the symptoms which are most troublesome to the patient, and success measured in terms of improvement in the woman's quality of life. Although objective evidence of improvement, using repeat cystometry, is desirable, this correlates poorly with changes in symptoms. In clinical practice, repeat cystometry is less important if significant symptomatic improvement is achieved. A follow-up cystometrogram is of use in women with persistent symptoms, and is important in the evaluation of treatment efficacy in clinical trials.

REFERENCES

1 Kinder RB, Mundy AR. Atropine blockade of nerve-mediated stimulation of the human detrusor. Br J Urol 1985; 57: 418–421.

2 Burnstock G, Dumsday B, Smythe A. Atropine resistant excitation of the urinary bladder: the possibility of transmission via nerve releasing a purine nucleotide. Br J Pharmacol 1972; 44: 51–61.

3 Gu J, Restorick JM, Blank M et al. Vasoactive intestinal polypeptide in the normal and unstable bladder. Br J Urol 1983; 54: 252–255.

4 The standardisation of terminology of lower urinary tract function. Br J Obstet Gynaecol 1990; Suppl 6: 1–16.

5 Female urinary incontinence. Proceedings of an educational course held at the Royal College of Obstetrics & Gynaecology, June 1989.

6 Castleden CM, Duffin HM. Factors influencing outcome in elderly patients with urinary incontinence and detrusor instability. Aging 1985; 14: 303.

7 Zoubek J, Bloom D, Sedman AB. Extraordinary urinary frequency. Pediatrics 1990; 85: 1112–1114.

8 Whiteside CG, Arnold GP. Persistent primary enuresis: a urodynamic assessment. Br Med J 1975; 1: 364–369.

9 Walters MD, Taylor S, Schoenfeld LS. Psychosexual study of women with detrusor instability. Obstet Gynecol 1990; 75: 22–26.

10 Norton KRW, Bhat AV, Stanton SL. Psychiatric aspects of urinary incontinence in women attending an outpatient clinic. Br Med J 1990; 301: 271–272.

11 Moore KH, Sutherst JR. Response to treatment of detrusor instability in relation to psychoneurotic status. Br J Urol 1990; 66: 486–490.

12 Webster JR. Combined video/pressure/flow cystometrography in female patients with voiding disturbances. Urology 1975; 5: 209–213.

13 Cardozo LD, Stanton SL, Williams JE. Detrusor instability following surgery for genuine stress incontinence. Br J Urol 1979; 51: 204–207.

14 Jeffcoate TNA, Francis WJA. Urgency incontinence in the female. Am J Obstet Gynecol 1966; 94: 604–609.

15 Kieswetter H. Mucosal sensory threshold of urinary bladder and urethra measured electrically. Urol Int 1977; 32: 437–439.

16 Wise BG, Cardozo LD, Cutner A, Benness CJ, Burton G. The prevalence and significance of urethral instability in women with detrusor instability. Br J Urol 1993; 72: 26–29.

17 Sutherst JR, Brown M. The effect on the bladder pressure of sudden entry of fluid into the posterior urethra. Br J Urol 1978; 50: 406–409.

18 Brading AF, Turner WH. The unstable bladder: towards a common mechanism. Br J Urol 1994; 73: 3–8.

19 Cardozo LD, Stanton SL. Genuine stress incontinence and detrusor instability: a review of 200 cases. Br J Obstet Gynaecol 1980; 87: 184–190.

20 Hilton P. Urinary incontinence during sexual intercourse: a common but rarely volunteered symptom. Br J Obstet Gynaecol 1988; 95: 377–381.

21 Sutherst JR, Brown MC. Comparison of single and multichannel cystometry in diagnosing bladder instability. Br Med J 1984; 288: 1720.

22 Griffiths CJ, Assi M, Styles RA, Ramsden PD, Neal DE. Ambulatory monitoring of bladder and detrusor pressure during natural filling. J Urol 1989; 142: 780–784.

23 Khullar V, Personal communication. 1994

24 Van Waalwijk van Doorn ESC, Zwiers W. Ambulant monitoring to assess the efficacy of oxybutynin in patients with mixed incontinence. Eur Urol 1990; 18: 49–51.

25 Holmes DM, Plevnik S, Stanton SL. Bladder neck electrical conductivity in female urinary urgency and urge incontinence. Br J Obstet Gynaecol 1989; 96: 816–820.

26 Ingleman-Sundberg A. Partial bladder denervation for detrusor dyssynergia. Clin Obstet Gynecol 1978; 21: 797–805.

27 Mundy AR. Long term results of bladder transection for urge incontinence. Br J Urol 1983; 55: 642–644.

28 Torrens MG, Griffith HB. The control of uninhibited bladder by selective sacral neurectomy. Br J Urol 1974; 46: 639–644.

29 Helmstein K. Treatment of bladder carcinoma by a hydrostatic pressure technique. Br J Urol 1972; 44: 434–450.

30 Dunn M, Smith JC, Ardran GM. Prolonged bladder distension as a treatment of urgency and urge incontinence of urine. Br J Urol 1974; 46: 645–652.

31 Pengelly AW, Stephenson TP, Milroy ESG, Whiteside CG, Turner-Warwick RT. Results of prolonged bladder distension as treatment for detrusor instability. Br J Urol 1978; 50: 243–45.

32 Turner-Warwick RT, Ashken MH. The functional results of partial subtotal and total cystoplasty with special reference to ureterocaecoplasty, selective sphincterotomy and cystocystoplasty. Br J Urol 1976; 39: 3–12.

33 Blaivas JG, Labib KB, Michalik SJ, Zayed AAH. Cystometric response to propantheline in detrusor hyperreflexia: therapeutic implications. J Urol 1980; 124: 259–262.

34 Gibaldi M, Grundhofer G. Biopharmaceutic influences on the anticholinergic effect of propantheline. Clin Pharmacol Ther 1975; 18: 457–461.

35 Cornella JL, Ostergard DR, Bent AE, Horbach NS. Prospective study utilising transdermal scopolamine in detrusor instability. Urology 1990; 25: 96–97.

36 Moisey CU, Stephenson TP, Brendler CB. The urodynamic and subjective results of treatment of detrusor instability with oxybutynin chloride. Br J Urol 1980; 52: 472–475.

37 Holmes DM, Montz FJ, Stanton SL. Oxybutynin versus propantheline in the treatment of detrusor instability in the female: a patient regulated variable dose trial. In: Proceedings of the fifteenth annual meeting of the International Continence Society, London, 1985; pp 63–64.

38 Thuroff JW, Bunke B, Ebner A et al. Randomized, double-blind multicenter trial on treatment of frequency, urgency, and incontinence related to detrusor hyperactivity: oxybutynin versus propantheline versus placebo. J Urol 1991; 145: 813–817.

39 Cardozo LD, Cooper D, Versi E. Oxybutynin chloride in the management of idiopathic detrusor instability. Br Med J 1987; 280: 281–282.

40 Baigre RE, Kelleher JP, Fawcett DP, Pengelly AW. Oxybutynin, is it safe? Br J Urol 1988; 62: 319–322.

41 Moore KH, Hay DM, Imrie AE, Watson A, Goldstein M. Oxybutynin hydrochloride (3 mg) in the treatment of women with idiopathic detrusor instability. Br J Urol 1990; 66: 479–485.

42 Briggs RS, Castleden CM, Asher MJ. The effect of flavoxate on uninhibited detrusor contractions and urinary incontinence in the elderly. J Urol 1980; 123: 665–666.

43 Chapple CR, Parkhouse H, Gardener C, Milroy EJG. Double-blind placebo-controlled, cross-over study of flavoxate in the treatment of idiopathic detrusor instability. Br J Urol 1990; 66: 491–494.

44 Tapp AJS, Fall M, Norgaard J et al Terodiline: a dose titrated, multicenter study of the treatment of idiopathic detrusor instability in women. J Urol 1989; 142: 1027–1031.

45 Bodner DR, Lindan R, Leffler E, Resnick MI. The effect of verapamil on the treatment of detrusor hyperreflexia in the spinal cord injured population. Paraplegia 1989; 27: 364–369.

46 Castleden CM, George CF, Renwick AG, Asher MJ. Imipramine, a possible alternative to current therapy for urinary incontinence in the elderly. J Urol 1981; 125: 318–320.

47 Cardozo LD. Sex and the bladder. Br Med J 1988; 296: 587–588.

48 Monson JP, Richards P. Desmopressin urine concentration test. Br Med J 1979; 1: 2420.

49 Ramsden PD, Hindmarsh JR, Price DA, Yeates WK, Bowditch JD. DDAVP for adult enuresis – a preliminary report. Br J Urol 1982; 54: 256–258.

50 Hilton P, Stanton SL. The use of desmopressin (DDAVP) in nocturnal urinary frequency in the female. Br J Urol 1982; 54: 252–255.

51 Knudsen UB, Rittig S, Pederen JB, Norgaard JP, Djaarhus JC. Long term treatment of nocturnal enuresis with desmopressin – influence on urinary output and haematological parameters. Neurourol Urodyn 1989; 8: 348–349.

52 Tapp AJS, Cardozo LD. The postmenopausal bladder. Br J Hosp Med 1986; 35: 20–23.

53 Fantl JA, Wyman JF, Anderson RL, Matt DW, Bump RC. Postmenopausal urinary incontinence: comparison between non-oestrogen supplemented and oestrogen supplemented women. Obstet Gynecol 1988; 71: 823–828.

54 Wise BG, Benness CJ, Cardozo LD, Cutner A. Vaginal oestradiol for lower urinary tract symptoms in postmenopausal women – a double-blind placebo-controlled study. In: Proceedings of the 7th International Congress on the Menopause, Stockholm, 1993: p 15.

55 Jeffcoate TNA, Francis WJA. Urgency incontinence in the female. Am J Obstet Gynecol 1966; 94: 604–618.

56 Frewen WK. An objective assessment of the unstable bladder of psychological origin. Br J Urol 1978; 50: 246–249.

57 Frewen WK. A reassessment of bladder training in detrusor dysfunction in the female. Br J Urol 1982; 54: 372–373.

58 Jarvis GJ. A controlled trial of bladder drill and drug therapy in the management of detrusor instability. Br J Urol 1981; 53: 565–566.

59 Holmes DM, Stone AR, Bary PR, Richards CJ, Stephenson TP. Bladder training 3 years on. Br J Urol 1983; 55: 660–664.

60 Cardozo LD, Abrams PH, Stanton SL, Feneley RCL. Idiopathic bladder instability treated by biofeedback. Br J Urol 1978; 50: 521–523.

61 Holmes DM, Plevnik S, Stanton SL. Bladder neck electric conductivity in female urinary incontinence and urge incontinence. Br J Obstet Gynaecol 1989; 96: 816–820.

62 Freeman RM, Baxby K. Hypnotherapy for incontinence caused by the unstable bladder. Br Med J 1982; 284: 1831–1834.

63 Philp T, Shah PJR, Worth PHL. Acupuncture in the treatment of bladder instability. Br J Urol 1988; 1: 490–493.

64 Klarskov P. Enkephalin inhibits presynaptically the contractility of urinary tract smooth muscle. Br J Urol 1987; 59: 31–35.

65 Murray KH, Feneley RCL. Endorphins – a role in lower urinary tract function? The effect of opioid blockade on the detrusor and urethral sphincter mechanisms. Br J Urol 1982; 54: 638–640.

66 Pigne A, Degausac C, Nyssen C, Barrat J. Acupuncture and the unstable bladder. In: Proceedings of the Fifteenth Meeting of the International Continence Society. 1985: pp 186–187.

67 Gibson JS, Pardley J, Neville J. Infra-red low power laser therapy on acupuncture points for treatment of the unstable bladder. In: Read by titles. The twentieth meeting of the International Continence Society, 1990: 146–147.

68 Griffiths J. Observations on the urinary bladder and urethra. Part 2. The nerves. Part 3. Physiological Journal of Anatomy and Physiology 1895; 29/61 254.

69 Fall M. Does electrostimulation cure urinary incontinence? J Urol 1984; 131: 664–667.

70 Plevnik S, Janez J, Vrtacnik P, Trasinar B, Vodusek DB. Short term electrical stimulation: home treatment for urinary incontinence. World J Urol 1986; 4: 24–26.

71 Ohlsson BL, Fall M, Frankenberg-Sommar S. Effects of external and direct pudendal nerve maximal electrical stimulation in the treatment of the uninhibited overactive bladder. Br J Urol 1989; 64: 374–380.

72 Jonasson A, Larsson B, Pschera H, Nylund L. Short-term maximal electrical stimulation – a conservative treatment of urinary incontinence. Gynecol Obstet Invest 1990; 30: 120–123.

73 Wise BG, Cardozo LD, Cutner A, Kelleher C, Burton G. Maximal electrical stimulation: an acceptable alternative to anticholinergic therapy. Int Urogynecol J 1992; 3(3): 270.

74 Warrel DW. Vaginal denervation of the bladder nerve supply. Urol Int 1977; 32: 114–116.

75 Lucas MG, Thomas DG. Endoscopic bladder transection for detrusor instability. Br J Urol 1987; 59: 526–528.

76 Higson RH, Smith JC, Whelan P. Bladder rupture: an acceptable complication of distension therapy? Br J Urol 1978; 50: 529–534.

77 Ewing R, Bultitude MI, Shuttleworth KED. Subtrigonal phenol injection for urge incontinence secondary to detrusor instability in females. Br J Urol 1982; 54: 689–692.

78 Blackford W, Murray K, Stephenson TP, Mundy AR. Results of transvesical infiltration of the pelvis with phenol in 116 patients. Br J Urol 1984; 56: 647–649.

79 Cameron-Strange A, Millard RJ. Management of refractory detrusor instability by transvesical phenol injection. Br J Urol 1988; 62: 323–325.

80 Rosenbaum TP, Shah PJR, Worth PHL. Transtrigonal phenol: the end of an era? Neurourol Urodyn 1988; 7: 294–295.

81 Wall LL, Stanton S. Transvesical phenol injection of pelvic nerve plexuses in females with refractory urge incontinence. Br J Urol 1989; 63: 465–468.

82 Bramble FJ. The treatment of adult enuresis and urge incontinence by enterocystoplasty. Br J Urol 1982; 54: 693–696.

83 Mundy AR, Stephenson TP. 'Clam' ileocystoplasty for the treatment of refractory urge incontinence. Br J Urol 1985; 57: 641–646.

84 McRae P, Murray KH, Nurse DE, Stephenson TP, Mundy AR. Clam enterocystoplasty in the neuropathic bladder. Br J Urol 1987; 60: 523–525.

85 Rosenbaum TP, Shah PJR, Rose GA, Lloyd-Davis RW. Cranberry juice helps the problem of mucus production in enterouroplastics. Neurourol Urodyn 1989; 8: 344–345.

86 Nurse DE, Mundy AR. Cystoplasty infection and cancer. Neurourol Urodyn 1989; 8: 343–344.

87 Stone AR, Davis N, Stephenson TP. Cancer associated with augmentation cystoplasty. Br J Urol 1987; 60: 236–238.

88 Pavlakis RW, Siroky MB, Goldstein I, Krane RJ. Neurologic findings in Parkinson's disease. J Urol 1983; 129: 80–83.

89 Malone-Lee JG, Sa'adu A, Lieu PK. Evidence against the existence of a specific Parkinsonian bladder. Neurourol Urodyn 1993; 12(4): 341–343.

90 Miller H, Simpson CA, Yeates WK. Bladder dysfunction in multiple sclerosis. Br Med J 1965; 1: 1265–1269.

20

Voiding difficulties and retention

INTRODUCTION

Women with voiding difficulty may present to a variety of medical practitioners. Unfortunately, the pathophysiology is poorly understood and therefore management is commonly inappropriate. Normal voiding requires co-ordinated relaxation of the pelvic floor and the urethral striated sphincter, which is usually followed by a detrusor contraction and complete evacuation of the urinary bladder. Defects in the complex neurological control mechanisms may be seen at many levels and differ from detrusor–sphincter dyssynergia as a consequence of traumatic spinal injury, where there is failure of urethral relaxation and co-ordinated voiding, to reflex inhibition of the voiding reflex in response to pain. Not only may the control mechanisms fail but also there may be structural and functional failure of the component parts, namely the bladder and urethra. The dominant position of urethral dilation and urethrotomy as the treatment of choice for the majority of patients is evidence of the lack of understanding of voiding dysfunction.[1]

SYMPTOMS

The symptoms encountered in patients with voiding difficulty may be considered in different categories. Women may complain of symptoms of difficulty with micturition; they may complain of other symptoms of the underlying cause of the voiding difficulty; or they may complain of the symptoms arising as a consequence of the voiding difficulty, such as recurrent urinary tract infection. The symptom which is diagnostic of voiding difficulty is complete inability to void with a full bladder. All other symptoms overlap with other diagnoses. Such retention may be acute or chronic. Acute urinary retention is usually very easy to diagnose unless there is some impairment of bladder sensation. It is defined as sudden painful inability to void over a 24-h period, requiring catheterization which yields at least 50% of the cystometric capacity.[2]

Chronic retention is much more difficult to define. The normal bladder, despite age changes, empties completely. Therefore, chronic retention occurs when the bladder fails to empty.[3] Authors have tried to identify specific volumes for the residual urine to confirm the underlying diagnosis. Such figures as 40 ml,[4] 100 ml[5] and 500 ml[6] have been proposed. Stanton[2] prefers to make this diagnosis if the patient fails to empty more than 50% of the bladder capacity on voiding. Apart from acute painful urinary retention other symptoms are not specific to voiding difficulty. The sensation of incomplete emptying is common in women with lower urinary tract dysfunction but is only objectively confirmed in 10% of those who complain of it.[7] Frequency and urgency of micturition is common in women with voiding dysfunction but no more so than in those women with normal voiding.[8] Women, unlike men, do not see how their peers void and therefore have little ability to compare the force or duration of their stream with those of others. Changes in such voiding parameters may be subtle and slow and avoid personal detection. Incontinence is, of course, seen with many conditions and would not lead one directly to the diagnosis of voiding difficulty.

Table 20.1 Symptoms of voiding difficulty

Poor stream
Intermittent stream
Prolonged voiding time
Double void
Post-micturition incontinence
Incomplete emptying
Hesitancy
Frequency
Nocturia
Urgency
Incontinence
Abdominal distension

Table 20.2 Symptoms of underlying disease

Polydipsia
Abdominal distension
Vulval mass
Pregnancy
Perianal pain
Peripheral paresthesia/anesthesia
Herpetic rash

PREVALENCE

The prevalence of voiding difficulty in the general population has yet to be determined. In selected groups of patients attending urodynamic clinics between 6.7%[8] and 14.5%[9] have urodynamically substantiated voiding difficulty.

ETIOLOGY OF VOIDING DIFFICULTY

The causes of voiding difficulty may be listed as follows:

- neurological
- myogenic
- iatrogenic
- obstructive
- inflammatory
- psychogenic
- resulting from aging.

Neurological

Different types of classification system have been used to describe voiding dysfunction. The aim of each classification system is accurately and logically to display the pathophysiology of the voiding difficulty and also to indicate the appropriate approach to treatment. Bors & Comarr,[10] Bradley,[11] Lapidus,[12] Krane & Siroky[13] and Wein[14] have all proposed classification schemes. None of these systems is perfect but they supply a framework. Patients may not fit exactly into one particular system as there may be mixed lesions or there may be secondary changes that further disrupt or alter voiding. The important ideal is that each patient should be thoroughly evaluated with an attempt made at classification. This requires an in-depth understanding of potential neurological injuries and subsequent secondary changes.

Anatomically, one can identify different levels of lesion that may result in voiding difficulty. Usually suprapontine lesions result in detrusor hyperreflexia, but if the area affected by a cerebrovascular accident or brain tumor is facilitatory to micturition then voiding difficulty ensues. Central nervous lesions produced by trauma or demyelination which are distal to the pons but proximal to the parasympathetic outflow may produce detrusor–sphincter dyssynergia with or without hyperreflexia. Detrusor–sphincter dyssynergia is where co-ordinated urethral relaxation followed by detrusor contraction does not occur and the bladder contracts and tries to empty against a closed urethral sphincter. More peripheral lesions at the sacral outflow such as those due to polio, herpes zoster infection,[15] HIV conversion[16] or a prolapsed intravertebral disc result in motor paralysis with some element of sensory loss. The afferent tracts may be damaged in diabetes, tabes dorsalis or pernicious anemia, resulting in poor bladder sensation which may subsequently result in bladder distension and direct detrusor injury.

Fowler & Kirby[17,18] have identified much more subtle abnormalities in women with voiding difficulty. Using concentric needle electromyographic (EMG) studies of the urethral sphincter mechanism they found that one-third of women with voiding difficulty in their study had evidence of denervation and in a further 40% a particular abnormality of decelatory bursts and complex repetitive discharges (CRD) was identified. Such discharges were defined as abnormal if they were widespread, spontaneous, present at more than one site and occurring at times other than at needle insertion. Although a hormonal etiology has been postulated,[19] this is far from proven. Webb et al[20] have obtained similar findings to those of Fowler & Kirby,[17,18] but they also extended their investigation to the anal sphincter, where there were CRDs. These authors found that most patients with CRDs also had abnormalities suggestive of denervation and reinnervation. They concluded that voiding difficulty in association with CRDs suggested a widespread disorder of pelvic innervation.

Myogenic

Direct detrusor injury with ischemia of the detrusor muscle and disruption of the detrusor muscle syncytium may occur in unrelieved urinary retention. In association with this there may be injury to the postsynaptic parasympathetic fibers. Although the history of acute retention may be easy to identify,[7] the onset of voiding difficulty following the unrelieved urinary retention may be more insidious. This form of injury may occur where there has been a temporary alteration in bladder sensation or motor function such as with epidural analgesia or spinal shock. It is important for the physician to be vigilant in such cases and positively look for evidence of retention and relieve this before permanent detrusor injury occurs.

Iatrogenic

Urinary retention after a whole variety of non-urological and urological interventions is well recognized. It may be seen in 52% of elderly patients after major joint surgery[21] and 30% of patients after open cholecystectomy.[22] A number of elements have been identified that are associated with a higher risk of postoperative retention:

- male gender
- increased age
- long operation times
- high doses of analgesic agents
- patient-controlled analgesia
- large amounts of intravenous fluid.

Opiates as a class of drug have long been recognized as a cause of urinary retention[25,26] and this effect may be reversed with naloxone.[27]

Epidural analgesia is associated with hypotonic detrusor function and appears to be one of the important factors that increases the risk of urinary retention post partum, although subsequent prolonged voiding difficulty may relate more to myogenic injury produced as a consequence of the retention. Other drugs that may result in voiding difficulty include tricyclic antidepressants, anticholinergic agents, antihistamines, ganglion blockers, α-adrenergic stimulants, phenothiazine and monoamine oxidase inhibitors.

Surgical procedures for urinary stress incontinence frequently produce short-term voiding difficulty and this is managed with suprapubic catheterization or intermittent self-catheterization. In a small number of patients, typically after a sling procedure, this voiding difficulty may be prolonged. There is certainly a case to be made when postoperative voiding difficulty is predicted by preoperative urodynamics that patients should be taught intermittent self-catheterization prior to their surgery.

Obstructive

Obstructive lesions which result in voiding difficulty may be intrinsic within the urethra and bladder neck or may be caused by external pressure on, or kinking of, the urethra. Intrinsic obstructive lesions are rare in women, implying that the common therapy of urethral dilation or 'recalibration' is inappropriate. The most frequent site of urethral obstruction viewed radiologically is the distal urethra,[1] although the caliber of the distal urethra must be small (10–12F) to produce a significant degree of obstruction.[1] Intrinsic bladder neck obstruction in the absence of dyssynergia is even less common, but occasionally occurs secondary to fibrosis as a consequence of surgery or schistosomiasis.[28]

Rarely, foreign bodies or calculi may be found within the urethra. Gross condylomata acuminata of the urethra or urethral meatus may be an intrinsic cause of obstruction.[29] Extrinsic causes include an incarcerated pelvic mass such as a retroverted gravid uterus, a fibroid uterus or rarely an ovarian tumor. Surprisingly, acute reduction in size of a large fibroid uterus in response to GNHRH analogs has been shown to cause urinary obstruction.[30] Kinking of the urethra is commonly seen with gross cystocele and uterovaginal prolapse. The patient may resort to digital replacement of the prolapse to enable her to void.[1]

The resolution of this kinking after vaginal surgery may account for the 10% of women who report de novo onset of urinary incontinence after vaginal repair for prolapse when established urethral sphincter incompetence has been masked by urethral kinking.

Inflammatory

Any painful lesion, whether surgical or pathological, may result in reflex inhibition of voiding and voiding difficulty. In the case of genital herpes[31] the pain may occur in association with sacral sensory loss. Common local lesions that may precipitate acute urinary retention are vulvovaginitis, cystitis, urethritis or a vulval abscess.

Psychogenic

For many years urinary retention in women was assumed to be hysterical or psychogenic.[32,33,34] With the advent of increasingly complex urodynamic investigations it is now possible to exclude the bulk of women from this diagnosis. Wheeler et al[35] showed that 15 of 60 women presenting with voiding difficulty had psychosocial problems thought to be significant in the genesis of voiding difficulty.

Resulting from ging

Elderly women tend to have a reduction in the power of the detrusor contraction and this may be associated with an inelastic urethra. The net result is that there may be a significantly greater residual urine in women over the age of 70 than in those under the age of 70.[36]

EXAMINATION

Clinical examination of a patient with voiding difficulty may reveal a tender or non-tender mass arising out of the pelvis which is dull to percussion. There may also be abnormalities secondary to the voiding difficulty, such as vulval excoriation if there is overflow incontinence. The underlying pathology may be revealed.

The bladder may be palpable abdominally when it contains between 150 and 300 ml of urine,[2,37] although this depends considerably on the obesity and co-operation of the patient. Bimanual examination usually reveals a bladder that contains more than 200 ml.[2] When examining the patient with voiding difficulty it is important to conduct a complete neurological examination as well as a detailed genitourinary examination. An understanding of the potential pathologies is essential for one to be able to interpret the relevance of abnormal findings.

INVESTIGATIONS

Investigations for patients presenting with symptoms and signs of voiding difficulty are designed to confirm the diagnosis, identify potential underlying pathologies and secondary changes and monitor treatment. The cardinal findings for the confirmation of voiding difficulty are a significant residual urine and a poor urine flow rate. The relevant investigations may be listed as follows:

- midstream specimen of urine
- uroflowmetry
- measurement of residual urine
- cystometry/videocystourethrography
- cystourethroscopy
- urethral pressure profilometry
- single-fiber electromyography
- miscellaneous.

Midstream specimen of urine

Either a midstream specimen of urine or a catheter sample of urine should be sent for microscopy, culture and sensitivity as urinary tract infection can precipitate acute urinary retention. More importantly, recurrent urinary tract infection is a recognized complication of prolonged voiding difficulty and is one of the indications for active management to avoid damage to the upper tract.

Uroflowmetry

Uroflowmetry is advocated as the simplest screening for voiding dysfunction.[1,2] However, although it is useful in the male, now that cheap portable ultrasound scanners are available, measurement of the post micturition residual urine probably supplies information of greater significance in women (*see below*).

The normal flow rate is dumb-bell in shape with a normal peak flow of greater than 15 or 20 ml/s[1,2] for a volume voided of at least 150 ml. In patients with voiding difficulty not only is there a reduced peak flow rate but also the voiding time is prolonged with intermittent voiding being a common feature. Whenever voiding studies are undertaken it is important that the patient should void in privacy and report that she has felt that the void was representative of her normal voiding.

Residual urine

After a representative void in privacy the presence of residual urine is of considerable significance. Bimanual examination of the bladder will reveal a residual urine of greater than 200 ml,[2] but exact quantification is difficult clinically. Ultrasound is a non-invasive, relatively simple technique for estimating residual urine volume. Although a large number of different formulae have been proposed, correlation with the volume of urine at catheterization is reasonable. Ultrasound machines are now available which are readily portable and can be used in the community.

Post-micturition catheterization supplies the most accurate information of the volume of retained urine but may be painful and can introduce infection.

Cystometry/video-cystourethrography

The most useful investigations in patients with voiding difficulty both confirm the diagnosis and give some indication of the underlying pathophysiology. Filling and voiding cystometry in conjunction with X-ray screening and electromyography (EMG) of the urethral sphincter probably provides the most complex assessment. Although single-channel cystometry is possible, it is not desirable as extrinsic pressures may be misinterpreted as detrusor activity. In a simplistic manner a low flow rate with a high detrusor pressure implies obstruction. A low flow rate with a low detrusor pressure implies a defect in the activity of the detrusor muscle. However, the bladder may decompensate after prolonged voiding against a stricture, resulting in low-flow, low-pressure voiding. The pathology may be primarily muscular or secondary to a lower motor neurone lesion. Urethral sphincter EMG in association with voiding cystometry will positively diagnose detrusor–sphincter dyssynergia, which on simple cystometry would be shown as high-pressure, low-flow voiding.

X-ray screening at the time of cystometry, with contrast medium instilled in the bladder, means that the internal aspect of the bladder can be inspected for trabeculation or sacculation, and ureteric reflux can be identified and assessed. Distal urethral meatal stenosis will be shown by a high-pressure, low-flow voiding pattern in association with ballooning of the proximal and mid-urethra on X-ray screening during the voiding phase.

Cystourethroscopy

This investigation is not particularly productive at identifying the etiology of voiding difficulty in the majority of patients. If the passage of the endoscope is difficult then one considers urethral stricture as a potential underlying cause. The diagnosis of bladder neck obstruction, however, cannot be made by using endoscopy alone.[38]

The finding of trabeculation within the bladder is relatively unhelpful because not only is this a feature of obstructive voiding but it is most commonly seen with detrusor instability. Occasionally, foreign bodies or calculi are identified by endoscopy.

Urethral pressure profilometry

Although one can generate quite striking urethral pressure profiles from patients with urethral strictures, the diagnosis is usually obvious, as one has difficulty inserting the urethral pressure catheter. Combined cystometry and urethral pressure measurements can be used to confirm dyssynergia although EMG is preferable.

Single-fiber electromyography

Fowler & Kirby[17,18] have shown that single-fiber EMG is useful in up to 40% of women presenting with voiding difficulty when the diagnosis of hysteria would previously have been made. They have identified specific deceleratory bursts and complex repetitive discharges which may indicate complex neuromuscular pathology within the pelvic floor.[20]

Others

With an understanding of the specific functional abnormalities identified by urodynamic investigations further tests may be used to look for specific underlying pathologies, although frequently the label 'idiopathic' is applied. Lumbar spine X-rays and myelograms may be used in selective cases where there is a clinical suspicion of nerve root compression. A glucose tolerance test may be indicated if the bladder is hypotonic and there is glycosuria on simple ward testing. A DMSO scan or intravenous urethrography may be used to assess the condition of the upper tract. Klarskov et al[39] found that in 18 women who presented with acute urinary retention, 10 had possible provocative situations: acute cystitis in 7, a large fluid intake in 2 and constipation in 1. In 14 patients there were also definitive underlying causes: infravesical obstruction in 2, infravesical obstruction and underactive detrusor in 3, and underactive detrusor alone in 9. The infravesical obstruction occurred as a consequence of urethral calculi, urogenital prolapse and urethral stricture.

TREATMENT

Treatment of established voiding difficulty can be complex, particularly if the voiding difficulty is combined with other lower urinary tract pathologies such as detrusor instability or genuine stress incontinence. It is important to avoid iatrogenic acute urinary retention because if this is prolonged then direct detrusor and postsynaptic parasympathetic injury may occur resulting in chronic voiding difficulty.

Prophylaxis

The importance of relieving acute urinary retention cannot be overstated. The recognition that iatrogenic voiding difficulty is common means that all physicians must be fully aware of the possibility. A number of elements have been identified which appear to increase the relative risk of postoperative retention: male gender, increased age, long operation times, high doses of analgesic agents, patient-controlled analgesia, large amounts of intravenous fluids and opiates.[22,23,24] In gynecology postoperative urinary retention is particularly common. Forty-five per cent of women after radical pelvic surgery[40,41] and over 60% after vaginal surgery for incontinence or cystocele[42] have difficulty resuming spontaneous voiding. In obstetrics epidural analgesia in association with operative or instrumental delivery is a potent cause of postpartum acute urinary retention.[19]

The use of prophylactic postoperative in-dwelling urethral or suprapubic catheterization is widespread, although intermittent catheterization to maintain a residual urine below 600 ml has been proposed.[5] More importantly, it is vital that junior medical staff, nurses and midwives should be aware of the complication of acute urinary retention after surgery or delivery and particularly that it may be relatively painless in someone with adequate analgesia. Protocols should be employed to encourage members of staff to look for this particular complication.

Relief of retention

Most medical and nursing students have been taught that rapid release of retained urine may result in hypovolemia and bleeding from ruptured submucosal vessels in the bladder. Although this is repeated in numerous medical and nursing textbooks, supporting evidence is scanty. In view of the lack of firm scientific data it is not surprising that there is an immense diversity of advice about the relief of urinary retention. In the absence of scientifically based protocols the advice of York[43] seems reasonable, with initial drainage of 1000 ml followed by 100–200 ml/h until the bladder is empty. If it is felt that a single episode of catheterization is required, then catheterization with a 12–14F urethral catheter is usually effective. Subsequently, a careful fluid balance should be maintained for 24 h, with bimanual post-micturition examination of the bladder after this time. If the single catheterization has failed, or is thought likely to fail on a temporary basis, then a size 14F indwelling urethral Foley catheter should be used for 48 h and then removed. For further episodes of retention after this one should resort to suprapubic catheterization. One must remember that catheterization is potentially dangerous, particularly in the elderly, and is associated with threefold increase in mortality in hospital.[44]

Drug therapy

The use of drugs for the treatment of voiding difficulty is disappointing and this can be explained by the following. The innervation of the bladder in normality and in disease is more complex than implied by the simple understanding that the parasympathetic nervous system predominates. The sympathetic (adrenergic) system has numerous receptors,[45] and there are interconnections between sympathetic and parasympathetic divisions with adrenergic and cholinergic receptors present in both divisions of the autonomic nervous supply.

Other neurotransmitters, such as vasoactive polypeptide, are found within the lower urinary tract and play some inhibitory role. Drugs designed to act on such a system should not only be designed to act on the one organ but also on specific parts of the innervation of that organ. Unfortunately, drugs currently available fail even to be specific to the bladder and have undesirable effects on other organs. This is usually dose-related. In the case of cholinergic agents there is some specificity for the bladder and bowel (muscarinic) rather than the heart (nicotinic).

The cholinomimetic agents bethanechol and carbachol, and the anticholinesterases physostigmine, neostigmine and distigmine bromide, are perhaps the most extensively researched agents that have been advocated to encourage bladder emptying. Although pharmacologically active in the tissue bath, these drugs are very disappointing in clinical practice even when patients with incomplete lower motor neurone lesions, myogenic injury or voiding difficulty after surgery in the absence of outlet obstruction have been selected.[46] The side effects are those of nausea, vomiting, sweating, blurred vision, bradycardia and intestinal colic. Bethanechol is more specific to muscarinic receptors than carbachol. The usual dose of bethanechol is 10–25 mg orally, half an hour before food, three to four times a day. Carbachol may be given orally (2 mg three times a day) or by subcutaneous injection (250 µg) when the bladder is assessed to be full. The subcutaneous injection may be repeated after half an hour. Distigmine bromide is prescribed at 5 mg/day.

In some instances of voiding difficulty there is functional outlet obstruction. Drugs acting on the central nervous system, autonomic ganglia or cholinergic receptors are helpful in these cases. Occasionally α-adrenergic-blocking drugs such as phenoxybenzamine, prazosin or phentolamine have been helpful. Unfortunately, potentially serious side effects may occur and some authors have advocated using the intravenous Regitine test[47] before commencing phenoxybenzamine. The usual dose of phenoxybenzamine is 10 mg twice daily. Its onset of action is slow and there may be some carry-over effect when stopped.[48]

The striated urethral sphincter may be influenced by drugs such as diazepam (Valium) or baclofen (Lioresal). Stanton et al[49] found valium to be of use for initiating voiding after suprapubic incontinence surgery. Other authors[48,50] have found baclofen useful in some patients with detrusor–sphincter dyssynergia.

The intravesical instillation of prostaglandin $F_{2\alpha}$ has been shown to stimulate detrusor contractions postoperatively in a double-blind placebo-controlled study,[51] and Bergman has advocated its use after vaginal hysterectomy.[52] In those patients with abnormal myotonic-like EMG activity of the urethral striated muscle,[17,18,19] botulinum toxin does not produce symptomatic relief.[53]

Surgery

Voiding difficulty due to extrinsic urethral obstruction from an impacted fibroid uterus or a large cystocele is best treated by acute relief and then surgical correction of the primary abnormality. Intrinsic urethral obstruction is rare in women.[31] Where urodynamic investigations have demonstrated urethral obstruction, effective relief may be achieved by urethral over-dilation or recalibration[54] under general anesthesia to a caliber of 35–40F. Overdilation under local anesthesia is difficult to achieve because of patient discomfort. Urethrotomy with longitudinal incisions of the epithelium and submucosa at 4, 7, and 12 o'clock using an Otis urethrotome has also been advocated.[2] An indwelling size 26F catheter is left on free drainage for 2–5 days after this procedure. Where the bladder neck has been demonstrated to be competent, urethral overdilation does not carry a risk of incontinence.[1] However, if the bladder neck is not competent then temporary incontinence or worsening of an existing problem may be seen. In women with voiding difficulty secondary to abnormal myotonic-like EMG activity of the urethral striated sphincter in association with CRDs[17,18] urethral dilation offers only temporary relief.

Urethral obstruction due to a calculus is readily treated by removal of that calculus. Condylomata acuminata may be treated by cryotherapy.[29]

Behavioral therapy

Reinforcement exerts a powerful influence on behavior which is dependent upon intermittent reinforcement at variable intervals.[55] Using this behavioral model some patients with voiding difficulty may be successfully treated. The patient records the time from the moment of trying to micturate to initiation. If the patient fails to void within a given time interval then she is instructed to leave the toilet and return in not less than 2 min. Using this technique and the slow introduction of unfamiliar toilets, successful resolution of voiding difficulty has been obtained[55] in patients with no obvious underlying neuromuscular disease.

Intermittent self-catheterization

Intermittent self-catheterization, introduced by Lapides et al[56] in 1972, has revolutionized the treatment of patients with intractable voiding difficulty. It usually requires the patient to be both reasonably dextrous and mobile although with additional equipment quadriplegics may be able to perform self-catheterization.[57] The patient is usually taught by a nurse or continence advisor using a clean technique. Initially, she is taught in the semi-recumbent position using a mirror but once she is proficient she may be able to do it by feel either sitting or standing over a toilet. The risk of urinary tract infection in patients with a chronic residual urine is dramatically decreased with intermittent self-catheterization. Intermittent self-catheterization is safe[58] and acceptable to both the elderly[59] and institutionalized.[60]

Other treatments

In those patients with spinal cord or cauda equina lesions the possibility of nerve-stimulating implants to allow successful bladder evacuation has been pioneered by Professor Giles Brindley.[61] The sacral anterior nerve root stimulator was developed using the baboon as the experimental animal.

It has now been used worldwide in patients with partial or complete cord lesions where the sacral segments of the cord have been left intact or nearly so. The stimulator is implanted in the subarachnoid space and incorporates the anterior nerve roots of S2, 3 and 4. A receiver is implanted over the left lower ribs and stimulation is achieved with a radio transmitter placed over the receiver unit. Depending on the type of stimulation, bladder contraction, rectal contraction or erection may be achieved. When the stimulator is implanted the posterior nerve roots may be cut to abolish reflex detrusor contractions, some detrusor–sphincter dyssynergia and some low compliance. In those patients in whom implantation was carried out the majority have subsequently become continent with remarkably reduced residual urines. Urinary tract infections are less frequent and ureteric reflux is often abolished. Insertion is not, however, without problems, including leakage of cerebrospinal fluid, mechanical failure, accidental damage to nerve roots and infection.

Unfortunately, there is a group of patients who will not be successfully treated by any of the techniques described and may require long-term urethral or suprapubic catheterization with all the inherent problems. It is now uncommon for a patient to be considered for urinary diversion.

CONCLUSION

Voiding difficulty in women is still poorly understood and commonly managed inappropriately. Unfortunately, successful curative treatment is rare, although symptomatic relief with avoidance of upper tract damage is possible in the vast majority.

REFERENCES

1 Farrar DJ, Osborne JL. Voiding dysfunction in women.
2 Stanton SL (ed) Clinical gynaecologic urology. Mosby, 1984.
3 Williams MP, Wallhagan M, Dowling G. Urinary retention in hospitalised elderly women. Journal of Gerontological Nursing 1993; 7–14.
4 Veneema RJ, Carpenter FG, Root WS. Residual urine is an important factor in the interpretation of cystometrograms. Journal of Urology 1952; 68: 237.
5 Smith NGK, Murrant JD. Post operative urinary retention in women: management by intermittent catheterisation. Age & Ageing 1990; 19: 337–340.
6 Anderson J, Grant J. Post operative retention of urine. A prospective urodynamic study. BMJ 1991; 302: 894–896.
7 Osborne JL. Urodynamics and the gynaecologist. Alec Bourne Lecture 1981.
8 Farrar DJ, Osborne JL, Stephenson TP et al. A urodynamic view of bladder outlet obstruction in the female. British Journal of Urology 1975; 47: 815–822.
9 Stanton SL, Ozsoy C, Hilton P. Voiding difficulties in the female: prevalence, clinical and urodynamic review. Obstet. Gynaecol 1983; 61(2): 144–147.
10 Bors E, Comarr AE. Neurological urology. Baltimore: University Park Press, 1971.
11 Raz S, Bradley WE. Neuromuscular dysfunction of the lower urinary tract. In: Harrison JH, Gitters RJ, Perimutter AD et al (eds) Campbell's urology, 4th edn. Philadelphia: WB Saunders, 1979.
12 Lapides J. Cystometry. JAMA 1967; 201: 618.

13 Krane RJ, Siroky MB. Classification of neuro-urologic disorders. In: Krane RJ, Siroky MB (eds) Clinical neuro-urology Little, Brown, Boston: 1979.

14 Wein AJ. Classification of neurogenic voiding dysfunction. J Urol 1981; 125: 605.

15 Richmond W. The genitourinary manifestations of herpes zoster: three case reports and review of the literature. Br J Urol 1974; 46: 193–200.

16 Zeman A, Donaghy M. Acute infection with human immunodeficiency virus presenting with neurogenic urinary retention. Genitourin Med 1991; 67: 345–347.

17 Fowler CJ, Kirby RS. Abnormal electromyographic activity (decelerating bursts and complex repetitive discharges) in the striated muscle of the urethral sphincter in 5 women with persistent urinary retention. Br J Urol 1985; 57: 67–70.

18 Fowler CJ, Kirby RS. Electromyography of urethral sphincter in women with urinary retention. Lancet 1986; 1: 1455–1457.

19 Fowler CJ, Christmas TJ, Chapple CR et al. Abnormal electromyographic activity of the urethral sphincter, voiding dysfunction and polycystic ovaries: a new syndrome. BMJ 1988; 297: 1436–1438.

20 Webb RJ, Fawcett PRW, Neal DE. Electromyographic abnormalities in the urethral and anal sphincters of women with idiopathic retention of urine. B J Urol 1992; 70: 22–25.

21 Michelson JD, Lotke PA, Steinberg ME. Urinary bladder management after total joint replacement surgery. N Eng J Med 1988; 319: 321–326.

22 Petross JG, Rimm EB, Robillard MA. Factors influencing urinary tract retention after elective open cholecystectomy surgery. Gynaecology & Obstetrics 1992; 174: 497–500.

23 Tammela T, Kontturi M, Lukkarinen O. Postoperative urinary retention. 1. Incidence and predisposing factors. Scan J Urol Nephrol 1986; 20: 197–201.

24 Petros JG, Bradley TM. Factors influencing postoperative urinary retention in patients undergoing surgery for benign anorectal disease. Am J Surg 1990; 159: 374–376.

25 Bromage PR. The price of intraspinal narcotic analgesia: basic constraints. Anesth Analg 1981; 60: 461–463.

26 Murray K. Acute urinary retention associated with sublingual buprenorphine. BMJ 1983; 286: 763–764.

27 Rawal N, Millefors K, Axelsson K, Lingardh G, Widman B. Naloxone reversal of urinary retention after epidural morphine. Lancet 1981; 11: 1411.

28 Turner-Warwick R, Whiteside CG, Worth PH, Milroy EJG, Bates CP. A urodynamic view of the clinical problems associated with bladder neck dysfunction and its treatment by endoscopic incision and transtrigonal posterior prostatectomy. Br J Urol 1973; 45: 44–59.

29 Cervigni M, Scotto V, Panei M, Sbiroli C. Acute urethral obstruction due to condylomata acuminata. Obstet Gynaecol 1991; 78(5): 970–971.

30 Friedman A. Acute urinary retention after gonadotrophic releasing hormone agonist treatment for leiomyomata uteri. Fertility & Sterility 1993; 59(3): 677–678.

31 Corey MD, Adams HG, Brown ZA, Holmes KK. Genital herpes simplex virus infections: clinical manifestations, course and complications. Ann Int Med 1983; 98: 958–972.

32 Margolis, GJ. A review of literature on psychogenic urinary retention. J Urol 1965; 94: 257–258.

33 Larson JW, Swensen WM, Utz DC et al. Psychogenic urinary retention in females. JAMA 1963; 184: 697–700.

34 Allen TD. Psychogenic urinary retention. South Med J 1972; 65: 302–304.

35 Wheeler JS, Culkin DJ, Walter JS, Flanagan RC. Female urinary retention. 1990; 35(5): 428–432.

36 Malone Lee J. Urinary incontinence. Reviews in Clinical Gerontology 1992; 2: 123–139.

37 Tanagho E. Physical examination of the genitourinary tract. In: Tanagho E, McCormick J (eds) Smith's general urology. San Mateo: Appleton & Lange, 1992.

38 Farrar D, Turner-Warwick R. Outflow obstruction in the female. In: Turner-Warwick R, Whiteside CJ, Clinical urodynamics. Urol Clin North Am 1979; 6: 217–225.

39 Klarskov P, Anderson JT, Asmussen CF et al. Acute urinary retention in women; a prospective study of 18 consecutive cases. Scand J Urol Nephrol 1987; 21: 29–31.

40 Fraser AC. The late effects of Wertheim's hysterectomy on the urinary tract. Br J Obstet Gynaecol 1966; 73: 1002–1007.

41 Smith PH et al. The urological complications of Wertheim's hysterectomy. Br J Urol 1969; 41: 685–688.

42 Cameron MD. Distigmine bromide (Ubretid) in the prevention of post operative retention of urine. Br J Obstet Gynaecol 1966; 73: 847–848.

43 York JL. What to do about acute urinary retention. Emerg Med Clin North Am 1991; 23(10): 88–96.

44 Platt R, Polk BF, Murdoch B, Rosner B. Mortality associated with nosocomial urinary

tract infection. N Eng J Med 1982; 307: 637–642.

45 El-Badawi A, Schenk EA. Dual innervation of bladder musculature. A histochemical study of distribution of cholinergic and adrenergic nerves. Am J Anat 1966; 119: 405.

46 Finkbeiner AE. Drug therapy for voiding disorders: theoretical and practical considerations. Controversies in Neurourology 261–275.

47 Olssen CA, Siroky MB, Krane RJ. The phentolamine test in neurogenic bladder dysfunction. J Urol 1977; 117–481.

48 Finkbeiner AE. Drug therapy for voiding disorders: theoretical considerations. In: Controversies in Neurourology 261–275.

49 Stanton SL, Cardozo LD, Kerr Wilson R. Treatment of delayed onset of spontaneous voiding after surgery for incontinence. Urology 1979; 13: 494–496.

50 Kiesswetter H, Schrober W. Lioresal in the treatment of neurogenic bladder dysfunction. Urol Int 1975; 30: 63.

51 Tammela T, Konturri M, Kaar K, Lukharinen O. Intravesical prostaglandin F2 for promoting bladder emptying after surgery for female stress incontinence. Br J Urol 1987; 60: 43–46.

52 Bergman A, Mushket Y, Gordon D, David MP. Prostaglandin prophylaxis and bladder function after vaginal hysterectomy: a prospective study. Br J Obs & Gynae 1993; 100: 69–72.

53 Fowler C, Betts C, Christmas T, Swash M, Fowler G. Botulinum toxin in the treatment of chronic urinary retention in women. B J Urol 1992; 70: 387–389.

54 Farrar D et al. A urodynamic view of bladder outlet obstruction in the female. B J Urol 1975; 47: 815–822.

55 Jammes J, Tigchelaar P, Rosenburger P. Habituation and urinary retention. JAMA 1975; 232 (12): 1264–1266.

56 Lapides J et al. Clean intermittent self catheterisation in the treatment of urinary tract disease. J Urol 1972; 107: 458–461.

57 Billau B, Howland D. Self-catheterisation for women with quadriplegia. The American Journal of Occupational Therapy 1991; 45: 366–369.

58 Diokno A, Sonda P, Hollander J, Lapides J. Fate of patients started on clean intermittent self catheterisation therapy 10 years ago. J Urol 1983; 129: 1120–1121.

59 Whitelaw S, Hammond J, Tregallas R. Clean intermittent self catheterisation in the elderly. B J Urol 1987; 60: 125–127.

60 Terpenning M, Allada R, Kaufmann C. Intermittent urethral catheterisation in the elderly. J AM Geriatric Soc 1989; 37: 411–416.

61 Blindley GS. Control of the bladder and urethral sphincters by surgically implanted electrical stimulation. In: Chisholm GD, Fair WB (eds) Scientific foundations of urology Chicago: Year Book Medical 1990: pp 336–339.

21 Prolapse

INTRODUCTION

The word 'prolapse' is derived from the Latin word meaning 'to fall'. A prolapse occurs when there is a defect in the pelvic floor sufficient to allow one or more of the pelvic viscera to fall through it. It is a common gynecological problem which, although not life-threatening, can severely adversely affect the quality of life of many women, especially during their climacteric years.

The human female pelvis and pelvic floor have undergone evolutionary changes to enable adoption of an erect posture whilst still allowing vaginal delivery of babies with large heads. The pelvic floor trauma accompanying childbirth weakens the vagina and allows subsequent 'pelvic relaxation'. This permanent damage may be asymptomatic initially, but with the withdrawal of estrogens at the time of the menopause, atrophy occurs and symptomatic prolapse may result.

As many women now spend a third of their lives in the post-menopausal state, an understanding of pelvic floor dysfunction and its correction is important in order to maintain normal bladder, bowel and sexual function.

TERMINOLOGY

The word 'procidentia' was first used in 1497 by Benedetti to describe genital organ prolapse. The term 'cystocele' was used in the 1600s to describe a herniation of the anterior vaginal wall and the term 'enterocele' was introduced in the 1700s to describe a herniation of peritoneum covered by vaginal epithelium.[1]

The same terminology is employed today and prolapse is classified according to the organ which has herniated into the vagina. Thus from anterior to posterior there can be a urethrocele, cystocele (these commonly occur together and are termed a cystourethrocele), uterovaginal prolapse, enterocele or rectocele. In addition, the perineal body may be deficient allowing gaping of the introitus with or without descent of the pelvic viscera. Various different terms for describing the severity of the prolapse have been advocated but these tend to be somewhat subjective. Cystocele and rectocele are usually termed mild, moderate or severe, the last being employed when the descending structure protrudes through the introitus.

Uterovaginal prolapse is normally graded as first degree when the cervix descends within the vagina but not as far as the introitus, second degree when it descends as far as the introitus but only through it on straining, and third degree (procidentia) when the whole of the uterus is outside the body and the vagina is completely inverted (Fig. 21.1).

Following hysterectomy, either abdominal or vaginal, the vaginal vault may prolapse or even invert producing an enterocele which is termed 'vault prolapse.' Any of the different types of prolapse can occur in isolation or in conjunction with descent of other structures. In addition, a cystourethrocele may be associated with stress incontinence due to urethral sphincter incompetence (genuine stress incontinence), as the same etiological factors are responsible for both. However, this is not universally true and both cystourethrocele and genuine stress incontinence can occur independently.

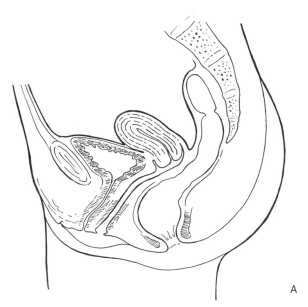

Fig. 21.1A Normally positioned pelvic anatomy

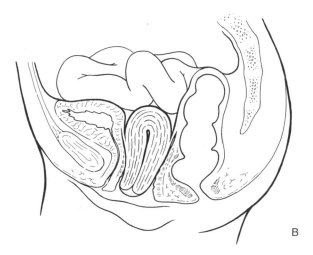

Fig. 21.1B Second degree utero-vaginal prolapse

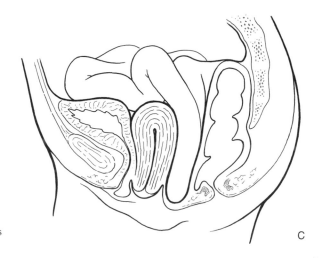

Fig. 21.1C Second degree utero-vaginal prolapse with an enterocele containing loops of small bowel

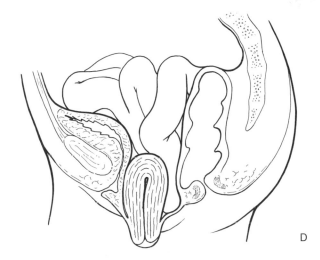

Fig. 21.1D   Procidentia

INCIDENCE

The majority of parous women have relative pelvic floor laxity and therefore asymptomatic prolapse is very common. It has been estimated that 50% of parous women have some degree of genital prolapse, and of these 10–20% are symptomatic.[2] Approximately 20% of all women awaiting major gynecological surgery have prolapse and this rises to 59% amongst elderly women. The incidence increases with age and in a series of 190 women with severe vaginal vault prolapse, 60% were over the age of 60 years.[3]

There is also thought to be a racial difference, prolapse being most common in Whites, less common in Asians and uncommon in Blacks.[4] However, more recent data reported by Bump[5] revealed that in North America interracial variations in prolapse did not exist and therefore the apparent difference may be due to underreporting by certain groups of women. Prolapse is uncommon in nulliparous women, only 2% of symptomatic prolapses occurring in women who have not had children.[4] In these cases the prolapse is almost always uterovaginal, presumably due to congenital weakness of the supporting structures. Although some degree of vault prolapse is common after a hysterectomy, severe symptomatic vault prolapse requiring surgical intervention occurs in fewer than 0.5% of women who have undergone hysterectomy.[6]

ANATOMY OF THE PELVIC FLOOR

The pelvic floor is composed of layers of muscle and fascia which act together to provide support for the pelvic viscera. Unfortunately, the pelvic floor in adult women is inherently weak, mainly due to their orthograde posture. In pronograde mammals the pubic symphysis is largely responsible for sustaining the weight of the pelvic viscera, whilst the caudal muscles, lying at right angles to the bony pelvis, are non-weight-bearing.[7] In dogs and cats, for example, the pelvic floor is a muscular organ which is responsible for movement of the tail but which does not have to support the pelvic viscera. However, in more advanced primates such as the chimpanzee and the human, the fascial layers of the pelvic floor are more developed in order to provide support for the pelvic contents. Thus in adult women the pelvic floor contains a greater proportion of fascia to muscle and this, when torn by parturition, may never regain the strength which is required to maintain the genital organs within the intra-abdominal cavity. Decreased cellularity and an increase in collagen fibres have been demonstrated in the pelvic connective tissue of 70% of women with uterovaginal prolapse as compared to 20% of normal women.[8,9]

The muscles of the pelvic floor are composed mainly of the levator ani and coccygei which arise on each side from the pelvic side wall and unite in the midline to form the anococcygeal raphe (Fig 21.2 and Fig 21.3). This striated muscle of the pelvic floor contains both slow twitch and fast twitch fibers. The slow twitch fibers provide tone over a long period of time, whereas the fast twitch fibers may be activated in response to stress or increases in intra-abdominal pressure. The urethra, vagina and rectum pass through a hiatus in the levator plate and each of these tracts has fibers of the levator muscle inserted into it (Fig. 21.3).

In a normal woman standing erect, the levator plate is nearly horizontal with the rectum, vagina and uterus resting on it (Fig. 21.4). When there is a rise in intra-abdominal pressure the pelvic floor contracts and pushes the pelvic viscera towards the pubic symphysis, thus increasing the closure pressure of the urethra.[10]

The pelvic fascia covers the pelvic floor and attaches to both the pelvic viscera and the bony skeleton. The uterosacral ligaments are condensations of pelvic fascia which help to maintain the cervix in a posterior position over the levator plate. The cardinal (lateral or transverse cervical) ligaments provide lateral support for the cervix and upper vagina. The round ligaments help to maintain the uterus in

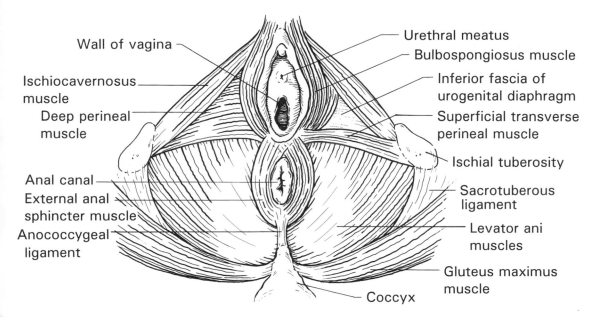

Fig. 21.2   Vaginal view of pelvic floor musculature

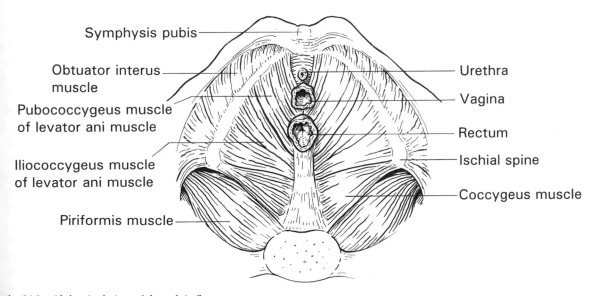

Fig. 21.3   Abdominal view of the pelvic floor

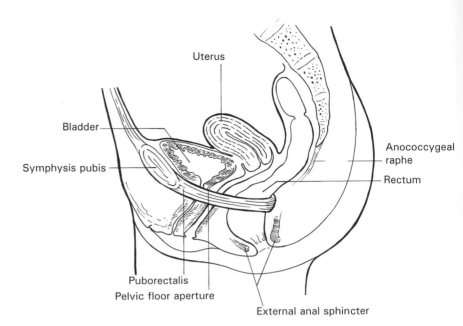

Fig. 21.4 Lateral view of female pelvic organs

anteversion whilst the pubourethral ligaments, which are largely composed of smooth muscle, are possibly important in the maintenance of continence.[11]

The pelvic floor may be permanently damaged by parturition or, less commonly, it may be congenitally weak.[12] This will initially cause the levator plate to become more oblique or vertical creating a funnel which allows the uterus, vagina and rectum to herniate through the levator hiatus. In women with severe prolapse, electromyographic studies of the perineal muscles have shown a 50% loss of motor units.[13] There is also good histochemical evidence of fascial denervation of the muscles in pelvic floor biopsies from patients with fecal incontinence and rectal prolapse.[14] In addition, partial denervation of the external anal sphincter has been demonstrated using single-fiber electromyography when a delayed pudendal nerve conduction time to the anal sphincter is shown in patients with fecal incontinence.[15,16] This delay in nerve conduction may be due to peripheral nerve injury resulting from denervation.

Studies from Manchester have identified pelvic floor denervation following parturition.[17,18,19] They have also shown gradual denervation of muscle with advancing years amongst nulliparous women without prolapse or stress incontinence. Parous women without prolapse or stress incontinence also had increased denervation with age and these women had considerably more denervation injury than nulliparous women. Those women who had stress incontinence, prolapse or both had significantly more denervation damage to their pelvic floor muscle than either of the other two groups. The electromyographic findings have been supported by the results of pudendal nerve terminal motor latency recordings, where delayed conduction to the pelvic floor and urethral sphincter has been demonstrated in women with prolapse and stress incontinence.

Histochemical examination of pelvic floor muscle biopsies showed changes in muscle fiber type and distribution and myopathic changes typical of denervation injury. The conclusions drawn from these studies are that partial denervation of the pelvic floor muscle is a normal part of the aging process; that it is increased by childbearing; and that it is significantly increased in women who have genitourinary prolapse and/or stress incontinence. However, it is still unclear why some women are affected more than others by giving birth to the same number of children.

Few studies have tried to assess the effect of pregnancy and childbirth on subsequent pelvic floor damage. Allen et al[19] asked women in their first pregnancy about urinary control. They carried out pelvic floor concentric needle electromyography at 36 weeks' gestation and again 8 weeks after delivery, and correlated changes with various obstetric events. After denervation of a motor unit, there may be reinnervation which produces changes in the amplitude, duration and number of phases in the motor unit potential. An increase in motor unit duration and polyphasicity are the most important indices of muscle denervation injury. At 8 weeks post partum a significant increase in motor unit duration was noted in postpartum women and this was considered to be indicative of denervation injury with subsequent reinnervation. The only obstetric factors which influenced the degree of denervation injury were the duration of pushing in the second stage of labor and the size of the baby. Women who were delivered by elective Caesarean section had no evidence of denervation injury. There was no relationship between denervation injury and the length of the first stage of labour, type of vaginal delivery or whether an episiotomy or epidural block were employed. In addition, pelvic floor muscle exercises post partum did not influence reinnervation of the pelvic floor or the power of pelvic floor contraction. However, Wilson and colleagues[20] have shown that intensive pelvic floor exercises performed from 3 months to 1 year post partum reduce the incidence of stress incontinence.[20]

Mechanical changes occurring in fascia during pregnancy have also been implicated in the genesis of pelvic floor weakness and urinary incontinence following pregnancy. Landon et al[21] tested this theory using rectus sheath fascia as a model, because its biochemical properties appear to be similar to those of pelvic floor fascia. They showed that rectus fascia becomes less elastic with age and that less energy is required to produce irreversible damage. These data correlate with the reduction in skin collagen content found in women after the menopause.[22] In pregnancy, fascia is more elastic and more likely to 'fail' than in the non-pregnant state.[21] This may be due to the endocrine environment in pregnancy. It may be that the increase in elasticity is responsible for the development of pelvic floor weakness and reduced fascial strength.

The muscle and fascial components of the pelvic floor work together to provide satisfactory support for normal function of the pelvic viscera. Changes occur in both components with increasing age and this is reflected in the increased incidence of prolapse and associated disorders seen in older women. This aging effect may be partly due to endocrine changes and the role of estrogens in this area has not yet been fully established. It appears that childbirth is the major cause of pelvic floor dysfunction,[23] but apart from carrying out elective Caesarean sections for all women, it is difficult to see how obstetric practice could make a significant difference. Certainly, the reduction in family size and improved nutrition of the population has helped to reduce the incidence of severe prolapse seen in clinical practice.

It is likely that some women have a predisposition to prolapse, but other factors have been implicated as precipitating causes. These include anything which increases intra-abdominal pressure, such as chronic cough, constipation with repeated straining at stool, intra-abdominal masses or ascites. Although many authors have included obesity there is no good evidence to show that this is the case.

Pelvic surgery may have a disruptive effect on the relationship of the pelvic viscera. Two operations in particular have been associated with the occurrence of a postoperative enterocele. The first of these is the Manchester repair, where the cardinal and uterosacral ligaments are plicated anterior to the cervical stump in order to maintain anteversion of the uterus, leaving a large hiatus posteriorly. The other operation which causes a problem is the Burch colposuspension, where the lateral vaginal fornices are fixed to the ipsilateral ileopectineal ligaments leaving a potential posterior vaginal defect. In one series, 9% of patients with an enterocele had previously undergone this type of retropubic urethropexy,[24] and in another report of 109 women with vaginal vault prolapse 43% had undergone a Burch type of colposuspension[25]. In a recent study of 113 women treated for genuine stress incontinence by means of a Burch colposuspension, over 25% required further surgery for prolapse. Although it was impossible to predict which women would do so, those with a large cystocele prior to surgery were more likely to develop a subsequent prolapse.[26]

It is often difficult to differentiate between the various underlying etiological factors in a patient who presents with a prolapse. For example, in one large series 37% had the onset of their symptom more than 37 years after a hysterectomy.[4] It is therefore difficult to know whether to blame the hysterectomy, the aging process, hormone deficiency following the menopause or the possibility of chronic increases in intra-abdominal pressure. However, in the same series 39% had the onset of their symptoms within 2 years of surgery. The possible etiological factors in the genesis of prolapse have been reviewed by Harris & Bent.[27]

CLINICAL PRESENTATION

The symptom of 'something coming down' is almost universal. Women may describe a lump in the vagina which is nearly always worse towards the end of the day, is relieved by lying down and may be totally asymptomatic when they get out of bed in the morning. Additional symptoms will depend upon the organ which has prolapsed into the vagina. In the case of a uterovaginal prolapse protrusion of the cervix through the introitus and a feeling of pressure are almost always present,[25] and in cases where there is a large prolapse which is predominantly outside the introitus, vaginal bleeding or discharge may be a secondary complication.

A cystocele or cystourethrocele often presents with urinary symptoms. Although stress incontinence may occur it is not a universal complaint in women with a cystourethrocele and more often they complain of voiding difficulties. Some women comment that they have to reduce the bulge digitally in order to pass urine normally, or that they are unable to empty their bladders completely despite straining. This may also be the case when there is significant uterovaginal prolapse.[28]

Increased frequency of micturition may occur in association with a large cystocele because of a persistent urinary residual or recurrent urinary tract infections. Unfortunately, correction of a cystocele may lead to urinary incontinence in women who did not suffer from leakage pre-operatively. Bergman et al[29] evaluated 67 women with a large cystocele but without urinary incontinence. Preoperatively they investigated them urodynamically, with and without a ring pessary in situ. With pessary correction, 35% showed signs of incipient stress incontinence with reduced urethral pressure transmission ratios. However, it is difficult to ensure that a ring pessary is not increasing outflow obstruction.

Although unusual, upper urinary tract problems may accompany severe prolapse and include recurrent urinary tract infection, hydro-ureter or hydronephrosis (Fig. 21.5). Dilatation of the collecting system is rare in mild prolapse, occurring in not more than 2% of cases. It becomes

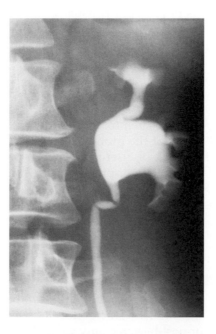

Fig. 21.5 Hydronephrosis secondary to a large prolapse

increasingly common with severe prolapse and has been identified in between 33% and 92% of patients presenting with complete procidentia. Renal ultrasound or possibly intravenous urography are useful investigations in such cases. The exact mechanism of upper urinary tract obstruction is uncertain but it may be due to kinking of the ureters or obstruction of the ureter between the fundus of the uterus and the levator hiatus.[30,31]

A rectocele may be asymptomatic even when it is quite large. If symptoms do occur they tend to be related to difficulty in defecation, tenesmus or coital discomfort. Less common symptoms occurring in association with prolapse are pelvic pain, urinary urgency and other less specific symptoms which are difficult to evaluate. Table 21.1 shows common symptoms associated with genital prolapse.

Table 21.1   Symptoms associated with genital prolapse in 109 women

Symptoms	Frequency (%)
Protrusion of tissue	> 90
Pressure	> 90
Impaired coitus	37
Difficulty voiding	33
Urinary incontinence	33
Difficulty walking	25
Difficulty defecating	25
Pelvic pain	17
Urinary frequency/urgency	14
Nausea	10
Low back pain	10
Mucosal irritation	10

From Addison et al 1988[25]

The diagnosis of prolapse is usually easy to make on clinical examination. There are a few differential diagnoses; these include a vaginal wall cyst, a prolapsed subendometrial fibroid and chronic uterine inversion. A procidentia can usually be diagnosed as soon as the woman opens her legs and any significant degree of cystocele or rectocele will be easy to recognize on parting the labia prior to digital vaginal examination (Fig. 21.6 and 21.7).

A Sims' speculum is helpful to identify the organ which has prolapsed and also the extent of the problem (Fig. 21.8). In order to provide some consistency it would be useful to have a universal grading system to demonstrate the severity of prolapse. One popular descriptive grading is given below.[32]

Cystocele: First degree – the anterior vaginal wall, from the urethra meatus to the anterior fornix, descends halfway to the introitus.
Second degree – the inferior bladder wall and its attached vaginal wall extend to the introitus.
Third degree – the entire urethra and bladder are outside the vagina. (This cystocele is usually part of a procidentia or post-hysterectomy vaginal vault prolapse.)

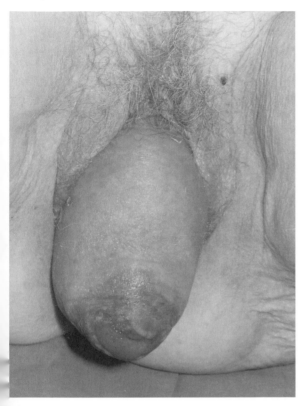

Fig. 21.6   A procidentia

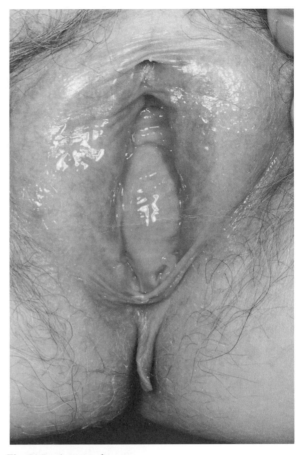

Fig. 21.7   A rectocele

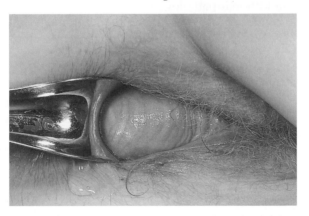

Fig. 21.8   Sims' speculum examination demonstrating a cystocele

Uterine or vaginal vault prolapse:	First degree – the cervix or vaginal apex descends halfway to the introitus.
	Second degree – the cervix or vaginal apex descends to the introitus or over the perineal body.
	Third degree (procidentia) – the cervix and body of the uterus lie totally outside the introitus or the vaginal vault is totally everted.

Enterocele: The presence and depth of the enterocele sac should be described anatomically with reference to the hymen, with the patient in the supine and standing positions during Valsalva' maneuver.

Rectocele: First degree – the saccular protrusion of the rectovaginal wall descends halfway to the introitus.
Second degree – the sacculation descends to the introitus.
Third degree – the sacculation protrudes outside the introitus.

An alternative 'APEX' classification has seen proposed by Genadry.[33] A, anterior wall; P, posterior wall; E, enterocele; and X, apex of vagina and cervix. The patient is examined in the erect position, at rest, and during Valsalva's maneuver with the labia spread open, and each component is graded depending on its displacement relative to the hymeneal ring, with grade I remaining above it and grade III beyond it. The staging system is as follows:

Stage I   + All grade I defects
Stage II   + All grade I and II defects with no more than two grade II defects
Stage III + Any grade III or three grade II defects
Stage IV   + Any two grade III defects or one grade III and three grade II defects.

Nowadays it is unusual to apply traction to the cervix in order to assess the degree of uterovaginal descent, although it may be necessary to reduce a cystocele with sponge-holding forceps for visualization of the cervix. It is important to carry out a careful examination to exclude any additional pathology such as a pelvic mass, and this will also allow the condition of the tissues to be identified. It may also be necessary to carry out a rectal examination in order to differentiate a rectocele from an enterocele; alternatively, this can be done by reversing the Sims' speculum to withdraw the anterior vaginal wall, digitally reducing the rectocele and feeling for a cough impulse above it. The International Continence Society has recently issued guidelines for the standardizations of terminology of female pelvic organ prolapse and pelvic floor dysfunction. A final draft of their document is shown in the appendix. This is likely to be adopted as the standard descriptive system for future research.

SPECIAL INVESTIGATIONS

Most women with a prolapse do not require any special investigations. However, if there are mixed or unusual findings in the history or on clinical examination, then certain additional tests should be undertaken. If urinary symptoms are present, it may be useful to give the patient a frequency/volume chart to complete in order to assess her drinking and voiding habits. Stress incontinence should be evaluated urodynamically prior to surgical intervention. This is important as a prolapse is generally easier to cure than stress incontinence and the first operation for stress incontinence is the most likely to cure the problem. Thus in women who complain of urinary incontinence or in whom this is demonstrated on clinical examination the minimum investigations would include a subtracted cystometrogram and measurement of urine flow rate. This will identify any lower urinary tract dysfunction which may alter the type of operation which is undertaken.

Women who complain of incomplete bladder emptying or straining to void should have their post-micturition urinary residual estimated either by ultrasound or 'in–out' catheterization in order to identify a large urinary residual. A midstream specimen of urine should be sent for culture and sensitivity to exclude a urinary tract infection prior to further investigation or treatment. In those patients who complain of urinary incontinence which cannot be demonstrated clinically or urodynamically, a pad test should be carried out to verify and quantify the problem, or else a pessary test may be performed to see whether reducing the cystocele will cause incontinence to occur.

If there is a large cystocele or procidentia then a renal ultrasound scan or an intravenous urogram should be performed to exclude upper urinary tract damage. If the symptoms of urgency and frequency of micturition are unusually severe for the degree of prolapse, a cystoscopy should be undertaken prior to surgical intervention. However, in the majority of cases, no investigations are needed before correction of a mild to moderate prolapse.

TREATMENT

The management of prolapse can be divided into general measures, non-surgical intervention, surgery and prophylaxis.

General measures

Around the time of the menopause there is a reduction in circulating estrogen levels which leads to genital atrophy as well as an increase in the symptoms of urogenital estrogen deficiency. Genital atrophy may be corrected by the use of estrogen replacement. Although this will not cure a pre-existent prolapse, it certainly improves the condition of the tissues and relieves the symptoms of vaginal soreness, itching and dryness which trouble so many postmenopausal women. There is also some evidence that estrogen therapy may help to improve a cystocele. We have shown that bladder base descent (as visualized during videocystourethrography) was improved in stress incontinent women who had been taking estrogen replacement therapy as compared to those who had been on placebo.

Physiotherapy

Physiotherapy has been advocated for the treatment of prolapse. Although there is evidence that pelvic floor exercises help and even cure some women with genuine stress incontinence, there is no real evidence to show that pelvic floor exercises are capable of curing a prolapse. Additional devices have been used to try to re-educate the pelvic floor. These include a perineometer, the most popular of which is the Bourne perineometer, and vaginal cones. The use of these adjunctive aids and devices is described in Ch. 37. We have found that pelvic floor exercises and cones are equally efficacious in the treatment of mild to moderate genuine stress incontinence but that cones are easier for women to use and compliance is likely to be better than with pelvic floor exercises alone.[34] If pelvic floor exercises or any other type of pelvic floor re-education is undertaken, it is mandatory that the physiotherapist or nurse continence advisor be enthusiastic, as this type of treatment needs to be carried out over a long period of time to produce any major benefit.

Electrical therapy

Electrical treatment such as faradism or interferential therapy is sometimes employed in women with prolapse in order to try to re-educate the pelvic floor. It is also used as a method of biofeedback to teach women which muscles they should contract. However, there is no good evidence that either of these methods of treatment is effective. They are fully described in the chapter on conservative treatment of genuine stress incontinence (Ch. 37). Shepherd et al[35] reported the results of a 6-month trial of an intravaginal electrical stimulation pessary, but showed that only 15 out of 68 patients studied actually completed the trial. They stated that this type of treatment was not really acceptable to British women. More recently, maximum electrical stimulation has been used as a conservative method of treatment for genuine stress incontinence but its place in the management of prolapse has yet to be evaluated.[36]

Intravaginal devices

Many women with prolapse fail to respond to simple measures or pelvic floor exercises. Although surgery is the definitive treatment, it is inappropriate for some women. These include the elderly who are unfit for surgery (although age in itself should not be a deterrent). In addition, there are women who do not wish to have an operation, and those who are pregnant or have recently had a baby in whom surgery would be undesirable. Nowadays, gynecological waiting lists tend to be long and a woman with a symptomatic prolapse may benefit from temporary conservative therapy whilst awaiting definitive treatment. Finally, it is sometimes difficult to be sure that the symptoms of which a woman complains are due to the prolapse and a pessary can be used as a therapeutic test.

The most commonly used pessary nowadays is a silicone or polythene ring pessary which comes in a wide variety of sizes (Fig. 21.9). It can be inserted into the vagina with minimal discomfort, usually digitally but sometimes using an introducer. A pessary should lie with one side in the posterior vaginal fornix and the other retro-pubically, thus creating an artificial levator shelf on which the intrapelvic organs can rest. These

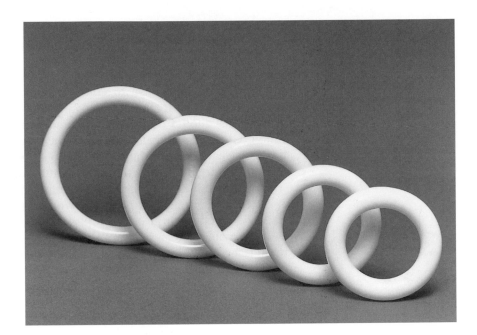

Fig. 21.9 Selection of ring pessaries

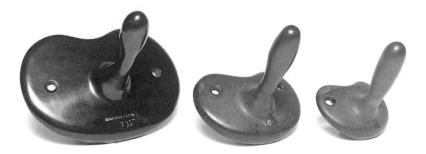

Fig. 21.10 Shelf pessaries

pessaries are not carcinogenic, as were the previous rubber ones, but they do sometimes cause vaginal discharge and this may be helped by concurrent local estrogen therapy. In addition, an ill-fitting ring pessary or one which has been in situ for too long may cause vaginal ulceration, which will only resolve when the pessary has been removed. Ring pessaries should be changed approximately every 6 months, and although they will never cure the problem, they may give sufficient relief for further treatment to be unnecessary. In the majority of cases the ring can be left in situ during sexual intercourse and does not cause a major problem. Severe uterovaginal prolapse or prolapse following hysterectomy may be better controlled with a shelf pessary (Fig. 21.10). These can be difficult to insert and remove and the stem can become encrusted.

Other intravaginal devices include sponge tampons which are removed, washed and reinserted, although their value has yet to be assessed. They have been advocated in cases of mild or exercise-induced stress incontinence rather than for prolapse alone.

Surgery

The definitive treatment for prolapse is surgery. Over 100 operations have been described, although fewer are in common use nowadays. Prior to any surgical operation it is important to assess the patient's general health and mental state, and if necessary ask the opinion of the anesthetist, who may wish to consider a regional block rather than a general anesthetic. If there is any evidence of urinary or vaginal infection, this should be investigated and treated prior to surgical intervention. Chronic medical conditions such as hypertension or diabetes should be treated, and if the patient has a chronic cough it may be worth considering surgery during the summer months.

Prophylactic measures have considerably decreased the morbidity associated with surgery for prolapse. Women at risk of thromboembolism should be given heparin or intraoperative dextran and it is wise to use either inflatable boots or thromboembolic deterrent (TED) stockings. Prophylactic antibiotics (especially metronidazole) are usually employed in order to minimize the risk of vaginal infection, and if a catheter is left in situ postoperatively a urinary antiseptic may be prescribed in addition.

Aims of surgery

It is no longer sufficient to alleviate a patient's symptoms of prolapse alone. For satisfactory sexual function it is important that a normal vaginal axis be restored and that vaginal length be maintained. In addition it is important to provide a permanent cure without the risk of subsequent urinary dysfunction. When surgery is undertaken, the patient must be correctly evaluated prior to her operation and the procedure tailored to suit the individual. It may not always be possible to cure all problems via one route, or even all at the same time. Unfortunately, even with expert surgery recurrences do occur and a recurrence rate of up to 25% has been quoted.[37]

Repair of a cystourethrocele

A cystocele or cystourethrocele may be repaired vaginally or abdominally, although most gynecologists use the vaginal route. It has been suggested[38] that a cystocele which develops from stretching of the anterior vaginal wall should be termed a 'pulsion' or 'distension' cystocele. This type of defect usually occurs after parturition and the lateral attachments of the vaginal wall remain intact whereas the central portion is overstretched. The cystocele which results from loss of lateral vaginal wall support is termed a 'displacement' or 'traction' cystocele. Most cystoceles involve a combination of distension and displacement elements. Surgical repair needs to take into account the type of defect which is present.

Anterior colporrhaphy

Gynecologists normally repair a cystocele or cystourethrocele vaginally, even if it is quite large. This is appropriate for a central defect (pulsion cystocele). The operation is normally performed under general anesthesia, although regional block is adequate and may be preferable in elderly women with chronic medical conditions. The patient is positioned supine with her ankles supported in stirrups and her hips abducted and flexed. Her buttocks should be beyond the edge of the operating table to facilitate the use of a Sims' (or similar) speculum. The vagina and perineum are cleaned with sterile solution and draped, and a 14F Foley catheter with a small balloon is inserted into the bladder to help to identify the position of the bladder neck and to drain the bladder throughout the operation.

Following a bimanual examination, a vaginal speculum is inserted and the cervix is grasped with a vulsellum. If the patient has previously undergone a hysterectomy, the vaginal vault is grasped with the vulsellum. A small pair of Kocher's forceps is positioned approximately 1 cm below the urethral meatus. The vaginal epithelium is either incised in the midline between the Kocher's forceps and the vulsellum or alternatively a diamond-shaped section of redundant anterior vaginal wall epithelium is excised using a scalpel. Either way the bladder is then dissected off the overlying vaginal epithelium using sharp and blunt dissection. The vaginal skin edges are grasped with Kocher's forceps to facilitate this dissection. When the whole of the cystocele has been mobilized, the bladder neck is identified by pulling gently on the Foley catheter. Even in women who are not complaining of incontinence, the repair usually begins at the urethrovesical junction, to try to avoid the recurrence or occurrence of stress incontinence postoperatively.

In women who do have a degree of genuine stress incontinence concurrent with their cystocele, it is appropriate to insert a 'Kelly' suture at this stage. This was originally described by Kelly in 1913 as the placement of a mattress suture under the urethrovesical junction for the correction of stress incontinence.[39] Alternatively, in women with more severe genuine stress incontinence and a large cystocele an endoscopically guided needle suspension such as a Stamey or Raz procedure can be carried out at this time.

If there is a very large cystocele a purse-string suture may be inserted to reduce it partially. Thereafter, the bladder neck and remainder of the cystocele are repaired by approximating the pubocervical fascia on each side of the midline, thus reducing the herniation of the bladder. The suture material is important. Catgut is absorbed too quickly and causes a tissue reaction, whereas Vicryl or Dexon (polyglycolic acid) are stronger and more appropriate for reconstruction of the fascial layers. The redundant vaginal epithelium is trimmed and the anterior vaginal wall is closed using interrupted polyglycolic acid sutures.

It is possible to carry out an anterior colporrhaphy on its own or it may be performed at the same time as a vaginal hysterectomy, in which case the hysterectomy is carried out first and the approximated cardinal ligaments are employed as the new vaginal vault instead of the cervix.

Occasionally, for women who are reluctant to undergo a hysterectomy but who have a second-degree uterovaginal prolapse, a Manchester or Fothergill repair may be appropriate. In this operation the cervix is amputated and the cardinal/uterosacral ligaments are approximated anterior to the cervical stump in order to antevert the uterus. The vaginal epithelium is reconstructed over the cervical stump and an anterior and posterior colporrhaphy are performed.

In many women who have a prolapse more than one 'compartment' requires repair and it is often preferable to carry out a posterior colpoperineorrhaphy at the same time as an anterior colporrhaphy in order to support the anterior vaginal wall with a firm posterior vaginal wall.

Abdominal repair of a cystocele

Retropubic operations such as the Burch colposuspension are effective in the treatment of a mild or moderate cystocele, although they may leave a high anterior vaginal wall defect. This is usually asymptomatic and does not therefore require further surgical intervention. Occasionally, it is necessary to repair a cystocele at the same time as performing an abdominal hysterectomy. This can be done after the uterus has been removed. The bladder is dissected off the anterior vaginal wall nearly to the level of the ureters. A full thickness midline wedge of anterior vaginal wall is excised and the vagina is closed longitudinally with an absorbable suture material. It is possible to unmask stress incontinence using this procedure, and therefore important to undertake appropriate evaluation of the patient prior to surgery.

Paravaginal repair

The paravaginal repair was first described by White in 1909[40] as a vaginal operation which he acknowledged could also be performed abdominally. In recent years, the paravaginal repair performed abdominally has been popularized by Richardson and colleagues[41,42] as an operation for the correction of cystourethrocele due to lateral detachment and also as a method of treatment for genuine stress incontinence in association with a cystocele. Through a Pfannenstiel or Cherney incision the retropubic space is opened and the bladder is drawn medially away from the pelvic side wall (as in the Burch colposuspension). With the surgeon's left hand in the patient's vagina, the lateral sulcus of the vagina is elevated together with its overlying pubocervical fascia and reattached to the pelvic side wall using a series of sutures at 1-cm intervals. The first suture should be about 1 cm in front of the ischial spine and ventrally the last stitch should be as close as possible to the pubic ramus. When all sutures have been placed they are tied. It is recommended that a permanent suture material be used and that the procedure be performed bilaterally. Richardson[43] quoted a satisfactory result of more than 95% in a series of over 800 paravaginal repairs.

Repair of a posterior vaginal wall prolapse

Posterior vaginal wall prolapse may be due to a rectocele, a lax or deficient perineum or a combination of both. Before undertaking a posterior colpoperineorrhaphy it is essential to talk to the patient about her expectations of the procedure. Even if she is not sexually active at present, she may wish to be so in the future and therefore a vagina of sufficient calibre and length to permit penetration should be the end result of surgical intervention. The posterior colpoperineorrhapy may be undertaken on its own or in combination with an anterior colporrhaphy and/or a vaginal hysterectomy. If a rectocele is asymptomatic it is usually best to avoid carrying out a posterior repair as this may lead to dyspareunia and postoperative urinary retention. However, women with a significant rectocele may complain of difficult defecation, tenesmus or a lump in the vagina, and those with a lax or deficient perineum may feel that sexual intercourse is unsatisfactory for them or for their partner.

The patient is positioned supine with her ankles supported in stirrups and her hips flexed and abducted. Her buttocks need to be positioned over the edge of the operating table in order for a Sims' speculum to be utilized. Two Allis tissue forceps are placed on the perineum, one on either side at the level of the hymeneal remnants. These two forceps are first approximated to confirm that the caliber of the introitus will be adequate, and then retracted laterally. Phenylephrine 0.005% in saline is injected to raise the posterior vaginal wall off the underlying tissues. Drawing the two Allis forceps laterally the old perineal scar tissue is excised, except when the perineum is so deficient that the anus might be injured.

A diamond-shaped incision is made with one apex into the vagina and the other into the perineum and thus the posterior fourchette together with the underlying scar tissue is excised. A subepithelial tunnel is made in the rectovaginal space using Fergusson's scissors. This dissection is extended to the apex of the rectocele. The vaginal epithelium is then incised longitudinally and the edges of the flaps grasped with small Kocher's forceps. The rectum can then be mobilized away from the vaginal epithelium using blunt and sharp dissection. When the rectocele has been completely freed, a small strip of skin is removed on either side. The dissection is extended laterally as far as is necessary to mobilize the perirectal fascia and expose the medial margins of the pubococcygeus muscles.

If the rectocele is very large or if there is an additional enterocele, one or more purse-string sutures may be inserted high up using Vicryl or Dexon. Thereafter, the pararectal and rectovaginal fascia from each side is approximated over the underlying rectum and this suture may incorporate the vaginal skin. In the lower part of the vagina the levator ani muscles are approximated in the midline to cover the rectocele and also increase support to the anterior vaginal wall. Care is taken not to create a constriction ring in the vagina due to overambitious levator approximation. The overlying vaginal skin is then repaired using continuous or interrupted Vicryl sutures.

A perineoplasty is finally performed placing deep sutures into the perineal muscles and fascia to build up the perineal body and this lengthens the vagina. The overlying perineal skin is closed using a subcuticular 3/0 Dexon or Vicryl suture.

When an anterior and/or posterior repair has been performed, it is common to insert a vaginal pack for the first 24 postoperative hours and to leave the Foley catheter in situ until the pack has been removed. Alternatively, if bladder neck sutures have been inserted or another incontinence procedure has been carried out a suprapubic catheter may be preferred and initially left on free drainage postoperatively.

Unfortunately, there have been few studies which have assessed the long-term success of vaginal repairs in the treatment of cystocele or rectocele. Early recurrence (or failure) is usually because not all of the defects have been repaired appropriately. Late recurrence is more likely to be due to weakness of the patient's supporting tissues, which increases with advancing age and estrogen deprivation after the menopause.

Complications associated with both anterior and posterior colporrhaphies are rare. The most likely problem is accidental injury to the underlying organ, namely the bladder, urethra or rectum. If these injuries are identified intraoperatively then they can be repaired in layers and the appropriate action taken. If the bladder or urethra is traumatized then continuous bladder drainage for 10 days with antibiotic cover is appropriate. If the rectum is injured a low-residue diet together with a stool softener should be administered postoperatively. Occasionally, hemorrhage or infection may occur in association with vaginal surgery. The latter can be minimized by the use of prophylactic antibiotics, which are now used routinely in many centers.

Urinary tract infection may occur in association with the use of an indwelling catheter, but this too should be minimized by the use of prophylactic antibiotics. Voiding difficulties postoperatively are relatively common after both anterior and posterior colporrhaphy. This may be predicted by preoperative urodynamics in women who have a low flow rate and low maximum voiding pressure. Initially, treatment should consist of insertion of a suprapubic catheter which can be clamped and released easily to encourage normal spontaneous voiding to occur per urethram. If voiding difficulties persist then clean intermittent self-catheterization should be instituted.

A few studies have looked at the effect of vaginal repairs on sexual function. Francis & Jeffcoate[44] found that about 50% of sexually active women had some sexual difficulties after a pelvic floor repair with or without vaginal hysterectomy. Fifty-five per cent of them reported loss of sexual desire or impotence which may have predated the surgery. The remaining women reported sexual difficulties due to shortening of the vagina, dyspareunia or fear of injury. More recently, Haase & Skibsted[45] reported on 55 sexually active women who underwent a variety of operations for stress incontinence and/or prolapse. Postoperatively 24% of them experienced improvement in sexual satisfaction, 67% reported no change and 9% said that their sex lives had deteriorated. Improvement often resulted from the cessation of urinary incontinence. Deterioration was always due to dyspareunia following a posterior colporrhaphy.

Treatment of uterovaginal prolapse

Nowadays the choice of surgery for uterovaginal prolapse lies between a vaginal hysterectomy and pelvic floor repair or a Manchester repair. It used to be stated that a vaginal hysterectomy was associated with greater risk of complications than a Manchester repair,[46] but nowadays with modern anesthesia and the use of prophylactic antibiotics this is probably no longer true. It is appropriate to perform a vaginal hysterectomy in conjunction with a pelvic floor repair in women who have completed their family, especially those who have concurrent benign uterine pathology such as small fibroids or menorrhagia. It is also advisable to remove the uterus in cases of severe uterovaginal prolapse or when an enterocele is present. Manchester repair has been performed in young women who do not wish to lose their fertility; however, the complications of this operation include infertility, increased risk of miscarriage and problems in labor. Thus in general it is more sensible for young women with uterovaginal prolapse to avoid surgery until after they have completed their family.

Vaginal hysterectomy is considered to be the operation of choice for uterovaginal prolapse. Relative contraindications are:

- a uterus larger than the size of a 12-week gestation (unless bisection or morcellation is undertaken)
- endometriosis
- pelvic inflammatory disease
- suspected malignancy.

In addition some gynecologists consider nulliparity, a narrow subpubic arch and a long narrow vagina to be contraindications as they reduce access and make the surgery more difficult.

The principles of vaginal hysterectomy are similar to those of abdominal hysterectomy and are fully described in textbooks of gynecological or pelvic surgery. The three major pedicles are taken in reverse order. The cardinal and uterosacral ligaments are clamped, cut and ligated first, followed by the uterine vessels and finally the tubo-ovarian and round ligament pedicles. The pelvic peritoneum is opened anteriorly and posteriorly prior to removal of the uterus and is reconstituted thereafter. In the majority of women it is possible to perform a bilateral salpingo-oophorectomy vaginally at this stage of the operation. The upper pedicles are identified and approximated in the midline to help to support the vault of the vagina. Finally, the uterosacral ligaments are approximated posteriorly in order to obliterate the potential enterocele space. The vaginal vault can be closed transversely unless an anterior colporrhaphy is to be performed for a cystourethrocele at the same time, in which case 'Y' closure of the vault is commonly undertaken. Intraoperative complications include bleeding and damage to the bladder or occasionally the ureter. Postoperatively the most common problem is a vault hematoma, which may cause a low-grade pyrexia or which may become infected and occasionally cause a pelvic abscess. Additional complications are those associated with any surgical procedure. Long-term complications are rare but include vault prolapse and dyspareunia.

Manchester (Fothergill) repair This operation aims to elevate the uterus by approximating and shortening the cardinal ligaments anterior to the cervical stump following amputation of the distal portion of the cervix. The operation is combined with an anterior colporrhaphy and a posterior colpoperineorrhaphy. Intraoperative complications are uncommon and are the same as those for anterior or posterior colporrhaphy. Long-term sequelae include problems of fertility and childbirth. Additionally, there is the risk of recurrence of the uterovaginal prolapse and a relatively high incidence of enterocele. This occurs because of the posterior defect created by bringing the cardinal and uterosacral ligaments anterior to the cervix.

The Le Fort operation This type of colpocleisis is rarely performed nowadays but is still sometimes used in the frail elderly. It involves total vaginal obliteration and is therefore only suitable when vaginal access to the pelvis is no longer required. This is useful as a 'last resort' because it is quick and easy to perform even under local anesthesia with minimal blood loss and very few complications. It is important that the patient and her partner understand that sexual intercourse will thereafter be impossible.

There is a relatively high incidence of stress incontinence post-operatively, presumably due to the fusion of the anterior and posterior vaginal walls causing descent of the bladder neck and proximal urethra. It is possible to carry out a simultaneous bladder neck plication but this complicates the operation.

To perform a Le Fort procedure the cervix is grasped with a Vulsellum and approximately 20 ml of local anesthetic with adrenaline is injected into the vaginal tissue beneath the epithelium. A Foley catheter with a small balloon is inserted into the bladder. A dilatation and curettage is performed to exclude uterine pathology. Two rectangular strips of vaginal skin are marked out using a scalpel and are excised from the anterior and posterior vaginal wall. Each section of skin is removed leaving enough vagina laterally to allow drainage channels for vaginal secretions.

The cut edge of the anterior vaginal wall is sewn to the cut edge of the posterior vaginal wall with interrupted polyglycolic acid sutures. The lateral margins of the rectangle are sutured with the cut inside the epithelial line on either side; this way the uterus and/or vaginal apex are gradually inverted. When the entire vagina has been pushed inside, the superior and inferior margins of the rectangle are sutured horizontally.

A perineorrhaphy can be performed at the same time to give posterior support and to narrow the introitus.

The usual precautions and prophylactic antibiotics are employed, and as most of the patients undergoing this procedure are elderly, with an increased risk of thromboembolism, prophylactic heparin should also be considered. Certainly, TED stockings and early mobilization are important.

Early complications include hematoma, infection and urinary symptoms, especially urinary retention. Later complications include urinary incontinence – 10.2% in one series[47] – but in general there is total cure of prolapse with a recurrence rate of 2–5%. This operation has largely been superseded by vaginal hysterectomy and pelvic floor repair.

Surgical treatment of an enterocele

An enterocele is, by definition, a herniation of the peritoneum with or without intraperitoneal contents. It typically arises from the pouch of Douglas, and may occur in conjunction with other types of prolapse or on its own.

Four different types of enterocele have been described. A congenital enterocele is rare but may arise in conjunction with neurological disorders such as spina bifida. A traction enterocele occurs secondary to uterovaginal descent. A pulsion enterocele results from prolonged increased intra-abdominal pressure, for example when there is a chronic cough or pelvic mass. Iatrogenic enterocele follows surgical procedures which alter the vaginal axis towards the vertical, and this is common following a Burch colposuspension or Manchester repair.

An enterocele can be repaired either vaginally at the time of a pelvic floor repair, abdominally at the time of hysterectomy or when bladder neck surgery is performed for urinary incontinence.

Vaginal approach With the patient in the lithotomy position a midline incision is made in the posterior vaginal wall, over the enterocele and extending up to the vaginal apex. It is extended down to the perineum if a rectocele is also present. The vaginal skin is dissected off the underlying enterocele sac and anterior wall of the rectum. The enterocele sac should be fully mobilized. It is sometimes difficult to differentiate between an enterocele and a rectocele and in order to do this a rectal examination can be performed. Sometimes it is difficult to differentiate the enterocele sac from a cystocele and a bladder sound may be helpful. When the enterocele sac has been fully mobilized it is opened and explored to ensure that no small bowel is adherent to the sac. Any excess peritoneum is excised and under direct vision two or three purse-string sutures of a long-term absorbable or non-absorbable material are used to close the neck of the sac. If the uterosacral or cardinal ligaments can be identified they are approximated to support the vault of the vagina. The posterior vaginal wall is then reconstructed in order to provide additional support.

If there is a hiatus between the two uterosacral ligaments at the time of vaginal hysterectomy, this can be obliterated prior to closure of the vaginal vault by approximation of the uterosacral ligaments in the midline. The sutures which are employed to do this may also incorporate the peritoneum and or the posterior vaginal wall epithelium.[48]

Abdominal approach An isolated enterocele can be dealt with by means of a Moschowitz procedure.[49] This is performed by inserting concentric purse-string sutures around the peritoneum in the pouch of Douglas. The first suture is positioned at the base of the hernia incorporating the posterior vaginal wall, the pelvic side wall, the serosa of sigmoid colon and the opposite pelvic side wall in turn. Usually three or four sutures are required. The purse-string sutures are tied so that no small defects remain which could trap small bowel or lead to an enterocele recurrence. It is possible to kink a ureter during this procedure so care must be taken. Alternatively, the pouch of Douglas may be obliterated with interrupted sutures inserted between the serosa of the sigmoid colon and the posterior vaginal wall.

Treatment of a recurrent prolapse

Vaginal vault prolapse is a complication of hysterectomy or other pelvic surgery and occurs in somewhere between 0.2% and 43% of cases,[50] although usually an incidence of below 5% is quoted.[51] It occurs equally commonly after abdominal or vaginal hysterectomy.[52] Vault prolapse can be notoriously difficult to treat, but reconstructive pelvic surgery has advanced considerably over recent years and now a number of surgical options are available. The most straightforward repair of this type of enterocele is performed vaginally by opening the vaginal vault, dissecting out the enterocele sac, and closing off the space. However, this commonly leads to narrowing and shortening of the vagina and dyspareunia is not uncommon thereafter.

Sacrospinous ligament fixation

This operation was originally described as the 'transvaginal sacrospinous colpopexy'.[53] In America it was popularized by Nichols.[54] Although the operation is usually performed for vault prolapse it can be undertaken at the same time as a vaginal hysterectomy in cases of uterovaginal prolapse.

With the patient in the lithotomy position the posterior vaginal wall is incised longitudinally from the introitus to the vault, exposing the recto-vaginal space. The epithelium is dissected laterally on both sides. The right ischial spine is palpated and exposed using sharp and blunt dissection by creating a space through the right rectal pillar. The sacrospinous ligament is palpated as it passes from the ischial spine to the lower part of the sacrum. A double permanent non-absorbable or long-term absorbable suture is placed through the ligament. This can be facilitated by use of a Miya hook ligature carrier.[55] Care is taken to avoid damage to the sacral plexus and sciatic nerve, which are located above the superior border of the sacrospinous ligament, and the pudendal vessels and nerve which course round the ischial spine. The sutures are loaded on to a loose needle and passed through the vaginal epithelium at the vaginal vault on each side of the midline and held for later tying. The enterocele is dissected out and obliterated with one or two purse-string sutures. The rectovaginal septum is reconstructed using polyglycolic sutures and the upper third of the vaginal epithelium is closed in the normal way. The sacrospinous sutures are then tied, rather like a pulley bringing the vaginal vault up to the sacrospinous ligament. A perineorrhaphy is performed and a vaginal pack and catheter are left in situ.

Richter & Albricht[56] reported a 96% cure rate for this type of surgery, but comment that urinary incontinence is not corrected by the operation. Shull et al[57] reported the outcome in 66 women who underwent sacrospinous colpopexy for vault prolapse following hysterectomy. They also achieved an excellent cure rate for vault prolapse (98%), but reported less success in the cure of anterior compartment defects (cystocele). It appears that the posterior fixation of the vaginal vault to the sacrospinous ligament predisposes to prolapse of the anterior vaginal wall in a similar way to ventral fixation (Burch-type colposuspension), predisposing to posterior vaginal wall (recto-enterocele) prolapse. In a recently reported series sacrospinous colpopexy has been undertaken in 40 women for vault prolapse following hysterectomy and 24 women with marked uterovaginal prolapse.[58] In those women with co-existent stress incontinence a long needle bladder neck suspension was performed at the same time. The authors reported 3 failures in the group treated for vault prolapse, all of whom underwent subsequent successful repeat sacrospinous colpopexy. In this series, too, the main long-term complication was cystocele formation and one patient complained of dyspareunia following surgery.

Abdominal sacrocolpopexy

Sacrocolpopexy using a strip of fascia or inorganic mesh (Mersilene or Gortex) is now the most popular method of dealing with a vaginal vault prolapse by the abdominal route.[59] This type of operation restores the normal anatomical relationships of the vagina and maintains good coital function. It can be combined with a colposuspension if genuine stress incontinence is present and a posterior colpoperineorrhaphy may need to be performed at the same time or more commonly on a subsequent occasion.

The sacrocolpopexy can be performed through a lower midline or Pfannenstiel incision. The apex of the prepacked vagina is identified and the overlying peritoneum is opened. The sacral promontory is then exposed in the midline and a retroperitoneal tunnel is created from the sacral promontory, slightly to the right of the midline, but medial to the right ureter, to join up with the incision at the vaginal apex. A strip of mesh is then sutured to the vaginal vault and posterior vaginal wall in several places using non-absorbable suture material (Ethibond). The sutures are left untied and the other end of the mesh is brought through the retroperitoneal tunnel and sutured to the periosteum overlying the sacral promontory, also with non-absorbable sutures, such that the vagina is on minimal tension. The sutures are then tied and the peritoneum closed over the vaginal vault and sacral promontory. Surgical complications include bleeding from the middle sacral artery; damage to the sigmoid colon, which has to be retracted to the left; and damage to the right ureter. When there is a large enterocele it may be difficult to tunnel retroperitoneally in the pouch of Douglas and it may therefore be necessary to close off the enterocele itself prior to performing the sacrocolpopexy.

Satisfactory correction of vaginal vault prolapse has been described using this operation[25] and the long-term results in a series of 147 patients have been reviewed, with a 93% 5-year success rate reported. A large series by Timmons et al[59] reports few failures and a low complication rate but emphasizes the importance of a broad attachment of the synthetic suspensory material to the prolapsed vaginal vault. In a recent series of 41 women undergoing 43 sacrocolpopexies the cure rate of vault prolapse was 88%.[60] There was no difference between failures and successes in terms of weight, parity, age, previous surgery, pulmonary history or difficulties with defecation. The most common complications were stress incontinence, urinary tract infections and persistent vaginal discharge.

Unfortunately, an associated cystocele or rectocele must still be corrected vaginally, although not necessarily at the same time as the sacrocolpopexy. Genuine stress incontinence may actually be made worse by this type of operation and urodynamic assessment prior to surgery is helpful in identifying those patients who will require additional surgery to the bladder neck. In women with a capacious vagina, it is possible to perform a Burch-type colposuspension at the same time as the sacrocolpopexy, but in older women with a narrow atrophic vagina where there is scarring from previous surgery, it may be easier to perform a vaginal vault suspension initially and later to correct genuine stress incontinence with an endoscopically guided bladder neck suspension or injectables. Early complications include urinary retention and infection. Late complications are few and include the possibility of erosion of the mesh through the vagina (which may necessitate its removal) or very rarely into the bladder or rectum.

Abdominoperineal repair   Zacharin & Hamilton[61] have described a complicated technique for the correction of a large enterocele. This operation is particularly useful in women with a weak pelvic floor in whom other procedures have failed or where there is recurrent vaginal vault prolapse. The Zacharin procedure really requires two operators. The abdominal surgeon opens the abdomen through a Pfannenstiel or lower midline incision, reflects the peritoneum around the pelvic brim and laterally identifies the levator muscles; meanwhile the vaginal surgeon opens the vagina and identifies the enterocele sac. Under direct vision the enterocele can be excised and once the ureters have been mobilized laterally, the levator muscles on either side can be brought together in the midline. Finally, the vagina is reconstructed and stitched on to the new levator plate. A long-term success rate of 93% cure has been described using this technique; however, it is time-consuming and requires two experienced operators.

PREVENTION

During recent decades, the incidence of prolapse has decreased because of smaller family size, shorter labors and an improvement in general health. In addition, the increased use of hormone replacement therapy is probably having a beneficial effect, although this has not as yet been evaluated. Those prolapses which do cause symptoms are usually less severe and few women present with procidentia. It is possible that the increasing use of Caesarean section (particularly elective Caesarean section) may further reduce the risk of prolapse, and although there is no real evidence that postnatal pelvic floor exercises are effective, it may be possible to reduce the incidence of prolapse associated with childbirth still further by appropriate teaching of antenatal pelvic floor exercises.

Any factor which increases intra-abdominal pressure should be avoided. The incidence of chronic bronchitis is decreasing and in general more attention is being paid to diet. It is to be hoped that the latter will reduce the problem of constipation, which has been incriminated as a major factor in the relatively high incidence of prolapse amongst Western women.

CONCLUSIONS

Prolapse is a common condition which affects many women, mostly those who have borne children. This is usually a condition which is easy to diagnose and the initial management is straightforward. However, treatment which fails presents a problem and the management of recurrent prolapse may be considerably more complicated. Where possible prophylactic measures should be employed in order to prevent the recurrence of prolapse and treatment should be modified to suit the individual's symptoms and requirements.

REFERENCES

1 Emge LA, Durfee RB. Pelvic organ prolapse: four thousand years of treatment. Clin Obstet Gynecol 1966; 9: 997.

2 Beck RP, Nordstrom L. A 25 year experience with 519 anterior colporrhaphy procedures. Obstet Gynecol 1991; 78: 1011–1018.

3 Symmonds RE, Williams TJ, Lee RA et al. Post hysterectomy enterocele and vaginal vault prolapse. Am J Obstet Gynecol 1981; 140: 852.

4 Nichols DH. Vaginal surgery. Baltimore: Williams & Wilkins, 1978.

5 Bump R. Racial comparisons and contrasts in urinary incontinence and genital prolapse. Neurourol Urodynam 1992; 11(4): 357–358.

6 Mattingly RF, Thompson JD. Telinde's operative gynecology. Philadelphia: JB Lippincott, 1985.

7 Smout CVF, Jacoby F. Gynecological and obstetrical anatomy and functional histology, 3rd edn. Baltimore: Williams & Willkins, 1953: pp 76–77.

8 Makinen J, Kahari V, Soderstrom K et al. Collagen synthesis in the vaginal connective tissue of patients with and without uterine prolapse. Eur J Obstet Gynecol Reprod Biol 1987; 24: 319.

9 Makinen J, Kiilholma P, Soderstrom K et al. Historic changes in vaginal connective tissue of patients with and without uterine prolapse. Arch Gynecol 1986; 239: 17.

10 DeLancey JOL. Anatomy of the pelvis. In: Thompson JD, Rock JA (eds) Telinde's operative gynecology, 7th edn. Philadelphia: JB Lippincott, 1992.

11 DeLancey JOL. The pubovesical ligament, a separate structure from the urethral supports ('pubo-urethral ligaments'). Neurourol Urodyn 1989; 8: 53–61.

12 Ulmsten U, Ekman G, Giertz G et al. Different biochemical composition of connective tissue in continent and stress incontinent women. Acta Obstet Gynecol Scand 1987; 66: 455.

13 Sharf B, Zilberman A, Sharf M et al. Electromyogram of pelvic floor muscles in genital prolapse. Int J Gynecol Obstet 1976; 14:2.

14 Parks A, Swash M, Urich H. Sphincter denervation, anorectal incontinence and rectal prolapse. Gut 1977; 18: 656–665.

15 Neill ME, Swash M. Increased motor unit fibre density in the external anal sphincter muscle in ano-rectal incontinence: a single fibre EMG study. J Neurourol Neurosurg Psychiatry 1980; 43: 343–347.

16 Kiff E, Swash M. Slowed conduction in the pudenal nerve in idiopathic (neurogenic) faecal incontinence. Br J Surg 1984; 71: 614–616.

17 Smith ARB, Hosker GL, Warrell DW. The role of partial denervation of the pelvic floor in the aetiology of genitourinary prolapse and stress incontinence. A neuro physiological study. Br J Obstet Gynaecol 1989a; 96: 24–28.

18 Smith ARB, Hosker GL, Warrell DW. The role of pudenal nerve damage in the aetiology of genuine stress incontinence of urine in women. A neurophysiological study. Br J Obstet Gynaecol 1989b; 96: 29–32.

19 Allen RE, Hosker GL, Smith ARB, Warrell DW. Pelvic floor damage and childbirth: a neurophysiological study. Br J Obstet Gynaecol 1990; 97: 770–779.

20 Wilson PD, Herbison GP, Borland M, Grant A. A randomised controlled trial of physiotherapy treatment of postnatal urinary incontinence. Proceedings of the 26th British Congress of Obstetrics & Gynaecology, 1992.

21 Landon CR, Smith ARB, Crofts CE, Trowbridge EA. Biomechanical properties of connective tissue in women with stress incontinence of urine. Neurourol Urodyn 1989; 8: 369–370.

22 Brincat M, Moniz CF, Studd JWW et al. Long term effects of the menopause and sex hormones on skin thickness. Br J Obstet Gynaecol 1985; 92: 256–259.

23 Sultan AH, Kamm MA, Hudson CN. Pudenal nerve damage during labour prospective study before and after childbirth. Br J Obstet Cynaecol 1994; 101: 22–28.

24 Burch JC. Urethrovaginal fixation to Cooper's ligament for correction of stress incontinence, cystocele and prolapse. Am J Obstet Gynecol 1967; 81: 281.

25 Addison WA, Livergood CH, Parker RT. Post hysterectomy vaginal vault prolapse with emphasis on management by transabdominal sacral colpopexy. Post Grad Obstet Gynaecol 1988; 8: 1.

26 Wiskind AK, Creighton SM, Stanton SL. The incidence of a genital prolapse following the Burch colposuspension operation. Neurourol Urodyn 1991; 10: 453–454.

27 Harris TA, Bent AE. Genital prolapse with and without urinary incontinence. J Reprod Med 1990; 35: 792–798.

28 Richardson DA, Bent AE, Ostergard DR The effect of uterovaginal prolapse on urethrovesical pressure dynamics. Am J Obstet Gynecol 1983; 146: 901.

29 Bergman A, Koonings PP, Ballard CA. Predicting post operative urinary incontinence development in women undergoing operation for genitourinary prolapse. Am J Obstet Gynecol 1988; 158: 1171.

30 Stabler J. Uterine prolapse and urinary tract obstruction. Br J Radiol 1977; 50: 493.

31 Hadar H, Meiraz F. Total uterine prolapse causing hydro-ureteronephrosis. Surg Gynecol Obstet 1980; 150: 711.

32 Beecham CT. Classification of vaginal relaxation. Am J Obst et Gynecol 1980; 136: 957.

33 Genadry RR. Urogynecology: editorial overview. Current Science. Current Opinion in Obstetrics and Gynecology 1993; 5: 437–439.

34 Haken J, Benness C, Cardozo LD, Cutner A. A randomised trial of vaginal cones and pelvic floor exercises in the management of genuine stress incontinence. Neurourol Urodyn 1991; 10: 393–394.

35 Shepherd AM, Blannin JP, Winder A. Proceedings of the 15th Annual Meeting of the International Continence Society, London: 1985; pp 224–225.

36 Plevnik S, Janez J, Vrtacnik P, Trsinar B, Vodusek D. Short term electrical stimulation: home treatment for urinary incontinence. World J Urol 1986; 4: 24–26.

37 Fergusson ILC. Genital prolapse in contemporary gynaecology. London: Butterworth, 1984: pp 211–218.

38 Benson JT. Cystocele: vaginal approach to cystocele repair. In: Benson JT (ed) Female pelvic floor disorders investigation and management. New York: Norton, 1992: pp 289–294.

39 Kelly HA. Incontinence of urine in women. Urol Cutan Rev 1913; 17: 291–297.

40 White GR, Cystocele, JAMA 1909; 53: 1707.

41 Richardson AC, Lyon JB, Williams NL. A new look at pelvic relaxation. Am J Obstet Gynecol 1976; 126: 568.

42 Richardson AC, Edmonds PB, Williams NL. Treatment of stress urinary incontinence due to paravaginal fascial defect. Obstet Gynecol 1981; 57: 357.

43 Richardson AC. Paravaginal repair. In: Benson JT (ed) Female pelvic floor disorders. New York: Norton, 1992: pp 280–287.

44 Francis WJA, Jeffcoate TNA. Dyspareunia following vaginal operations. Br J Obstet Gynaecol 1961; 68: 1.

45 Haase P, Skibsted L. Influence of operations for stress incontinence and/or genital descensus on sexual life. Acta Obstet Gynaecol Scand 1988; 67: 659.

46 Warrell DW. Prolapse and urinary incontinence. In: Dewhurst's textbook of obstetrics and gynaecology, 4th edn. London: Churchill Livingstone, 1985: pp 680–689.

47 Goldman J, Ovadia J, Feldberg D. The Neugebauer – Le Fort operation: a review of 118 partial colpocleises. Eur J Obstet Gynecol Reprod Biol 1985; 12: 31.

48 McCall ML. Posterior culdoplasty. Obstet Gynecol 1957; 10: 595.

49 Moschowitz AV. The pathogenesis, anatomy and cure of prolapse of the rectum. Surg Gynecol Obstet 1912; 15: 7.

50 Cruikshank SH. Sacrospinous fixation – should this be performed at the time of vaginal hysterectomy? Am J Obstet Gynecol 1991; 162: 1611–1619.

51 Scott R. Prophylactic sacrospinous fixation discouraged. Am J Obstet Gynecol 1992; 166: 1022.

52 Morley GN, Delancy JO. Sacrospinous ligament fixation for eversion of the vagina. Am J Obstet Gynecol 1988; 158: 872–879.

53 Richter K. Die chirurgische anatom der vaginae fixatio sacrospinalis vaginalis. Ein Beitrag zur operativen Behandlung des Scheidenblindsack-prolapses. Geburtshilfe Frauenheilkd 1968; 28: 32–327.

54 Nichols DH. Sacrospinous fixation for massive eversion of the vagina. Am J Obstet Gynecol 1982; 142: 901–904.

55 Miyazaki FS. Miya hook ligature carrier for sacrospinous ligament suspension. Obstet Gynecol 1987; 70: 286–288.

56 Richter K, Albrich W. Long term results following fixation of the vagina in the sacrospinal ligament by the vaginal route (vaginaefixatis sacrospinalis vaginalis). Am J Obstet Gynecol 1981; 141: 811.

57 Shull BL, Capen CV, Riggs MW, Kuehl TJ. Pre-operative and post operative analysis of site-specific pelvic support defects in 81 women treated with sacrospinous ligament suspension and pelvic reconstruction. Am J Obstet Gynecol 1992; 166: 1764–1771.

58 Carey M, Slack M. Transvaginal sacrospinous colpopexy for vault and marked uterovaginal prolapse. Brit J Obstet Gynaecol 1994; 101: 536–540.

59 Timmons MC, Addison WA, Addison SB, Cavenar MG. Abdominal sacral colpopexy i 163 women with post hysterectomy vaginal vault prolapse and enterocele: evolution o operative techniques. J Reprod Med 1992; 37: 323–327.

60 Valaitis SR, Stanton SL. Sacrocolpopexy: a retrospective study of a clinician's experience. Brit J Obstet Gynaecol 1994; 101: 518–522.

61 Zacharin RF, Hamilton N. Pulsion enterocele: long term results of an abdominoperitoneal technique. Obstet Gynaecol 1980; 55: 141–145.

22 Urinary tract infection

EPIDEMIOLOGY

Age

Lower urinary tract infections (UTIs) in normal women are a common health problem throughout the world. Six million visits a year to medical practitioners to manage urinary tract infections have been recorded in the United States.[1] The sex distribution and prevalence of UTIs are based on the age of the individual. Up to the age of one year they are more prevalent in boys than in girls,[2] and if a girl under 1 has bacteriuria then it is likely she will have an abnormality in her urinary tract.[3] Approximately 5% of girls will have a UTI while they are between the ages of 1 and 18[3] and this proportion increases in such a way that the prevalence of UTIs in adult women is 50 times that in males and that 20–30% of adult women have at least one urinary tract infection per year.[4] In the elderly the prevalence may be as high as 50%, especially if the woman is institutionalized.[5]

Recurrent urinary tract infection

These can be conveniently divided into relapses and reinfection. Relapses account for about 20% of recurrent UTIs[6] and are usually associated with pyelonephritis or an anatomical abnormality. Reinfection accounts for 80% of recurrent infections. These are not associated with physical abnormalities[7] but appear to be a reinfection from perineal flora.[8] There is a strong link with sexual intercourse, with 75–90% of women relating their infection to coitus.[9,10] Contraceptive diaphragm use is also a risk factor for recurrent UTIs.[11]

Special circumstances

Pregnancy

Five per cent of pregnant women will have bacteriuria if screened in the first trimester. This increases with parity and age but does not increase with gestation.[12,13,14] The two main problems with bacteriuria in pregnancy are a 25% rate of ascending pyelonephritis[12,13] and an association with premature labour.[15]

Hospital infections

Approximately 40% of all nosocomial infections are urinary tract infections and two-thirds of these are in patients with urinary catheters.[16] There is some evidence that there is a much higher mortality rate among patients who are catheterized and are bacteriuric than among those who have bacteriuria without a catheter.[17]

CLINICAL

Lower urinary tract infections are mostly a problem of women. The bacteria ascend from the urethra[18] and cause an inflammatory response in the bladder lining. There is typically an IgA response[19] in the epithelium and polymorphonuclear leucocytes are noted in the urine. However, the level of inflammation is quite variable and hence the symptoms are variable. The classic symptoms are dysuria, frequency, urgency and suprapubic pain. The patient is often febrile and is tender in the lower abdomen. If the ureters and kidneys are involved, loin pain and tenderness in the renal angles are often present.

If untreated most lower urinary tract infections will resolve, although it may take several months.[20] Certainly, if there is no adherence to the bladder wall the bacteria are usually voided out.[21] Most women have episodes of bacteriuria, especially after intercourse[22] and these usually clear up within days.[23] However, if treated with antibiotics the infection resolves much faster[21] and hence there is considerably less morbidity.

DIAGNOSIS

The problem with the diagnosis of UTIs is that of all the patients with the typical symptoms of dysuria, frequency and suprapubic pain most will have pyuria but only about half will have bacteriuria.[24] Diagnostic testing is therefore aimed at rapid identification of women with bacteriuria as these require antibiotic sensitivities and treatment. Dipstick testing can be used but is an indirect test for bacteria. Some sticks indicate whether break down products such as nitrite are present, while others will test for the absence of glucose. Because they are indirect tests false positives can occur.

Modern laboratory techniques now try to 'screen' urine sent to a laboratory to be tested for bacteriuria so that those without bacteria are reported quickly while those with can be processed. The bacteria can be detected quickly by a number of techniques such as measuring the dissipation of light by the bacteria present, counting bacteria directly using a Coulter counter, detecting antigens by an ELISA technique or detecting bacterial ATPase.[25]

Resistance is now a common problem, especially in nosocomial infection so once bacteria are detected it becomes more important to determine antibiotic sensitivities than to identify the bacteria themselves.[25] This is achieved by simple plating techniques and each laboratory uses routine screens based on local resistance. Some forms of resistance can quickly be detected by indirect tests. For example β-lactamase activity can be detected by nitrocefin hydrolysis activity[25] and gene probes are now available for particular types of resistance such as trimethoprim resistance.

Identification of the actual microbe is important in recurrent UTIs and in very ill immunosuppressed patients. Probes for genes that cause bacteria-specific enzymes such as ureases and β-galactosidases are available and enable rapid identification but their cost prohibits routine use in the management of UTI.

Significant bacteriuria

A major problem with microbiological analysis of urine is contamination. Techniques such as bladder aspiration and catheterization are painful but give contaminant-free urine. Midstream urine can be very reliable if collected properly but can be contaminated with vaginal, rectal or skin bacteria. Landmark work by Kass[26] found that in women with pyelonephritis, counts of bacteria >10^5/ml were confirmed as urinary tract infections on later specimens, but when the count was <10^5/ml infection was not present in later specimens and it was presumed that contamination had occurred. However, many women with dysuria and frequency will have bacteria counts less than 10^5 yet will improve with treatment.[27] Stamm et al[28] have shown that if 10^9 cfu/ml, is used as the sole criterion for significant bacteriuria the specificity is high (0.99) but the sensitivity is low (0.51). If 10^2 cfu/ml is used then the specificity is an acceptable 0.85 and the sensitivity is 0.95. It is important not to take the bacteria count in isolation as other factors such as the presence of mixed bacteria or the presence of normal vaginal flora in the urine may also indicate contamination.

If a catheter specimen is taken then a colony count above 10^2 cfu/ml represents an infection that if left untreated will continue to multiply.[29] The presence of any bacteria in a bladder aspirate will identify infection.[30]

Urethral syndrome

Up to 50% of women with dysuria and frequency will not have significant bacteriuria.[24] Various theories have been advanced for this phenomenon. Stamm et al[28] felt that low levels of bacteriuria associated with pyuria could be explained by inflammation of the urethra. Unfortunately, this study has been criticized for patient selection and measurement reasons.[31] Some authors felt it may be hard to culture bacteria such as the 'fastidious' lactobacilli and this may be an explanation for reduced bacterial counts,[32] but this is contested.[32] *Mycoplasma* and *Ureaplasma* can now be cultured from simple culture swabs so a periurethral swab is indicated in women with urethral symptoms. However, there is no strong correlation between symptoms and culture results and therefore treatment gives varying results. Chlamydial urethral infections can give symptoms so a urethral brushing should be carried out to test for this. It is important to treat partners if the woman has *Chlamydia*, *Mycoplasma* or *Ureaplasma*.

Location of infection

The site of UTI can be important as treatment can be better targeted if this is first located. Clinically, patients with pyelonephritis present with renal angle pain and tenderness. However, if it is important to prove upper urinary tract infection then ureteric catheterization is the best test.[25] Other tests, such as the urine concentration test, neomycin bladder wash-out test and urine concentration test using desmopressin, check for renal involvement but are tedious and unpleasant tests. It was hoped that the use of monoclonal antibodies towards various parts of the renal parenchyma would localize infection easily but there is not enough specificity to use the tests clinically. Tests such as the antibody-coated bacteria test are difficult to interpret.[34] Even the localization of urethral infection is difficult unless samples are taken directly from the urethra.[35]

TREATMENT

Asymptomatic bacteriuria

There are three main treatment groups that need to be considered: young girls, pregnant women and elderly women. In young girls there is a high incidence of associated renal tract abnormality and there is evidence that on-going infection predisposes to renal scarring.[36] In pregnant women there is a 25% incidence of pyelonephritis if a urinary tract infection occurs, as already stated.[12,13] Therefore in young girls and pregnant women treatment is indicated in asymptomatic bacteriuria. There have been no long-term studies looking at the outcome of asymptomatic bacteriuria in the elderly, so treatment depends on the patient's past history, medical status and likelihood to comply with treatment.

Urinary tract infection

Uncomplicated UTIs are caused by *Escherichia coli* in 80–90% of cases, by *Staphylococcus saprophyticus* in a further 10–20% and occasionally by *Proteus mirabilis* or *Klebsiella*.[6,18,37] Antibiotic resistance varies widely depending whether infection was acquired in the community or in an institution, but also varies throughout individual countries, therefore individual clinicians need to be aware of the resistance patterns of *E. coli* and *Staphylococcus* in particular.

Bailey & Abbott have demonstrated the efficacy and lack of side effects of a single 3-g dose of amoxycillin when treating *E. coli* and *Staphylococcus* but it is less successful in women with a *Proteus* or *Klebsiella* infection.[38,39] Philbrick & Bracikowski have reviewed papers looking at single-dose trimethoprim or co-trimoxazole and have shown that it is more effective than single-dose amoxycillin.[40] Other studies have also shown good results for single-dose doxycycline (300 mg) and pivmecillinam (600 mg)[41] and nitrofurantoin (100–200 mg).[42,43] It would seem that symptoms disappear just as quickly with single-dose therapy and that recurrence is no more frequent than when prolonged therapy is used.[40,44] Single-dose therapy is therefore the treatment of choice in community-acquired un-complicated UTIs. There are at present no large randomized trials studying single-dose therapy in hospitalized patients.

Recurrent urinary tract infection

It is now established beyond doubt that prophylactic, low-dose, rotating antimicrobial therapy decreases recurrent infections by 95% when compared with placebo.[22,45] The prophylactic use of urinary antiseptics such as methenamine mandelate and methenamine hippurate used alone are effective but are not as good as antimicrobials.[46] The most studied regimen of rotating medication is trimethoprim, nitrofurantoin and norfloxacin[46] and this has worldwide efficacy with very few side effects. Patients have been studied for as long as 5 years and no increase in infection, resistance or side effects observed.[47] However, if medication is stopped then infection rates will return to those prior to treatment, as there appears to be no long-term benefit from prophylactic treatment once it is ceased.[22]

As intercourse appears to be a precipitating factor in up to 90% of recurrent infections[9,10] another method of treatment is to use antimicrobials prophylactically after intercourse, although there are few studies looking at its efficacy.[48,22] A third strategy for treatment of recurrent infection is based on the fact that 85% of women can identify symptoms of infection with accuracy and therefore could treat themselves with single-dose medication.[22]

CONCLUSIONS

Urinary tract infection is a common occurrence that is generally easy to diagnose, investigate and treat. Modern laboratory techniques can give rapid results and antibiotic therapy will usually give quick relief. Children, pregnant women, women with recurrent UTIs and the elderly require more active management.

REFERENCES

1 National Centre for Health Statistics: 1985 Summary. National ambulatory medical care survey. Adv Data 1985; 128: 1–8.
2 Abbott GD. Neonatal bacteriuria: a prospective study in 1460 infants. Br Med J 1972; 1: 267–269.
3 Kunin CM. Detection, prevention and management of urinary tract infections, 4th edn. Philadelphia: Lea and Febiger, 1987: pp 57–124.
4 Sanford JP. Urinary tract symptoms and infection. Ann Rev Med 1975; 26: 485–905.
5 Boscia JA, Kaye D. Asymptomatic bacteriuria in the elderly. Infect Dis Clin North Am 1987; 1: 893–903.
6 Hooton TM. The epidemiology of urinary tract infection and the concept of significant bacteriuria. Infection 1990; 18: (Suppl 2) S40–S43.
7 Stamm WE. Recent developments in the diagnosis and treatment of urinary tract infections. West J Med 1982; 137: 213–220.
8 McGeachie J. Recurrent infection of the urinary tract: reinfection or recrudescence? Br Med J 1966; 1: 952–954.
9 Nicolle LE, Harding GKM, Preiksaitis J, Ronald AR. The association of urinary tract infection with sexual intercourse. J Infect Dis 1982; 146: 579–583.
10 Leibovici L, Alpert G, Laor A, Kalter-Lebovici O, Danon YL. Urinary tract infections and sexual activity in young women. Arch Int Med 1987; 147: 345–347.
11 Fihn SD, Johnson C, Roberts P et al. Association between diaphragm use and urinary tract infection. JAMA 1985; 254: 240–245.
12 Kass EH. Bacteriuria and pyelonephritis of pregnancy. Arch Intern Med 1960; 105: 194–198.
13 Norden CW, Kass EH. Bacteriuria of pregnancy. A critical appraisal. Ann Rev Med 1968; 19: 431–470.
14 Williams JD. Bacteriuria in pregnancy. In: Asscher AW, Brumfitt W (eds) Microbial diseases in nephrology. Chichester: Wiley, 1986: pp 159–181.

15 Naeye RL. Causes of the excessive rates of perinatal mortality and prematurity in pregnancies complicated by maternal urinary tract infections. New Engl J Med 1979; 300: 819–823.

16 Haley RW, Hooton TM, Culver DH et al. Nosocomial infections in US hospitals, 1975–76. Estimated frequency by selected characteristics of patients. Am J Med 1981; 70: 947–959.

17 Kreger BE, Craven DE, Carling PC, McCabe WR. Gram-negative bacteremia: III Reassessment of aetiology, epidemiology and ecology in 612 patients. Am J Med 1980; 68: 332–343.

18 Kunin CM. Detection, prevention and management of urinary tract infection. Philadelphia: Lea and Febiger. 1987, pp 57–124.

19 Kraft JK, Stamey TA. The natural history of symptomatic recurrent bacteriuria in women. Medicine 1977; 56: 55–60.

20 Mabeck CE. Treatment of uncomplicated urinary tract infection in non-pregnant women. Postgrad Med J 1972; 48: 69–75.

21 Sobel JD, Kaye D. Host factors in the pathogenesis of urinary tract infections. Amer J Med 1984; 76: 122–130.

22 Nicolle LE. The optimal management of lower urinary tract infection. Infection 1990; 18: (Suppl 2) S50–52.

23 Nicolle LE, Harding GKM, Preiksaitis J, Ronald AR. The association of urinary tract infection with sexual intercourse. J Infect Dis 1982; 146: 579–583.

24 Mond NC, Percival A, Williams JD, Brumfitt W. Presentation, diagnosis and treatment of urinary tract infections in general practice. Lancet 1965; 1: 514–516.

25 Brumfitt W, Hamilton-Miller JMT. Urinary infection in the 1990's: the state of the art. Infection 1990; 18: (Suppl 2) S34–S39.

26 Kass EH. Asymptomatic infections of the urinary tract. Trans Ass Amer Physicians 1956; 69: 56–64.

27 Stamm WE. Quantitative urine cultures revisited. Eur J Clin Microbiol 1984; 3: 279–281.

28 Stamm WE, Counts GW, Running KR, Fihn S, Turck M, Holmes KK. Diagnosis of coliform infection in acutely dysuric women. N Engl J Med 1982; 307: 463–468.

29 Stark RP, Maki DG. Bacteriuria in the catheterised patient. What quantitative level of bacteriuria is relevant? N Engl J Med 1984; 311: 560–564.

30 Monzon OT, Ory EM, Dobson HL. A comparison of bacterial counts of urine obtained by needle aspiration of the bladder, catheterisation and midstream voided methods. N Engl J Med 1958; 259: 764.

31 Smith GW, Brumfitt W, Hamilton-Miller JMT. Diagnosis of coliform infection in acutely dysuric women. New Engl J Med 1983; 309: 1393–1394.

32 Maskell R. Are fastidious organisms an important cause of dysuria and frequency? – the case for. In: Asscher AW, Brumfitt W (eds) Microbial diseases in nephrology. Chichester: Wiley, 1986, pp 1–18.

33 Hamilton-Miller JMT, Brumfitt W, Smith GW. Are fastidious organisms an important cause of dysuria and frequency? The case against. In: Asscher AW, Brumfitt W (eds) Microbial diseases in nephrology. Chichester: Wiley, 1986, pp 19–30.

34 Mundt KA, Polk BF. Identification of site of urinary tract infections by antibody-coated bacteria assay. Lancet 1979; 2: 1172–1175.

35 Helmholtz HF. Determination of the bacterial content of the urethra: a new method with the results of a study of 82 men. J Urol 1950; 64: 158–166.

36 Jacobsen SH, Eklof O, Eriksson CG, Lins LE, Tidgren B, Winberg J. Development of hypertension and uraemia after pyelonephritis in childhood: 27-year follow-up. Br Med J 1989; 299: 703–706.

37 Rubin RH. Infections of the urinary tract. Scient Am Med 1984; 23: 1–12.

38 Bailey R, Abbott GD. Treatment of urinary tract infections with a single dose of amoxicillin. NZ Med J 1976; 84: 324–325.

39 Bailey RR. Studies to compare various antibacterial regimens in hospital and domiciliary practice. In: Bailey RR (ed) Single dose therapy of urinary tract infection, 1st edn. Sydney: ADIS Health Science Press, 1983: pp 7–15.

40 Philbrick JT, Bracikowski JP. Single dose antibiotic treatment for uncomplicated urinary tract infections: less for less? Arch Intern Med 1985; 145: 1672–1678.

41 Bailey RR, Peddie BA, Chambers PF et al. Single dose doxycycline, cefuroxime and pivemecillam for treatment of bacterial cystitis. NZ Med J 1982; 95: 699–700.

42 Gossius G. Single dose nitrofurantoin therapy for urinary tract infections in women. Curr Therap Res 1984; 35: 925–931.

43 Bailey RR. Review of published studies on single dose therapy of urinary tract infections. Infection 1990; 18: (Suppl 2) S53–56.

44 Bailey RR, Keenan TD, Elliott JC, Peddie BA, Bishop V. Treatment of bacterial cystitis

with a single dose of trimethoprim, co-trimoxazole or amoxicillin compared with a course of trimethoprim. NZ Med J 1985; 98: 387–389.

45 Nicolle LE, Ronald AR. Recurrent urinary tract infection in adult women: diagnosis and treatment. Infect Dis Clin North Amer 1987; 1: 793–806.

46 Harding GK, Nicolle LE, Thomson M, Ronald AR. Placebo controlled trial of norfloxacin for the prophylaxis of recurrent urinary tract infection. 28th Interscience Conference on Antimicrobial Agents and Chemotherapy. American Society for Microbiology 1988. Abstract 194.

47 Nicolle LE, Harding GK, Thomson M, Kennedy J, Urias B, Ronald AR. Efficacy of continuous low-dose trimethoprim-sulfamethoxazole prophylaxis for urinary tract infection. J Infect Dis 1988; 157: 1239–1242.

48 Vosti KL. Recurrent urinary tract infections: prevention by prophylactic antibiotics after sexual intercourse. J Amer Med Assoc 1975; 231: 934–940.

23

Frequency, urgency and painful bladder syndromes

Many women complain of urinary frequency, urgency or the 'painful bladder syndrome'. The severity of these symptoms varies from mild to very distressing and the symptoms of frequency and urgency may occur alone, together, or in conjunction with other lower urinary tract symptoms. A careful history, examination and investigation are required in order to determine the underlying cause and institute appropriate management.

Diurnal frequency is defined as the passage of urine every 2 hrs, or more than seven times a day. Nocturia is the interruption of sleep more than once each night for micturition. However, in elderly women voiding two or more times a night may be considered normal. Those who void several times a night because of broken sleep or insomnia are not suffering from true nocturia. Urinary urgency is the strong and sudden desire to void, which if not relieved may result in urinary incontinence. Bungay et al[1] found that approximately 20% of women admit to urinary frequency and that this prevalence does not alter greatly with age. The same study found that 15% of women suffer from the symptom of urgency.

Those patients with the painful bladder syndrome complain of bladder pain and irritative bladder symptoms (frequency, urgency, nocturia and dysuria) and have negative urine cultures. These symptoms can be quite disabling. In some cases the etiology may be known or suspected, but in the majority the pathogenesis is uncertain. Known causes of the 'painful bladder syndrome' include radiation cystitis, cyclophosphamide cystitis and systemic diseases affecting the bladder.

Other causes of this syndrome which will be discussed include the urethral syndrome, sensory urgency and interstitial cystitis. These conditions are generally poorly understood and vaguely defined, and have unclear pathogenesis and largely empirical treatments.

The known causes of frequency and urgency may be listed as follows:

- large fluid intake
- habit
- pregnancy
- diuretic therapy
- urinary tract infection
- detrusor instability
- bladder mucosal lesion
- bladder calculus
- urethritis
- diabetes insipidus
- small bladder capacity
- pelvic mass
- previous pelvic surgery
- chronic urinary residual
- radiation cystitis
- upper motor neurone lesion
- urethral syndrome
- urethral diverticulum
- impaired renal function
- diabetes mellitus.

ASSESSMENT

A detailed urinary and gynecological history is required. Information should also be sought regarding any neurological symptoms, medications taken and drinking habits. Gynecological examination will exclude pregnancy, a pelvic mass and chronic large residual urine. A simple neurological examination is performed with particular regard to the S2,3 and 4 nerve roots.

A midstream urine specimen should be sent for culture and sensitivity in all patients (including culture for *Mycoplasma* and *Ureaplasma*), and urine obtained for cytological examination. Diabetes mellitus should be excluded by appropriate investigation. Vaginal and urethral swabs are taken, including swabs for *Chlamydia*. If tuberculous cystitis is suspected then three early morning urine samples should be sent for acid-fast bacillus culture. A urinary diary should be completed for at least several days and provides useful information on drinking habits and voided volumes.

Where the assessment detailed above has not revealed an obvious cause for the symptoms, further investigation by cystourethroscopy or cystometry should be considered. Endoscopy can be performed under local or general anesthesia and may reveal urethritis, a urethral diverticulum, a bladder polyp or calculus or interstitial cystitis. Bladder base biopsy is essential for the diagnosis of interstitial cystitis. Subtracted cystometry may detect detrusor instability or sensory urgency and ultrasound can be used to assess urinary residual volume accurately.

INTERSTITIAL CYSTITIS

Interstitial cystitis is an enigmatic and disabling condition associated with chronic inflammation of the bladder. Although it was first described by Skene in 1887,[2] its etiology remains poorly understood and its management confusing. Interstitial cystitis occurs more frequently in women then men, with a predominance of 10:1.[3] The typical presentation is of a woman aged between 40 and 60 years with the symptoms of urinary frequency, urgency and bladder pain. The true incidence of interstitial cystitis is uncertain due to subjective diagnostic criteria. However, in the United States, it is estimated that there are approximately 50 000 diagnosed cases with as many as five times that number undiagnosed. For some reason, this condition has a higher profile and is more widely diagnosed in the United States than in the United Kingdom. What is apparent, though, is the significant impact that interstitial cystitis can have on a person's quality of life. A survey presented as part of an National Institute of Health consensus conference on interstitial cystitis found that 40% of affected women were unable to work because of their disease, 58% were unable to have intercourse and 55% had considered suicide.

Etiology

Many theories have been proposed for the etiology of interstitial cystitis but none has been widely accepted. Suggested causes (for which there is little current support) include infection, lymphatic obstruction and endo-crinological and psychosomatic disorders. No micro-organism has been identified in these patients, although some suggest that fastidious organisms may play a role. Perineural leucocytic infiltration has been observed within the bladder wall lesions of women with interstitial cystitis. There is, however, no other evidence for a neurogenic etiology.

An autoimmune theory has some credibility, and a relationship between interstitial cystitis and systemic lupus erythematosus was observed over 50 years ago.[4] There is an increased incidence of this and other collagen diseases in women with interstitial cystitis. Many patients also have increased serum antinuclear antibodies[5] and the presence of antibladder antibodies has been identified in the serum of these patients.[6] However, these immunological responses may be a secondary phenomenon oc-curring after bladder damage rather than a primary cause of interstitial cystitis. Evidence against an immunological cause is the relief of all symp-toms following a urinary diversion without cystectomy[7] and the recurrence of interstitial cystitis in the intestinal segments of colocystoplasties.[8]

The glycosaminoglycan (GAG) layer on the transitional epithelium of the bladder is thought to have a protective function.[9] If it is deficient, micro-organisms or carcinogens obtain access to the bladder wall and cause inflammation.[10] Parsons[11] suggested that similar deficiencies allow unspecified urinary components to reach the inner layers of the detrusor muscle, leading to the symptoms and histological appearances of interstitial cystitis. However, Collan[12] was unable to demonstrate GAG layer deficiencies in patients with histologically confirmed interstitial cystitis using immunoflourescence and electron microscopy.

Diagnosis

The diagnosis of interstitial cystitis is made in patients with suggestive symptoms and typical cystoscopic findings. There is some degree of subjectivity in the diagnosis. The bladders in these women are 'irritable' and the symptoms can be severe and disabling. The common symptoms include frequency, urgency, nocturia, dysuria and suprapubic or perineal pain. Micturition usually improves the discomfort, while it is often exacerbated by drinking caffeine and alcohol.[13] Some women experience urge incontinence. Criteria which generally exclude the diagnosis of interstitial cystitis may be listed as follows:

- <18 years old
- bladder tumor
- radiation cystitis
- tuberculous cystitis
- bacterial cystitis
- cyclophosphamide cystitis
- vaginitis
- urethral diverticulum
- lower genital tract malignancy
- active genital herpes
- bladder calculus
- diurnal frequency <5 times
- nocturia <2 times
- (detrusor instability).

The onset of the disease may be acute but a gradual development of symptoms is more common. The disease is usually progressive and spontaneous remissions are uncommon.

The findings of physical examination are most often normal, although anterior vaginal wall tenderness may be present on pelvic examination. Microhematuria may be present and urine cytology is normal. Cystometry usually reveals a decreased bladder capacity and low bladder compliance may be evident.

Cystoscopy is the most important diagnostic test and should be performed under general anesthesia using a rigid cystoscope. This enables an accurate assessment of true bladder capacity. Bladder filling should be by passive gravity filling with a pressure head of approximately 80 cmH_2O. The bladder capacity under anesthesia is usually less than 400 ml. The bladder is left distended for 1–2 min once capacity is reached and then drained. The terminal fluid is typically blood-tinged. The bladder is refilled as the features of interstitial cystitis are more likely to be present on a second distension. These include subepithelial petechial hemorrhages (glomerulations), splotchy hemorrhages and linear cracking of the mucosa. Ulcers and scarring may be present in patients with late-stage interstitial cystitis. Bladder base biopsies are mandatory to confirm the diagnosis and exclude conditions such as carcinoma in situ tuberculosis and schistosomiasis.

The histological appearances of biopsies from patients with interstitial cystitis are generally non-specific. Evidence of chronic inflammation is usually present with submucosal edema and vasodilatation being consistent features. Fibrosis may be present, as may infiltration with round cells, plasma cells and eosinophils. Increased numbers of mast cells are present in up to 50% of cases (more than 20 cells/mm^2 of detrusor muscle tissue); although some workers feel that this finding is helpful in establishing the diagnosis, the presence of mast cells may not be specific to interstitial cystitis. A decrease in bladder perfusion in women with interstitial cystitis has been demonstrated by laser Doppler flowmetry.[14]

Treatment

Many therapeutic modalities have been tried in the treatment of interstitial cystitis with varying degrees of success. As the etiology remains poorly understood, the treatment of this condition is largely empirical. There are also few well-controlled, prospective studies from which to determine the most appropriate therapy. Suggested treatment regimens may grouped as systemic, local or surgical.

Systemic treatment

The following systemic therapies may be beneficial in interstitial cystitis.

Antihistamines Mast cells are present in increased numbers in the bladders of women with interstitial cystitis. The release of histamine from these cells may result in pain, inflammation and subsequent fibrosis. One study[15] reported improvement in symptoms in a small group of patients and further assessment of this therapy would be worthwhile.

Heparin This may be administered subcutaneously or instilled into the bladder. It has an anti-inflammatory action and also mimics some of the characteristics of the GAG layer of the bladder. In an uncontrolled study, Parsons et al[16] subcutaneously injected heparin for 1 week and this provided good symptomatic improvement. Alternatively, 10 000 IU heparin in 10 ml sterile water may be instilled into the bladder by the patient using a self-catheterizing technique. This is performed several times each week and can be continued indefinitely.

Pentosan polysulfate This oral medication is a synthetic analog of sulphonated glycosaminoglycan. It augments the normal protective mucus layer of the bladder. Reports on efficacy are conflicting. However, benefits in some placebo-controlled trials have been demonstrated.[16,17] Significant improvement can be expected in approximately 50% of patients with moderate disease. The activity was lower in those with severe disease. The usual dose is 100 mg three times daily and side effects are low.

Antidepressants Amitriptyline has analgesic properties as well as anticholinergic and antihistaminic effects. Given in doses of 25–75 mg at night, it improved pain and frequency in an uncontrolled study.[18] These medications may also help patients cope with their symptoms by improving sleep and minimizing the depression which can accompany chronic disorders.

Anti-inflammatories and immunosuppressants These agents should improve interstitial cystitis if it is an inflammatory disorder with an autoimmune basis. However, the results are variable and unpredictable. There are no good studies on the use of steroids and the high doses used have resulted in frequent side effects. Badenoch[19] reports an improvement in 70% of patients; however, relapse rates are high and duration of remission unpredictable. Walsh[20] suggests that the response to steroids is unpredictable, while Messing & Stamey[7] report that improvement is likely only with high-dose regimens. Azathioprine, an immunosuppressant, has had some good results.[21] Benzydamine has analgesic and anti-inflammatory properties and has had dramatic results in some patients.[22] Hexamine hippurate (Hiprex), a urinary antiseptic, has been used with some success at a dose of 1 twice daily (Cardozo, unpublished observations).

Local treatment

Bladder distension Many patients have a dramatic improvement in symptoms following cystodistension. Unfortunately, this is short-lived in most. The benefit is presumed to be secondary to ischemic damage to afferent nerve plexuses or stretch receptors within the bladder wall. A number of different techniques are used. Dunn[23] reported symptomatic cure in over 60% of patients at a mean of 14 months after distension for 3 hrs under anesthesia. Bladder pressure was increased to the level of systolic blood pressure throughout this time. Other authors distend the bladder for different periods of time and at different pressures. Regional anesthesia can be used for this procedure. Bladder rupture may occur in a small number of patients but can usually be managed conservatively.

Instillation therapy Dimethyl sulphoxide (DMSO), an industrial solvent, has been shown to be beneficial in the management of interstitial cystitis. The treatment regimen is easy to perform, is inexpensive and can be administered as an out-patient procedure. The substance has a number of pharmacological actions including local analgesia, anti-inflammatory activity and bacteriostasis. The patient is catheterized and 50 ml of a 50% solution of DMSO is instilled into the bladder. This is retained for 15–30 min before the bladder is emptied by voiding. The treatment is performed every 1 or 2 weeks and four to six treatments may be required to achieve the maximum response. Patients who self-catheterize can administer DMSO themselves at home. Cataracts should be excluded prior to commencing therapy. A significant improvement can be expected in 50–80% of cases with early interstitial cystitis.[24,25,26]

Oxychlorosene may also be instilled into the bladder for the treatment of interstitial cystitis. General anesthesia is required and several instillations may be necessary. A subjective success rate of 70% has been found[27] and treatment is associated with cystoscopic evidence of healing of bladder lesions.

Functional electrical stimulation has been used successfully in uncontrolled trials. Either an intravaginal device may be used, or transcutaneous electrodes can be applied to the lower abdomen. Bladder pain seems to respond better than the symptom of urinary frequency. Prolonged treatment may be required.

Surgical treatment

The surgical management of interstitial cystitis is frequently indicated and is reserved for those cases which have failed to respond to conservative management. The available methods can generally be grouped into either endoscopic or open procedures. Endoscopic surgery involves fulguration or resection of ulcers and is usually combined with other conservative therapies. Early reports of the use of the Nd: YAG laser are encouraging. Local injection of hydrocortisone or heparin around the ulcerated areas may be of benefit.

Open surgery is used as a last resort and the available options include partial cystectomy, augmentation cystoplasty, cystolysis and urinary diversion with or without cystectomy. Partial cystectomy is probably a poor option, as the disease may recur in the bladder remnant. Augmentation cystoplasty or substitution cytoplasty, where the supratrigonal portion of the bladder is removed, are generally the procedures of choice, particularly if the bladder is severely contracted. Cystolysis involves division of the sensory pathways to the upper part of the bladder and may be appropriate where the bladder is not contracted.

SENSORY URGENCY

Sensory urgency is a diagnosis made after urodynamic assessment. Such patients have symptoms of frequency, urgency and sometimes urge incontinence and have no cystometric evidence of detrusor instability. It is thought to be due to a 'hypersensitive' bladder, although there are no generally agreed cystometric parameters which define this increased sensitivity. Some authors require the first sensation of filling to occur at less than 100 ml and the bladder capacity to be less than 400 ml before the diagnosis can be made. Because the diagnostic criteria are rather vague, the incidence of sensory urgency is unclear, but this diagnosis is made in approximately 10% of women investigated in our unit.[28] The etiology of sensory urgency is poorly understood. However, psychological factors may be involved and the women have been shown to be more anxious than those with genuine stress incontinence.[29] It is also probable that some do in fact have detrusor instability that was undetected at the time of laboratory urodynamics. Ambulatory testing may be appropriate further investigation in some patients.

Diagnosis requires a detailed history and examination, a urinary diary and cystometric examination. Once the diagnosis has been made on cystometry, cystoscopy and biopsy should be performed to exclude interstitial neoplastic conditions of the bladder wall, or other intravesical pathology. Most patients with sensory urgency respond to treatment with bladder retraining.[30] Anticholinergic therapy, for instance with propantheline, can be used in addition to bladder retraining or in those in whom retraining in not effective. A combination of diazepam and anticholinergics has been reported as giving reasonable results, either alone[31] or together with bladder retraining.[32]

THE URETHRAL SYNDROME

Introduction

The urethral syndrome is not a distinct clinical entity. No universally accepted definition exists, and the term has been described as a 'waste-basket' diagnosis by Karam.[33] Other terms used to describe the urethral syndrome include 'abacterial cystitis' and the 'dysuria-pyuria syndrome.' The syndrome was first described in 1934 by Folsom & Alexander,[34] who stated that 'any pain within two feet of the female urethra which does not seem to be adequately accounted for should be suspected of being due to the urethral syndrome'.

Over the past 10 years there have been more than 50 scientific papers published relating to the urethral syndrome. However, its etiology remains obscure and is almost certainly multifactorial. Favoured treatment modalities have varied results, although those most successful are often aimed at a specific etiological factor.

Lower urinary tract symptoms in women are a common reason for medical consultation and in the absence of obvious infection or local pathology treatment can prove unsatisfactory and frustrating for both the patient and her physician.

Definition

Urethral syndrome has been defined by Stamm et al[35] as acute dysuria and frequent micturition in women whose midstream urine was either sterile or contained less than 10 micro-organisms per ml. The symptom complex additionally includes urgency, a feeling of incomplete emptying, suprapubic and lower back pain and perineal pain. Less commonly difficulty in voiding and a feeling of pressure or pain in the lower abdomen are described. Summit & Ling[36] have described 8 patients who were referred for evaluation of chronic pelvic pain and whose symptoms were found to result from urethral syndrome secondary to chronic urethritis.

Whatever definition is adopted, significant bladder bacteriuria and macroscopic pathological conditions of the lower urinary tract must be absent.

Incidence

It has been reported, as long ago as 1970, that the prevalence of lower urinary tract symptoms in general practice in the United Kingdom is 22%.[37] More recent data are not available but it is suggested that up to 5 million consultations a year take place in the United States for lower urinary tract symptoms (Health Statistics USA, 1977), of which 25% may fulfil the criteria for diagnosis of urethral syndrome.

Etiology

The etiology of urethral syndrome remains poorly understood. Research suggests that almost certainly more than one pathogenic factor is involved in the development of lower urinary tract symptoms in the absence of bacterially proven cystitis. Suggested etiologies include:

- bacterial infection (often with a growth of <10 bacteria/ml)
- atypical infection (e.g. *Chlamydia*, *Mycoplasma*)
- senile atrophy
- psychosomatic causes
- trauma
- allergy/hypersensitivity
- inflammatory causes.

Infection

Infection, either bacterial or atypical, probably accounts for most cases of the urethral syndrome and has been most thoroughly studied.

Bacterial Traditionally, the criteria used to interpret a urine culture are those developed by Kass.[38] He emphasized that a colony count higher than 100 000 (10/ml) from a midstream specimen of urine indicates true bacteriuria and was able to distinguish women with asymptomatic bacteria or pyelonephritis from those with contaminated specimens.

Kass himself suggested that there may be exceptions to his rule. These included patients in whom the rate of urine flow is rapid or the number of bacteria discharged is small and cases where on testing, the urine has been present in the bladder for an insufficient time to allow growth of the bacteria to significant numbers. Indeed it has subsequently been shown that 20–40% of women with lower urinary tract symptoms have as few as 10 bacteria/ml. Studies in general practice in the United Kingdom[39,40] have shown that 40–50% of women with lower urinary tract symptoms will have significant bacteriuria and up to 30% will have sterile urine. This suggests various possibilities:

1. That an infective agent other than a bacterium is responsible for the symptoms in this group of patients.
2. That non-infective lower urinary tract pathology exists.
3. That Kass's criterion may be incorrect in this group of patients.

Brooks,[41] in a study of 138 patients with lower urinary tract symptoms, found that 49% had bacterial cystitis. However, a bacterial count of less than 10/ml was found in 34% compared with 9% of a control group. It is possible that when applied to the urethral syndrome, a bacterial count of 10/ml is too high a cut-off value. Infectious urethral syndrome may be considered as cystitis with low bacterial counts.

The paraurethral glands of the posterior urethra (Skene's glands) have been suggested as a possible site of deep-seated infection. To substantiate this some workers have attempted to culture the initial 5–10 ml of voided urine (the VB1 fraction), assuming that this represents a culture of urethral flora. However, Finn[42] has failed to correlate microbiological growth from the VB1 fraction to the presence of symptoms in women with the acute urethral syndrome.

Atypical infection Good evidence exists implicating *Chlamydia* as a potential pathogen in the urethral syndrome. The symptoms of non-gonococcal urethritis in men are similar to those of the urethral syndrome. Like the urethral syndrome this disease too may run a protracted course. Its diagnosis relies on the observation of greater than 10 leucocytes per high-power field on microscopic examination of a urethral smear. The findings of sterile pyuria in a significant number of women with the urethral syndrome suggests that the two conditions may be similar.

Stamm et al,[43] in a study of 59 patients, isolated coliforms from 24 but not in significant numbers; however, all 24 had pyuria. Three patients grew *Staphylococcus saprophyticus*. Of the remaining group of 32 women, there were 16 with and 16 without pyuria. Ten of those patients with pyuria had confirmation of chlamydial infection.

Weil et al[44] examined urethral swabs in 22 women suffering from the urethral syndrome and an age-matched control group with no urinary symptoms. *Chlamydia trachomatis* was isolated in 59% of those women with the urethral syndrome compared with 13% of the control group.

Other studies have failed to corroborate these findings. Gillespie et al[45] compared 41 patients with urethral syndrome to 42 control patients. No difference was found in the incidence of infection with *Chlamydia trachomatis*, lactobacilli or other fastidious organisms. The numbers of leucocytes in the urine were also similar in both groups. Tait[46] identified a possible microbiological cause in only 4 of 31 patients.

Masket et al[47] studied 20 patients presenting to a Sexually Transmitted Disease Clinic either as contacts of non-specific urethritis or complaining of urinary symptoms. Ten yielded positive culture of *Chlamydia*. Interestingly, only 3 admitted on direct questioning to any urinary symptoms and of these, 2 had coliform urinary infections and *Gardnerella vaginalis* was isolated from the third.

Ureaplasma urealyticum and *Mycoplasma hominis* have been implicated in the pathogenesis of urethral syndrome;[48] however, recent work by Stamm et al[49] found a similar prevalence of *Mycoplasma hominis* amongst women with cystitis and asymptomatic women. Nevertheless, these two organisms should probably be included as etiological agents in the infective spectrum of this disorder.

Urethral obstruction and spasm

Early investigators supported the idea of obstruction secondary to stenosis of the urethra as causal of the urethral syndrome. However, obstructive lesions of the urethra and bladder neck remain rare in women and in spite of one paper by Richardson & Stonington[50] suggesting an increased amount of elastic tissue in the distal urethra in patients with urethral syndrome, the theory of urethral obstruction is becoming less favoured.

Hole[51] measured urethral caliber in a group of women with lower urinary tract symptoms and found no significant difference when compared to a control group. This has not prevented urethral dilatation achieving some note as a therapeutic measure.

Spasm of the external urethral sphincter secondary to poor voiding habits has been suggested as a potential cause of urethral syndrome.[52,53] This has led to the use of urodynamic techniques, including urethral pressure profiles, for investigative purposes.

Urodynamic studies in the urethral syndrome

Various urodynamic anomalies have been found when these studies have been applied to patients with urethral syndrome. Barbalia & Meares[54] studied 18 women with urethral syndrome using urodynamic synchronous video pressure/flow studies and electromyography of the external urethral sphincter. In comparison with an age-matched control group, the most striking finding was a significantly higher than normal maximum urethral closure pressure. Other findings included low urinary flow rates, instability and intraurethral narrowing. In this study detrusor–sphincter or primary sphincter spasm was not observed. The author does, however, state that spasm of the external urethral sphincter cannot be excluded as a cause of urethral syndrome in some patients, but suggests that an autonomically mediated spasm of the smooth muscle sphincter may explain the urodynamic findings and this is reinforced by a favourable response in 4 patients treated with α-blocking agents.

Urodynamic assessment was also performed by Lipsky,[55] whose findings in 43 patients appear to substantiate urethral obstruction as a predominant feature of urethral syndrome. He described two types of obstruction. The first was seen in postmenopausal women who appeared to have a narrow distal urethra; the second was seen in younger women when the cause was suspected as incomplete relaxation or indeed spasm of the external urethral sphincter.

In a study of 6 women, Kaplan et al[52] found intermittent urinary flow accompanied by external sphincter spasm when they carried out evaluation using uroflowmetry and electromyography. In these women diazepam therapy resulted in clinical improvement.

Summit & Ling[36] performed uroflowmetry in patients who complained of postcoital voiding dysfunction and in whom pelvic examination revealed urethral and subtrigonal tenderness. Six demonstrated prolonged and intermittent voiding patterns.

Weil et al[56] evaluated urethral pressure profiles in 427 women with lower urinary tract symptoms. Urethral instability (defined as a variation of urethral pressure greater than 15 cm H_2O) was found in 16.4% of patients. The comparison of urinary symptoms and urodynamic data between patients with urethral instability and those with stable urethrae showed that urethral instability was related to frequency, nocturia, urgency and a history of urethral syndrome. In 27% of these patients urethral instability was also associated with detrusor instability.

The role of urodynamic and radiographic studies has been questioned by Mabry et al,[57] who evaluated 105 patients and analyzed the necessity for a complex urological work-up. No significant urodynamic anomalies were found. The cost-effectiveness of urodynamic studies in urethral syndrome is questioned.

Nevertheless, we feel that urodynamic tests should be selectively performed in patients who are suspected to have outflow obstruction or detrusor instability. Uroflowmetry is a simple, non-invasive test that can be performed to confirm symptoms of voiding dysfunction and cystometry should especially be performed in patients complaining of severe urgency or urge incontinence.

Estrogen deficiency

The urethra is derived from the urogenital sinus and therefore responds to female sex hormones in the same way as genital organs. Conditions of estrogen deficiency may lead to thinning of the stratified squamous epithelium of the lower urinary tract. This may predispose to infection.

Bent et al[58] evaluated in detail 100 women over the age of 60 who had lower urinary tract symptoms. The five primary diagnoses were: urethral syndrome in 20%, along with genuine stress incontinence in 21% and detrusor instability in 19%. In spite of this only 7% were clinically diagnosed as suffering from estrogen deficiency. In a study of 329 women with senile urethritis, Youngblood et al[59] showed that addition of 0.1 mg diethylstilbestrol to a regimen of standard furacin suppositories produced significant improvement compared to a group treated with placebo and furacin. A further study by the same author[60] confirmed the initial impression when the same treatment was given to 20 women with senile urethritis, and an observed change in cell type from basal cells to squamous cells was seen in urethral smears.

In a randomized study comparing antibiotic therapy alone and in combination with local estrogen therapy, the addition of estrogen proved of little value.[61]

Both oral and topical estrogen therapy have been shown to reduce the incidence of urinary tract infection in postmenopausal women, presumably by strengthening physical host defences and by restoration of local flora. Additionally, estrogen supplementation can reduce the symptoms of frequency, urgency and dysuria.

Psychological causes

It is difficult to establish whether the psychological and psychiatric symptoms exhibited by women presenting with the urethral syndrome are a matter of cause or effect. Carson[62] reviewed 160 patients with urethral syndrome. Evaluation included urinalysis, urine culture, cystoscopy and excretion urography and in 56 of the patients a psychological evaluation using the Minnesota Multiphasic Personality Inventory (MMPI). Of all evaluated parameters, only the MMPI had significant positive findings. Patients with urethral syndrome had higher scores for hysteria and hypochondriasis when compared with scores of age-matched controls.

In a larger study performed by Rees & Farhoumand,[63] 342 women were asked to complete a psychiatric questionnaire and subsequently underwent formal psychiatric review. These patients were found to have significantly more psychiatric problems than the general population.

Kaplan & Steege[64] have suggested that there may be a sexual component to urethral syndrome and advocates sexual and psychological evaluation in addition to routine medical investigation. He considers that multiple painful medical procedures such as cystoscopy and urethral dilatation may only succeed in reinforcing the conditioned vaginal muscle contraction and worsen any vaginismus.

Inflammatory causes

Tait et al[46] studied 31 women with recurrent urethral syndrome. All had undergone extensive microbiological, cytological and histological investi gations. A possible microbiological cause was identified in only 4 of 31 patients and urethral cytology was normal in all patients. Cystoscopic appearances in 26 suggested trigonitis and bladder biopsies showed squamous metaplasia in 15 patients. There was lymphocytic infiltration of the lamina propria in 29 patients. This supports an inflammatory etiology of urethral syndrome. Further studies may be warranted.

Other causes

An inflammatory reaction in the urethra may be precipitated by physical or chemical irritation. The distressing symptom of postcoital dysuria follows anterior vaginal trauma during intercourse. Allergy to the rubber of a sheath or diaphragm, contraceptive foam or gel and vaginal deodorants have all been described.

Diagnosis

The urethral syndrome remains a diagnosis of exclusion. The overall significance of the syndrome remains uncertain; these patients do not die of their disease although significant morbidity may result. Certainly, more serious causes of urinary frequency, dysuria and suprapubic discomfort must be excluded. A systematic approach in the evaluation of these patients with a view to making a clinical diagnosis should provide a greater likelihood of success for any particular treatment.

Local causes of lower urinary tract symptoms, including candidal or herpetic vulvovaginitis and urogenital atrophy, should be excluded. Often these patients complain of external dysuria rather than internal dysuria. The latter is more characteristic of urethral syndrome.

Careful examination of the external genitalia will rule out local pathology such as urethral carcuncle, cystocele, uterine prolapse and local dermatoses. Naked eye examination of the urethral mucosa may suggest inflammation or hypo-estrogenism. Pelvic examination should also be performed.

A midstream specimen of urine should be obtained for culture and microscopic examination. When a sexually transmitted disease is suspected, urethral and cervical swabs should be taken for culture of *Neisseria gonorrhoeae* and *Chlamydia trachomatis*.

Cystoscopy may be used in some patients to exclude other pathology of the bladder; urethral or bladder diverticulum, carcinoma in situ or frank carcinoma and interstitial cystitis may all cause symptoms common to the urethral syndrome. Summit & Ling[35] performed cystourethrography in either patients with chronic pelvic pain. Findings included urethral edema, exudate and cystic inclusions in the urethral wall. All patients stated that the procedure reproduced their symptoms of pelvic pain.

Urodynamic assessment is probably indicated in those patients with urethral syndrome who exhibit voiding dysfunction suggestive of urethral stenosis or with incontinence of urine.

Treatment

Commonly, advice is given to increase fluid intake 'in order to flush out infecting organisms'. This may result in worsening of urinary frequency and may indeed exacerbate other symptoms, such as incontinence. A sensible fluid intake should be in the order of 1.5 l/24 h. Advice should be given concerning the use of local irritants such as perfumed soaps and in some cases biological washing powders. Vaginal douches should be avoided as they only irritate the urethra further. It may be helpful to empty the bladder immediately following intercourse and similarly adequate lubrication with a non-allergenic substance should be ensured if required.

A useful stratification, depending upon the results of urinalysis and culture, has been described by Bashi.[65] Four groups of patients are recognized:

1. Bacteriuria (usually coliform) greater than 10/ml and pyuria. Diagnosis: acute cystitis.
2. Bacteriuria of less than 10/ml and pyuria. These patients cannot be clinically differentiated from those with acute cystitis and should be considered to have urethral syndrome secondary to infection with urinary pathogens such as coliforms.
3. Sterile urine and pyuria. These patients are likely to have urethral syndrome secondary to urethral pathogens. Atypical organisms seem likely.
4. Sterile urine and no pyuria. These patients are considered to have urethral syndrome of undetermined etiology.

Acute cystitis can be treated with the appropriate antibiotics according to sensitivity. Those patients in group 2 in whom the bacterial count is less than 10/ml may also be treated with appropriate broad-spectrum antibiotics.

In those patients who have sterile pyuria and who are sexually active or in whom a chlamydial contact is suspected, a 10-day course of tetracycline or doxycycline would be effective in relieving symptoms. A double-blind randomized trial comparing the efficacy of doxycycline versus a placebo in the treatment of acute urethral syndrome[66] showed that doxycycline was significantly more effective than placebo in the improvement of the symptoms of dysuria and frequency. However, in women with acute urethral syndrome and no pyuria, no benefit was seen with doxycycline versus placebo.

In postmenopausal patients, a trial of local estrogen therapy may be warranted. It is now clear that estrogen supplementation will result in a reduction in irritative symptoms in a significant number of patients.

Urethral dilatation and urethrotomy have both been used in the treatment of this disease. In a study by Darling & McClean[67] a group of 10 patients were followed up, having previously received one of three treatments: urethral dilatation, internal urethrotomy or urethrolysis. This study suggests that urethral dilatation was as good as internal urethrotomy in patients with urethral syndrome, but the cure rate was only 25%. However, no urodynamic assessment was made in patients to confirm prior outflow obstruction. In a more recent study by Bergman et al,[68] 60 patients with a diagnosis of urethral syndrome were randomly assigned to receive either placebo, tetracycline or three successive urethral dilatations. A 75% improvement was noted in the urethral dilatation group, which was significantly higher than that in placebo or tetracycline groups. Urodynamic assessment was performed in these patients and, as one might expect, in the group treated with serial urethral dilatation, an increase in uroflowmetry was noted. It would therefore seem reasonable to retain urethral dilatation for those patients in whom urethral stenosis is confirmed by urodynamic assessment. Recently, the CO_2 laser has been used to treat a variety of soft tissue disorders encountered by the urogynecologist, including distal urethral stenosis caused by a fibroelastic band of tissue. Rosenzwieg & Bhatia[69] have used the laser to destroy this abnormal tissue band, thereby increasing the caliber of the urethral meatus and improving symptoms of urethral syndrome.

Cryocautery of the urethra under local anesthetic has been used with some effect, probably by damaging the sensory nerve fibers which supply the urethra. Sand et al,[70] in a prospective, randomized, crossover trial comparing urethral dilation and massage to urethral cryosurgery using a specifically designed urethral cryoprobe, found a 91% symptomatic improvement with cryocautery.

Bladder retraining may be helpful to reduce troublesome frequency and urgency. However, it is unlikely to improve the dysuria or urethral discomfort associated with urethral syndrome.

Conclusions

The urethral syndrome is an elusive disease that defies categorization and is therefore difficult to treat effectively. The term 'urethral syndrome' implies both unknown causation and a solely urethral origin for symptoms. Perhaps this term should be abandoned in favour of specific etiological diagnoses. With greater understanding of the pathophysiology of lower urinary tract infections and the innervation of both bladder and urethra, it would seen reasonable to carry out further research toward a better understanding of the urethral syndrome and its etiology and a more effective treatment rationale.

REFERENCES

1 Bungay G, Vessey MP, McPherson CK. Study of symptoms in middle life with special reference to the menopause. Br Med J 1980; 281: 181–183.
2 Skene AJC. Diseases of the bladder and urethra in women. New York: William Wood, 1887.
3 Oravisto KJ. Epidemiology of interstitial cystitis. Ann Chir Gynaecol. 1975; 64: 75.
4 Fister GM. Similarity of interstitial cystitis (Hunner's ulcer) to lupus erythematosus. J Urol 1938; 40: 37.
5 Oravisto KJ. Interstitial cystitis as an autoimmune disease: a review. Eur Urol 1980; 6: 10.
6 Jokinen EJ, Alfthan OS, Oravisto KJ. Antitissue antibodies of interstitial cystitis. Clin Exp Immunol 1972; 11: 333.
7 Messing EM, Stamey TA. Interstitial cystitis: early diagnosis, pathology and treatment. Urology 1978; 12(4): 381.
8 McGuire ES, Lytton B, Carnog SL. Interstitial cystitis following colocystoplasty. Urology 1973; 2: 28.
9 Parsons CL, Stauffer C, Schmidt JD. Bladder surface glycosaminoglycans: an efficient mechanism of environmental adaptation. Scince, 208: 605, 1980.
10 Hanno PM, Parsons CL, Shrom SH, et al: The protective effect of heparin on experimental bladder infection. J. Surg. Res., 25: 324, 1978.

11 Parsons CL, Schmidt JD, Pollen JY. Successful treatment of interstitial cystitis with sodium pentosan polysulfate. J. Urol., 130: 51, 1983.

12 Collan Y, Alfthan O, Kivilaasko E, and Oravisto KL. Electronic microscopic and histological findings in urinary bladder epithelium in interstitial cystitis. Eur. Urol., 2: 242, 1976.

13 Koziol JA, Clark DC, Gittes RF, Tan EM. The natural history of interstitial cystitis: a survey of 374 patients. J Urol 1993; 149: 465–469.

14 Irwin P, Galloway NT. Impaired Bladder Perfusion in interstitial cystitis: a study of blood supply using laser doppler flowmetry. J Urol 1993; 149: 890–892.

15 Simmons JL. Interstitial cystitis: an explanation for the beneficial effect of an antihistamine. J Urol 1961; 85(2): 149.

16 Parsons CL, Benson G, Childs SJ. A quantavely controlled method to study prospectively interstitial cystitis and demonstrate the efficacy of pentanopolysulfate. J Urol 1993; 159(3): 845–848.

17 Parsons CL, Mulholland SG. Successful therapy of interstitial cystitis with pentanopolysulfate. J Urol 1987; 138: 513.

18 Hanno PM, Buehler J, Wein AJ. Use of amitriptyline in the treatment of interstitial cystitis. J Urol 1989; 141: 849.

19 Badenoch AW. Chronic interstitial cystitis. Br. Med J. 43: 793, 1971.

20 Walsh A. Interstitial Cystitis. In Harrison JH, Gittes RF, Perlmutter AD, Stamey TA, Walsh PC. (Eds): Campbells Urology. 4th Ed. Philadelphia, W.B. Saunders Co. 1978. pp 693–707.

21 Oravisto KJ, Alfthan OS. Treatment of interstitial cystitis with immunosuppression and chloroquine derivatives. Eur Urol 1976; 2: 82.

22 Walsh A. Interstitial cystitis: observations on diagnosis and treatment with anti-inflammatory drugs, particularly benzydiamine. Eur Urol 1977; 3: 216.

23 Dunn M. Interstitial cystitis: treated by prolonged bladder distension. Br J Urol 1977; 49: 641–645.

24 Sant GR. Intravesical 50% dimethyl sulfoxide in treatment of interstitial cystitis. Urology 1987; 29 (suppl): 17.

25 Mathews P, Barker S, Phillip PA. Prospective study of intravesical DMSO in treatment of chronic inflammatory bladder disease. J Urol 1986; 135: 187.

26 Perez-Marrero R, Emerson LE, Feltis JT. A controlled study of dimethyl sulfoxide in interstitial cystitis. J Urol 1988; 140: 36.

27 Wishard WN, Nourse MH, Mertz JHO. Use of Clorpactin WCS-90 for relief of symptoms due to interstial cystitis. J Urol 1957; 77: 420.

28 Benness CJ, Barnick CG, Cardozo LD. Is there a place for videocystourethrography in the assessment of lower urinary tract dysfunction. Neurourol Urodyn 1989; 8: 299–300.

29 Macaulay A, Stanton S, Holmes D. Micturition and the mind: psychological factors in the aetiology of urinary disorders in women. Br Med J 1987; 294: 540–543.

30 Jarvis GJ. The management of urinary incontinence due to primary vesical sessory urgency by bladder drill. Br J Urol 1982; 54: 374.

31 Frewen WK. Urgency incontinence. J Obstet Gynaecol Br Commonw. 1972; 79: 77.

32 Ferrie BG, Smith JS, Logan D. Experience with bladder training in 65 patients. Br J Urol 1984; 56: 482.

33 Karram MM. The painful bladder: urethral syndrome and interstitial cystitis. Curr Opin Obstet Gynecol. 1990; 2: 605–611.

34 Folsom and Alexander. J Urol 31: 731. 1934.

35 Stamm WE, Wagner KF, Amsel R et al. Causes of the acute urethral syndrome in women. N Engl J Med 1980; 303: 409–415.

36 Summitt RL, Ling FW. Urethral syndrome presenting as chronic pelvic pain. J Psychosom Obstet Gynecol 1991; 12: 77–86.

37 Waters EW, Elwood PC, Asscher AW, Abernathy M. Clinical significance of dysuria in women. Br Med J 1970; 11: 754.

38 Kass EH. Asymptomatic infections of the urinary tract. Trans Assoc Am Physicians 1956; 69: 56.

39 Steensberg J, Bartels ED, Bay-Neilson H, Fance E, Hede T. Epidemiology of urinary tract diseases in general practice. Br Med J 1969; 11: 390.

40 Gallagher DJ, Montgomery J, North JDK. Acute infections of the urnary tract. Br Med J 1965; 1: 622.

41 Brooks D, Mauder A. Pathogenesis of the urethral syndrome in women and its diagnosis in general practice. Lancet 1977; 2: 893.

42 Finn SD, Stamm WE. Sem Urol 1: 121, 1983.

43 Stamm WE, Running K, McKevitt M et al. Treatment of the acute urethral syndrome. N Engl J Med 1981; 394: 956–958.

44 Weil A, Gaudenz R, Burgener L, Schultz B. Isolation of chlamydia trachomatis from women with urethral syndrome. Arch Gynecol 1981; 230: 329–333.

45 Gillespie WA, Henderson EP, Linton KB, Smith PJB. Microbiology of the urethral (frequency and dysuria) syndrome. A controlled study with 5-year review. Br J Urol 1989; 64: 270–274.

46 Tait J, Peddie BA, Bailey RR et al. Urethral syndrome (abacterial cystitis) – search for a pathogen. Br J Urol 1985; 57: 552–556.

47 Maskell R, Pead PJ, Pead L, Balsdon MJ. Chlamydial infection and urinary symptoms. Br J Vener Dis 1984; 60: 65.

48 Taylor-Robinson D, Tully JG, Furr PM et al. Urogenital mycoplasma infections of man: A review with observations on a recently discovered mycoplasma. Isr J Med Sci 1981; 17: 524–530.

49 Stamm WE, Running K, Hale J, Holmes KK. Etiologic role of Mycoplasma hominis and Ureaplasma urealyticum in women with the acute urethral syndrome. Sex Trans Dis 1983; 10: 318.

50 Richardson FH, Stonington OG. Urethrolysis and external urethroplasty in the female. Surg Clin North Am 1969; 49: 1201.

51 Hole R. The calibre of the adult female urethra. Br J Urol 1972; 44: 68.

52 Kaplan WE, Firlit CF, Schoenberg HW. The female urethral syndrome: external sphincter spasm as etiology. J Urol 1980; 124: 48–49.

53 Raz S, Smith RB. External sphincter spasticity syndrome in female patients. J Urol 1976; 115: 443.

54 Barbalias GA, Meares EMJ. Female urethral syndrome: clinical and urodynamic perspectives. Urology 1984; 23: 208–212.

55 Lipsky H. Urodynamic assessment of women with urethral syndrome. Urology 1976; 15: 207.

56 Weil A, Miege B, Rottenberg R, Krauer F. Clinical significance of urethral instability. Obstet Gynecol 1986; 68: 106–110.

57 Mabry EW, Carson CC, Older RA. Evaluation of women with chronic voiding discomfort. Urology 1981; 18: 244–246.

58 Bent AE, Richardson DA, Ostergard DR. Diagnosis of lower urinary tract disorders in postmenopausal patients. Am J Obstet Gynecol 1983; 145: 218–222.

59 Youngblood VH, Tomlin EM, Davis JB. Senile urethritis in women. J. Urol. 78, 150 (1957).

60 Youngblood VH, Tomlin E, Williams JO, Kemmelsteil D. Exfoliative cytology of the senile female urethra. J Urol 1958; 79: 110.

61 Parziani S, Constantini E, Petroni PA, Ursini M, Porena M. Urethral syndrome: clinical results with antibiotics alone or combined with estrogen. Eur Urol 1994; 26: 115–119.

62 Carson CC, Segura JW, Osborne DM. Evaluation and treatment of the female urethral syndrome. J Urol 1980; 124: 609–610.

63 Rees DLP, Farhoumand N. Psychiatric aspects of recurrent cystitis in women. Br J Urol 1977; 49: 651.

64 Kaplan DL, Steege JF. The urethral syndrome: sexual components. Sex Disabil 1983; 6: 78–82.

65 Bashi SA, Q. The urethral syndrome. Int Urol Nephrol 1988; 20: 367–374.

66 Stamm 1985.

67 Darling MR, McClean PA. The female urethral syndrome: a comparison of three different methods of treatment. J Ir Med Assoc 1977; 70: 338–339.

68 Bergman A, Karram MM, Bhatia NN. Urethral syndrome. A comparison of different treatment modalities. J Reprod Med 1989; 34: 157.

69 Rosenzweig BA, Bhatia NN. The use of carbon dioxide laser in female urology. J Gynecol Surg 1991; 7: 11–16.

70 Sand PK, Bowen LW, Ostergard DR, Bent A, Panganiban R. Cryosurgery versus dilation and massage for the treatment of recurrent urethral syndrome. J Reprod Med 1989; 34(8): 499–504.

24 Urethral problems

The female urethra is a complex muscular tube between 30 and 50 mm in length. It has the dual functions of aiding in the maintenance of continence and acting as a urinary conduit during micturition. Normal functioning of the lower urinary tract requires a healthy urethra and bladder and appropriate integration of their actions. A wide range of abnormalities may affect the urethra and give rise to symptoms. The spectrum of these urethral problems may be listed as follows:

- congenital abnormalities
- urethral caruncle
- urethritis
- urethral diverticulum
- urethral instability
- fistulae/trauma
- urethral syndrome
- urethral prolapse
- senile urethritis
- urethral stenosis
- urethrocele.

Those of these conditions which are not covered in detail elsewhere in the book will be discussed in this chapter.

STRUCTURE AND FUNCTION

The structure of the urethra has been the subject of considerable debate over the years, particularly with regard to the presence or otherwise of an internal urethral sphincter. Whereas most women are continent at the level of the urethrovesical junction, there is no definable anatomical sphincter at this level. Continence at the level of the urethrovesical junction is probably maintained by the presence of considerable elastic fibers which are present there.[1] The wall of the urethra is composed of several layers. The outermost layer is the striated urogenital sphincter muscle (rhabdosphincter). This surrounds a thin circular layer of smooth muscle, which in turn surrounds a longitudinal layer of smooth muscle (Fig. 24.1). A richly vascular submucosa exists between the smooth muscle and urethral mucosa. Except during the passage of urine, the

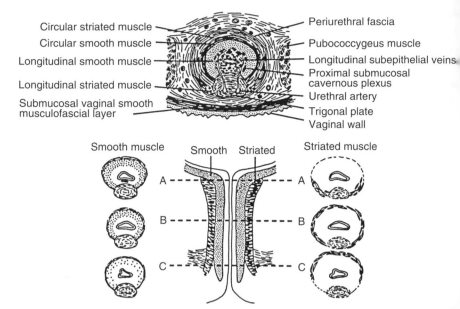

Circular striated muscle
Circular smooth muscle
Longitudinal smooth muscle
Longitudinal striated muscle
Submucosal vaginal smooth musculofascial layer

Periurethral fascia
Pubococcygeus muscle
Longitudinal subepithelial veins
Proximal submucosal cavernous plexus
Urethral artery
Trigonal plate
Vaginal wall

Smooth muscle   Smooth   Striated   Striated muscle

Fig. 24.1 Urethral anatomy

anterior and posterior walls of the urethra are in close apposition, with the urethral epithelium forming extensive folds.

The fibres of the striated urogenital sphincter are mainly slow twitch type, giving rise to constant urethral tone. They also provide a back-up continence mechanism for those women with an incompetent bladder neck. In contrast, the longitudinal smooth muscle layer of the urethra probably shortens the urethra during micturition. The usual level of continence in the female is not the mid-urethra, the level of maximum resting pressure, but at the bladder neck.[2] There is a strong association between bladder neck competence and urodynamic diagnosis in women with lower urinary tract symptoms.[3]

A number of changes occur to the urethra with aging. There is gradual decrease in the amplitude of urethral vascular pulsations with increasing age. After the menopause they rarely exceed 5 cmH$_2$O.[4] The urethral closure pressure also gradually falls. After peaking at age 20 years it declines, with a steeper fall occurring after the menopause.[5] Estrogen deficiency leads to decreased urethral connective tissue and thinning of the urethral epithelium. Anatomical supports of the urethrovesical junction weaken with age.

CARUNCLE

Urethral caruncles are probably the most common urethral lesion and occur more often in older women. They appear as a red mass at the meatus, usually at the 6 o'clock position. Usually asymptomatic, they may give rise to 'spotting' and are occasionally painful. Estrogen deficiency is probably involved in the pathogenesis of many urethral caruncles. They are very vascular and are covered by transitional epithelium. If they not respond to local estrogen therapy, then biopsy is indicated to exclude more serious pathology. Following this they can be treated by excision or cautery. Thirty per cent of caruncles will recur.

URETHRAL MUCOSAL PROLAPSE

This occurs predominantly in older women but may also present in girls aged 5–10 years. In the younger age group Black girls seem to be particularly affected. Urethral prolapse resembles a caruncle but the whole of the circumference of the urethra is involved. Urethral prolapse usually has a congested or bluish colour and appears as a tumor mass with a central meatus. Although not usually painful, urethral prolapse may give rise to bleeding, dysuria or watery discharge. All should be biopsied to exclude malignancy. If large or symptomatic, then treatment should be by excision or cautery.

NEOPLASIA

Although urethral neoplasia is uncommon in women, all urethral lesions should be biopsied. When it does occur, a urethral neoplasm is most often an epidermoid carcinoma. Less common types include adeno-carcinoma, sarcoma and melanoma. Neoplasia is generally a problem of the elderly, with 90% occurring in women over the age of 50 years. Presenting symptoms include frequency, dysuria and hematuria. Inspection will indicate either a mass or ulceration. Where the lesion occurs in the distal third of the urethra, cure is more likely to be achievable.

CONGENITAL ANOMALIES

The main congenital anomalies in women which affect the urethra are bladder exstrophy and epispadias. Bladder exstrophy occurs in 1 in 30 000 live-born females and is due to incomplete fusion of the mesonephric tubules. There is a variable degree of severity of the abnormality with the mild forms seen as epispadias in women.

In epispadias the urethra has a deficient dorsal aspect and may be associated with a bifid clitoris. The urethral sphincter is usually absent and the bladder neck incompetent, resulting in incontinence. The upper urinary tracts need to be assessed by ultra-sound or radiology and bladder compliance and capacity should be assessed by cystometry. Urethral repair and bladder neck reconstruction usually result in satisfactory function. Patients with mild epispadias occasionally reach adulthood before diagnosis, when they present with incontinence.

Complete bladder exstrophy is at the other extreme; it is recognized at birth and requires complex reconstructive surgery. There is divergence of the recti and pubic bones, with the abdominal wall being open exposing

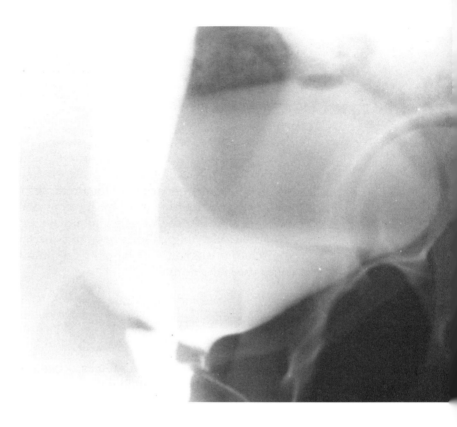

Fig. 24.2   Ectopic ureter

the pelvic viscera. The urethra is open along its entire length and the clitoris is bifid. The long-term results of reconstruction may be complicated by continuing bladder neck incompetence, persistent low bladder capacity, ureteric reflux and recurrent lower urinary tract infections. Urinary diversion is sometimes required.

Ectopic ureters may enter the urethra and usually do so below the level of the bladder neck, resulting in incontinence (Fig. 24.2). This diagnosis should be considered in children with continual incontinence but with an otherwise normal voiding pattern. Diagnosis usually requires examination under anesthesia followed by radiological studies and the appropriate surgery.

URETHRAL INSTABILITY

The unstable urethra is characterized by sudden drops in urethral pressure which may be associated with urine loss. Incontinence will occur if the uninhibited urethral relaxation results in a urethral pressure less than the prevailing bladder pressure. The existence of this condition as a true clinical entity remains controversial and the International Continence Society has not as yet formally defined the condition. The definition of urethral instability varies between authors, with the suggested diagnostic criteria varying from a pressure fall of 15 cm H_2O[6] to 20 cm H_2O[7] or even 25 cm H_2O.[8] It has also been suggested that rather than have an absolute cut-off, a fluctuation of greater than 33% of the resting maximum urethral pressure might be more appropriate to regard as abnormal.[9]

Urethral instability is probably quite uncommon and its diagnosis requires observing the urethral pressure for at least several minutes during filling cystometry, and monitoring its fluctuations. In most studies the fall in urethral pressure is followed by a detrusor contraction. Less often the urethral pressure falls and incontinence occurs while the detrusor pressure remains constant. Tapp et al[9] found no difference in clinical symptoms when comparing women with and without significant variations in maximum urethral closure pressure. Artefactual pressure fluctuations are common and need to be excluded. The typical symptoms of urethral instability are urgency and urge incontinence. The most appropriate therapy for this condition is still unclear and further studies are required in this area.

URETHROCELE

The urethra is fused to the lower 4 cm of the vagina. Descent of this portion of the anterior vaginal wall is called a urethrocele or dislocation of the urethra. It rarely occurs in isolation and is most often associated with bladder descent, when it is termed a cystourethrocele. A urethrocele can easily be seen on vaginal examination when the posterior vaginal wall is retracted with a Sims' speculum. It may be associated with genuine stress incontinence.

URETHRITIS

Urethritis refers to inflammation of the urethra. This may be due to an infectious agent or chemical irritation. The associated symptoms are urethral discomfort, frequency, urgency and dysuria. When these are due to infection, the responsible micro-organism may be sexually transmitted and can include *Chlamydia, Neisseria gonorrheae, Trichomonas*, herpes simplex virus and the human papilloma virus. Organisms which are typically found in acute bacterial cystitis, such as *Escherichia coli*, may also cause urethritis. Midstream urine assessment in patients with urethritis typically shows evidence of pyuria and bacteria on microscopy; however, culture usually results in the growth of $< 10^5$ cfu. Where urethritis is suspected, appropriate cultures should be taken and the patient and her partner treated. Genital herpes infection, particularly a primary attack, may result in acute urinary retention and require the use of a catheter. Use of irritating agents such as perineal deodorants and perfumes, bubble baths and colored toilet paper may result in chemical urethritis. This can be determined by a careful history and cessation of use of the offending product will result in symptomatic improvement.

URETHRAL SYNDROME

The urethral syndrome refers to a constellation of common lower urinary tract symptoms occurring in the absence of bacteriuria. The symptoms vary greatly between patients but the most common are urinary frequency, urgency and dysuria. Less common features include suprapubic and perineal discomfort, hesitancy and a sensation of incomplete bladder emptying. The etiology and pathogenesis of the urethral syndrome are still incompletely understood and the diagnosis is basically one of exclusion. Significant bacteriuria is usually defined as $> 10^5$ cfu/ml in freshly voided urine. Using these criteria, only 40–50% of the patients with the symptoms of frequency and dysuria will have significant bacteriuria.

Many etiological factors have been implicated in the pathogenesis of the urethral syndrome. Infection is thought to be an important cause by many investigators, and it is likely that in some women bacterial counts of $< 10^5$ are indicative of infection. One theory is that fecal organisms may colonize the urethra, without extending up into the bladder, and give symptoms of the urethral syndrome. Infection with fastidious organisms is also a popular concept. In particular, *Chlamydia trachomatis* has been isolated from many of these women[10], most commonly in those of low socioeconomic status. However, its exact role in the pathogenesis of the urethral syndrome remains uncertain. Other fastidious organisms which have been implicated are *Ureaplasma urealyticum* and *Mycoplasma hominis*, although the evidence for the involvement of these is not strong.

Obstructive lesions of the urethra and bladder neck are thought by some to be the fundamental abnormality. Early writers suggested urethral stenosis was the cause of the urethral syndrome and recommended dilatation. However, bladder neck obstruction is uncommon in women, the diagnostic criteria are inconsistent and histological studies showing periurethral fibrosis are not reproducible. As urethral dilatation may result in incontinence, or actually cause fibrosis and obstruction, this treatment should be used with caution.

Increased elastic tissue in the distal urethrovaginal septum has been suggested as a cause of the urethral syndrome and urethrolysis to free the urethra improves symptoms in some of these women.[11] Urodynamic evaluation of women with the urethral syndrome demonstrates a subgroup of patients in whom urethral spasm may be important.

The urethra contains estrogen receptors and is an estrogen-sensitive tissue. Postmenopausal estrogen deficiency may give rise to irritative bladder symptoms and there is good evidence that these will often respond to estrogen replacement therapy.[12] Also impaired vaginal lubrication in postmenopausal women may result in bladder irritation and can be prevented by the use of vaginal lubricants and estrogen therapy. It would appear that psychological factors may play a role in some women with the urethral syndrome. Psychosomatic symptoms and relationship problems are more common than in matched controls. Moreover, those with the urethral syndrome have higher scores for hysteria and hypochondriasis on personality assessment. Symptoms of the urethral syndrome often commence after sexual intercourse, particularly in nulliparous women, and are probably related to trauma to the bladder base from penile thrusting.

Careful evaluation of the patient is required so that an accurate diagnosis can be made and obvious organic pathology is not overlooked. Physical examination will exclude a pelvic mass or large urethral diverticulum. It is necessary to obtain cultures from the urethra, bladder and introitus. Pyuria may be observed on urine microscopy. Urine cytology should be negative for malignant cells. Cystourethroscopy is indicated and will usually reveal no abnormality, although inflammation of the urethra and trigone may be seen. Uroflowmetry and urethral pressure profilometry will identify those few patients with significant urethral obstruction.

Treatment for the urethral syndrome is usually symptom-specific. The initial therapy should address the most prominent symptom, and subsequent therapy should utilize the least invasive options first. In patients who have pyuria, or in whom *Chlamydia* has been isolated, doxycycline is often effective in relieving symptoms.[13] Where urethral stenosis is present, urethral dilatation is temporarily effective and recurrences may be treated by Otis urethrotomy. In postmenopausal women a trial of estrogen therapy is indicated and will often be beneficial. Vaginal administration is most appropriate and continuous therapy may be required.

When urethral spasm is found in women with the urethral syndrome, skeletal muscle relaxants such as diazepam or phenoxybenzamine, either alone or in combination, may achieve good results. Alternatively, neuro-stimulation therapy can be used with either surface or percutaneous stimulation of sacral routes.[14] This treatment fatigues urethral striated smooth muscle, leading to resolution of symptoms.

Many other treatment plans have been advocated for patients with the urethral syndrome, including urethral dilatation and massage, freezing or cauterizing the bladder, periurethral steroid and anesthetic injections, bladder instillations (e.g. DMSO) and a variety of surgical procedures. Further clinical trials are needed to determine the clinical efficacy of these procedures.

URETHRAL DIVERTICULA

The incidence of this condition in women is unclear but is probably of the order of 3%.[15] Patients with a urethral diverticulum may be asymptomatic or complain of a variety of symptoms. These include recurrent cystitis, frequency, dysuria, dyspareunia, urinary incontinence and voiding difficulties. The classic symptom, which is not always present, is that of post-micturition dribble. Urethral diverticula should be considered in all women with chronic lower urinary tract symptoms unresponsive to standard therapy. On clinical examination a suburethral mass may be palpable, the urethra is usually tender and it may be possible to express pus from the urethra. Occasionally a stone may develop within the diverticulum (Figs 24.3, 24.4). Commonly no abnormalities may be found on physical assessment.

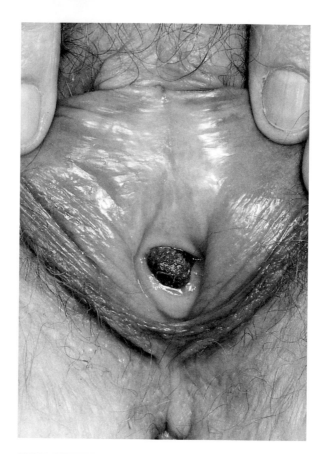

Fig. 24.3 Calculus within a urethral diverticulum

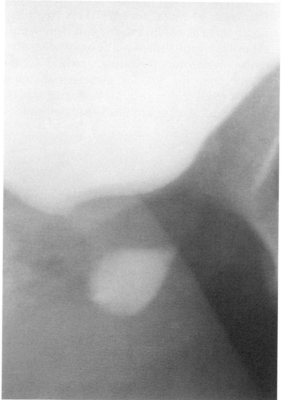

Fig. 24.4 Micturating cystogram showing a urethral diverticulum

Urethral diverticula are occasionally congenital but most are acquired. They may arise secondary to birth trauma, infection or instrumentation. The most popular theory for the development of diverticula is of repeated infection and obstruction of periurethtral glands, resulting in the formation of cystic structures. They develop primarily in the posterior wall of the distal urethra. Diverticula can have quite complex anatomy and may be multiple. Urethroscopy will sometimes detect a diverticulum if it is large and has an open neck but many will be missed. Radiographic screening for diverticula can be achieved by a voiding cystourethrogram or positive pressure double-balloon urethrography. This latter technique using a Trattner catheter is highly effective (Fig 24.5). Diverticula may be demonstrated by vaginal ultrasound. Urethral pressure profilometry may show a characteristic 'dip' on the urethral pressure profile which can be helpful in determining the most appropriate surgical procedure by indicating whether the diverticulum is distal or proximal to the maximum urethral closure pressure.

Asymptomatic diverticula should be left alone as the surgery can be difficult and occasionally results in a urethrovaginal fistula. For the symptomatic diverticulum which is distal to the maximum urethral closure pressure point, marsupialization or the Spence procedure[16] is appropriate. This simple procedure involves placing one blade of the scissors in the urethra and the other in the vagina. The scissors divide the floor of the diverticulum and the overlying vaginal epithelium, including the posterior urethra distal to the diverticulum. Redundant tissue is excised and a running, locking suture provides hemostatis. Alternatively, diverticulectomy is performed as a vaginal procedure. The urethra is then reconstructed in layers, using fine sutures, and avoiding superimposition of suture lines whenever possible. Failure to remove the whole sac, including its neck, may result in recurrence of the diverticulum. Unfortunately total diverticulectomy may result in a urethral stricture at the point of excision, and therefore subtotal diverticulectomy may be preferred.

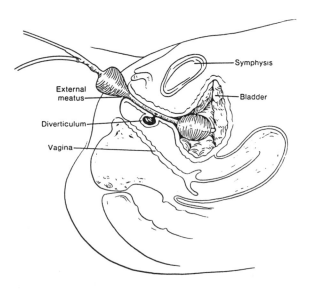

Fig. 24.5   Trattner catheter used to demonstrate a urethral diverticulum.

DRAINPIPE URETHRA

This refers to a urethra which is fixed, rigid and non-functioning. It no longer functions adequately as a sphincter and stress incontinence is usually present. It has also been termed a 'type III urethra.' Radiological studies will indicate an open bladder neck at rest in the absence of a detrusor contraction. The maximum urethral closure pressure is typically low (<30 cmH_2O) in these women. A drainpipe urethra may be secondary to previous bladder neck surgery, radiation or advanced age. Treatment of incontinence in these women can be difficult and usually requires surgery. Procedures which may be of benefit include a suburethral sling, periurethral collagen injection or insertion of an artificial sphincter.

REFERENCES

1 Gosling J. The structure of the bladder and urethral in relation to function. Urol Clin North Am 1979; 6:31.
2 Turner-Warwick RT, Brown ADG. A urodynamic evaluation of urinary incontinence in the female and its treatment. Urol Clin North Am 1979; 6: 203–216.
3 Benness CJ, Cutner A, Cardozo LD. Bladder neck competence in women with lower urinary tract symptoms. Int Urogyn J 1990; 3: 173.
4 Asmussen M. Intraurethral pressure recordings. Scan J Urol Nephrol 1976; 10: 1–6.
5 Huisman AB. Morphologie van de vrouwelijke urethra. Thesis, Groningen, The Netherlands, 1969.
6 Ulmsten U, Henriksson L, Iosif S. The unstable female urethra. Am J Obstet Gynecol 1982; 144: 93–97.
7 Kulseng-Hanssen S. Prevalence and pattern of unstable urethral pressure in one hundred and seventy four gynecological patients referred for urodynamic investigation. Am J Obstet Gynecol 1983; 146: 895–900.
8 Cardozo LD, Versi E. Urethral Instability in normal postmenopausal patients. Proceedings of the 15th Annual Meeting of the ICS, London. 1985; 115–116.
9 Tapp AJS, Cardozo LD, Versi E, Studd JWW. The prevalence of variation of resting urethral pressure in women and its association with lower urinary tract function. Brit J Urol 1988; 61: 314–317.
10 Stamm W, Wagner KF, Amsel R. Causes of acute urethral syndrome in women. N Engl J Med 1980; 304: 409–413.
11 Richardson FH. External urethroplasty in women: technique and clinical evaluation. J Urol 1969; 40: 694.
12 Walter S, Wolf H, Barlebo H et al. Urinary incontinence in post menopausal women treated with estrogen: a double-blind clinical trial. Urol Int 1978; 33: 135–143.
13 Stamm W, Running K, McKevitt J. Treatment of the acute urethral syndrome. N Engl J Med 1981; 304: 956.
14 Schmidt RA. The urethral syndrome. Urol Clin North Am 1985; 12: 349–354.
15 Anderson MJF. The incidence of diverticula in the female urethra. J Urol 1967; 98: 96.
16 Spence H, Duckett J. Diverticulum of the female urethra: clinical aspects and presentation of a simple operative technique for cure. J Urol 1970; 104: 432–437.

25

Congenital abnormalities

The formation of the urinary and genital systems is very closely linked and to gain a full understanding of congenital abnormalities of the region it is important to understand the developmental embryology (Ch. 2). Although the abnormalities appear to be diverse they can usually be explained by a study of the embryology.

RENAL ABNORMALITIES

Formation of the mature kidney requires the original presence of the nephrogenic ridge on the dorsolateral aspect of the coelomic cavity and the presence of a ureteric bud from the Wolffian duct. If there is no metanephric blastema or no ureteric bud then kidney formation cannot occur.[1]

Bilateral renal agenesis

Complete bilateral agenesis was described by Potter.[2] It is associated with oligohydramnios, low birth weight, characteristic facies (prominent crease under eyes, blunted nose, ears appearing to be low set, large ear lobes) and severe pulmonary hypoplasia. There is a high incidence of genital abnormalities.[1] Forty per cent are born dead and the rest die quickly due to respiratory problems.

Unilateral renal agenesis

Unilateral renal agenesis occurs in 1 in 1200 births.[3] It is appears to be a problem associated with an absent ureteric bud as the ipsilateral gonad (from the adjacent mesenchyme) is almost always present and normal and there is a high incidence of mesonephric duct abnormalities. Depending on the timing of the abnormal embryonic development a unicornate, bicornuate or normal uterus can be present.[4] One-third of women with unilateral renal agenesis have an abnormality of the genital tract and 43% of women with genital abnormalities have unilateral renal agenesis.[5] There do not appear to be any problems associated with having a single kidney.

Renal ectopia

This phenomenon has an incidence of about 1 in 900.[6] The pelvic kidney is against the sacrum or near the sacral promontory and the lumbar kidney is near the second lumbar vertebra. They occur in these sites with similar frequencies.[7] The ureter is in its usual site and the kidney itself is often smaller and misshapen. The nephrogenic tissue migrates cephalad between the 4th and 8th week so the problem must occur at this time. There is a 15–45% incidence of genital abnormalities, especially bicornuate and unicornate uteri.[8] An ectopic kidney is more likely to have calculus formation due to malrotation and poor drainage and is slightly more prone to blunt trauma. (Fig 14.6)

Horseshoe kidney

This renal fusion disorder occurs in 1 in 400 people. The renal masses are fused so that the kidneys are malrotated. There is a high incidence of other abnormalities including skeletal, cardiac and neurological abnormalities. Many have no symptoms but the kidneys are prone to hydronephrosis, infection and calculus formation.[9] Horseshoe kidneys have a higher incidence of tumor formation.[10]

URETERAL DUPLICATION, ECTOPIA AND URETEROCELE

Duplication and ectopic ureter

The ureter forms from a urethral bud which branches from the wolffian duct. The ureteral bud eventually enters the urogenital sinus at a different site from the Wolffian duct. The ureteral bud grows cephalad with renal tissue around it to form a kidney. If the bud divides duplication occurs and if the incorporation of the bud into the urogenital sinus is at fault an ectopic ureter can form. Ureteral duplication can be incomplete or complete (Fig 14.7). In the incomplete type the upper pole is often small and virtually non-functioning. In complete duplication the upper pole ureter enters caudal and medial to the lower pole ureter. The lower pole ureter enters higher and more medial (Weigert–Meyer law). This makes the intravesical tunnel shorter so that reflux and urinary tract infections occur more often.[11]

The term 'ectopic ureter' describes a ureter that does not drain into the bladder. It can be single but is usually duplicated. It can drain into the trigone, bladder neck or urethra (Fig 24.4). If there is no drainage into the bladder (bilateral single ectopic ureter) the bladder does not form. This is a very unusual condition. The most common presentation is a duplication with ectopia. If the ectopic ureter drains into the bladder neck or urethra then incontinence occurs. If the Wolffian duct (mesonephric) has not degenerated then an ectopic ureter can drain into the vagina via Gartner's duct. The normal sites for ectopic ureters to drain are urethra (35%), vestibule (34%), vagina (24%), cervix or uterus (5%) and Gartner's duct (< 1%).[12]

The management of duplications and ectopia is based on symptoms and renal function. If incontinence is occurring in a woman with a duplication then the ureter can be excised or reimplanted. If chronic infection, renal scarring or deterioration of renal function occurs despite prophylactic antibiotics then an anti-reflux procedure is indicated, or division of the distal ureter if the problem is associated with a ureter draining from a small upper pole. If the upper pole is scarred and is a focus for infection then it can be removed.

Ureterocele

A simple ureterocele is a cystiform dilatation of the terminal submucosal ureter draining into the bladder.[13] If the ureterocele is associated with an ectopic ureter it is called an ectopic ureterocele and is almost always associated with an ipsilateral duplication. It will therefore affect the ureter draining the upper pole of the kidney. The embryology of a ureterocele is uncertain.

It may present as a vaginal mass causing pain and obstruction of the urethra or vagina or it may be asymptomatic. If the ureterocele is not causing reflux or obstructing then observation is indicated. If renal damage is occurring then excision and an anti-reflux procedure are indicated. The management of ectopic ureteroceles is more controversial. Some surgeons do the entire operation as a single procedure while others will stage the bladder and renal reconstruction.[14,15]

VESICOURETERIC REFLUX

It is uncertain why some children have vesicoureteric reflux (VUR). It may be because of a more lateral positioning of the ureteric orifice[16] or bladder instability.[17] There are five grades of reflux:

1. into ureter only
2. into ureter, renal pelvis and calyces
3. mild to moderate dilatation of the ureter and renal pelvis with minimal blunting of fornices
4. moderate dilatation and tortuosity of the ureter and blunting of the fornices.
5. gross dilatation and tortuosity of the ureter with absence of the papillary impressions.[18]

The incidence of VUR is 0.4–1.8%.[19] There is an inverse relationship with age, with the younger children having a higher incidence of VUR. If children with urinary tract infection are investigated, up to 60% of infants less than a year old will have reflux and a similar figure is achieved if young children with bacteriuria are examined.[20] There is a strong familial element with 8–43% of siblings having VUR if it has been identified in another sibling.[21]

There is a high rate of spontaneous resolution. Bellinger & Duckett have shown that over a 3-year period the resolution rates for the different grades are: 1, 87%; 2, 63%; 3, 53%; 4, 33%.[22]

The main problem with VUR is that it predisposes to urinary tract infections and this makes the likelihood of renal scarring and kidney damage much greater. After the first urinary tract infection 4% of children will have renal scarring and after the second infection 17% will have renal scarring.[23] The rate of renal scarring is increased with the grade of reflux or if the child is very young.

The management of VUR is aimed at preventing infections that will damage the kidneys. As 80% of VUR will resolve spontaneously when the grade of reflux is low, antimicrobial prophylaxis and routine urine culture and annual ^{99m}Tc-dimercaptosuccinic acid (DMSA) scans are appropriate. If the VUR is grade 4 or 5 or multiple infections are occurring despite antibiotic prophylaxis, of if renal scarring is progressing, or the reflux is finally not improving, then an anti-reflux procedure is indicated.

BLADDER EXSTROPHY, EPISPADIAS, CLOACAL AND UROGENITAL ABNORMALITIES

Bladder exstrophy and epispadias and cloacal exstrophy

These rare abnormalities occur when the cloacal membrane fails to form and: (1) part of the bladder or urethra is left exposed (epispadias) Fig 24.3 ; (2) the whole bladder's wall is exposed to the anterior abdominal wall (bladder exstrophy) Fig 14.3; or (3) the urorectal septum fails to form so that bowel is also exposed and the symphysis pubis is separated.

Classic exstrophy and cloacal exstrophy can easily be recognized but female epispadias may be hidden by the labia. The clitoris is usually bifid and the urethra is gaping with a defect in the dorsal surface. Management of these conditions is based on closure of the defect (now normally closed soon after birth), preservation of renal function and the control of urinary and or fecal incontinence.[24]

Cloacal and urogenital sinus abnormalities

The cloaca divides into the urogenital sinus and into the hindgut. The sinus interacts with the müllerian tubercle to form the sinovaginal plate which then becomes the vagina.

Normal Sexuality

If the sexual differentiation has been normal three types of lesion can occur.

1 Vaginal obstruction If the obstruction is distal then often it is only a membrane up against the hymen. This can present as hydrocolpos in the younger child or hematocolpos in the pubescent girl. The vagina may be full of fluid at birth due to secretions stimulated by the maternal hormones. This can obstruct the urethra and the bladder overfills and overflows.

A large abdominal mass (the bladder) can be the presenting symptom and inspection of the vulva will show a tense membrane protruding. Management is simple excision. An ultrasound scan should be performed to exclude vesico uretric reflux (VUR). If the obstruction is complete vaginal atresia is present. This is associated with a high rate of renal and ureteric ectopia.

2 Persistent urogenital sinus abnormality The vagina and urethra open through one outlet as the distal vagina does not develop. Unless there is associated hydrocolpos the urethra will drain and the child is usually continent. Therefore there is no urgency to separate the vaginal and urinary tissues and this can be done later when the patient is able to use dilators to keep the vagina open.

3 Persistent cloacal abnormality The vagina, rectum and urethra all open into a single orifice and hence the child is incontinent of feces and urine. There are often other serious abnormalities such as hydrocolpos, sacral agenesis, pelvic floor dysfunction and urethral reflux. Some surgeons feel that the gastrointestinal, urinary and vaginal tissues should be separated early in the child's life to reduce sepsis.[25] Others feel that a colostomy can be formed and a more extensive operation can be performed later.[26]

Intersexuality

If the fetus has had abnormal hormonal stimulation either due to an intersex state, hermaphroditism, congenital adrenal hyperplasia or excessive exogenous hormones, then abnormalities of the urogenital sinus will present as enlarged external genitalia and a variety of müllerian tract abnormalities. Electrolyte status must be quickly ascertained in congenital adrenal hyperplasia and rapid chromosomal analysis should be undertaken so that the sex of the child can be quickly identified. External genitalia can be surgically corrected when the child is a little older.

The understanding of congenital urogenital abnormalities is based on the embryological development of the urinary and genital tract. There are many close associations and family history is often significant. The management of the urological problem often involves gynecological practice so that often it is most appropriate that a urogyecologist is involved in treatment.

REFERENCES

1 Ashley DJ, Mostofi FK. Renal agenesis and dysgenesis. J Urol 1960; 83: 211.
2 Potter EL. Bilateral renal agenesis. J Pediatr 1946; 29: 68.
3 Shieh CP, Hung CS, Wei CF, Lin CY. Cystic dilatations within the pelvis in patients with ipsilateral renal agenesis or dysplasia. J Urol 1990; 144: 324.
4 Magee MC, Lucey DT, Fried FA. A new embryological classification for uro-gynaecologic malformations: the syndromes of mesonephric duct induced müllerian deformities. J Urol 1979; 121: 265.
5 Thompson DP, Lynn HB. Genital anomalies associated with solitary kidney. Mayo Clin 1966; 4 : 538.
6 Abeshouse BS, Bhisistkul I. Crossed renal ectopia with and without fusion. Urol Int 1959; 9: 63.
7 Dretler SP, Olsson CA. Pfister RC. The anatomic radiologic and clinical characteristics of the pelvic kidney, and analysis of 86 cases. J Urol 1971; 105: 623
8 Downs RA, Lane JW, Burns E. Solitary pelvic kidney: its clinical implications. Urology 1973; 1: 51.
9 Pitts WR, Muecke EC. Horseshoe kidneys: a 40 year experience. J Urol 1975; 113: 743.
10 Buntley D. Malignancy associated with horseshoe kidney. Urology 1976; 8: 146.
11 Kelias PP. Anomalies of the urinary tract. In: Kelias PP, King LR, Belman AB (eds) Clinical Pediatric Urology. 2nd edn, vol II. Philadelphia: WB Saunders. 1985: pp 635–725.
12 Ellerker AG. The extravesical ectopic ureter. Br J Surg 1957; 45: 344.
13 Churchill BM, Abara EO, McLorie GA. Ureteral duplicaiton, ectopy and ureteroceles. Pediatric Clinics of North America 1987; 34 (5): 1273–1289.
14 Kroovan RL, Perlmutter AD. A one stage surgical approach to ectopic ureterocele. J Urol 1979; 122: 367.
15 Churchill BM, Sheldon CA, Ghazal G et al. The ectopic ureterocele: a proposed practical classification based on renal unit jeopardy. AUA abstracts, AUA Meeting, Atlanta GA May 1985.
16 Stephens FD. Correlation of urethral position orifice position with renal morphology. Trans Am Assoc GU Surg 1977; 68: 53–55.
17 Koff SA, Lapides J, Piazza DH. Association of urinary tract infection and reflux with uninhibited bladder contractions and voluntary sphincteric obstruction. J Urol 1979; 122: 373–376.

18 Report of the International Reflux Study Committee: Medical versus surgical treatment of primary vesicoureteral reflux: a prospective international reflux study in children. J Urol 1981; 125: 277–283.

19 Bailey RR. Vesicoureteric reflux in healthy infants and children. In: Hodson JJ, Kinkaid-Smith P (eds) Reflux nephropathy. New York: Masson. 1979: pp 59.

20 Kollerman MW, Ludwig H. The current status of vesicoureteral reflux: a review. Monogr Urol 1984; 5: 155–173.

21 Van den Abbeele AD, Treves ST et al. Vesicoureteral reflux in asymptomatic siblings of patients with known reflux: radionuclide cystography. Pediatrics 1987; 79 (1): 147–153.

22 Bellinger MF, Duckett JW. Vesicoureteral reflux: a comparison of non-surgical and surgical management. Contrib Nephrol 1984; 39: 81–93.

23 Winberg J, Anderseon HJ, Bergstrom T, Jacobsson B, Larson H, Lincoln K. Epidemiology of symptomatic urinary tract infection in childhood. Acta Paediatr Scand 1974; S252: 1–20.

24 Jeffs RD. Exstrophy, epispadias, and cloacal and urogenital sinus abnormalities. Pediatric Clinics of North America. 1987; 34: 5: 1233–1257.

25 Raffensperger JG, Ramenofsky ML. The management of a cloaca. J Pediatr Surg 1973; 8: 647–657.

26 Bill AH. Clinical aspects of female patients with high anorectal agenesis. Surg Gynecol Obstet 1972; 135: 411–416.

Nocturnal enuresis

Enuresis is defined as the involuntary discharge of urine.[1] Unfortunately, the term is often used rather loosely to describe night-time bed-wetting. The correct term is nocturnal enuresis and daytime wetting is called diurnal enuresis. If the child has never had night-time control then it is primary nocturnal enuresis, and if there has been a period of control followed by relapse it is secondary.

EPIDEMIOLOGY

As night-time incontinence is normal in young children it is difficult to get accurate prevalence figures. Studies use different criteria for wet nights, patient groups that often include diurnal enuresis and data that include primary and secondary enuresis combined.[2] The prevalence appears to be about 25% at age 4, 15% at age 5 and 10% at age 7.[3,4,5,6] The resolution rate is approximately 15% per year so that only 1% of adolescents have nocturnal enuresis at age 15.[7] A high proportion of these affected adolescents and adults have urodynamic abnormalities.[8] Levels of adult nocturnal enuresis are difficult to establish but appear to be between 1% and 2%.[3,9]

In the first year of life a child voids about 20 times a day, and this then decreases to about 11 times a day at 3 years old. The mean volume voided increases by a factor of four.[1,10]. The reduction in frequency is due to the increase in bladder capacity as the child grows being greater than the rise in urine output.[8,10]

There are four events that appear to be important in the development of night-time urine control.

1. Increase in bladder capacity.
2. Voluntary control over the urethral sphincter. This is part of the normal order of development and occurs by 3 years of age.[1,11]
3. Voluntary control over the spinal micturition reflex.[11,12]
4. The onset of the circadian rise of antidiuretic hormone (ADH) and the subsequent decrease in nocturnal urine volume. This occurs by about age 3–4.[13,14]

ETIOLOGY

There are many theories to explain the cause of nocturnal enuresis. However, it is clear that most children with nocturnal enuresis are perfectly normal children with no obvious neurological, urological or psychological problems. The main theories for nocturnal enuresis are discussed below.

Bladder capacity

A number of authors have demonstrated decreased bladder capacity in enuretic children.[12,15,16,17] However, various methods were used to measure bladder capacity and all were indirect measurements. When more direct methods such as cystometry are used enuretic children have the same cystometric capacity as normal children.[7,18,19] There is no increase in bladder capacity after the successful treatment of enuresis.[20]

Bladder stability

Sleep studies have shown increased bladder activity in nocturnal enuretics compared with normal children, particularly in stages III and IV of sleep.[21,8] In children with diurnal enuresis there is a high incidence of bladder instability. A study of 204 enuretic children undergoing cystometry and EEG showed that 70% had normal cystometry during sleep. Some of the children had EEG changes associated with enuresis without any cystometric changes.[2,22] The data is therefore conflicting but there does appear to be some association between bladder instability and nocturnal enuresis although perhaps not a direct causal one.[1]

Family history

Enuretic children often have a family history of enuresis.[23,24] Compared with normal children, enuretic children are three times more likely to have a parent who has enuresis.[25] Twin studies have shown a high rate of enuresis in the other twin if the first twin has enuresis.[26]

Sleep

Many parents perceive that deep sleep is a major cause of enuresis.[24,27] However, studies have shown that bed-wetting can occur in any sleep stage and is just as likely to occur in an arousal phase as in deep sleep.[21,28,29,30] Recent studies suggest that the problem may lie in disruption of arousal thresholds rather than the level of sleep itself.[2,22,31]

Psychological factors

Early studies showed increased emotional problems in children with enuresis. However, in these studies, the enuresis was often diurnal rather than nocturnal and the patient selection was often biased.[32] Many recent papers have shown children with nocturnal enuresis to have no increase in emotional disturbance.[27,33,34] Techniques such as psychotherapy are of little use in the treatment of enuresis.[2] Enuresis does, however, appear to increase if an event that causes significant anxiety occurs.[35] This is especially so between the age of 2 and 4 years, which is a critical time for the development and maturation of the urinary control system.[36]

Developmental delay

Nocturnal enuresis could be seen as just a delay in the normal maturation of the continence mechanisms. The above evidence points to this, as does the association between encopresis and enuresis. In addition, a higher than expected proportion of children with delays in walking and talking have nocturnal enuresis.[7] However, against this theory of developmental delay is the physiological evidence that once pathways form they should not decay. Hence by the time a child has achieved night-time dryness at least once the pathways must have matured.[37]

Urinary tract abnormality

Children with nocturnal enuresis do not have a higher incidence of urinary tract abnormality.[1,7,24,38] However, children with diurnal enuresis have a higher incidence of abnormalities and these cases need to be investigated.[36]

Antidiuretic hormone

Antidiuretic hormone or vasopressin increases at night[13] and therefore urine concentration increases and urine volume decreases. Enuretics seem to have higher nocturnal urine volumes and also have reduced secretion of ADH compared with normal controls.[39,40] The higher urine volumes themselves are not the cause of enuresis and its is noteworthy that treatment with synthetic ADH (desmopressin (DDAVP)) is only moderately successful.[1]

Other factors

Urinary tract infections are not a common cause of primary nocturnal enuresis. About 1–2% of children with primary enuresis will have a urinary tract infection but when the infection is treated the bed-wetting will usually not improve.[7,38] However, children with urinary tract infections will often present with secondary diurnal enuresis and treatment will cure the problem.[41]

Constipation has some association with diurnal enuresis but not particularly with nocturnal enuresis.[42] There are anecdotal reports of children having secondary enuresis when exposed to allergens such as dust mites or certain foods and plants.[2] Children with combined sleep apnea and enuresis will often lose their enuresis once the airway obstruction is relieved.[43]

ASSESSMENT

As the vast number of children with nocturnal enuresis have no obvious abnormality and can be expected to become dry spontaneously there is little indication for extensive testing. A careful history should be taken, including the onset of toilet training and its success or otherwise. A careful note should be taken of the pattern of incontinence and any techniques used by the child to improve continence. It is important to get an assessment of whether the child feels there is a problem and if the child is suitably mature. Examination should include a careful assessment of the neurological system, as well as excluding occult spina bifida. Rectal sphincter tone and perineal sensation and reflexes should be specifically examined and lower limb neurological abnormalities and gait problems investigated.

The only investigations that are warranted in nocturnal enuresis are urinalysis, microscopic analysis and urine culture. If after this assessment the child has monosymptomatic nocturnal enuresis then no further investigation is necessary. If there is infection present or there is a daytime problem as well, then imaging the urinary tract with ultrasound is indicated. If the ultrasound findings are normal and the child has day- and night-time wetting and symptoms of urgency and frequency, then urodynamic studies would be the next investigation. However, most clinicians would try an anticholinergic treatment before embarking on urodynamic studies. The number of children needing these advanced investigations is very small.[1]

TREATMENT

Most children will have had some form of home treatment before presenting to the doctor. This can range from fluid reduction, star charts, positive and negative reinforcement through to routine night-time toileting. Often the first part of 'treatment' is to explain to the parents and the child the true nature of the problem and to make sure that previous misconceptions are removed. It is very important to indicate that the problem is not a pathological entity. The child must be given confidence that he or she does not have a major problem, that it is common and that most children become dry spontaneously.

The assessment of different treatments for nocturnal enuresis is difficult as there is a placebo effect of up to 68% and the spontaneous resolution rate is about 15%.[7,44] Treatment is divided into behavior modification and pharmacological support.

Behavior modification

Enuresis alarms

This is the most effective treatment for nocturnal enuresis. There are many good randomized trials demonstrating an efficacy of about 75%. There is a relapse rate of 20–40%.[45,46,47] There does not appear to be any difference in efficacy between the different alarm types.[48,49] Alarms vary from aluminum sheets in the bed connected to a bell alarm through to small detectors in pyjamas connected by radio to buzzer systems. The modern alarms are low voltage and only have current running when the alarm is activated so there is little risk of serious problems. The main drawbacks are failing to awaken the child, false alarms, alarm failure and waking the rest of the family.[2]

The most common reason why treatment fails is lack of parental co-operation and understanding.[1] Treatment takes up to 4 months. The child needs to awake as soon as the alarm rings and needs to be motivated to continue. If the parents are not involved or do not understand the principle of the treatment then this system will often fail. Although the relapse rate is 20–40%, repeating the treatment will often result in cure.[50]

Compared with drug treatments (imipramine and DDAVP) the cure rates are higher (alarm 85%; DDAVP, 70%) and there is a ten times higher relapse rate with DDAVP.[51] The combination of enuresis alarm and DDAVP gives a very good cure rate.[52]

Bladder training

This is based on the theory that reduced bladder capacity is a cause of enuresis. Children are taught to hold urine for progressively longer and longer so as slowly to increase the bladder capacity. Initial studies showed improvement but only about 20% were cured.[53] Later studies have been unable even to show this level of improvement.[47]

Dry bed training

'Lifting' children at night so they can urinate and therefore keep the bladder volume small does not cure enuresis.[54] However, if a programed awakening schedule is used then a conditioning effect can occur. It is time-consuming and demanding on parents but can give good results.[55] Parents often try fluid restriction at night-time but it usually does not work.[2]

Psychotherapy

Although there is little evidence to support the theory that enuresis is a psychological disorder psychotherapy is still used to treat enuresis. Studies show a cure rate of 10–20%.[45] A placebo effect may explain this.

Responsibility reinforcement

Methods of getting the child to take responsibility, such as star charts, rewards and punishment have mixed success and depend on the child being motivated.[54] Certainly, negative reinforcement is both cruel and unsuccessful. In extreme cases it can even evolve into child abuse.[56]

Hypnotherapy

Although only small trials have been undertaken, hypnosis appears to be successful[54,57] but very time-consuming.

Pharmacological treatment

A large number of drugs have been used to treat nocturnal enuresis but only DDAVP and tricyclic antidepressants have been shown to have benefit in treating monosymptomatic nocturnal enuresis.

DDAVP

This is an analog of the pituitary antidiuretic hormone (ADH or vaso-pressin). As noted previously, enuretic children produce less ADH at night and therefore theoretically DDAVP should improve enuresis. Early studies showed improvement[58] and since then good placebo-controlled trials have shown a 50% cure rate.[59] After treatment, unfortunately, there is a high relapse rate. If treatment is continued for a longer period of time or reduced in a tapered fashion then the relapse rate is lower.[60] Children with high urine output at night or a family history of nocturnal enuresis often respond well to DDAVP.[61,62]

If used correctly there are few side effects. The most common are headache, abdominal pain, nausea and nasal congestion and bleeding. Some children gain weight, which is then lost when therapy is stopped.[59] If the treatment is used inappropriately electrolyte imbalance and hyponatremia and eventually convulsions can occur. While it can be taken for long periods of time it is an expensive drug and this often precludes long-term therapy. Originally DDAVP was available as snuff, but is now most readily available as a nasal spray. Long-term use of the spray can lead to very sore nasal passages. Recently, it has become available in some countries in tablet form.

Tricyclic antidepressants

Imipramine is the most commonly used drug in this category. Such drugs are thought to act as a weak anticholinergic and an antispasmodic and to alter the action of noradrenaline on the α- and β-receptors.[1] Most studies have shown a cure rate of approximately 50% and an improvement in another 20%.[63] Given that most children with nocturnal enuresis do not have an unstable bladder it is surprising that imipramine does work. As anticholinergics do not seem to work,[43] one of the other known actions or an unknown action must be the mechanism of cure. The major problem with the tricyclic antidepressants is their sedating side effects. Most clinicians try to avoid these drugs if possible.[64] Once the medication is stopped the enuresis returns.

Anticholinergic drugs

In children with monosymptomatic nocturnal enuresis there is little evidence that these drugs work.[43,65] If the child has other symptoms such as urgency and frequency or urodynamically proven instability then anticholinergic treatment can be very successful.[65] If cystometry is normal then these drugs are of no benefit. If the drugs are to be used the dose must be related to the weight of the child.

Other drugs

There are many drugs that have been tried. Non-steroidal anti-inflammatories have been tried with mixed success, but most other medications do not seem to work at all.[2]

Resource and support groups

These groups can be a valuable part of treatment. Not only do they provide libraries for books and equipment but they often provide sources for donations and research funds. Importantly these groups can co-ordinate support and self-help groups which can be very valuable for parents and children.

REFERENCES

1 Koff SA. Enuresis. In: Walsh P, Gittes B, Perlmutter A, Stamey T (eds) Campbell's urology. Philadelphia: WB Saunders, 1992: pp 1621–1633.
2. While S. Primary nocturnal enuresis. In: Children. Background and treatment. Scan J Urol Nephrol 1994; Suppl.
3 Thorne FC. Incidence of nocturnal enuresis after the age of five. Am J Psychiatry 1944; 686–689.
4 Cederbland M, Rahim SI. Epidemiology of nocturnal enuresis in a part of Khartoum. Sudan II. The intensive study. Acta Paediatr Scand 1986; 75: 1021–1027.
5 Feehan M, McGee R, Stanton W, Silva PA. A 6 year follow-up of childhood enuresis: prevalence in adolescence and consequences for mental health. J Paediatr Child Health 1990; 26: 75–79.
6 Bloom DA, Seeley WW, Ritchey ML, McGuire EJ. Toilet habits and continence in

children: an opportunity sampling in search of normal parameters. J Urol 1993; 149: 1087–1090.

7   Forsythe WI, Redmond A. Enuresis and spontaneous cure rate: study of 1129 enuretics. Arch Dis Child 1974; 49: 259–263.

8   Koff SA. Estimating bladder capacity in children. Urology 1983; 21: 248.

9   Wrist LG, Foldspang A, Elving LB, Mommsen S. Social context, social abstention and problem recognition correlated with adult female urinary incontinence. Danish Medical Bulletin 1992; 39: 565–570.

10 Goellner MH, Ziegler EE, Fomon SJ. Urination during the first three years of life. Nephron 1981; 28: 174.

11 Lapides J, Sweet RB, Lewis LW. Role of striated muscle in urination. J Urol 1957; 77: 247.

12 Muellner SR. Development of urinary control in children. JAMA 1960; 172: 1256.

13 George CP, Messeril FH, Gennest J et al. Diurnal variation of plasma vasopressin in man. J Clin Endocrinol Metab 1975; 41: 332–338.

14 Winter JS, Hughes IE, Rayes FI, Famin C. Pituitary-gonadal relations in infancy: serum gonadal streoid concentrations in man from birth to two years of age. J Endocrinol Metab 1976; 42: 679–686.

15 Hallman N. On the ability of enuretic children to hold urine. Acta Paediatr 1950; 39: 87.

16 Esparanca M, Gerrard JW. Nocturnal enuresis: studies in bladder function in normal children and enuretics. Can Med Assoc J 1969a; 101: 324.

17 Starfield B. Functional bladder capacity in enuretic and non-enuretic children. J Pediatr 1967; 5: 777–781.

18 Norgaard JP. Urodynamics in enuretics I: Reservoir function. Neurourol Urodyn 1989; 8: 199–211.

19 McGuire EJ, Savastano JA. Urodynamic studies in enuresis and nonneurogenic bladder. J Urol 1984; 132: 299–302.

20 Berg I, Forsythe I, McGuire R. Response of bedwetting to the enuretic alarm. Arch Dis Child 1982; 57: 394–396.

21 Broughton RJ. Sleep disorders: disorders of arousal? Science 1968; 159: 1070.

22 Watanabe H, Azuma Y. A proposal for a classification system of enuresis based on overnight simultaneous monitoring of electroencephalography and cystometry. Sleep 1989; 12(3): 257–264.

23 Frary LG. Enuresis: a genetic study. Am J Dis Child 1935; 49: 553.

24 Hallgren B. Enuresis: a clinical and genetic study. Acta Psychiatr Neurol Scand 1957; (Suppl.) 114: 1.

25 Javelin MR, Moilanen I, Kangas P et al. Aetiological and precipitating factors for childhood enuresis. Acta Paediatr Scan 1991; 80: 361–369.

26 Bakwin H. Enuresis in twins. Am J Dis Child 1971; 121(3): 222–225.

27 Butler RJ, Redfern EJ, Forsythe WI. The child's construing of nocturnal enuresis: a method of inquiry and prediction of outcome. J Child Psychol Psychiatry 1990; 31: 447–454.

28 Ritvo ER, Ornitz EM, Gottlieb F et al. Arousal and non-arousal enuretic events. Am J Psychiatry 1969; 126: 115–122.

29 Mikklesen EJ, Rappapot JL, Nee L, Gruenau C, Mendelson W, Gillin JC. Childhood enuresis I. Sleep patterns and psychopathology. Arch Gen Psychiatry 1980; 37(10): 1139.

30 Inoue M, Shimojima H, Shiba H et al. Rhythmic slow wave observed on nocturnal sleep encephalogram in children with idiopathic nocturnal enuresis. J Sleep 1987; 10(6): 570–579.

31 Norgaard JP, Hansen JH, Nielsen JB, Rittig S, Djurhuus JC. Nocturnal studies in enuretics. A polygraphic study of sleep-EEG and bladder activity. Scand J Urol Nephrol Suppl 1989; 125: 73–78.

32 Werry JS. Emotional factors and enuresis nocturna. Dev Med Child Neurol 1965; 7: 563–564.

33 Butler RJ, Brewin CR, Forsythe WI. Maternal attributions and tolerance for nocturnal enuresis. Behav Res Ther 1986; 24: 307–312.

34 Warzak WJ. Psychological implications of nocturnal enuresis. Clin Pediatr 1993; Spec Ed 38–40.

35 Miller FJ, Court SD, Walton NG, Knox EG. Growing up in Newcastle upon Tyne. London: Oxford University Press, 1960.

36 MacKeith RC. A frequent factor in the origins of primary nocturnal enuresis: anxiety in the third year of life. Dev Med Child Neurol 1968; 10: 465.

37 MacKeith RC. Is maturation delay a frequent factor in the origins of primary nocturnal enuresis? Dev Med Child Neurol 1972; 14: 217.

38 Jarvelin MR, Huttunen NP, Sepanen U, Moilanen I. Screening of urinary tract

abnormalities among day and nightwetting children. Scand J Urol Nephrol 1990; 24: 181–189.

39 Norgaard JP, Pedersen EB, Djurhuus JC. Diurnal antidiuretic hormone levels in enuretics. J Urol 1985; 134: 1029–1031.

40 Rittig S, Knudsen UB, Sorensen S, Djurhuus JC, Norgaard JP Abnormal diurnal rhythm of plasma vasopressin and urinary output in patients with enuresis. Am J Physiol 1989; 56: 664–671.

41 Stansfield JM. Enuresis and urinary tract infection. In: Kolvin I, MacKeith RC, Meadows SR (eds) Bladder control and enuresis. London: Heinemann, pp 102–103.

42 O'Regan S, Yasbeck S, Hamberger B, Schieck E. Constipation a commonly unrecognised cause of enuresis. Am J Dis Child 1986; 140: 260–261.

43 Miller K, Atkin B, Moody ML. Drug therapy for nocturnal enuresis. Current treatment recommendations. Drugs 1992; 44: 47–56.

44 Mishra PC, Agarwal VK, Rahman H. Therapeutic trial of amtriptyline in the treatment of nocturnal enuresis – a controlled study. Indian Pediatr 1980; 17: 279.

45 DeLeon G, Mandell AJ. A comparison of conditioning and psychotherapy and the treatment of functional enuresis. J Clin Psychol 1966; 22: 326–330.

46 McKendry JB, Stewart DA, Kahnna F, Netley C. Primary enuresis: relative success of three methods of treatment. Can Med Assoc J 1975; 113: 953–955.

47 Moffatt ME, Kato C, Pless IB. Improvements in self concept after treatment of nocturnal enuresis: randomised controlled trial. J Pediatr 1987; 110: 647–652.

48 Goel KM, Thomson RB, Gibb EM, McAinsh TF. Evaluation of nine different types of enuresis alarms. Arch Dis Child 1984; 59: 748–753.

49 Butler RJ, Forsythe WI, Robertson J. The body worn alarm in the treatment of childhood enuresis. BJCP 1990; 44(6): 237–241.

50 Doleys DM. Behavioural treatments for nocturnal enuresis in children: a review of the recent literature. Psychol Bull 1970; 1: 30.

51 Wagner W, Johnsson SS, Walker D, Carter R, Wittner J. A controlled comparison of two treatments for nocturnal enuresis. J Pediatr 1982; 101: 302–307.

52 Sukhai RN, Mol J, Harris AS. Combined therapy of enuresis alarm and desmopressin in the treatment of nocturnal enuresis. Eur J Pediatr 1989; 148: 465–467.

53 Muellner SR. Development of urinary control in children: a new concept in cause, prevention and treatment of primary enuresis. J Urol 1960; 84: 714–716.

54 Butler RJ. Nocturnal enuresis: psychological perspectives. Bristol: Wright, 1987.

55 Street E, Broughton L. The treatment of childhood nocturnal enuresis in the community. Child: Care, Health and Development 1990; 16: 365–372.

56 Kempe CH, Helfer RE. Helping the battered child and his family. Oxford: Lippincott, 1972.

57 Olness K. The use of self-hypnosis in the treatment of childhood nocturnal enuresis. Clin Pediatr (Phila) 1975; 14: 273–279.

58 Dimson S. Desmopressin as a treatment for enuresis. (letter). Lancet 1977; 1: 1260.

59 Klauber GT. Clinical efficacy and safety of desmopressin in the treatment of nocturnal enuresis. J Pediatr 1989; 114: 719–722.

60 Miller K, Goldberg S, Atkin B. Nocturnal enuresis: experience with long term use of intranasally administered desmopressin. J Pediatr 1989; 114 (4 pt 2): 723–726.

61 Hunsballe JM, Hansen TK, Rittig S, Norgaard JP, Pedersen EB, Djurhuus JC. Pathogenic differences in nocturnal enuresis – polyuric and non-polyuric bedwetting. Abstract. 2nd ICCS Rome, 1993.

62 Hogg RJ, Husman D. The role of family history in predicting response to desmopressin in nocturnal enuresis. J Urol 1993; 150: 444–445.

63 Blackwell B, Currah J. The psychopharmacology of nocturnal enuresis. In: Kolvin I, MacKeith RC, Meadow SR (eds) Bladder control and enuresis. London: Heinemann, pp 231–257.

64 Hindmarch I, Alford C, Barwell F, Kerr JS. Measuring the side effects of psychotropics: the behavioural toxicity of antidepressants. J Psychopharm 1992; 6: 198–203.

65 Kass EJ, Diokono AC, Montealegre A. Enuresis: principles of management and result of treatment. J Urol 1979; 121: 794–796.

27 Genitourinary fistulae

Genitourinary fistulae reported in 4000-year-old mummies are almost certainly of obstetric origin. When Faith Howard performed her own vaginal hysterectomy in 1670, a second major etiology of this distressing condition was introduced. Although H. Van Roonhyse described vaginal repair of fistulae in 1672, it was not until George Hayward in 1839 and J. Marion Sims in 1852[1] reported successful surgical repair that relief from this condition was possible. Unfortunately, in the developing world there are still large numbers of women outcast by their society who do not have direct access to surgical treatment. The most common simple genitourinary fistulae are vesicovaginal (42%), ureterovaginal (34%), urethrovaginal (11%) and vesicocervical (3%).[2] There are other rare forms of genitourinary fistulae, such as vesico-ovarian[3] or vesicouterine. More complex mixed fistulae include vesicouterovaginal, vesicouterouterine, vesicovaginorectal and vesicosalpingovaginal.

VESICOVAGINAL FISTULAE

In developed countries the most common etiology of vesicovaginal fistulae is gynecological surgery, accounting for between 44% and 74% of cases.[4,5] Total abdominal hysterectomy for benign gynecological disease is the most common surgical procedure that results in such fistula (Fig. 27.1), although it may be seen after anterior repair, vaginal hysterectomy, radical hysterectomy, laparoscopic pelvic surgery, urological surgery, radiotherapy, pelvic malignancy, pelvic trauma and even sexual intercourse.[6] Obstetric injury in the developed world resulting in vesicovaginal fistula is now remarkably rare,[7] although it is the primary cause in the developing world (Fig. 27.2). The reasons why vesicovaginal fistula may follow abdominal hysterectomy include anatomical distorsion by fibroids, endometriosis or previous surgery; failure to recognize a direct bladder injury at the time of surgery; inappropriate suture placement at the vaginal cuff for closure or hemostasis; and lack of surgical expertise.

Prevention of such surgical injury is of prime importance and rests with appropriate surgical training; immediate detection of vesical injury aided on occasion by instillation of indigo carmine or methylene blue into the bladder; a two-layered watertight closure of the defect once identified; and appropriate prolonged vesical drainage. Predisposing

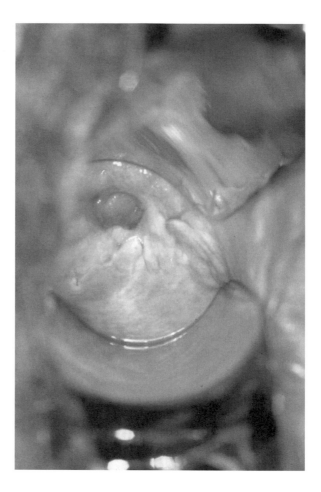

Fig. 27.1 Small vesicovaginal fistula anterior to the vaginal vault, presented with urinary leakage per vaginam 11 days after an apparently uncomplicated hysterectomy for fibroids
(With permission from Paul Hilton)

factors to vesical injury include obesity, pelvic inflammatory disease, endometriosis, previous pelvic surgery, diabetes, hypertension and atherosclerosis.

The typical presenting symptom of vesicovaginal fistula is continuous incontinence both day and night. Presentation may occur within days of surgery or may be delayed for up to 20 years after radiotherapy. In some cases it is difficult to distinguish the loss as a consequence of a vesicovaginal fistula from other causes of urinary incontinence. Indeed, if the fistula is small one may be misled into thinking that the vaginal loss is simply physiological or an infective vaginal discharge. In association with the loss of urine there may be excoriation of the vulva and thighs. Large fistulae can be easy to see in the left lateral position with the Sims speculum. Urine may be found pooling in the vagina and there is absence of urinary loss from the urethral meatus on coughing or straining, but a trickle of urine is seen coming from the introitus. On occasion, of course, more than one etiology for the urinary incontinence may exist. Confirmation of a vesicovaginal fistula can be obtained by instilling coloured dye, such as indigo carmine or methylene blue, into the bladder and seeing it discharge vaginally. Some authors believe that sterile milk is

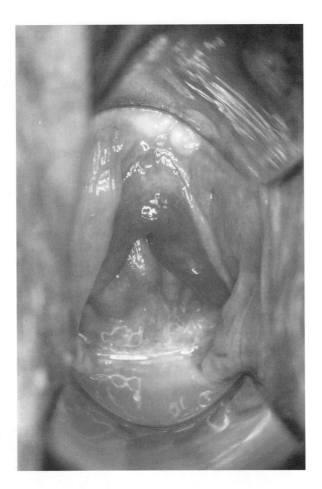

Fig. 27.2 Large vesicovaginal fistula, with pooling of urine in the vagina, following obstructed labour (With permission from Paul Hilton)

more useful for clear identification of the site of the fistula as it does not stain the vaginal tissues.[5]

The three-swab test[7] or its modification[8] help one to locate the site of a small fistula. In this test gauze swabs 10 cm square are inserted sequentially into the vagina. Methylene blue is then instilled into the bladder. The swabs are removed half an hour later with the site of fistula being suggested by the most heavily stained swab. Although highly suggestive of a vesicovaginal fistula, a positive result is not diagnostic as vaginal loss of methylene blue may be seen with ureteric reflux and a ureterovaginal fistula. If any of the swabs are wet but not stained with methylene blue then this is suggestive of a ureterovaginal fistula. The swab should be wrung out and the fluid sent for estimation of urea and creatinine. Once a diagnosis of vesicovaginal fistula has been made or strongly suggested by these clinical investigations, all patients should undergo a micturating cystogram (Fig. 27.3), intravenous urography (Figs. 27.4 and 27.5), cystourethroscopy and inspection of the vagina under general anaesthetia. If more than one fistula is located then the patient should also undergo a retrograde study.[9] If there is a suggestion of a pelvic malignancy then the fistula should be biopsied. Rarely, small vesicovaginal fistulae may heal spontaneously with prolonged bladder drainage,[10,39] but if healing has

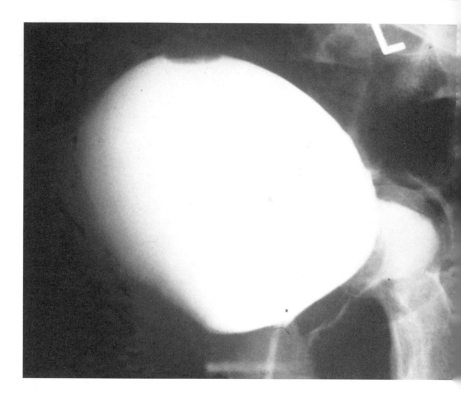

Fig. 27.3   Micturating cystogram showing contrast medium leaking out of the bladder, on the left, due to a vesicovaginal fistula (With permission from Paul Hilton)

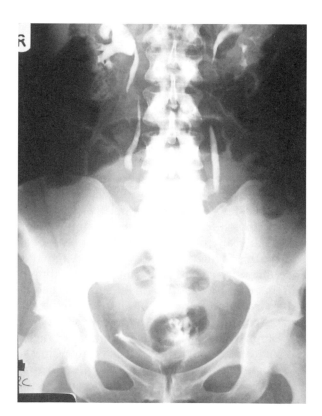

Fig. 27.4   Intravenous urogram showing contrast extravasating into the pelvis (With permission from Paul Hilton)

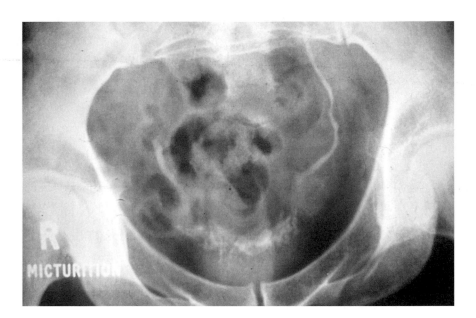

Fig. 27.5 Intravenous urogram (post-micturition film) showing contrast medium within the pelvis, outside the urinary tract

not occurred after 3–4 weeks, there is little point in continuing with this management course. Falk & Orkin[12] have reported the successful fulguration of small fistulae via a cystocope and others have been successful using Fibrinogen injected directly into the fistula.[13,14] Aycinem has forced a metal screw through the fistula tract creating raw edges and has achieved successful outcomes.[15] Once the diagnosis has been made the bladder may be drained with a urethral catheter. Sometimes it is necessary to put a second catheter through the fistula vaginally to ensure that the patient is acceptably dry.[16]

Alternatives to this are a modified vaginal diaphragm with an attached Foley catheter that is placed vaginally over the fistula to allow controlled vaginal drainage of urine,[17,18] or adequate pads with frequent changes in those where catheterization is not suitable. In the latter one sometimes encounters problems with perineal irritation. In those women who are postmenopausal, estrogen therapy either by local application or systemic administration will improve the vaginal tissues. Antibiotics will be required in 50% of cases to treat concurrent urinary tract infections. Oral corticosteroids have been used to facilitate early repair in the belief that edema and fibrosis around the fistula will be reduced.[19] However, this must be weighed against the potential detrimental effect on wound healing.[20]

Still one of the most controversial areas surrounding vesicovaginal fistula repair is its timing. The tradition has been to allow 3–6 months before surgical correction so that there is complete resolution of inflammation and edema that relates to the original insult, the area of devascularization is completely demarcated and there is clear delineation of fibrotic tissue. When the fistula is inspected and there is epithelialization of the tract with surrounding viable tissue, then surgery should be attempted. This approach has many supporters.[2,21,22,23] One drawback is that it exacerbates the patient's inevitable distress which results from both the incontinence and the change in lifestyle that ensues. Early repair, particularly if the injury is due to surgical trauma, has found increasing popularity and its proponents cite their own good surgical results.[24,25,26]

Adherence to surgical principles is the most important element in obtaining successful cure for patients with vesicovaginal fistula. These include the stipulation that the tissues should be in optimal condition, free of infection, inflammation and cancer; that there should be wide exposure of the fistula and surrounding area; that there should be extensive mobilization of all layers; that there should be excision of fibrous tissue; that the closure should be layered using absorbable sutures, which cause minimal tissue reaction; and that there should be interposition of flaps or grafts where the repair is tenuous. Many authors include in their basic surgical principles wide excision of the fistulous tract with freshening of the edges.[27,28] However, it has been argued that this is unnecessary for successful repair and simply enlarges the defect and may jeopardize the ureter.[29] In most instances the surgical approach to the repair of the vesicovaginal fistula, be it vaginal or abdominal, is determined by the experience and training of the surgeon. On the whole gynecologists tend to repair vesicovaginal fistulae vaginally and urologists tend to repair them abdominally, with some experts performing combined procedures.[31] In certain instances the abdominal or combined approach is more appropriate and these would include large or multiple fistulae, poor vaginal access, ureteric involvement where other urological procedures would be required, recurrent fistulae and the presence of poor quality tissues, perhaps as a consequence of radiotherapy.[21,11] Vaginal surgery has the advantage that it is a relatively minor procedure which is well tolerated without an abdominal wound and this results in a short recovery time. On occasion, however, there may be some loss of functional vaginal length and stress incontinence may ensure as a consequence of altered mobility of the bladder neck.[2]

When a vaginal repair is to be performed the patient is usually placed in the dorsal lithotomy position, although the inverted lithotomy position with the patient face down on the operating table has been used to improve access to the anterior vaginal wall.[30] A small Foley catheter is passed through the fistula from the vagina and, with the balloon inflated, gentle traction is applied[11,2,5] to improve access to the fistula. With the fistula tract so delineated a vaginal incision is made. This may be a vertical incision of the vaginal wall extending around the fistula, or a J-shaped incision starting posterior to the fistula with the curve of the 'J' running around the anterior aspect of the fistula.

The vaginal skin is undercut, separating the bladder from the vagina at least 1.5–2 cm from the fistula.[11,22] At this point most authors would excise the fistula and debride the edges, although this does not appear to improve success.[11] If there is excessive tension on the vaginal skin longitudinal releasing incisions may be made 3–4 cm lateral to the midline 3–0 Dexon is used for the first row of sutures to close the bladder. The sutures may be inserted so that they invert the edges of the fistula into the bladder or the knots of this layer may be left to lie internally. The sutures should be interrupted. A second layer of interrupted sutures using 3–0 Dexon is then used to close the perivesical fascia. It is commonly recommended that this be at right angles to the original suture line. The vagina is then closed in an interrupted layer. An alternative incision is a circumferential incision[2] around the fistula. The vaginal epithelium is then denuded leaving the fistula tract exposed centrally. The tract is then excised and the bladder and vagina are closed in three layers as previously described. If the fistula is close to the ureter, to save ureteric reimplantation one may leave the fistula tract intact with a ureteric catheter in place. In such circumstances safe closure of the defect is possible without impinging on the ureter.

Occasionally, when the repair is considered tenuous or the tissues are devitalized, an improvement of vascularity is possible with the interposition of a well-vascularized flap. For the vaginal closure this is relatively easy using a pad of labial fat as described by Martius.[28,32] Here a 5-cm incision is made along the lateral border of the labium majora and the fibrofatty tissue is exposed. This is then tunnelled to the vaginal incision and the fibrofatty tissue is sutured over the bladder closure. The vaginal skin is then closed over the graft. An alternative described by Ingleman-Sundberg[29] uses the gracilis muscle once detached from the medial condyle of the femur. Excellent surgical results are obtained.

The Latzko procedure[33,34] is an alternative vaginal operation. This is considered to be easy, fast and less traumatic.[2] The posterior vaginal wall becomes the posterior wall of the bladder with the aim of eventual re-epithelialization with transitional epithelium. First an elliptical incision is made around the fistula. The fistula is left intact and a partial colpocleisis is performed. Excellent results can be obtained.[37] The Latzko procedure can also be performed in combination with a Martius flap, gracilis flap or indeed a fascia lata patch.[35] The vaginal approach for simple vesicovaginal fistula results in cure of over 90% of cases.[36,37,38,39,40]

For the abdominal repair of vesicovaginal fistula the patient is positioned supine on the operating table with the legs apart and supported to allow access to the vagina. Some authors recommend packing the vagina, but this precludes the possibility of inserting a finger into the vagina to aid abdominal localization of the fistula tract, dissection and mobilization. The incision of choice is a subumbilical midline cut which can always be extended upwards if mobilization of the omentum is required. The Pfannenstiel incision is inadequate for such surgery, although as a compromise in the 'scar conscious' a Turner-Warwick suprapubic 'V' incision[42] or a Turner-Warwick suprapubic cross incision is an alternative to the midline. The abdominal repair of vesicovaginal fistula may be transvesical extraperitoneal or supravesical intraperitoneal. The transvesical route is similar in concept to the vaginal repair. The bladder is opened at the dome and the fistula identified. The bladder muscle is dissected off the vagina operating through the bladder and all fibrous or devitalized tissue is excised. The vagina and bladder are then closed in layers.

Commonly this technique has the drawback of affording poor access to the site of the fistula. Most surgeons therefore choose the supravesical intraperitoneal technique, although actual practice varies. O'Conor[39] led the way with bisection of the bladder to the level of the fistula after initial mobilization. The bladder is then dissected off the vagina and all devitalized tissue removed. The vagina and bladder are closed in separate layers. Turner-Warwick recommends that this posterior bladder incision is not in the midline but curved laterally to achieve a tension-free closure if there is induration librosis or radiation injury. Ureteric catherization is often required to protect the ureters. Some authors do not bivalve the bladder in this manner but use the transperitoneal approach to separate the bladder from the vagina at the site of the fistula, with a cystotomy being used to aid in this dissection.[2] As with the vaginal repair a flap of tissue may be interposed between vagina and bladder, thus supplying an alternative blood supply and lymphatic drainage to poor tissues. A number of different flaps have been proposed, such as a peritoneal flap,[40] gracilis muscle[41] and an epiploic appendix from the sigmoid colon; however, by far the most popular graft is that of the omentum, which has been expounded by Turner-Warwick.[43] In 33% of cases[43] the omental apron is long enough to reach the perineum once it is mobilized from the transverse colon. The blood supply to the omentum comes from the gastroepiploic arch on the greater curvature of the stomach. The right component is dominant and indeed the right side is lower than the left. In 30% of cases sufficient length of omentum is gained by just dividing the left gastroepiploic pedicle and the branches of the splenic vessel. In the remaining 40% the short gastric branches need to be ligated, thus dislocating the omentum from the greater curvature of the stomach. These vessels are divided above the gastroepilpoic arch, thereby maintaining the vascularity of this pedicle. Once one has commenced dividing the short gastric branches one should continue to the gastroduodenal origin, as traction may easily tear an undivided branch. The omentum so mobilized is an excellent tissue to interpose between the vagina and vesical surfaces of the fistula. Tissue flaps are of greatest use in recurrent fistulae, post-irradiation fistulae and large and complex fistulae.

The mainstay of postoperative management is continuous gravitational urinary drainage. This may be accomplished either by a urethral or suprapubic catheter or a combination. If catheters are combined then the urethral catheter may be removed at day 5 and all catheters are usually removed 10–14 days after the operation,[33,39,44] although a shorter duration of drainage of 24–72 h has been recommended.[37] Broad spectrum antibiotics are prescribed intravenously for 48 h and then orally until all catheters are removed. In postmenopausal patients preoperative oestrogen are continued and occasionally anticholinergic agents may be required to relieve bladder spasm.

Using either the abdominal or vaginal route for simple vesicovaginal fistula treatment, a cure rate of 90% or over should be expected. Even in difficult postradiation vesicovaginal fistulae high cure rates are possible if the appropriate operation with tissue interposition is chosen. Apart from surgical failure, urinary incontinence secondary to bladder neck incompetence and ureteric obstruction may be seen as postoperative complications.

URETHROVAGINAL FISTULAE

Urethrovaginal fistula is less common than the vesicovaginal fistula, although the two may coexist. In developing countries the major etiological factor is childbirth, which results in ischemic necrosis of the bladder, bladder neck and urethra. The defects so caused may be massive. The urethrovaginal fistula in the developed world is usually a consequence of anterior repair with or without a vaginal hysterectomy, urethral diverticulectomy (Fig. 27.6) or bladder neck suspension procedures. The site of the fistula usually dictates symptoms. Where the fistula is distal to the point of maximal urethral pressure there may be no symptoms, or there may be the symptom of spraying of urine or post-micturition incontinence as the vagina empties urine that has entered during voiding. As the site of the fistula progresses towards the bladder neck, urinary stress incontinence or recurrent urinary tract infection may become more predominant. When the fistula is proximal to the urethral sphincter mechanism, continuous incontinence is inevitable. The surgical repair of the urethrovaginal fistula is often difficult,[12] as there may be considerable loss of tissue and extensive surrounding fibrosis. In essence the repair is a three-layer repair after the vaginal wall has been mobilized

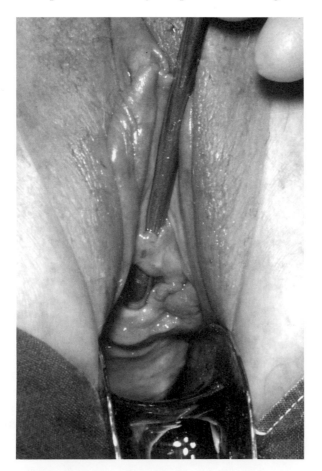

Fig. 27.6 Urethrovaginal fistula following the repair of a urethral diverticulum (with permission from Paul Hilton)

from the urethra or bladder. A urethral Foley catheter is sometimes use
ful to aid in closure of the urethral defect. One should aim for a two
layered closure of the urethra before the vaginal wall closure. If this i
not possible then it is recommended that a flap be inserted between th
vagina and urethra.[32] Either a gracilis muscle flap or a labial flap as de
scribed earlier may be used, and this improves the chance of successfu
return of continence. Overall one would expect a cure rate for urethro
vaginal fistula repair of between 73 and 100%.[45,46] This is certainly lowe
than seems possible with the vesicovaginal fistula and occasionally tw
or more attempts at closure are necessary.[55,54]

OTHER FISTULAE

Ureteric injury occurs in between 0.5 and 1% of all pelvic operations.[47] C
these, fistula formation is seen in 50% of patients.[48] Gynecologica
procedures, in particular abdominal hysterectomy, are the most commonl
implicated. Frequently, the gynecological surgery is complicated b
endometriosis, infection or malignancy. Indeed, the commonly use
Pfannenstiel incision itself with its limited surgical access may contribut
towards a number of postoperative fistulae. Only 20–30% of injuries ar
recognized at the time of surgery. The most common site of injury is th
distal part of the ureter as it passes under the uterine artery.[47] If injury
suspected during surgery, then the ureter may be cannulated retr
gradely at open cystotomy or by a cystoscopy. Alternatively, the patie
may have an intravenous bolus of indigo carmine or methylene blu
with Mannitol. The leak rapidly becomes obvious. In 10% of cas
hematuria maybe seen. When injury is not noted at surgery it may tak
days or even weeks before the patient presents. Prior to the vaginal loss
urine the patient may have an ileus, a fever or loin pain if there is
urinoma or an element of obstruction. The diagnosis is usually obviou
once a urinary leak has established. Confirmation may be achieved wit
dye studies: the vagina is packed and red carmine is instilled in the bladd
and indigo carmine given intravenously. The colour of the pack w
indicate the type of fistula.[51] An intravenous urogram must be performe
if a ureterovaginal fistula is suspected. This investigation will identi
upper tract obstruction and also drainage of contrast from the ureter in
the vagina will be seen. Retrograde pyelography may be helpful to clari
the diagnosis and plan management.

The treatment of ureterovaginal fistula has changed since Gross
1885 reported 12 cases cured of ureteric fistulae by a nephrectomy.
Indeed, conservative management with nephrostomy and/or double
stenting may result in closure of up to 50% of fistulae with maintenan
of upper tract function.[50] Retrograde ureteral stent placement can
difficult. This should be attempted with a nephrostomy as soon as t
fistula is diagnosed so that prompt drainage of urine is possible and t
upper tract is preserved.[11] As with a vesicovaginal fistula, there are tho
who advocate early recourse to surgical repair[25,44] and those w
recommend some delay to allow for spontaneous healing and an improv

ment in the viability of the tissues under question. If a conservative approach is taken it is important that renal function be assessed regularly as reduction of vaginal drainage may be a reflection of obstruction and not cure. The type of surgical repair would depend on the site of injury. As 90% of injuries are low a urethroneocystostomy is usually combined with an antireflux procedure. If the injury is higher or a considerable amount of the ureter has been lost, then a psoas hitch or an Ocherbland-Boari flap may be required.[52] If this surgical repair is not suitable then there are numerous alternatives including kidney mobilization, ileal ureteric substitution, renal autotransplantation or transreterostomy. Occasionally, a nephrectomy is the most suitable option, or on the physically unfit laparoscopic ligation of the ureter above the fistula may be performed.

More unusual fistulae may be seen between bladder and ovary,[3] bladder and fallopian tube,[53] and more commonly bladder and uterus. The last two usually result from vaginal hysterectomy or Caesarean section respectively.[54] Jobert de Lamballe in 1852[55] described covering the cervix with vaginal tissue to direct the menstrual flow into the bladder. Surgical treatment now follows the standard principles of excision of the tract and layered closure of viable tissue. In the case of a fistula between the bladder and fallopian tube or bladder and ovary, the operation of choice is probably salpingo-oophorectomy. Spontaneous closure of vesicouterine fistulae may be seen following induced amenorrhea[2] or after prolonged urinary catheter drainage.

Genitourinary fistulae represent a disaster to the patient. We must endeavor to ensure adequate and appropriate training for all concerned in obstetric management and pelvic surgery. Once the condition has developed then sympathetic treatment is of paramount importance. Adherence to standard surgical principles will usually result in an excellent outcome.

REFERENCES

1 Sims. JM. The treatment of vesicovaginal fistula. Am J Med Sci 1852; 23: 59.
2 Jonas U,Petri E. Genitourinary fistula. In: Stanton SL (ed) clinical gynaecological urology. Mosby, 1984.
3 Carl P. Vesico-ovarian fistula in suppurative ovarian inflammation and salpingitis. J Urol 1990; 143: 352.
4 Everett HS, Mattingly RF. Urinary tract injuries resulting from pelvic surgery. Am J Obstet Gynaecol 1956; 71: 502–514.
5 Goodwin WE, Scardino PT. Vesicovaginal and ureterovaginal fistulas: a summary of 25 years experience. J Urol 1980; 123: 370–374.
6 Sharma SK, Madhusudnan P, Kumar A, Bapna BC. Vesicovaginal fistulas of uncommon aetiology. J Urol 1987; 137: 289.
7 Moir JC. Vesicovaginal fistulae as seen in Britain. Br J Obst Gynaecol Brit. Commonwealth 1973; 80: 598.
8 Gannon M. The three swab test using knots for urovaginal fistula. Surgery, Gynaecology & Obstetrics 1980; 170: 171.
9 Blandy JP, Badenoch DF, Fowler CG, Jenkins BJ, Thomas N. Early repair of iatrogenic injury to the ureter or bladder after gynaecological surgery. J Urol 1991; 146: 761.
10 Zimmern PE, Leach CE. Vesicovaginal fistula repair. Probl Urol 1991; 5: 171.
11 Gerber G, Schoenberg H. Female urinary tract fistulas. J Urol 1993; 149: 229–236.

12 Falk HC, Orkin LA. Non surgical closure of vesicovaginal fistulas. Obstet Gynaecol 1957; 9: 538.

13 Pettersson S, Hedelin H. Jansson I, Teger-Nilsson A. Fibrin occlusion of a vesicovaginal fistula. Lancet 1979; 1: 933.

14 Hedelin H, Nilson A, Teger-Nilsson A, Thorsen G. Fibrin occlusion of fistulas postoperatively. Surg Gynaecol & Obstet 1982; 154: 366.

15 Aycinena JF. Small vesicovaginal fistula. Urology 1977; 9: 543.

16 Magee MC. The changing social implications of vesico vaginal fistulas; linking vesical catheters – a useful adjunct. J Urol 1979; 122: 260–262.

17 Banfield P et al. A modified contraceptive diaphragm for relief of uretero-vaginal fistula. Br J Obstet Gynaecol 1991; 98: 101–102.

18 Landes R. Simple transvesical repair of vesico vaginal fistula. J Urol 1979; 122: 604–606.

19 Collins CG, Pent D, Jones F. Results of early repair of vesico vaginal fistula with preliminary cortisone treatment. Am J Obstet Gynaecol 1960; 80: 1005.

20 Symmonds R. Verhutung und Behandlung von Urogenital-fisteln. Extracta Gynaecol 1980; 4: 103–116.

21 Wein AJ. Vesicovaginal fistula. In: Resnick MI, Kursh E (eds) Current therapy in genitourinary surgery. Philadelphia: BC Decker, 1987: pp 209–213.

22 O'Conor VJ. Review of experience with vesicovaginal fistula repair. J Urol 1980; 123: 367.

23 Persky L, Rabin R. Experiences with vesicovaginal fistulas. Am J Surg 1973; 125: 763.

24 Persky L, Herman B, Guerrier K. Non-delay on vesicovaginal fistula repair. Urology 1979; 13: 273.

25 Blandy J, Badenocu D, Fowler C, Jenkins B & Thomas N Early. Repair of iatrogenic injury. To tie ureter or bladder after gynecological surgery J Urol 1991; 146: 761.

26 Zimmern P, Hadley H, Staskin D, Raz S. Genitourinary fistulae: vaginal approach for repair of vesicovaginal fistulae. Clin North Am 1985; 12: 361–367.

27 Barnes R, Hadley H, Johnston O. Transvaginal repair of vesicovaginal fistulae. Urology 1977; 10: 258.

28 Martius H. Die operative Wiederherstellung der vollkommen fehlenden Harnrohre und des Schiessmushels derselber. Zentralbl Gynak 1928; 52: 480.

29 Ingleman-Sundberg A. Pathogenesis & operative treatment of urinary fistulae in irradiated tissue. In: Youssef AF (ed) Gynaecological urology. Springfield, Illinois: Charles C Thomas, 1960: p 263.

30 Hamlin RHJ, Nicholas EC. Reconstruction of urethra totally destroyed in labour. BMJ 1969; 1: 147.

31 Marshall VF, Vesidovaginal fistulas on the urological service 1979; J urol 121: 25–29.

32 Birkhoff JD, Wechler M, Romas N. Urinary fistulas: vaginal repair using a labial fat pad. J Urol 1977; 117: 595.

33 Staskin DR. Vesicovaginal fistula. In: Glenn JF (ed) Urologic surgery, 4th edn. Philadelphia: JB Lippincott, 1991: pp 474–483.

34 Radar ES. Post hysterectomy vesicovaginal fistula: treatment by partial colpocleisis. J Urol 114: 389–390.

35 Hribar Der interessante Fale: Verschluss einer Vesicovaginal fistel mit Hilfe eines aufgeklebten Patches. Altern Urologie 1977; 8: 221–223.

36 Käser O. The Latzko operation for vesicovaginal fistulae. Acta Obstet Gynaecol Scand. 56: 427–431.

37 Trancer ML. The post total hysterectomy (vault) vesicovaginal fistula. J Urol 1980; 123: 839.

38 Gonzalez R, Fraley EE. Surgical repair of post hysterectomy vesicovaginal fistula. J Urol 1976; 115: 660–663.

39 O'Conor VJ Jr. Review of experience with vesicovaginal fistula repair. J Urol 1980; 123 367.

40 Petri E, Hohenfellner R. Zur Therapie komplizieter Blasenscheidenfistlen. Gynakologe 1981; 14: 177–182.

41 Fleishmann J, Picha G. Abdominal approach for gracilis muscle interposition and repair of recurrent vesicovaginal fistulas. J Urol 1988; 140: 552.

42 Turner-Warwick R, Worth P, Milsoy E, Duchett J, The suprapubic V-incision Brit J Urol 1974; 46: 39–45.

43 Turner-Warwick R. The use of omentum pedical graft in the urinary tract reconstruction. J Urol 1976; 116: 341–347.

44 Badenoch DF, Tiftaft R, Thackar D, Fowler CJ, Blandy JP. Early repair of accidental injury to the ureter or bladder following gynaecological surgery. Brit J Urol 1987; 59: 516.

45 Gray LA. Urethrovaginal fistulas. Am J Obstet Gynaecol 1968; 101: 28.

46 Keettel W, Sehring F, de Prosse C & Scott Surgical management of urethrovaginal and vesidovaginal fistulas. Amer J. Obstet Gynac 1978; 131: 425.

47 Mattingley RF, Barkowf HI. Acute operative injury to the lower urinary tract. Clin Obstet Gynaecol 1978; 5: 123–149.

48 Higgins CC. Ureteral injuries during surgery. A review of 87 cases. JAMA 1967; 199: 82–88.

49 Gross SW. Nephrectomy: its indications & contraindications. Am J Med Sci 1885; 90: 79.

50 Turner WH, Cranston DW, Davies AH, Fellows CJ, Smith JC. Double J stents in the treatment of gynaecological injury to the ureter. Journal of the Royal Society of Medicine 1990; 83: 623–624.

51 Raghavaiah NV. Double-dye test to diagnose various types of vaginal fistulas. J Urol 1974; 112: 811–812.

52 Ocherbland NF. Re-implantation of the ureter into the bladder by a flap method. J Urol 1947; 57: 845.

53 Turner B, Ekbladh L, Edson M. Vesicosalpingovaginal fistula. Urology 1976; 8: 49.

54 Lenkovsky Z, Pode D, Shapiro A, Caine M. Vesicouterine fistula: a rare complication of Caesarean section J Urol 1988; 139: 123.

55 de Lamballe J. Traité des fistules vesico-uterines, vesico-utero-vaginales. Cited in Bardescon N. Ein neues Vefahren fur die Operahin der tiefen Blasen-uters-Schiedenfisteln. Zentralbl Gynaekol 1900; 6: 170–182.

Section 5 Special Problems

28

The urinary tract in pregnancy

Pregnancy is a time when many bodily systems undergo both anatomical and functional alterations and the urinary tract is no exception. The upper urinary tract, kidneys and ureters undergo dilatation and renal function is altered. The lower urinary tract has changes in its own right and these are further influenced by altered renal function. Superimposed on the physiological changes that occur are abnormalities which take place due to pathological states of pregnancy and from labor.

UPPER URINARY TRACT

The kidneys increase in size by 1 cm in length in normal pregnancy. Dilatation of the renal calyces, renal pelvis and ureters also takes place.[1,2] Dilatation is more marked on the right than the left and this may be due to dextrorotation of the uterus, which applies increased pressure on the right side of the urinary tract. In addition, the sigmoid colon protects the left ureter from undue pressure. There is also an increase in renal parenchymal volume. This functional dilatation which occurs is thought to be due to the muscle-relaxing effect of the raised progesterone level. It has implications for pregnant women as stasis of urine in the upper urinary tract predisposes to pyelonephritis in those women with asymptomatic bacteriuria. Due to the dilatation which occurs, it is important not to undertake radiological studies of the upper tract until 4 months post partum as otherwise results may be erroneous.

Functional changes occur in the kidneys during pregnancy. There is an increase in renal plasma flow and glomerular filtration rate. There is an increase of about 50% occurring shortly after conception with a further rise in the second trimester.[3,4] In the third trimester there is a reduction, but levels remain above prepregnancy values.[5] These changes alter blood biochemistry and must be considered in the interpretation of renal function tests. Normal plasma creatinine, urea and urate values are below the normal range for the non-pregnant woman and plasma osmolality also falls. Values should be judged according to the gestation at which they are measured. Indeed, creatinine clearance is increased in pregnancy and an apparently normal value may signify pathology.

Urinary tract infection

True bacteriuria is defined as a pure growth of at least 10^5 organisms from a clean midstream specimen of urine[6] or any growth from a sample obtained by suprapubic aspiration.[7] Ideally, two specimens should be obtained to exclude contamination. Antiseptic solutions should not be used to clean the vulva prior to collection as this will result in false negative results.[8]

The prevalence of asymptomatic bacteriuria is no different in the pregnant from in the non-pregnant female population and is between 2 and 10%.[9] It is not the asymptomatic bacteriuria which is a problem but rather the development of acute pyelonephritis, which is more common in pregnancy and may result in adverse pregnancy outcome.

Up to 40% of women with asymptomatic bacteriuria in pregnancy will develop a symptomatic urinary tract infection.[10] For this reason all pregnant women should be screened for asymptomatic bacteriuria. To send a specimen for culture is time-consuming and expensive, and therefore alternative screening methods have been developed.[11,12] Reagent strip testing for nitrites, leucocyte esterase, protein and blood in the urine has a positive predictive value of 10.5% for urinary tract infection. More importantly, it has a negative predictive value of 99.3%. Looking at protein and blood as the sole screening method has a positive predictive value of 19.7% and a negative predictive value of 98.1%.[12] Those women with a positive screen would then have a midstream specimen of urine sent for full culture and sensitivity.

About 2% of those women with initial negative cultures will develop bacteriuria later in pregnancy. This, however, constitutes a significant number as it is 2% of the 95% of pregnant women with initially clear urine, i.e. about 30% of cases of significant bacteriuria.[13] Thus even if an initial specimen is clear, it is important to retest any women with either symptoms or with blood or protein in the urine on dipstick testing.

Since acute pyelonephritis may be associated with fetal problems, it is important that all cases of asymptomatic bacteriuria should be treated. Sensitivity should be obtained prior to treatment but the choice of antibiotic is limited by the potential harmful effects on the fetus. Single-dose treatment probably has a higher failure rate and treatment should therefore be for 14 days.[14,15] A specimen of urine should be re-examined 1 week after treatment as up to 20% of women will have persistent bacteriuria. In those in whom initial treatment was successful there is a recurrence rate of up to 15% and these women must have monthly specimens tested throughout pregnancy.[15] If repeated recurrence is a problem, then full investigations should be undertaken 4 months post partum. These women may require long-term prophylactic treatment for the remainder of the pregnancy.

Acute cystitis

This occurs in about 1% of pregnant women[16] and 60% will have an initial negative screen. Symptoms are similar to those normally experienced in pregnancy, making diagnosis form symptomatology alone difficult. When identified these women should receive a full course of antibiotic treatment and be followed up as for asymptomatic bacteriuria.

Acute pyelonephritis

The prevalence is approximately 1–2% of pregnant women. Screening for asymptomatic bacteriuria will prevent 70% of cases.[17] Patients may be pyrexial with rigors and severe loin tenderness. They may have nausea and vomiting and often appear systemically unwell. They may also complain of uterine contractions and be in premature labor. Treatment should be with intravenous antibiotics, rehydration and analgesia. Treatment should initially be empirical while cultures are awaited. However, the differential diagnosis of other causes of pyrexia and abdominal pain must be sought.

Urinary calculi

Despite urinary stasis, obstruction and infection which would all make urinary calculi appear likely to be more common in pregnancy, the rate differs little from that in the non-pregnant population.[18] The prevalence is approximately 0.3%. The stones are normally single and predominantly calcium in composition. They are often difficult to diagnose and the main differential diagnosis is acute pyelonephritis. Demonstration of a dilated upper renal tract by ultrasound is unhelpful and radiological investigations are relatively contraindicated, but a single plain abdominal X-ray may be necessary and due to the calcium composition will identify many of the calculi. Initial treatment is intravenous fluids with adequate analgesia. Antibiotics are sometimes necessary as infection may develop due to stasis. Conservative management should be employed wherever possible during pregnancy.

LOWER URINARY TRACT

Studies of the lower urinary tract in pregnancy have been few. Subjective studies have reported the incidence of lower urinary tract symptoms and their changes during pregnancy. In addition, several authors have retrospectively assessed the effects of pregnancy on lower urinary tract symptoms. Objective studies have examined the lower urinary tract radiologically, using frequency/volume charts, urodynamically and with electromyography during pregnancy and post partum. There have also been reports on lower urinary tract dysfunction at some time interval after pregnancy and inferences have been drawn from these.

Symptoms

Lower urinary tract symptoms are very common in pregnancy. To date most studies have been concerned with the prevalence of abnormal voiding patterns and stress incontinence. More recently, other symptoms such as urgency, urge incontinence/and symptoms of voiding difficulties have been explored.

Voiding patterns

There are no standardized definitions of voiding patterns and most studies are not comparable due to differing definitions. Early reports suggest that diurnal frequency occurs in about 50% of women in the first trimester and speculate that during this time it is due to pressure on the bladder and thereafter due to recurrent urinary residuals often accompanied by infection.[19,20] Francis[21] questioned 400 women personally and found that the onset of frequency usually occurred in the first trimester, but once present it tended to get worse and did not resolve as was previously thought (Table 28.1). In addition, she found that 81% of women experienced frequency of micturition at some stage in pregnancy and that the prevalence was the same in both nulliparous and multiparous women.

Table 28.1 The prevalence of frequency in pregnancy according to Francis 1960a[21]

Early pregnancy	Mid pregnancy	Late pregnancy
59.5%	61%	81%

In the study by Stanton et al[22] the prevalence of frequency, nocturia and combined frequency and nocturia in 181 women was recorded. Questions were asked by a nurse in the antenatal clinic. The women were grouped according to parity for each of the gestations studied. Frequency was defined as at least 7 daytime voids and nocturia as at least 2 night-time voids. Diurnal frequency and combined diurnal and nocturnal frequency were significantly more common in nulliparous women at 38 weeks' and 40 weeks' gestation. In agreement with Francis[21] they found a steady increase throughout pregnancy. Table 28.2 gives a summary of their results for all women.

Table 28.2 The prevalence of frequency according to Stanton et al 1980[22]

	Before Preg.	Booking	32/40	36/40	38/40	40/40	Post Natal
Day	16%	45%	61%	72%	76%	85%	17%
Night	4%	22%	37%	46%	57%	64%	6%
Combined	1%	12%	27%	32%	43%	54%	1%

Parboosingh & Doig,[23] who defined nocturia as night-time voiding during 3 nights in a week, found a prevalence in the first trimester of 58%, in the second trimester of 57% and in the third trimester of 66%. However, this was a cross-sectional study with different women being questioned in each trimester.

We used the same definitions as Stanton et al[22] and found a similar prevalence of frequency (43%), nocturia (34%) and combined frequency and nocturia (18%) in early pregnancy.[24,25] Although abnormal voiding patterns appear to be very common in pregnancy and worsen as pregnancy progresses, it is an increase in the actual number of voids which a patient will complain of and in our study 91% of women complained of an increase in the number of voids in a 24-hr period (Table 28.3). Furthermore, Black women complained of less frequency and more nocturia than their White counterparts (Table 28.4), and this may further explain differences between previous studies where race was not taken into account.

Table 28.3   Voiding patterns prior to and during early pregnancy. Median values are given with interquartile ranges beneath in brackets

	Prepregnancy	Pregnancy
No. of day time voids	4 (3–4)	6 (5–8)
No of night-time voids	0 (0–0)	1 (0–2)
No. of voids per 24 h	4 (3–5)	7 (5–10)

From Cutner 1993[25]

Table 28.4   Prevalence of frequency, nocturia and combined frequency and nocturia during pregnancy by race and parity

	Black	White	Black	White
	Nullip (n = 53)	Nullip (n = 68)	Parous (n = 71)	Parous (n = 56)
Frequency	28%*	51%*	38%	55%
Nocturia	35%	22%	51%**	27%**
Combined Frequency and Nocturia	6%	15%	31%	20%

*p <0.05; **p <0.01
From Cutner 1993.[25]

We questioned 119 women prior to pregnancy (retrospectively) and at 20 weeks', 28 weeks' and 36 weeks' gestation and post partum (prospectively) about voiding patterns.[25] Figure 28.1 demonstrates the prevalence of frequency and nocturia at each visit. Differences between each visit are significant except between 20 weeks' and 28 weeks' gestation. In addition the prevalence is significantly greater post partum than prior to pregnancy. Those women who suffered a greater increase in the number of voids both during the day and at night were significantly less likely to return to their prepregnancy state. This may suggest that abnormal voiding is a learnt phenomena.

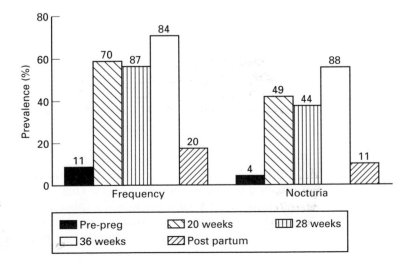

Fig. 28.1   Prevalence of frequency and nocturia according to gestation. (From Cutner A 1993. The lower urinary tract in pregnancy. MD Thesis, University of London, with permission.)

Thus, although increased frequency of micturition appears to be very common in pregnancy and tends to worsen with increasing gestation, the literature so far has been inconsistent because of the different definitions which have been employed. It is a change in the number of day-or night-time voids which a woman will complain of, so to use predefined limits is misleading as to the true prevalence of these symptoms. Finally, most studies have only examined the effect of parity and not racial origin on the prevalence of abnormal voiding patterns in pregnancy.

Causes

Malpas et al[26] performed radiological examination of the lower urinary tract in 32 pregnant women. They found distortion of the fundus of the bladder by the enlarged uterus and suggested that this pressure was likely to result in urinary frequency. This is in agreement with the findings of Hundley et al,[27] who cystoscoped 50 pregnant women and observed a characteristic saddle-shaped fundus to the bladder due to the enlarged uterus.

Francis[21] carried out radiological visualization in 83 pregnant women and confirmed distortion of the fundus of the bladder due to the gravid uterus. However, she rejected the idea of pressure leading to increased voiding patterns as it would not explain the high prevalence of nocturia, since pressure would be relieved in the recumbent position. However, a report of changes in lower urinary tract function after the treatment of uterine fibroids with gonadotropin-releasing hormone analogs has shown a significant reduction in urinary frequency, although there were no objective changes in bladder function.[28]

Both Francis[21] and Parboosingh & Doig[23] have studied urine output in a series of women in each trimester of pregnancy (Table 28.5). These

Table 28.5 The average urine output in pregnancy per 24 h in the studies by Francis (1960a)[21] and Parboosingh & Doig (1973a)[23]

	First Trimester	Second Trimester	Third Trimester	Non-Pregnant
	(n = 53)	(n = 68)	(n = 71)	(n = 56)
Francis	1.9 l	2.0 l	1.8 l	1.5 l
Parboosingh & Doig	1.3 l	1.3 l	1.3 l	1.1 l

were largely cross-sectional studies and compared values to those in non-pregnant normal controls. They concluded that the increased fluid intake and urine output alone was sufficient to explain the prevalence of frequency in pregnancy.

In addition, Parboosingh & Doig[23,29] suggested that with regard to nocturia it is increased nocturnal sodium excretion which results in increased urine production at night. This increased urine production in the first and second trimester would explain the prevalence of nocturia. In the third trimester urine production was reduced. However, the authors found a reduction in the volume of the first morning void and suggest that this would account for the high prevalence of nocturia in the third trimester despite the reduction in urine production.

We studied women in early pregnancy and in on-going pregnancy[25] and found a significant correlation between the number of voids and urine output. In addition, our results suggest that nocturia may be a result of more hours spent in bed and a decreased functional bladder capacity. Although we found little correlation between lower urinary tract symptoms and urodynamic findings in pregnancy,[30,31] we did find that women with low compliance had a significantly altered first desire to void and bladder capacity[25] (Table 28.6).

Table 28.6 First sensation and bladder capacity according to urodynamic diagnosis. Median values given with interquartile ranges below. Only significant differences are shown.

Parameter	Normal	Low Compliance	Phasic DI
First sensation (ml)	180 150–250 (n = 34)	150 100–150 (n = 23)	160 100–250 (n = 18)
		[p <0.05]	
Bladder capacity (ml)	420 400–475 (n = 34)	400 300–450 (n = 23)	450 350–500 (n = 18)
		[p <0.05]	[p <0.05]

From Cutner 1993[25]

The cystometric capacity of the pregnant bladder has been assessed by several authors. Muellner[32] performed 86 simple cystometrograms in pregnant women. He found that the bladder capacity gradually increased from 12 weeks' to 32 weeks' gestation where he found a surprisingly high average capacity of 1300 ml. There was also evidence of bladder atony in the third trimester. He claimed that there was a return to normal bladder tone by 6 weeks post partum. These findings were confirmed by Youssef,[33] who carried out similar studies in 10 pregnant women. Indeed, early animal studies looking at the effect of pregnancy on bladder muscle suggest that pregnancy reduces its tone and increases the bladder capacity.[34]

Francis[21] carried out 50 cystometrograms in pregnant women and found no difference in the bladder capacity in the first trimester compared to the normal non-pregnant state and no correlation between bladder capacity and frequency. Indeed, in each trimester she found women with large bladder capacities who complained of frequency and vice versa. However, she found a reduced bladder capacity in the third trimester and no evidence of bladder hypotonia but rather evidence of increased detrusor irritability in late pregnancy with unstable detrusor contractions.

Although the findings of these studies are contradictory, most of the data are cross-sectional and the relative change rather than absolute values may be of importance. In a longitudinal study, we found no significant differences in either the first desire to void or bladder capacity at 28 weeks' gestation, at 36 weeks' gestation or post partum (Table 28.7).[25]

Table 28.7   First desire to void and bladder capacities at each visit (n = 21)

	28 weeks' gestation	36 weeks' gestation	Postpartum
	First desire to void (ml)		
Median	190	250	200
(Mean)	(206)	(244)	(242)
Interquartile Range	100–300	200–300	175–300
Range	50–500	75–450	100–450
	Bladder capacity (ml)		
Median	475	430	440
(Mean)	(441)	(426)	(441)
Interquartile Range	400–500	350–500	400–490
Range	175–650	200–700	300–550

From Cutner 1993[25]

It may be that a combination of pressure effects, altered urine production and a relative change in bladder capacity leads to the development of frequency and nocturia. However, it is likely that large individual variations make most of the studies to date unreliable.

Prevention and treatment

If the causes are those that we have postulated, then there is no treatment in pregnancy and the patient who is troubled merely needs reassurance. However, if there is a marked increase in these symptoms antenatally or failure for symptoms to resolve post partum, then she should be investigated for the presence of a lower urinary tract infection. In addition, we have demonstrated[25] that those women who suffer a marked increased in their voiding pattern in pregnancy are less likely to return to their pre-pregnancy state. It would be interesting to determine whether bladder drill antenatally would improve postnatal symptoms in this group of women.

STRESS INCONTINENCE AND URGE INCONTINENCE

There is much debate as to whether pregnancy itself or labor results in stress incontinence. Although there have been several retrospective and a few prospective studies looking at this subject, it is important to appreciate that stress incontinence is merely a symptom and not synonymous with urethral sphincter incompetence.

Francis[35] found a 67% prevalence of stress incontinence in pregnancy, and it was significantly more common in multiparous women. In her study stress incontinence did not appear for the first time in the puerperium but rather during pregnancy itself. In addition, she found the time of onset of this symptom was equally distributed among the three trimesters but once present it gradually became more severe (Table 28.8).

Stanton et al[22] looked at the prevalence of stress incontinence in 181 women and in agreement with Francis[35] they found that it rarely occurs for the first time postnatally. The prevalence for nulliparous, multiparous

Table 28.8   Time of onset and prevalence of stress incontinence according to Francis 1960b[35]

	First Trimester	Second Trimester	Third Trimester
Time of onset	30%	31%	39%
Percentage with symptoms	16.5%	33.5%	55%

Table 28.9   Prevalence of stress incontinence according to Stanton et al 1980[22]

	Before Preg.	Booking	32/40	36/40	38/40	40/40	Post Natal
Nulliparous	0%	6%	30%	35%	39%	34%	6%
Multiparous	10%	27%	41%	42%	41%	38%	11%
Combined	6%	17%	36%	39%	40%	36%	8%

and all women is shown in Table 28.9. Analysis of their figures using a Fisher's two-tailed test reveals only a significant difference for parity before pregnancy and at the booking visit.

We looked at a multitude of lower urinary tract symptoms in early pregnancy via both direct questioning and visual analog scores[24,25] (Fig. 28.2). Both methods of questioning revealed a similar prevalence of stress incontinence to that reported by Stanton et al,[22] but we also demonstrated a significant difference in the prevalence of this symptom between White nulliparous and White multiparous women. The same symptoms were asked about at several stages of pregnancy in 119 women[25] and the prevalence on direct questioning can be seen in (Fig. 28.3). Again results for stress incontinence are similar to those of Stanton et al.[22]

Several retrospective studies have been carried out to try to ascertain whether pregnancy itself or childbirth leads to the development of stress incontinence. Beck & Hsu[36] questioned 1000 women attending a gynecological out-patient clinic and found that 31% admitted to stress incontinence. Of these, 82% said that it first occurred antenatally. This study

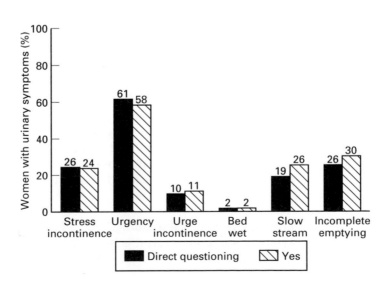

Fig. 28.2   Percentage of women with urinary symptoms on direct questioning and visual analog scores (VAS). (From Cutner, 1993[25])

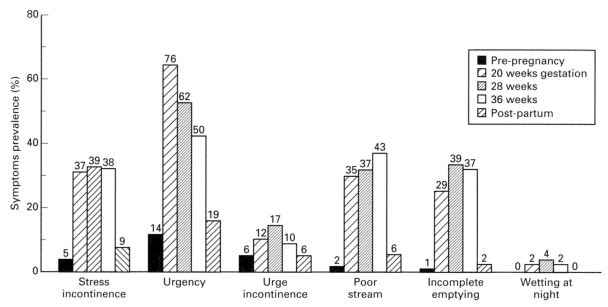

Fig. 28.3   Prevalence of symptoms in pregnancy on direct questioning. Actual numbers are shown above each bar. (From Cutner A 1993. The lower urinary tract in pregnancy. MD Thesis, University of London, with permission.)

is in agreement with other retrospective studies[37,38] that demonstrate that stress incontinence rarely occurs for the first time in the puerperium. More recently, Viktrup et al[39] have suggested that stress incontinence as a symptom may occur for the first time in the puerperium in those women undergoing a vaginal delivery. Again this was a retrospective study.

All these studies demonstrate a relatively high prevalence of stress incontinence in relation to pregnancy. They suggest that most cases are reversible, with only a small minority remaining incontinent long-term, and that very few cases originate following delivery.

Stanton et al[22] examined the prevalence of urge incontinence and hesitancy in pregnancy. Urge incontinence reached a peak prevalence of 19% in multiparous women. In our studies we found a prevalence of urgency of up to 60% and urge incontinence of about 10% in early pregnancy[24,25,30] (Fig. 28.2). The results for on-going pregnancy are shown in Fig. 28.3. Although these studies suggest the possibility of detrusor instability, again symptoms do not correlate with urodynamic diagnoses. The women were also asked to grade the severity of their lower urinary tract symptoms on a visual analog score. The correlation coefficient between the grading of each lower urinary tract symptom at 36 weeks' gestation and at post partum was calculated (Table 28.10). The results demonstrate that those women with severe symptoms in pregnancy are likely to be affected after delivery.

Causes

From the relatively few studies which have looked at lower urinary tract symptoms in pregnancy, it is obvious that functional changes must have occurred. However, it is well known that symptomatology and function

Table 28.10   Correlation between visual analogue scores at 36 weeks' gestation and postpartum (Spearman correlation coefficients)

	Correlation	Significance
Stress incontinence	0.24	p <0.005
Urgency	0.18	p <0.05
Urge incontinence	0.40	p <0.001
Poor stream	0.17	p <0.05
Incomplete bladder Emptying	0.25	p <0.005

From Cutner 1993[25]

correlate poorly in non-pregnant women.[40–45] Indeed, this lack of agreement has been confirmed in pregnancy.[25,30,31]

Anatomical studies have tried to determine the causes of stress incontinence. The first report of changes in the lower urinary tract as a result of pregnancy and labor is from sagittal dissections of two women, one who died in late pregnancy and the other in late labor. (Fig. 28.4)[46] The findings are discussed in a paper by Malpas et al.[26] The latter authors performed radiological studies in pregnancy and found changes in the urethrovesical junction (Fig. 28.5). In late pregnancy the urethra joined the bladder at right angles but in labor the bladder base was lifted

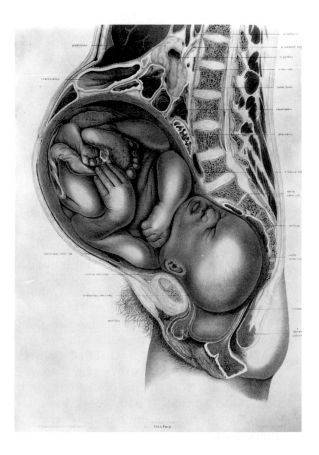

Fig. 28.4   The position of the bladder and urethra during labor. (From Braune W 1872. Atlas of Topical Anatomy. Leipzig: Veit, with permission.)

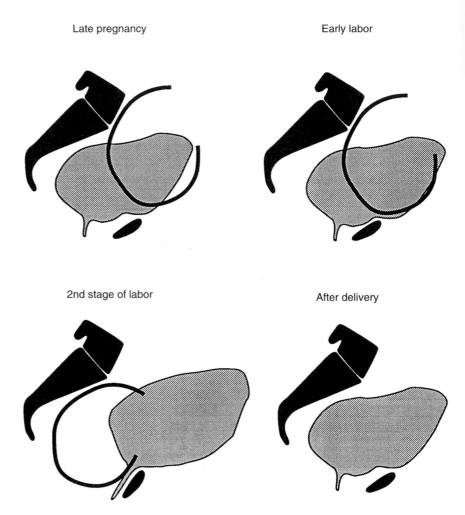

Late pregnancy

Early labor

2nd stage of labor

After delivery

Fig. 28.5 Movements of the bladder in labor (Modified from Malpas P, Jeffcoate TNA, Lister UM 1949. The displacement of the bladder and urethra during labour. J Obstet Gynaecol Br Empire 56: 949–960, with permission.)

upwards giving the impression that the urethra was elongated. In women who were examined postnatally the anatomy had returned to normal. These changes in the position of the bladder neck suggest that stretching of supporting structures as a result of labor may lead to damage and weakening of the sphincter mechanisms. This view is supported by Kantor et al.[47] Other reports of postpartum cystoscopy have revealed evidence of bladder trauma post partum.[48,49,50]

Landon et al[51] compared tensile properties of rectus sheath fascia in 24 women undergoing Caesarean section with that of 96 non-pregnant women having an abdominal operation. They found that pregnant fascia had a reduced tensile strength, which may account for the development of stress incontinence in pregnancy. Although post partum the fascia will regain its previous strength, it may be that in cases of permanent stress incontinence it has already undergone irreversible damage by overstretching.

These anatomical studies do not explain the high prevalence of stress incontinence antenatally with recovery in most cases post partum. Francis[35] found loss of the posterior urethrovesical angle in those women who complained of stress incontinence antenatally and cites this as the cause of stress incontinence. However, the posterior urethrovesical angle is no longer considered to be important in the maintenance of continence.

A few studies have examined the lower urinary tract by means of urethral pressure profilometry. Iosif et al assessed 14 women without stress incontinence[52] and 12 with stress incontinence[53] during pregnancy and post partum. In the continent women there were progressive increases in maximum urethral closure pressure, maximum urethral pressure, functional urethral length and urethral length with increasing gestation. Post partum these parameters returned to their early pregnancy values. The increases in maximum urethral closure pressure and functional urethral length were not apparent in the incontinent group and in addition most parameters were significantly reduced compared to the continent group (Fig. 28.6 and 28.7). In both groups there was an increase in bladder pressure with progression of pregnancy, and they concluded that the increases in urethral parameters are necessary to maintain continence because of the raised bladder pressures which occur in pregnancy.

Van Geelan et al[54] repeated similar work in 43 pregnant women. In addition estradiol, progesterone and 17-hydroxyprogesterone levels were measured at each visit. They failed to show increases in the maximum urethral closure pressure or functional urethral length with increasing gestation. However, they did not divide women into those with and those without stress incontinence and this may have led to different results. They also failed to show any correlation between hormone changes and urethral pressure profile measurements. Summaries of the changes in maximum urethral closure pressure and functional urethral length in all three studies are shown in Fig. 28.6 and 28.7.

It is important to realize that none of these papers examined the transmission of intra-abdominal pressure to the urethra. This is important in understanding urethral function.[55,56] There are, however, two reports on the effects of pregnancy on pressure transmission ratios in the French

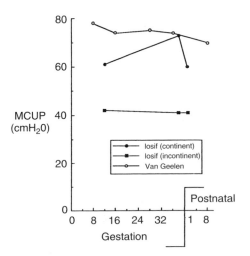

Fig. 28.6   Change in maximum urethral closure pressure (MUCP) with increasing gestation

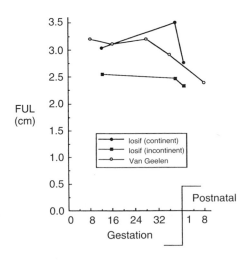

Fig. 28.7   Change in functional urethral length (FUL) with increasing gestation

literature, both by the same authors.[57,58] The first was a prospective study of 27 women studied at two gestations and again post partum.[57] The second was a retrospective study of 178 incontinent women.[58] The authors concluded that there was hypertransmission in the first trimester of pregnancy and that increasing parity leads to be cumulative reduction in pressure transmission. Furthermore, they suggested that obstetric trauma in multiparous women may lead to far worse deterioration in urethral function than similar events in first pregnancies.

We compared urethral pressure profile parameters in early pregnancy between those women with and without the symptom of stress incontinence[25] (Fig. 28.8). With regards to the maximum urethral closure pressure and maximum urethral pressure, our findings are in agreement

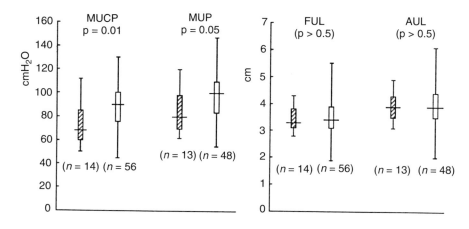

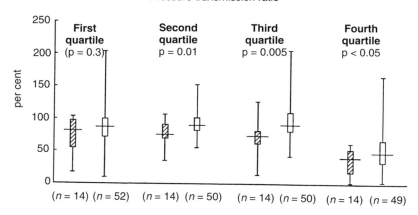

Fig. 28.8 Urethral pressure profile parameters in those women with and without stress incontinence on visual analog scores. Median values, interquartile ranges and ranges are shown. MUCP, maximum urethral closure pressure; MUP, maximum urethral pressure; FUL, functional urethral length; AUL, anatomical urethral length. (From Cutner 1993[25])

with those of Iosif et al.[52,53] In addition, we found significant differences in pressure transmission ratios. There were also differences in parameters between Black and White women (Fig. 28.9). This is consistent with the fact that Black women suffer genuine stress incontinence to a lesser degree than White women at all ages. When we looked at women during pregnancy and followed them up post partum, we found the functional urethral length and anatomical urethral length to be significantly greater in pregnancy. It is possible that increased functional urethral length in pregnancy results in improved pressure transmission to the proximal urethra, preventing the leakage of urine on stress. However, it must be remembered that the symptom of stress incontinence is taken to signify

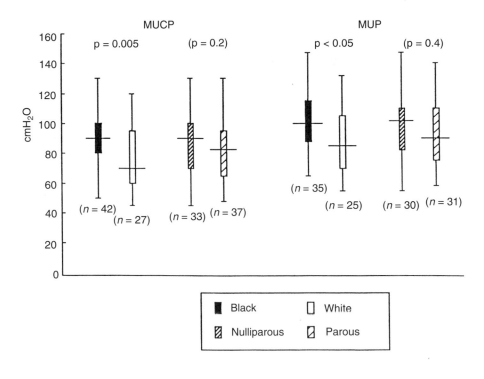

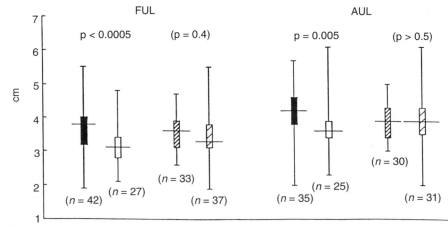

Fig. 28.9 Urethral pressure profile parameters according to race and parity. Median values, interquartile ranges and ranges are shown. MUCP, maximum urethral closure pressure; MUP, maximum urethral pressure; FUL, functional urethral length; AUL, anatomical urethral length. (From Cutner 1993[25])

genuine stress incontinence, although the diagnosis of this condition had not been determined by any objective urodynamic criteria.

Further indirect evidence of effects of delivery on lower urinary tract function has been presented. Tapp et al[59] compared two groups of women referred for urodynamic investigation. The first group had urodynamically proven genuine stress incontinence and the second group no evidence of urethral sphincter incompetence. There were no significant differences with regard to parity, number of vaginal deliveries or birth weight of the heaviest child between the two groups.

Electromyography has been used to examine the effects of vaginal delivery on denervation of the sphincter mechanism. Snooks et al[60] compared pelvic floor innervation in women who had a vaginal delivery to that in those who underwent a Caesarean section. They found evidence of pelvic floor denervation in women who delivered vaginally but not in the Caesarean section group. The same authors[61] compared similar groups both ante partum and post partum and confirmed that vaginal delivery results in pelvic floor denervation. Their conclusion that stretching of the bladder base during delivery results in damage agrees with that proposed by the earlier radiological studies.[26,47]

Allen et al[62] examined 96 nulliparous women at 36 weeks' gestation and again 2–5 days and 2 months after vaginal delivery. Concentric needle electromyography of the pelvic floor showed evidence of denervation in 80% of primigravid women post partum. In severe cases it was associated with incontinence. The only factor in labor that was associated with severe damage was a long active (pushing) second stage.

In the study already described, van Geelan et al[54] found significantly reduced urethral pressure profile parameters in postpartum primiparous women who had undergone vaginal delivery when compared to normal nulliparous controls. They found no difference when primiparous women who underwent Caesarean section were compared to the normal control group; however, the Caesarean section group consisted of only 6 women.

Iosif et al[63] carried out urethral function tests in 62 women who complained of stress incontinence during pregnancy. All women were examined 7–14 days post partum and had undergone a vaginal delivery. Twenty-seven of these women had severe stress incontinence which persisted post partum, whereas the other 35 had no postpartum urinary problems. They found decreased maximum urethral closure pressures and functional urethral lengths in those women in whom incontinence persisted post partum, and concluded that stress incontinence in pregnancy is physiological in many women, but in those in whom it persists, it is due to damage of the sphincter mechanism caused by delivery.

Beneficial effects of epidural analgesia have been demonstrated in two papers.[64,65] Both found that there was a lower prevalence of stress incontinence in women who had a forceps delivery under epidural analgesia than in those who had been given a pudendal block. They suggest that an epidural affords protection by enabling relaxation of the pelvic floor at the time of delivery.

Our symptom data[25] have demonstrated that those women affected badly with stress incontinence at the end of pregnancy are more likely to be affected postnatally. We also found that those women with a long first stage of labor were more likely to suffer from this symptom postnatally. There was no correlation with the length of the second stage.

In addition, the urethral pressure profilometry data revealed[25] a correlation between the length of the first stage and deterioration in urethral parameters postnatally. We found that the maximum urethral closure pressure, maximum urethral pressure, functional urethral length and anatomical urethral length were significantly greater in Black women than in White women postnatally. This would support the argument that susceptibility antenatally results in postnatal manifestation of sphincter damage in those women with adverse delivery factors.

Until recently only one author[66] had performed subtracted provocative cystometry in pregnant women. Clow investigated 25 women, 15 of whom developed stress incontinence in pregnancy. Three of these had detrusor instability and the bladder became stable in these women in the puerperium. Kerr-Wilson et al[67] performed subtracted cystometry 48 h post partum and again 4 weeks later. Out of the 20 women studied, 4 had detrusor instability on the first test and in 3 of these it had resolved by the second visit.

Recently, we have demonstrated the occurrence of detrusor instability in pregnancy.[25,30,31] The prevalence in early pregnancy is shown in Fig. 28.10. We found that women with low compliance had a significantly reduced first sensation and bladder capacity compared to women with a stable bladder and a significantly reduced bladder capacity compared to women with phasic detrusor instability. In addition, those women with phasic detrusor instability had a significantly greater prevalence of urethral instability than women in the low compliance and stable groups. These findings suggest that low compliance and phasic detrusor instability have a different etiology in pregnancy, the former being an effect of uterine pressure and the latter due to inherent irritability. The cause of the latter may be related to high progesterone levels.[68]

The prevalence of detrusor instability both during pregnancy and after delivery as derived from longitudinal data is shown in Fig. 28.11. We found the prevalence antenatally to be significantly greater than that post partum.[25] It would thus appear that detrusor instability is an entity in pregnancy with improvement once the pregnancy is complete.

Thus it can be seen that stress incontinence is a common transient feature in pregnancy but most studies suggest that it resolves postpartum. The effects of pregnancy and mode of delivery on its genesis remain uncertain. From our own observations, race is an important factor which has not always been taken into account. Those studies which only examined the women post partum are misleading as it may be the relative

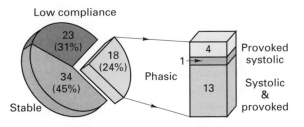

Fig. 28.10   The prevalence of detrusor instability in early pregnancy. DI, detrusor instability. (From Cutner A, 1993. The Urinary Tract in Pregnancy. MD Thesis, University of London.)

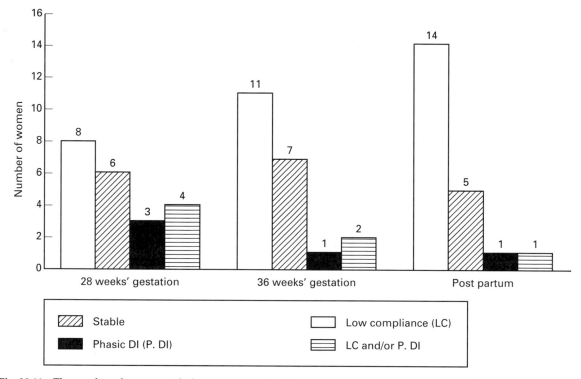

Fig. 28.11 The number of women with detrusor instability (DI) on each occasion. (From Cutner A 1993. The lower urinary tract in pregnancy. MD Thesis, University of London, with permission.)

change which is of paramount importance rather than exact values. Some studies cite urethral sphincter incompetence as the cause of stress incontinence in pregnancy, whilst our own work has demonstrated evidence of an increased prevalence of detrusor instability.

It would thus appear that stress incontinence in pregnancy and the postpartum period may be due to two different pathological processes with detrusor instability as the cause during pregnancy and genuine stress incontinence in the postpartum period.

Prevention and treatment

If antenatal stress incontinence is physiological and has no long-term sequelae, then reassurance is all that is required. However, this transient symptom may be a marker for possible long-term problems. It would now appear irrefutable that in susceptible women a protracted labour results in permanent genuine stress incontinence, and if we were able to identify this group of women, an elective Caesarean section might be justified. However, to subject all women with antenatal stress incontinence to an abdominal delivery would lead to an unacceptably high Caesarean section rate, as in some cases incontinence is due to detrusor instability and in others it will merely be transient.

When the equation of morbidity and mortality of elective Caesarean section versus an intended vaginal delivery is compared, one must also include the effects of an emergency Caesarean section and the late morbidity and mortality of an incontinence operation. If all parameter were included, then an elective Caesarean section in an 'at risk' group may be justified. At the present time there is one small group where elective Caesarean section should be advised. These are women who have undergone an effective incontinence procedure prior to pregnancy.[69]

The present trend of 'natural labor', with long first stages and no time limit for the second stage, may need to be questioned in the future if it is found that there is an unacceptably high prevalence of urethral sphincter damage. It is possible that a more liberal use of episiotomy and earlier recourse to forceps delivery will help to prevent some cases of sphincter damage. This is only speculation and further work is necessary before such a policy could be instituted.

A simple, non-invasive preventive measure may be the more formal teaching of pelvic floor exercises. However, if a muscle is already damaged, then pelvic floor training is unlikely to be effective. It has been shown that the institution of antenatal pelvic floor exercises results in better pelvic floor tone postnatally.[70] Whether this prevents the later development of prolapse or genuine stress incontinence is unknown.

Anticholinergic therapy for detrusor instability in pregnancy could not be justified and the rigors of bladder drill would be unacceptable to patients for a temporary condition. However, incontinence persisting postnatally should be investigated. To subject a person to incorrect treatment because a diagnosis has not been made is disheartening. We would recommend waiting at least 6 weeks before treating detrusor instability as it may recover spontaneously.

VOIDING DIFFICULTIES

Urinary retention in pregnancy is an uncommon event and usually due to an impacted retroverted uterus, classically occurring at 16 weeks' gestation. The cause is probably the result of the pelvic tumor (enlarged uterus) preventing the normal opening mechanisms of the internal urethral meatus. Treatment is catheterization and then manual correction of the uterus into an anteverted position using a ring or Hodge pessary. Subsequently, voiding difficulties must be looked out for as overdistension may have resulted in detrusor damage and require long-term catheterization until recovery occurs.

We found that symptoms of voiding difficulties were fairly common, with up to 25% of women complaining of a poor stream and 30% of incomplete bladder emptying in early pregnancy (Fig. 28.2).[24,25,31] The prevalence was similar in later pregnancy (Fig. 28.3)[25,31].

Although we have found a high prevalence of symptoms of voiding difficulties in pregnancy, it would appear that their cause is merely a function of small volumes of urine being passed.[25] We found no difference in the peak flow rate or average flow rate between those women with and without the symptom of a slow stream or incomplete bladder emptying once the volume voided was taken into account. In a similar way to Haylen et al,[71] we have calculated equations for the peak flow rate and average flow rate in pregnancy as a function of the volume voided (Fig. 28.12 and 28.13) and produced centile graphs from the 400 women studied.

Fig. 28.12 Equations for peak flow rate and average flow rate in pregnancy. (From Cutner A 1993. The lower urinary tract in pregnancy. MD Thesis, University of London, with permission.)

Ln (peak flow rate) − 0.140 + 0.587 × Ln (volume)
[Root mean square error = 0.358]

Square root (average flow rate) = −1.140 × 0.957 × Ln (volume)
[Root mean square error = 0.560]

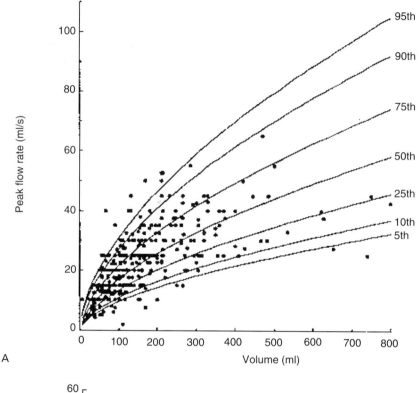

A

Fig. 28.13A Nomogram for peak flow rates in pregnancy with the centiles demonstrated on the right-hand side. **B** Nomogram for average flow rates in pregnancy with the centiles demonstrated on the right-hand side. (From Cutner A 1993. The Urinary Tract in Pregnancy. MD Thesis, University of London.)

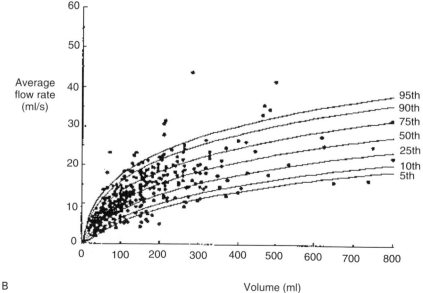

B

Absent Bladder Sensation

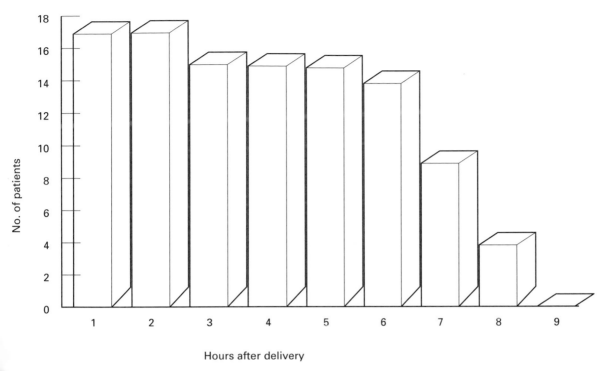

Fig. 28.14

Several studies have tried to determine the effects of delivery on both detrusor and urethral function. Vaginal delivery is often cited as resulting in detrusor hypotonia and the need for catheterization.

Weil et al[72] assessed 27 primigravid women urodynamically 2–5 days post partum. They were divided into 3 groups: vaginal delivery without epidural analgesia, vaginal delivery with epidural analgesia, and lower segment Caesarean section. The Caesarean section group had a lower bladder capacity compared to the other two groups and the epidural group had a greater prevalence of hypotonic bladders and larger bladder capacities than either of the other two groups. There was no difference between the groups with regard to maximum urethral closure pressure or functional urethral length. Evidence of increased bladder capacity after vaginal delivery with the risk of overdistension is confirmed by the earlier findings of Bennetts & Judd[49] and Shutter.[19] The effect of epidural analgesia on bladder dysfunction post partum is disputed by Crawford[73] and Grove.[74] Both the latter studies cite instrumental delivery as a cause of postpartum bladder dysfunction. Indeed, Kerr-Wilson et al[67] suggest that the avoidance of prolonged labor in combination with a practice of early catheterization avoids the problems of postpartum overdistension of the bladder. In a later study, Kerr-Wilson & McNally[75] identified a high prevalence of postpartum retention in women who were not routinely catheterized after a Caesarean section under epidural.

Tapp et al[76] have also examined the effect of epidural analgesia on postpartum voiding. Thirty-three women who delivered vaginally with a cephalic presentation were investigated by abdominal ultrasound for residual urine on day 2 and again at 5 days post partum. Those women who had residual urines at day 5 were reassessed at 6 weeks post partum. They found that women who had epidural analgesia had a significantly larger residual urine on day 2 and day 5 than those women who had other analgesia.

More recently we[77] have demonstrated that after epidural analgesia, the bladder takes up to 8 h to regain its sensation (Fig. 28.14) and within this time period more than 1 l of urine may be produced. This would result in detrusor damage.

All these studies probably used the traditional method of epidural analgesia with intermittent top-ups. Nowadays there are variations in the type of drug given and whether it is given intermittently or as a continuous infusion resulting in the advent of mobile epidurals. Future studies will need to describe the type of epidural, as this may be relevant to bladder sensation.[78]

Postpartum retention may have long-term sequelae. Versi & Barnick[79] reported 6 women who developed acute retention post partum. Two patients had permanent voiding difficulties, 2 required self-catheterization 6 months postpartum and 2 had altered bladder sensation although were voiding normally. Five of the 6 patients had epidural analgesia, and 4 had an instrumental delivery. Four of the patients had residual urine volumes in excess of 1 l when catheterized. However, this small retrospective study does not preclude the possibility that these patients may have had an underlying neuropathy rather than retention secondary to labor which resulted in their voiding difficulties.

Care of the bladder following delivery requires particular vigilance. Attention should be paid to those patients at risk of developing retention including those who have had a traumatic delivery, prolonged labor, epidural analgesia or Caesarean section. Voiding alone is not an adequate indication of bladder function since it may be incomplete, leading to increasingly large residuals of urine. Input/output charts are generally inadequate following delivery as a diuresis may occur and women are encouraged to increase their fluid intake to promote breast-feeding. Ideally with an epidural, an indwelling catheter should be inserted and left in situ for 12 h after the last top-up.

If a woman is resistant to catheterization, then at least her output should be carefully monitored to ensure that she is voiding at least 200 ml urine at more than 2-hourly intervals. Frequent small volumes of urine indicate incomplete voiding. If necessary a disposable catheter can be passed to ensure the bladder is empty. If a women is unable to void after delivery she should not be left more than 6 h before a catheter is passed to avoid overdistension of the bladder. If a second catheterization is required then it is advisable to leave an indwelling catheter in position for 48 h. If after this voiding is still unsatisfactory, then a suprapubic catheter is recommended together with investigations for possible underlying causes of retention. Cholinergic agents such as bethanecol may also speed up the return of detrusor function.

In short, epidural analgesia and traumatic vaginal delivery may lead to the development of acute urinary retention. Its sequelae of long-term voiding difficulties post partum are preventable by a policy of early catheterization if retention is suspected.

SUMMARY

Lower urinary tract symptoms antenatally are almost universal and in most cases transient. Retention of urine is one of the few conditions which must be treated in the antenatal period as otherwise there will be long-term consequences. Women who have undergone a successful anti-incontinence procedure should have an elective Caesarean section. In labour, there should be liberal use of catheterization to prevent long-term consequences. Most cases of incontinence are transient and investigation can be delayed until at least 6 weeks post partum. However, if the patient complains of a continuous leak, then investigation is mandatory to exclude retention with overflow or urinary fistulae.

REFERENCES

1 Fainstat T. Ureteral dilatation in pregnancy: a review. Obstet Gynecol Surv 1963; 18: 845–849.
2 Peake SL, Roxburgh HB, Langlois S. Ultrasonic assessment of hydronephrosis of pregnancy. Radiology 1983; 128: 167–170.
3 Davison JM, Hytten FE. Glomerular filtration during and after pregnancy. J Obstet Gynaecol Br Comm 1974; 81: 588–595.
4 Davison JM, Noble MCB. Serial changes in 24-hour creatinine clearance during normal menstrual cycles and the first trimester of pregnancy. Br J Obstet Gynaecol 1981; 88: 10–17.
5 Davison JM, Dunlop W, Ezimokhai M. Twenty four hour creatinine clearance during the third trimester of normal pregnancy. Br J Obstet Gynaecol 1980; 87: 106–109.
6 Kass EH. Bacteriuria and the diagnosis of infections of the urinary tract. AMA Archives Int Med 1957; 100: 709–714.
7 McFadyen IR, Eykryn SJ, Gardner NHN et al. Bacteriuria of pregnancy. J Obstet Gynaecol Br Comm 1973; 80: 385–405.
8 Roberts AP, Robinson RE, Beard RW. Some factors affecting bacterial colony counts in urinary infection. BMJ 1967; 1: 400–403.
9 Norden CW, Kass EH. Bacteriuria in pregnancy – a clinical reappraisal. Annual Rev Med 1968; 19: 431–470.
10 Whalley PJ. Bacteriuria in pregnancy. Am J Obstet Gynecol 1967; 97: 723–738.
11 Robertson AW, Duff P. The nitrite and leucocyte esterase for the evaluation of asymptomatic bacteriuria in obstetric patients. Obstet Gynecol 1988; 71(1): 878–881.
12 Etherington IJ, James DK. Reagent strip testing of antenatal urine specimens for infection. Br J Obstet Gynaecol 1993; 100: 806–808.
13 Davison J. Renal disease. In: De Swiet M (ed) Medica disorders in obstetric practice. Ch. 7. Blackwell Scientific Publications, pp 306–407.
14 McNeely SG Jr. Treatment of urinary tract infection during pregnancy. Clin Obstet Gynecol 1988; 31(2): 480–487.
15 Leveno KJ, Harris RE, Gilstrap LC et al. Bladder versus renal bacteriuria during pregnancy: recurrence and treatment. Am J Obstet Gynecol 1981; 139: 403–406.
16 Harris RE, Gilstrap LC, Pretty A. Single dose antimicrobial therapy for asymptomatic bacteriuria in pregnancy. Obstet Gynecol 1982; 58: 546–548.

17 Little P. The incidence of urinary tract infection in 5000 pregnant women. Lancet 1966; 1: 925–928.

18 Cumming DC, Taylor PJ. Urologic and obstetric significance of urinary calculi in pregnancy. 1979; 53(4): 505–508.

19 Shutter HW. Care of the bladder in pregnancy, labor and the puerperium. JAMA 1922; 79: 449–453.

20 Stevens WE, Arthurs E. The female bladder. JAMA 1924; 83: 1656–1663.

21 Francis WJA. Disturbances of bladder function in relation to pregnancy. J Obstet Gynaecol Br Empire 1960a; 67: 353–366.

22 Stanton SL, Kerr-Wilson R, Harris GV. The incidence of urological symptoms in normal pregnancy. Br J Obstet Gynaecol 1980; 87: 897–900.

23 Parboosingh J, Doig A. Studies of nocturia in normal pregnancy. J Obstet Gynaecol Br Commonw 1973a; 80: 888–895.

24 Cutner A, Carey A, Cardozo LD. Lower urinary tract symptoms in early pregnancy. Journal of Obstetrics and Gynaecology 1992; 12: 75–78.

25 Cutner A. The lower urinary tract in pregnancy. MD Thesis, University of London, 1993.

26 Malpas P, Jeffcoate TNA, Lister UM. The displacement of the bladder and urethra during labour. J Obstet Gynaecol Br Empire 1949; 56: 949–960.

27 Hundley JM Jr., Siegel IA, Hachtel FW, Dumler JC. Some physiological and pathological observations on the urinary tract during pregnancy. Sur Gynecol Obstet 1938; 66: 360–379.

28 Langer R, Golan A, Neuman M, Schneider D, Bukovsky I, Caspi E. The effect of large uterine fibroids on urinary bladder function and symptoms. Am J Obstet Gynecol 1990; 163: 1139–1141.

29 Parboosingh J, Doig A. Renal nyctohemeral excretory patterns of water and solutes in normal human pregnancy. Am J Obstet Gynecol 1973b; 116: 609–615.

30 Cutner A, Cardozo LD, Benness CJ. Assessment of urinary symptoms in early pregnancy. B J Obstet Gynaecol 1991; 98: 1283–1286.

31 Cutner A, Cardozo LD, Benness CJ. Assessment of urinary symptoms in the second half of pregnancy. International Urogynecology Journal 1992; 3: 30–32.

32 Muellner SR. Physiological bladder changes during pregnancy and the puerperium. J Urol 1939; 41: 691–695.

33 Youssef AF. Cystometric studies in gynecology and obstetrics. Obstet Gynecol 1956; 8: 181–188.

34 Langworthy OR, Brack CB. The effect of pregnancy and the corpus luteum upon vesical muscle. Am J Obstet Gynecol 1939; 37: 121–125.

35 Francis WJA. The onset of stress incontinence. J Obstet Gynaecol Br Empire 1960b; 67: 899–903.

36 Beck RP, Hsu N. Pregnancy, childbirth, and the menopause related to the development of stress incontinence. Am J Obstet Gynecol 1965; 91: 820–823.

37 Iosif S. Stress incontinence during pregnancy and in the puerperium. Int J Gynaecol Obstet 1981; 19: 13–20.

38 Iosif S, Ingemarsson I. Prevalence of stress incontinence among women delivered by elective caesarian section. Int J Gynaecol Obstet 1982; 20: 87–89.

39 Viktrup L, Lose G, Rolf M, Barfoed K. The frequency of urinary symptoms during pregnancy and puerperium in the primipara. Int Urogynecol J 1993; 4: 27–30.

40 Cantor TJ, Bates CP. A comparative study of symptoms and objective urodynamic findings in 214 incontinent women. Br J Obstet Gynaecol 1980; 87: 889–892.

41 Cardozo LD, Stanton SL. Genuine stress incontinence and detrusor instability: a review of 200 patients. Br J Obstet Gynaecol 1980; 87: 184–190.

42 Jarvis GJ, Hall S, Stamp S, Millar DR, Johnson A. An assessment of urodynamic examination in incontinent women. Br J Obstet Gynaecol 1980; 87: 893–896.

43 Ouslander J, Staskin D, Raz S, Su H-L, Hepps K. Clinical versus urodynamic diagnosis in an incontinent geriatric population. J Urol 1987; 137: 68–71.

44 Shepherd AM, Powell PH, Ball AJ. The place of urodynamic studies in the investigation and treatment of female urinary tract symptoms. J Obstet Gynaecol 1982; 3: 123–125.

45 Versi E, Cardozo LD, Anand D, Cooper D. Symptoms analysis for the diagnosis of genuine stress incontinence. Br J Obstet Gynaecol 1991; 98: 815–819.

46 Braune W. Atlas of topographical anatomy. Leipzig: Veit, 1872.

47 Kantor HI, Miller JE, Dunlap JC. The urinary bladder during labor. Am J Obstet Gynecol 1949; 48: 354–365.

48 Funnell JW, Klawans AH, Cottrell TLC. The postpartum bladder. Am J Obstet Gynecol 1954; 67: 1249–1256.

49 Bennetts FA, Judd GE. Studies of the post-partum bladder. Am J Obstet Gynecol 1941; 40: 419–427.
50 Seski AG, Duprey WM. Postpartum intravesical photography. Obst Gynecol 1961; 18: 548–556.
51 Landon CR, Crofts CE, Smith ARB, Trowbridge EA. Mechanical properties of fascia during pregnancy: a possible factor in the development of stress incontinence of urine. Contemp Rev Obstet Gynaecol 1990; 2: 40–46.
52 Iosif S, Ingemarsson I, Ulmsten U. Urodynamic studies in normal pregnancy and in puerperium. Am J Obstet Gynecol 1980; 137: 696–700.
53 Iosif S, Ulmsten U. Comparative urodynamic studies of continent and stress incontinent women in pregnancy and in the puerperium. Am J Obstet Gynecol 1981; 140: 645–650.
54 van Geelen JM, Lemmens WAJG, Eskes TKAB, Martin CB. The urethral pressure profile in pregnancy and after delivery in healthy nulliparous women. Am J Obstet Gynecol 1982; 144: 636–649.
55 Beck RP, Maughan GB. Simultaneous intraurethral and intravesical studies in normal women and those with stress incontinence. Am J Obstet Gynecol 1964; 89: 746–753.
56 Farghaly SA, Shah J, Worth P. The value of the intraurethral pressure transmission ratio in the assessment of female stress incontinence. Arch Gynecol 1985; Suppl 237: 366. Abstract.
57 Le Coutour X, Jouffroy C, Beuscart R, Renaud R. Influence de la grossesse et de l'accouchement sur la fonction de clôture cervico-urétrale. 1. Etude prospective chez 27 femmes. (The influence of pregnancy and delivery on closure of the bladder neck and urethra. 1. A prospective study carried out on 27 women). J Gynecol Obstet Biol Reprod 1984a; 13: 771–774.
58 Le Coutour X, Jouffroy C, Beuscart R, Renaud R. Influence de la grossesse et de l'accouchement sur la fonction de clôture cervico-urétrale. 2. Etude rétrospective des conséquences tardives du traumatisme obstétrical. (The influence of pregnancy and delivery on closure of the bladder neck and urethra. 2. A retrospective study of the late effects of obstetric trauma). J Gynecol Obstet Biol Reprod 1984b; 13: 775–779.
59 Tapp A, Cardozo L, Versi E, Montgomery J, Studd J. The effect of vaginal delivery on the urethral sphincter. Br J Obstet Gynaecol 1988b; 95: 142–146.
60 Snooks SJ, Swash M, Setchell M, Henry MM. Injury to innervation of pelvic floor sphincter musculature in childbirth. Lancet 1984; 2: 546–550.
61 Snooks SJ, Swash M, Henry MM, Setchell M. Risk factors in childbirth causing damage to the pelvic floor innervation. Int J Colorect Dis 1986; 1: 20–24.
62 Allen RE, Hosker GL, Smith ARB, Warrell DW. The role of pregnancy and childbirth in partial denervation of the pelvic floor – an update. Neurourol Urodyn 1988; 7: 237–239.
63 Iosif S, Henriksson L, Ulmsten U. Postpartum incontinence. Urol Int 1981h; 36: 53 58.
64 Schuessler B, Hesse U, Dimpfl Th, Anthuber C. Epidural anaesthesia and avoidance of postpartum stress urinary incontinence. Lancet 1988; 1: 762.
65 Dimpfl Th, Hesse U, Schussler B. Incidence and cause of postpartum urinary stress incontinence. European Journal Of Obstetrics and Gynecology and Reproductive Biology 1992; 43: 29–33.
66 Clow WM. Effect of posture on bladder and urethral function in normal pregnancy. Urol Int 1975; 30: 9–15.
67 Kerr-Wilson RHJ, Thompson SW, Orr JW, Davis RO, Cloud GA. Effect of labor on the postpartum bladder. Obstet Gynecol 1984; 64: 115–118.
68 Cutner A, Burton G, Cardozo LD, Wise BG, Abbott D, Studd J. Does progesterone cause an irritable bladder? International Urogynecology Journal 1993; 4: 259–261.
69 Cutner A, Cardozo LD, Wise BG. The effects of pregnancy on previous incontinence surgery. Br J Obstet Gynaecol 1991b; 98: 1181–1183.
70 Nielsen CA, Sigsgaard I, Olsen M, Tolstrup M, Danneskiold-Samsoee B, Bock JE. Trainability of the pelvic floor. A prospective study during pregnancy and after delivery. Acta Obstet Gynecol Scand 1988; 67: 437–440.
71 Haylen BT, Ashby D, Sutherst JR, Frazer MI, West CR. Maximum and average flow rates in normal male and female populations – the Liverpool nomograms. Br J Urol 1989; 64: 30–38.
72 Weil A, Reyes H, Rottenberg RD, Beguin F, Hermann WL. Effect of lumbar epidural analgesia on lower urinary tract function in the immediate postpartum period. Br J Obstet Gynaecol 1983; 90: 428–432.
73 Crawford JS. Lumbar epidural block in labour: a clinical analysis. Brit J Anaesth 1972; 44: 66–74.
74 Grove LH. Backache, headache, and bladder dysfunction after delivery. Brit J Anaesth 1973; 45: 1147–1149.

75 Kerr-Wilson RHJ, McNally S. Bladder drainage for caesarean section under epidural analgesia. Br J Obstet Gynaecol 1986; 93: 28–30.
76 Tapp AJS, Meir H, Cardozo LD. The effect of epidural analgesia on post-partum voiding. Neurourol Urodyn 1987; 6: 235–237.
77 Khullar V, Cardozo LD. Bladder sensation after epidural analgesia. Neurourol Urodyn 1993; 12(4): 424–425.
78 Russell R, Reynolds F. Epidural analgaesia: not just one technique. Br J Obstet Gynaecol (Letter) 1993; 100: 1155–1156.
79 Versi E, Barnick C. Post-partum urinary retention. Proceedings of the 17th Annual Meeting of the International Continence Society, Bristol, 1987; pp 218–219.

29 Lower urinary tract dysfunction and the menopause

INTRODUCTION

In England and Wales there are approximately 10 million climacteric or postmenopausal women[1] and therefore almost 1 in 5 of the population is potentially at risk of the symptoms of estrogen deficiency and a candidate for hormone replacement therapy (HRT).

At approximately 40 years of age the frequency of ovulation declines, and this initiates a period of waning ovarian function – the climacteric. The major manifestations of the climacteric are a result of decreased ovarian estrogen production. Dwindling ovarian function results sequentially in reduced ovulation, menstrual irregularities, the menopause and finally generalized atrophy of all estrogen-sensitive tissues.

It is not surprising, in view of their common embryological origin, that the female genital and urinary tracts are both sensitive to the effects of female sex steroids. Estrogen and progesterone receptors are present in the vagina, urethra, bladder and pelvic floor,[2,3,4,5] and symptomatic, cytological and urodynamic changes in the lower urinary tract have been demonstrated during the menstrual cycle, in pregnancy and following the menopause.[6,7,8,9]

Deteriorating ovarian function at the time of the menopause results in an increased incidence of urinary symptoms, including dysuria, frequency, nocturia, urgency and incontinence as well as the development of recurrent urinary tract infection. These symptoms are common and distressing, but may be reversible with exogenous estrogen replacement therapy.

EPIDEMIOLOGY

Over the years increased life expectancy has led to a rise in the number of the postmenopausal women. At present women spend a third of their lives in the estrogen-deficient postmenopausal state.[10] The prevalence of conditions occurring more frequently after the menopause is therefore also likely to increase, with a similar expansion in health care expenditure.

Epidemiological studies have attempted to document the prevalence of postmenopausal urinary incontinence. Many women are, however, reluctant to admit to incontinence and therefore the true extent of this distressing condition is probably underestimated.

Table 29.1 Prevalence of incontinence amongst women residing independently in the community

Study	Prevalence (%)
Milne et al 1972[11]	
65 + years	34
Thomas et al 1980[12]	
25–64 years	18
65 + years	23
Yarnell et al 1981 (women only)[13]	
25–64 years	46
65 + years	49
Vetter et al 1981[14]	14
Medical, epidemiologic and social aspects of aging study 1986[15] (65 + years)	30
Iosif & Bekassey 1984[16] (61 + years)	29
Market Opinion Research International (MORI) survey 1990[17]	14

The prevalence of urinary incontinence increases with age (Table 29.1), although there are many reasons apart from the menopause why this should be so. Bladder and urethral function become less efficient with age,[18,19] and Malone Lee[19] has shown that elderly women have a reduced flow rate, an increased urinary residual, higher end filling cystometric pressures (and maximum filling pressure), reduced bladder capacity and lower maximum voiding pressures. Additionally, whereas younger women excrete the bulk of their daily fluid intake before bedtime, as a result of many factors including congestive cardiac failure and drugs this pattern reverses in the elderly, nocturia becoming more common with advancing age.

The major causes of urinary incontinence amongst women of all ages are listed below:

- genuine stress incontinence (GSI)
- detrusor instability (DI) (detrusor hyperreflexia)
- overflow incontinence
- fistulae (vesicovaginal, uterovaginal, urethrovaginal)
- congenital
- urethral diverticula
- temporary (e.g. urinary tract infection, fecal impaction, drugs)
- functional (e.g. immobility)
- GSI + DI (mixed incontinence).

The impaired physical status of some elderly women results in additional causes of incontinence not frequently encountered by younger women. These may be listed as follows:

- dementia
- urinary tract infection
- fecal impaction
- decreased mobility
- acute illness/acute confusional state
- drugs (e.g. diuretics, hypnotics)
- change of environment (e.g. hospitalization)
- heart failure
- estrogen deficiency
- metabolic abnormalities
- endocrine abnormalities (e.g. diabetes)
- renal problems.

Although urinary incontinence is common in the postmenopausal years, prevalence data do not clearly indicate the role of estrogen deficiency. In their large postal survey of almost 10 000 British women, Thomas et al[12] showed that the prevalence of incontinence increased with age but not specifically at the time of the menopause, whereas Iosif & Bekassy[16] found that 70% of incontinent elderly Swedish women related the onset of their symptoms to their last menstrual period. Jolleys[20] found that the prevalence of stress incontinence reached a peak at the age of 50 years and declined thereafter (Fig. 29.1). Kondo et al[21] studied 1105 Japanese women and

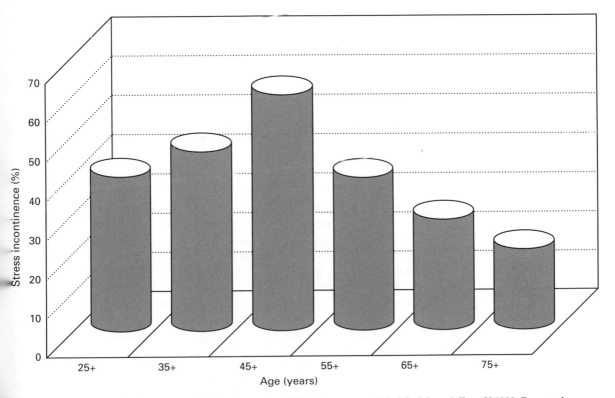

Fig. 29.1 The prevalence of stress incontinence amongst 833 British women. (Modified from Jolleys V 1988. Reported prevalence of urinary incontinence in women in general practice. Br Med J 296: 1300–1302, with permission.)

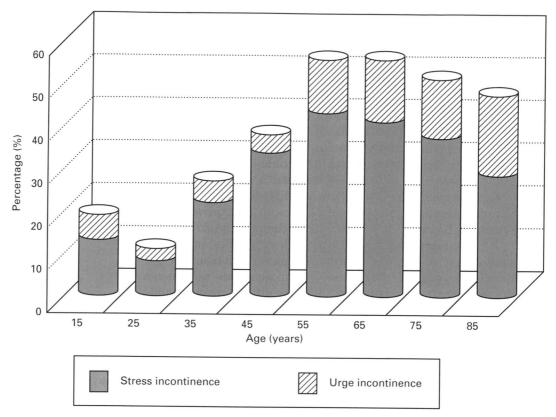

Fig. 29.2   The prevalence of stress and urge incontinence amongst 1105 Japanese women. (Modified from Kondo A, Kato K, Saito M, Otani T 1990. Prevalence of hand washing urinary incontinence in females in comparison with stress and urge incontinence. Neurourol Urodynam 9: 330–331, with permission.)

found that whereas the incidence of stress incontinence decreased after the age of 55 years, that of urge incontinence increased with age (Fig. 29.2).

An analysis of both urinary symptoms and urodynamic findings amongst climacteric women was performed at the Dulwich menopause clinic.[22] Two hundred and twenty-eight women referred for various climacteric complaints completed a detailed urinary symptom questionnaire and underwent urodynamic investigations comprising pad testing, uroflowmetry, videocystourethrography, cystometry and urethral pressure profilometry. Symptoms of stress incontinence occurred in over 50% of women and of urge incontinence in 26%. In only 60% of women were the findings of urodynamic investigations normal. Despite the common finding of urinary symptoms and urodynamic abnormalities no correlation was seen with the timing of the menopause.

There is little evidence that stress incontinence is a result of the menopause, whereas urge incontinence and other irritative bladder symptoms may be. Although urinary symptoms are common in climacteric and postmenopausal women, and the lower urinary tract is known to be estrogen-sensitive, a causal relationship to the menopause is difficult to demonstrate.

Unfortunately, epidemiological data are difficult to collect and incontinence in the elderly may be attributable to many other known factors. A measure of the importance of estrogen deficiency can, however, be gauged by the improvement in symptoms, cytology and urodynamic assessment following estrogen replacement therapy.

MECHANISM OF CONTINENCE

For continence to exist the urethral closure pressure must exceed the intravesical pressure at all times except during micturition. Estrogens may improve continence by increasing urethral resistance, raising the sensory threshold of the bladder, increasing α-adrenoreceptor sensitivity in the urethral smooth muscle,[22,23] or possibly by a combination of all three. In addition, estrogen therapy has been shown to increase the number of intermediate and superficial cells in the vagina of postmenopausal women[24] and similar changes have been demonstrated in the urethra and bladder.[25]

Although the use of estrogen therapy for the relief of postmenopausal urinary disorders remains controversial, it has been used extensively for this indication with varying degrees of success. Unfortunately, those studies which have been performed vary in many important respects, namely the type, route, dose and mode of administration of estrogen as well as the assessment of treatment efficacy. This heterogeneity has further complicated an already complex picture.

A recent meta-analysis of 166 articles published in English from 1969 to 1992 included only 6 controlled and 17 uncontrolled trials of estrogen therapy for the treatment of female urinary incontinence.[26] Meta-analysis found an overall significant subjective improvement in incontinence symptoms for all subjects following estrogen therapy, but no evidence of objective improvement.

HORMONE REPLACEMENT THERAPY

There are many reasons for offering postmenopausal and climacteric women estrogen replacement therapy apart from its beneficial effect on the lower urinary tract. Hot flushes, vaginal dryness, headaches, dyspareunia, loss of libido, poor memory, insomnia and depression are all relieved by estrogen replacement. Of greater long-term benefit is prophylaxis against ischemic heart disease (IHD), stroke, thrombosis and osteoporosis.[27]

To achieve all of these potential benefits estrogen replacement must be administered via a route and in a dose sufficient to achieve adequate systemic estrogen levels. As a consequence significant endometrial stimulation results and it has therefore become established practice to give cyclical or continuous progestogen each month to prevent the development of endometrial hyperplasia[28] and atypia.[29] This policy has proved effective in removing the excess risk of endometrial carcinoma associated with unopposed estrogen replacement therapy,[30] but unfortunately has resulted in unwanted side effects, i.e. cyclical bleeding and progestogenic psychological and physical symptoms. Withdrawal bleeding is currently the greatest problem with systemic hormone replacement therapy and even with continuous combined therapy one-third of women will discontinue treatment within the first 6 months because of irregular bleeding.[31]

Estrogen replacement therapy: types of estrogen available

There are two basic types of estrogen: synthetic and natural. Synthetic estrogens (e.g. ethinylestradiol and mestranol) give rise to substances in the plasma which have potent estrogenic activity, but which are structurally dissimilar to the estrogens produced by the ovary. The natural estrogens are estradiol, estrone and estriol. Although these are often synthesized for HRT, regardless of the method of manufacture they are structurally identical to estrogens produced by the ovary. Synthetic estrogens possess significantly greater potency than natural estrogens, particularly with respect to the production of hepatic coagulation and fibrinolytic factors and the suppression of follicle-stimulating hormone. This relative potency is a result of their longer half-life, the prolonged nuclear retention time and the absence of binding to sex-hormone binding globulin (SHBG). Only free unbound estrogen is biologically active and enters cells binding to cystoplasmic receptors in target tissues. The steroid receptor complex is translocated into the nucleus resulting in the synthesis of mRNA and subsequently both intra- and extracellular proteins. Although the biological activity of each estrogen is modified by many other factors, including absorption, protein binding and enzyme metabolism, their potency theoretically depends on their nuclear retention time. In this respect estriol, with a nuclear retention time of 1–4 h, is a weak estrogen, and estradiol, with a retention time of 6–8 h, is a stronger estrogen. However, with high doses and frequent administration of estriol the effects are the same as with other estrogens.

Although the potency of synthetic estrogens makes them ideal for hormonal contraception, natural estrogens result in fewer side effects and are consequently preferable for HRT. The estrogens used in various different preparations are shown in Table 29.2.

Table 29.2 Routes of administration of estrogen replacement therapy

Route	Proprietary name	Generic name
Oral	e.g. Premarin	Conjugated equine estrogen
	Progynova	Estradiol valerate
	Ovestin	Estriol
Transdermal	e.g. Estraderm	Estradiol
Subcutaneous		Estradiol
Transcutaneous	e.g. Oestragel	Estradiol
Local/topical		
Vaginal cream	e.g. Premarin	Conjugated equine estrogen
	Ovestin	Estriol
Vaginal tablets	e.g. Vagifem	Estradiol
Pessaries	e.g. Orthogynest	Estriol
Vaginal ring	e.g. Estring	Estradiol

Risk/benefits of estrogen replacement

Unfortunately, many women still remain suspicious of HRT despite its many obvious benefits. It is clear that estrogen replacement therapy markedly reduces the risks of postmenopausal IHD, and a meta-analysis of 31 published articles found an overall risk ratio for IHD of 0.56 (95% confidence intervals 0.5–0.61) amongst estrogen users.[32] This reduction in risk is numerically the most significant long-term effect of HRT because IHD is the greatest cause of death amongst postmenopausal women. The benefits of estrogen therapy are conferred through lipid changes, i.e. there is an increase in high density lipoprotein and a reduction in low density lipoprotein cholesterol, but estrogen also exerts a direct atheroma-inhibiting action on the arterial wall independent of blood cholesterol.[33] Color flow Doppler imaging has demonstrated that estrogen increases peripheral blood flow in the internal carotid artery.[34] Estrogen may also work by modifying carbohydrate metabolism and body fat distribution, both of which are related to the risk of IHD.

A history of thrombosis is often regarded as a contraindication to HRT, although worldwide experience with HRT has not shown any increased incidence of thrombosis; indeed, HRT actually reduces the risk of stroke.[35]

There is little question as to the benefit of estrogen replacement in the management of postmenopausal osteoporosis. Not only has estrogen been shown to prevent the acceleration of bone loss which normally accompanies the menopause[36] and reduce the risk of subsequent fracture,[37] but it has also been shown to increase bone density in those already manifesting postmenopausal osteoporosis.[38]

There is great disparity amongst studies which have sought to investigate the relationship between HRT and breast cancer incidence. Meta-analysis of 28 published studies yields a slightly greater risk ratio for estrogen users of 1.07, although this was not statistically significant.[39] Undoubtedly, the use of estrogen replacement therapy should result in closer screening of users and therefore the detection of more early stage cancer with a better prognosis.[40]

Routes of estrogen administration

All estrogens when given in a sufficient dosage to relieve systemic symptoms of estrogen deficiency have a significant metabolic effect.[41]

The major routes of administration of estrogen therapy are shown in Table 29.2. One of the main benefits of non-oral delivery is that any potential thrombotic tendency is minimized by the avoidance of first pass hepatic metabolism. Additionally, more stable 24-h estradiol profiles are achieved (Fig. 29.3) and more physiological hormone profiles, maintaining the 2:1 estradiol:estrone ratio which is normal for premenopausal women.[42] The inconvenience and skin irritation associated with estrogen patches, and the small (3%) risk of tachyphylaxis (supraphysiological estrogen levels) associated with implants, are outweighed by the benefits of these for many women.

In order to increase compliance with estrogen replacement therapy amongst women with urogenital complaints the use of low-dose topical estrogen has been advocated. Low-dose estradiol has been applied in the

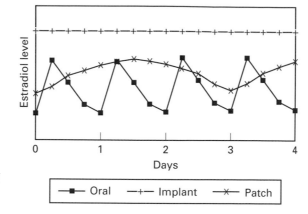

Fig. 29.3 Short-term variability in estradiol levels with oral, patch and implant therapy. (Modified from Smith RN, Studd JWW 1993. Recent advances in hormone replacement therapy. British J Hospital Medicine 49(11): 799–809, with permission.)

form of a sustained release vaginal tablet or vaginal ring and estriol pessaries or cream have been used, but significant absorption can take place through the vaginal epithelium and substantial systemic estrogen levels are achieved following administration of more potent treatments.

Minimal systemic estrogen levels are found with the majority of low-dose preparations, and hence unwanted withdrawal bleeding and the risk of endometrial hyperplasia and atypia do not appear to be a problem. Unfortunately, low-dose topical therapy is insufficient to prevent osteoporosis or IHD and may be better suited for older women, or those unwilling to accept or unsuitable for systemic HRT. Additionally, it appears that prolonged usage (greater than 1 year) of low-dose topical therapy is required for maximal benefit and that symptoms recur on discontinuing treatment.[43]

Iosif[43] reported a series of 48 women receiving treatment with 0.5-mg estriol suppositories for 1–10 years. Vabra curettage showed the majority to have an inactive, atrophic endometrium with only 7 (15%) having a weakly proliferative endometrium after prolonged treatment. None of the women had evidence of hyperplasia or atypia. Mettler & Olsen[44] assessed the effect of long-term low-dose estradiol vaginal tablets (25 mg 17b-estradiol) on the endometrium. Fifty-one women received once- or twice-weekly treatment for up to 2 years. All 9 women completing 2 years of treatment had an inactive atrophic endometrium and only 3 cases of weak endometrial proliferation were found after 1 year's treatment.

In addition, by avoiding the enterohepatic circulation and exerting a mainly local effect, low-dose topical estrogen replacement therapy is virtually free from systemic side effects.

Estrogens in undiagnosed incontinence

Early studies of the effect of estrogens on lower urinary tract dysfunction predated urodynamic studies and were largely subjective and uncontrolled. The first report was from Salmon et al,[45] who treated 16 women with dysuria, frequency, urgency and incontinence for 4 weeks using intramuscular estrogen therapy. Symptomatic improvement was seen in 12 women and treatment was discontinued. Symptoms recurred and were again relieved by intramuscular estrogen therapy.

Thirty years later, Musiani[46] gave 110 stress incontinent women quinestradol (which is no longer available), and reported a cure rate of 33% and an improvement rate of 39%. Schleyer-Saunders[47] used estradiol implants to treat 100 postmenopausal women with undiagnosed urinary incontinence and found that 70% were significantly improved, reducing the need for surgery.

Estrogen therapy for urge incontinence

There have been few controlled studies reported in the literature despite the presence of a large placebo response in the treatment of urge incontinence. Samsioe et al[25] entered 34 women aged 75 years into a double-blind, placebo-controlled crossover study of oral estriol 3 mg daily for 3 months. Despite the lack of objective assessment they found that urge incontinence and mixed incontinence were improved by estriol, although in women with stress incontinence there was no difference between estriol and placebo. Unfortunately, we have not been able to reproduce their results.

We have recently reported the results of a double-blind placebo-conrolled randomized multicenter study of oral estriol 3 mg/day in the treatment of 64 postmenopausal women with 'the urge syndrome'.[48] Women who entered the trial underwent urodynamic assessment and were divided into those with sensory urgency and those with DI. Treatment was for 3 months, after which patients were fully assessed both subjectively and objectively and side effects were recorded. Patient compliance was confirmed by a significant improvement in the maturation index of vaginal wall smears with estriol compared to placebo. Although estriol produced both subjective and objective improvement in urinary symptoms, particularly urgency and nocturia, it was not significantly better than placebo.

Iosif[43] has shown that urogenital atrophy, a late manifestation of estrogen deficiency, is only completely relieved after a year of treatment with 0.5-mg estriol suppositories, and that symptoms recur with discontinuation of treatment. It is likely that our study used too low a dose, the wrong route of administration or an inappropriate estrogen, and it is unclear whether low-dose topical therapy, which improves genital atrophy without significant endometrial stimulation, is sufficient to treat urinary symptoms. Indeed, it is possible that estrogen is actually no better than placebo for the management of postmenopausal women with this condition, although Fantl et al[49] have suggested that estrogen supplementation raises the sensory threshold of the bladder.

In view of our disappointing results using estriol in the management of postmenopausal urinary urgency, we have recently assessed the efficacy of sustained release 17β-estradiol vaginal tablets (Vagifem) (Benness et al, unpublished data). These are well absorbed from the vagina and have been shown to induce maturation of the vaginal epithelium within 14 days.[50]

In a randomized study 110 postmenopausal women suffering from urgency received either 25 mg 17β-estradiol or matching placebo each day for 6 months. All underwent urodynamic investigations and were divided into three groups: (1) those with detrusor instability, (2) those with sensory urgency and (3) those in whom urodynamic findings were normal. At the end of the treatment period the only significant difference between active and placebo therapy was the improvement in the symptom of urgency in those women with a diagnosis of sensory urgency, which responded better to estradiol than placebo. It is possible that localized atrophy causes or aggravates sensory urgency, and therefore topical estrogen therapy is useful for its management.

Eriksen & Rasmussen[51] showed, in a 12-week double-blind randomized placebo-controlled trial, that treatment with 25-μg 17β-estradiol tablets significantly improved lower urinary tract symptoms of frequency, urgency, urge and stress incontinence compared to placebo. Unfortunately, they did not select women on the basis of their urinary symptoms and the study lacked the benefit of objective urodynamic assessment.

Estrogen therapy for stress incontinence

The main parameter which has been used to assess the efficacy of estrogen therapy in the management of women with stress incontinence is urethral pressure profilometry. Caine & Raz[52] showed that 26 out of 40 (65%) women with stress incontinence had increased maximum urethral pressures and symptomatic improvement whilst taking conjugated oral estrogen. Rud[53] treated 24 stress incontinent women with high doses of oral estradiol and estriol in combination. He found a significant increase in transmission of intra-abdominal pressure to the urethra as well as an increase in maximum urethral pressure. Seventy per cent of women were symptomatically improved; however, high doses of estrogen were employed over a short period of time and other studies have not all reported the same changes in urethral pressure profilometry.

Walter et al[54] randomly allocated 29 incontinent, postmenopausal women with stable bladders to either estradiol and estriol or placebo (4 months' cyclical treatment). They found a significant improvement in urgency and urge incontinence (7 out of 15 (47%) with estrogen therapy) but no improvement in stress incontinence. They were unable to demonstrate a change in urethral pressure profile parameters. Similarly, Wilson et al[55] entered 36 women with urodynamically proven GSI into a double-blind, placebo-controlled study of cyclical oral estrone for 3 months and showed no difference in the subjective response, urethral pressure profile parametes or quantity of urine loss.

The only study to date which has shown a significant objective improvement in GSI using estrogen therapy was reported by Walter et al.[56] In a randomized, placebo-controlled study using estriol 4 mg daily they showed that 9 out of 12 women (75%) preferred estriol to placebo and that there was a significant objective decrease in urine loss with estriol compared to placebo. However, the numbers in this study were small and it is the only one in the literature to report this effect!

Combination therapies

Estrogens alone appear helpful for the symptoms of urgency and urge incontinence but not for stress incontinence, although there have been promising reports of combination therapy using an estrogen and an α-adrenergic agonist. Beisland et al[57] treated 24 menopausal women with GSI using phenylpropanolamine (50 mg twice daily orally) and estriol (1 mg/day vaginally) separately and in combination. They found that the combination cured 8 women and improved a further 9, and was more effective than either drug alone. Hilton et al[58] reported the results of a double-blind, placebo-controlled study using estrogen (oral or vaginal), alone or with phenylpropanolamine, in 60 postmenopausal women with urodynamically proven GSI. They found that the symptoms of frequency and nocturia improved more with combined treatment than with estrogen alone, and that stress incontinence improved subjectively in all groups but objectively only the combined group. It is likely that the effect of phenylpropanolamine on α-adrenergic receptors in the urethra is potentiated by the concomitant use of estrogen replacement therapy in postmenopausal women.

Estrogen therapy for atrophic vaginitis

Universal atrophy of estrogen-dependent tissues occurs following the menopause. Estrogen target organs include the breast, uterus, fallopian tubes, ovaries, vagina, vulva, the terminal urethra and trigone of the bladder. Symptoms of genital atrophy may not arise until many years after the menopause but they are thought to be very common (Table 29.3).

Table 29.3 Symptoms of urogenital atrophy

Vaginal	Vaginal dryness, vaginal 'burning', pruritis, dyspareunia, prolapse
Urinary	Urgency, frequency, dysuria, urinary tract infections, incontinence, voiding difficulties

The changes of genital atrophy include a progressive decrease in vascularity with fragmentation of elastic tissues, fusion and hyalinization of collagen fibers, and diminution of cellular cytoplasmic volume. The glycogen content of vaginal epithelial cells decreases and as a result colonization by lactobacilli decreases. As a consequence vaginal pH increases, encouraging colonization by streptococci, staphylococci and coliforms. The vaginal wall appears thin and dry, with absent rugae, and similar atrophic changes are seen in the urethra and trigone of the bladder.

Cytological studies have shown changes in the maturation index of atrophic vaginal epithelium. Above the epithelial basement membrane lie the basal cells, in the next layer the parabasal cells, and on the surface the superficial cells. With diminished estrogen exposure epithelial maturation is reduced and more parabasal cells are seen. Conversely, following estrogen replacement more superficial cells are seen, as well as a reversal of other atrophic changes.

In their study of 61-year-old Swedish women, Iosif & Beckassy[16] reported one or more vaginal symptoms in over 50% of subjects, and the prevalence of these symptoms increased with age. Amongst a group of women aged 56–69 years treated with intravaginal estrogen, Hilton & Stanton[59] reported that 22.3% complained of local vaginal discomfort.

Although in our study vaginal estradiol gave little benefit in the treatment of urinary symptoms, it has been shown to be useful in the management of atrophic vaginitis.[51] In a placebo-controlled study of 164 women, 78.8% of the Vagifem group and 81.9% of the placebo group had moderate to severe vaginal atrophy prior to treatment. After 12 weeks' therapy only 10.7% of the Vagifem group but 29.9% of the placebo group had the same degree of atrophy.[51]

Low-dose local therapy appears to be most beneficial in the management of symptoms due to vaginal atrophy, and recently a 55-mm diameter silicone vaginal ring releasing 5–10 µg estradiol/24 h for a minimum of 90 days has been evaluated.[60] Its efficacy, safety and acceptability have been assessed in 222 postmenopausal women with symptoms and signs of vaginal atrophy. Maturation of the vaginal epithelium, measured cytologically, significantly improved during treatment, as did symptoms of vaginal dryness, pruritus vulvae, dyspareunia and urinary urgency. Cure or improvement of atrophic vaginitis was recorded in more than 90% of subjects and the majority of the women found this form of treatment acceptable even during sexual intercourse.[60] Unfortunately, there has so far been no placebo-controlled trial of this device, which may be having an effect on the vaginal epithelium merely by its presence in the vagina.

Estrogens in the treatment of recurrent urinary tract infection

A possible application for estrogen therapy in postmenopausal women with lower urinary tract dysfunction is in the treatment and prophylaxis of recurrent urinary tract infections. Atrophic changes in the vagina reduce colonization by lactobacilli, increasing vaginal pH and encouraging overgrowth by Gram-negative uropathogens. Estrogen therapy has been shown to reverse atrophic changes and reduce the incidence of postmenopausal urinary tract infections.

Brandberg et al[61] treated 41 elderly women with recurrent urinary tract infections with oral estriol and showed that their vaginal flora was restored to the premenopausal type, and that they required fewer antibiotics. In an uncontrolled study, Privette et al[62] evaluated 12 women who experienced frequent urinary tract infections. They were all found to have atrophic vaginitis and had suffered a mean of 4 infections per patient per year. Treatment consisted of a combination of short-term douche and antibiotic for 1 week together with long-term estrogen therapy. Follow-up was for 2–8 years and during that time there were only 4 infections in the entire group.

Kjaergaard et al[63] studied 23 postmenopausal women with recurrent urinary tract infections. The women were treated with vaginal estradiol or placebo for 5 months, following which there was improvement in vaginal cytology in the estradiol group only, but no difference in the number of urinary tract infections or patient satisfaction between the two groups. Kirkengen et al[64] randomized 40 elderly women with recurrent urinary tract infections to receive either oral estriol 3 mg daily for 4 weeks followed by 1 mg daily for 8 weeks or matching placebo. There was no difference between estriol and placebo after the first treatment period, but following the second treatment period estriol was significantly more effective than placebo at reducing the incidence of urinary tract infections.

More recently, in the largest study of its type to date, Raz[65] randomized 93 postmenopausal women with recurrent urinary tract infections to receive either intravaginal estriol cream or placebo, and showed a significant reduction in the incidence of urinary tract infections with active treatment. Even estriol, a weak estrogen with minimal systemic effects, is effective in the prevention of recurrent urinary tract infections in women, suggesting that this is an important therapeutic role for estrogen replacement therapy in postmenopausal women.

Effects of progesterone on the urinary tract

Cyclical progestogens are used in conjunction with estrogen replacement therapy in postmenopausal women to prevent endometrial hyperplasia and atypia attributable to unopposed estrogen therapy.

Progesterone produces relaxation of the smooth muscle of the uterus by inducing α-adrenergic receptor formation. Since the urinary and genital tracts share a common embryological origin and progesterone receptors have been demonstrated in the bladder and urethra,[5] a similar mechanism of action on the lower urinary tract would be expected.

Raz et al[66] have shown in female rats that progesterone facilitates β-adrenergic activity in the ureters, producing pronounced ureteral relaxation on exposure to adrenaline which could be reversed by β-blockers. They[67] have also studied the effects of progesterone on the urethra of pregnant dogs, and showed similar facilitation of β-adrenergic receptors to that seen in the ureter. Zderic et al[68] have shown that strips of bladder tissue from pregnant rabbits generate 50% less tension than controls in response to calcium when exposed to bethanechol (a parasympathomimetic). Levin et al[69] have shown similar results, and these suggest that progesterone may also have an anticholinergic effect on the bladder.

Progestogenic action on the smooth muscle of the urethra and bladder may therefore be by facilitation of β-adrenergic relaxation and blunting of α-adrenergic contraction as well as anticholinergic effects.

The effect of progesterone on the lower urinary tract has been most extensively studied during pregnancy, when a physiologically elevated serum progesterone level affects the ureters, bladder and urethra. During pregnancy physiological hydroureter is attributed to both the smooth muscle relaxant effects of progesterone[70] and obstruction by the gravid uterus. Langworth & Brack[71] noted that during the course of experiments on vesical activity of healthy cats they had to exclude pregnant animals from the study as their bladder capacities were significantly increased. Similar studies were performed on pregnant rabbits and again it was found that there was an almost 50% increase in the bladder capacity of these pregnant animals.

Youssef[72] performed supine cystometrograms on 10 women throughout pregnancy, and noted an increase in bladder capacity and compliance. These changes have also been demonstrated following the administration of exogenous progesterone and during the luteal phase of the normal menstrual cycle.[73]

There are few studies of the effects of pregnancy or exogenous progestogen administration on the urethra. It is known that over 35% of pregnant women complain of stress incontinence at some time during their pregnancy and it has been suggested that this is related to progesterone levels.[74] Van Geelen et al[75] evaluated 43 pregnant women with urethral pressure profilometry, and also measured serum 17-hydroxy-progesterone levels. They found no change in the maximum urethral closure pressure despite increasing levels of 17-hydroxyprogesterone and concluded that progesterone does not significantly alter the tone of the urethra.

Rud[76] studied the effect of progesterone on the urethra of continent and incontinent women and found no change in maximal urethral closure pressure, but did find a decrease in urethral pressure transmission during the cough profile. Benness et al[77] evaluated 14 postmenopausal women on continuous estrogen and cyclical progestogen and in 10 patients noted increased incontinence by pad testing during the progestational phase of the cycle. Eight of their patients had GSI, and in 7 of these urethral incompetence was worse on progesterone. Raz[78] has shown, however, that in continent women there is no change in the urethral pressure profile and no incontinence following the addition of the progestogen component to HRT. Progesterone may therefore inhibit the urethral closure mechanism by decreasing both the pressure transmission ratio and periurethral blood flow, and this is most profound in women with compromised urethral function who are already incontinent.

Burton et al[79] questioned 217 women with premature ovarian failure on continuous estrogen and cyclical progesterone therapy. He found an increase in the symptom of urgency during the progesterone phase of their cycle but no change in the incidence of urge incontinence or stress incontinence. These findings are in conflict with the expected action of progesterone on the lower urinary tract, but this was a questionnaire study with no objective measurements, and the women included were not complaining of lower urinary tract symptoms.

The clinical value of progesterone in patients with urinary complaints awaits evaluation. It may play a beneficial role in HRT in women with DI through its proposed β-adrenergic and anticholinergic properties. It may, however, offset the beneficial effects of estrogen in postmenopausal women with GSI,[77,80] although in continent postmenopausal women this effect would appear to be minimal.

CONCLUSION

To date there have been few appropriate placebo-controlled studies using both subjective and objective parameters to assess the efficacy of estrogen therapy for the treatment of urinary incontinence. Further confusion arises from the heterogeneity of different investigations and consequently the best treatment in terms of dose, type of estrogen and route of administration is unknown.

Systemic estrogen replacement therapy offers many potential benefits to climacteric and postmenopausal women in addition to its effect on the lower urinary tract. The risks of correctly administered and monitored treatment are relatively small and many of the benefits of systemic therapy do not apply to low-dose topical therapy.

Clear evidence exists to suggest that recurrent urinary tract infections can be prevented or even treated by the use of estrogen therapy.

Systemic estrogen replacement appears to alleviate the symptoms of urgency, urge incontinence, frequency, nocturia and dysuria, and low-dose topical estrogen is effective in the management of atrophic vaginitis. Although the latter appears to be free from side effects, prolonged usage is required and symptoms often recur on discontinuing treatment. It is at present unclear whether low-dose therapy has sufficient effect on the lower urinary tract to treat urinary incontinence.

There is no conclusive evidence that estrogen alone cures stress incontinence, although in combination with an α-adrenergic agonist there may be a place for estrogen therapy in the conservative management of GSI.

Estrogen supplementation definitely improves the quality of life of many postmenopausal women and therefore makes them better able to cope with other disabilities.

The clinical value of progesterone and progestogens in women with urinary complaints awaits further evaluation. They may be of benefit to women with DI and conversely of detriment to women with GSI.

Undoubtedly, estrogen replacement therapy is of enormous therapeutic value to postmenopausal women; however, in the management of urinary disorders it may be primarily an adjunct to other methods of treatment.

REFERENCES

1 Central Statistical Office. Annual Abstract of Statistics, no 127. London: HMSO, 1991.
2 Cardozo LD. Role of estrogens in the treatment of female urinary incontinence. JAGS 1990; 38: 326–328.
3 Iosif S, Batra S, Ek A, Astedt B. Estrogen receptors in the human female lower urinary tract. Am J Obstet Gynaecol 1981; 141: 817–820.
4 Batra SC, Fosil CS. Female urethra, a target for estrogen action. J Urol 1983; 129: 418–420.
5 Batra SC, Iosif LS. Progesterone receptors in the female lower urinary tract. J Urol 1987; 138: 1301–1304.
6 Van Geelen JM, Desburg WH, Thomas CMG, Martin CB. Urodynamic studies in the normal menstrual cycle: the relationship between hormonal changes in the menstrual cycle and urethral pressure profiles. Am J Obstet Gynaecol 1981; 141(4): 384–392.
7 Tapp AJS, Cardozo LD. The postmenopausal bladder. Br J Hosp Med 1986; 35: 20–23.
8 McCallin PE, Stewart Taylor E, Whitehead RW. A study of the changes in cytology of the urinary sediment during the menstrual cycle and pregnancy. Am J Obstet Gynaecol 1950; 60: 64–74.
9 Solomon C, Panagotopoulous P, Oppenheim A. Urinary cytology studies as an aid to diagnosis. Am J Obstet Gynaecol 1958; 76: 57–62.
10 American National Institute of Health Population Figures. US Treasury Department. NIH.
11 Milne JS, Williamson J, Maule MM. Urinary symptoms in older people. Modern Geriatrics 1972; 2: 198.
12 Thomas TM, Plymat KR, Blannin J. Prevalence of urinary incontinence. British Medical Journal 1980; 281: 1243.

13 Yarnell JWG, St Leger AS. The prevalence and severity of urinary incontinence in women. J Epidemiol Comm Health 1981; 35: 71.

14 Vetter NJ, Jones DA, Victor CR. Urinary incontinence in the elderly at home. Lancet 1981; 2: 1275.

15 Diokno AC, Brook BM, Brown MB. Prevalence of urinary incontinence and other urological symptoms in the non institutionalised elderly. J Urology 1986; 136: 1022.

16 Iosif CS, Bekassy Z. Prevalence of genito-urinary symptoms in the later menopause. Acta Obstet Gynecol Scand 1984; 63: 257–260.

17 Health Survey Questionnaire: Market and Opinion Research International (MORI). 1990; 95 Southwark Street, London SE1 OHX.

18 Rud T, Anderson KE, Asmussen M, Hunting A, Ulmsten U. Factors maintaining the urethral pressure in women. Invest Urol 1980; 17: 343–347.

19 Malone-Lee J. Urodynamic measurement and urinary incontinence in the elderly. In: Brocklehurst JC (ed) Managing and measuring incontinence. Proceedings of Geriatric Workshop on Incontinence, July 1988. Geriatric Medicine, 1989.

20 Jolleys JV. Reported prevalence of urinary incontinence in women in general practice. Br Med J 1988; 296: 1300–1302.

21 Kondo A, Kato K, Saito M, Otani T. Prevalence of hand washing urinary incontinence in females in comparison with stress and urge incontinence. Neurourol and Urodynam 1990; 9: 330–331.

22 Versi E, Cardozo LD. Estrogens and lower urinary tract function. In: Studd JWW, Whitehead MI (eds) The menopause. Blackwell Scientific, 1988: pp 76–84.

23 Kinn AC, Lindskog M. Estrogens and phenylpropanolamine in combination for stress urinary incontinence in postmenopausal women. Urol 1988; 32: 273–280.

24 Smith PJB. The effect of estrogens on bladder function in the female. In: Campbell S (ed) The management of the menopause and post-menopausal years. MTP, pp 291–298.

25 Samsioe G, Jansson I, Mellstrom D, Svandborg A. Occurrence, nature and treatment of urinary incontinence in a 70 year old female population. Maturitas 1985; 7: 335–342.

26 Fantl JA, Cardozo LD, Ekberg J, McClish DK, Heimer G. Estrogen therapy in the management of urinary incontinence in postmenopausal women. A meta-analysis. Obstetrics and Gynaecology (In press).

27 Smith RJN, Studd JWW. Recent advances in hormone replacement therapy. British J Hospital Medicine 1993; 49(11): 799–809.

28 Sturdee DW, Wade-Evans T, Paterson MEL, Thom M, Studd JWW. Relations between bleeding pattern, endometrial histology and estrogen treatment in menopausal women. British Medical J 1978; 1: 1575.

29 Paterson MEL, Wade-Evans T, Sturdee DW, Thom MH, Studd JWW. Endometrial disease after treatment with estrogens and progestogens in the climacteric. British Medical J 1980; 1: 822–824.

30 Persson O, Adami HO, Bergkvist L et al. Risk of endometrial cancer after treatment with estrogens alone or in combination with progestogens; results of a prospective study. British Medical J 1989; 298: 147–151.

31 Magos AL, Brincat M, Wardle P, Schlesinger P, O'Dowd T. Amenorrhoea and endometrial atrophy with continuous oral estrogen and progestogen therapy in post menopausal women. Obstet Gynaecol 1985; 65: 496–499.

32 Stampfer MJ, Colditz GA. Estrogen replacement therapy and coronary heart disease: a quantitative assessment of the epidemiological evidence. Prev Med 1997; 20: 47–63.

33 Hough JL, Zilversmit DB. The effect of 17b-estradiol on aortic cholesterol content and metabolism in cholesterol fed rabbits. Arteriosclerosis 1986; 6: 57–63.

34 Gangar KF, Vyas S, Whitehead M, Crook D, Meire H, Campbell S. Pulsatility index in the internal carotid artery in relation to transdermal estradiol and time since the manopause. Lancet 1991; 338: 839–842.

35 Paganini-Hill A, Ross RK, Henderson BE. Postmenopausal estrogen treatment and stroke; a prospective study. British Medical J 1988; 297: 519–522.

36 Lindsay R, Cosman F. Estrogen in prevention and treatment of osteoporosis. Ann NY Acad Sci 1990; 592: 326–333.

37 Keil DP, Felson DT, Anderson JJ, Wilson DWF, Moskowitz MA. Hip fractures and use of estrogens in postmenopausal women. N Engl J Med 1987; 317: 1169–1174.

38 Studd JWW, Savvas M, Watson N, Garnett T, Fogelman J, Cooper D. The relationship between plasma estradiol and the increase in bone density in post menopausal women after treatment with subcutaneous hormone implants. Am J Obstet Gynecol 1990; 163: 1474–1479.

39 Dupont WD, Page DL. Menopausal estrogen replacement therapy and breast cancer. Arch Internal Med 1991; 151: 67–72.

40 Hunt K, Vessey M, McPherson K. Mortality in a cohort of long term users of hormone replacement therapy: an updated analysis. Br J Obstet Gynaecol 1990; 97: 1080–1086.

41 Hammond CB, Maxson WS. Current status of estrogen therapy for the menopause. Fertil Steril 1982; 37: 5–25.

42 Smith RNJ, Studd JWW. Hormone replacement therapy: a review. J Drug Dev 1992; 4: 235–244.

43 Iosif CS. Effects of protracted administration of estriol on the lower genitourinary tract in postmenopausal women. Arch Gynaecol Obstet 1992; 251: 115–120.

44 Mettler L, Oslen PG. Long term treatment of atrophic vaginitis with low dose estradiol vaginal tablets. Maturitas 1991; 14: 23–31.

45 Salmon UL, Walter RI, Gast SH. The use of estrogens in the treatment of dysuria and incontinence in postmenopausal women. Am J Obstet Gynecol 1941; 42: 845–847.

46 Musiani U. A partially successful attempt at medical treatment of urinary stress incontinence in women. Urol Int 1972; 27: 405–410.

47 Schleyer-Saunders E. Hormone implants for urinary disorders in postmenopausal women. J Am Geriar Soc 1976; 24: 337–339.

48 Cardozo LD, Rekers H, Tapp A et al. Estriol in the treatment of postmenopausal urgency – a multicentre study. Maturitas (In press).

49 Fantl JA, Wyman JF, Anderson RL, Matt DW, Bump RC. Postmenopausal urinary incontinence: comparison between non-estrogen supplement and estrogen-supplemented women. Obstet Gynecol 1988; 71: 823–826.

50 Nilsson K, Heimer G. Low dose estradiol in the treatment of urogenital estrogen deficiency – a pharmacokinetic and pharmacodynamic study. Maturitas 1992; 15: 121–127.

51 Eriksen PS, Rasmussen H. Low-dose 17 beta estradiol vaginal tablets in the treatment of atrophic vaginitis: a double-blind placebo controlled study. European Journal of Obstetrics and Gynaecology and Reproductive Biology 1992; 44: 137–144.

52 Caine M, Raz S. The role of female hormones in stress incontinence. Proceedings of the 16th Congress of the International Society of Urology, Amsterdam 1973.

53 Rud T. The effects of estrogens and gestagens on the urethral pressure profile in urinary continent and stress incontinent women. Acta Obstet Gynecol Scand 1980; 59: 265–270.

54 Walter S, Wilf H, Barlebo H, Jansen H. Urinary incontinence in postmenopausal women treated with estrogens: a double-blind clinical trial. Urol Int 1978; 33: 135–143.

55 Wilson PD, Faragher B, Butler B, Bullock D, Robinson EL, Brown ADG. Treatment with oral piperazine estrone sulphate for genuine stress incontinence in post menopausal women. Br J Obstet Gynaecol 1987; 94: 568–574.

56 Walter S, Kjaergaard B, Lose G et al. Stress urinary incontinence in postmenopausal women treated with oral estrogen (estriol) and alpha adrenoceptor-stimulating agent (phenylpropanolamine): a randomised double blind placebo controlled study. International Urogynecology Journal 1990; 12: 74–79.

57 Beisland HO, Fossberg E, Moer A, Sander S. Urethral sphincteric insufficiency in postmenopausal females: treatment with phenylpropanolamine and estriol separately and in combination. Urol Int 1984; 39: 211–216.

58 Hilton P, Tweddel AL, Mayne C. Oral and intravaginal estrogens alone and in combination with alpha adrenergic stimulation in genuine stress incontinence. International Urogynaecology Journal 1990; 12: 80–86.

59 Hilton P, Stanton SL. The use of intravaginal estrogen cream in genuine stress incontinence. Br J Obstet Gynaecol 1983; 90: 940–944.

60 Smith P, Heimer G, Lindskog M, Ulmsten U. Estradiol-releasing vaginal ring for treatment of post menopausal urogenital atrophy. Maturitas 1993; 16: 145–154.

61 Brandberg A, Mellstrom D, Samsioe G. Peroral estriol treatment of older women with urogenital infections. Lakartidningen 1985; 82: 3399–3401.

62 Privette M, Cade R, Peterson J, Mars D. Prevention of recurrent urinary tract infections in postmenopausal women. Nephron 1988; 50: 24–27.

63 Kjaergaard B, Walter S, Knudsen A, Johansen B, Barlebo H. Treatment with low-dose vaginal estradiol in postmenopausal women. A double-blind controlled trial. Ugeskrift For Laeger 1990; 152: 658–659.

64 Kirkengen AL, Andersen P, Gjersoe E, Johannessen GA, Johnsen N, Bodd E. Estriol in the prophylactic treatment of recurrent urinary tract injections in post menopausal women. Scand J Prime Health Care 1992; 10: 139–142.

65 Raz R, Stamm WE. A controlled trial of intravaginal estriol in post menopausal women with recurrent urinary tract infections. New England J Medicine 1993; 329(11): 753–756.

66 Raz S, Ziegler M, Laine M. Hormone influences on the adrenergic receptors of the urethra. Br J Urol 1972; 44: 405–410.

67 Raz S, Ziegler M, Laine M. The role of female hormones on stress incontinence. 26th Congrès de la Société International d'Urologie, Amsterdam 1973.

68 Zderic SA, Plzak JE, Duckett JW, Snyder HM, Wein AJ, Levin RM. Effect of pregnancy on rabbit urinary bladder physiology. Effect of extracellular calcium. Pharmacol 1990; 41: 124–129.

69 Levin RM, Tong YC, Wein AJ. Effect of pregnancy on the autonomic response of the rabbit urinary bladder. Neurourol and Urodynam 1991; 10: 313–316.

70 Van Wagenen G, Jenkins RH. An experimental examination of factors causing ureteral dilatation of pregnancy. J Urol 1939; 42: 1010–1020.

71 Langworth OR, Brack CB. The effect of pregnancy and the corpus luteum on vesical function. Am J Obstet Gynaecol 1939; 37: 121–125.

72 Youssef AF. Cystometric studies in gynaecology and obstetrics. Obstet Gynaecol 1956; 8: 181–188.

73 Gritsch E, Brandsfetter F. Phasen Sphinktero-Zystometrie. Zentralbl Gunaekol 1954; 39: 1746–1750.

74 Stanton SL, Kerr-Wilson R, Harris GV. The incidence of urological symptoms in normal pregnancy. Br J Obstet Gynaecol 1980; 87: 897–900.

75 Van Geelen JM, Lemmens WAJG, Eskes TKAB, Martin LB Jr. The urethral pressure profile in pregnancy and delivery in healthy nulliparous women. Am J Obstet Gynecol 1982; 144: 636–649.

76 Rud T. The effect of estrogens and gestagens on the urethral pressure profiles in urinary continent and stress incontinent women. Acta Obstet Gynaecol Scand 1980; 59: 265–270.

77 Benness C, Gangar K, Cardozo LD, Cutner A, Whitehead M. Do progestogens exacerbate incontinence in women on HRT? Neurourol and Urodynam 1991; 10: 316–318.

78 Raz S, Ziegler M, Laine M. The effect of progesterone on the adrenergic receptors of the urethra. Br J Urol 1973; 45: 131–135.

79 Burton G, Cardozo LD, Abdalla H, Kirkland A, Studd JW. The hormonal effects on the lower urinary tracts in 282 women with premature ovarian failure. Neurourol and Urodynam 1992; 10: 318–319.

80 Olah KJ, Bridges N, Farrer D. The conservative management of genuine stress incontinence. Int Urogynaecol J 1991; 2: 161–167.

INTRODUCTION

Elderly women have a high prevalence of bladder dysfunction. In particular, urinary incontinence is common among older women and is endemic in nursing homes. It often results in stigmatization and social isolation. Although age-related changes predispose to urinary incontinence, it is not a part of normal aging, and contrary to public opinion most cases of urinary incontinence can be cured or improved. This problem is a significant cause of disability and dependency among the elderly and urinary incontinence is often cited as the precipitating factor in long-term institutionalization.[1] The conclusions in a recent Consensus Development Conference Statement[2] organized by the government of the United States of America indicated that every person with urinary incontinence is entitled to evaluation and consideration for treatment. Disturbingly, they also found that most health care professionals ignore urinary incontinence and do not provide adequate diagnosis and treatment.

The changing demographic pattern is of significant importance (Fig. 30.1). Over the past 40 years the main growth in the population has been

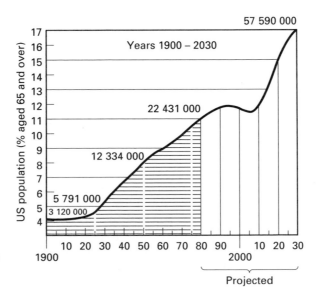

Fig. 30.1 Population over 65 years of age (From US Census Bureau 1981, Springer-Verlag 1984, with permission.)

amongst the elderly and it is estimated that by the year 2000 nearly 1 in 10 individuals will be over the age of 60 years. This growth rate is greatest in the most elderly with the number of over 75s increasing by 18% over the next 20 years and the number of over 85s increasing by as much as 38%. The significance of these numbers is compounded for the urogynecologist as the ratio of women to men in the latter group will be 2:1.

Urinary incontinence is also a costly problem both to the individuals concerned and to the community. The estimated annual cost of urinary incontinence in the United States is more than 10 billion dollars.[3] Unfortunately this problem, with its large psychosocial cost to those involved, has all too often been ignored by the women, their families and their physicians. This is generally due to ignorance and embarrassment and the mistaken viewpoint that urinary problems, particularly incontinence, are an inevitable accompaniment to old age.

The discussion of bladder dysfunction in elderly women warrants special attention for a number of reasons. As well as having the highest prevalence of disorders of the lower urinary tract, this group of women has a different spectrum of bladder dysfunction and all aspects of management, from investigation through to the different modalities of therapy, have significant variations from those used in their younger counterparts. As in younger women, urinary dysfunction and incontinence in the elderly can usually be significantly improved if not cured. It is therefore encouraging that research into these problems of the elderly female has been growing in recent years. However, much remains to be done and in some areas reliable data are still scarce.

Physicians should be able to identify and appropriately assess urinary incontinence in elderly women as it may be a manifestation of a subacute or reversible process either inside or outside the lower urinary tract. Incontinence is always a sign of some underlying disorder, the correction of which may restore bladder control. The initial investigation includes a targeted history and physical examination, urinalysis and simple tests of lower urinary tract function. Potentially reversible conditions that may be causing or contributing to the incontinence should be sought and treated. These include delerium, urinary tract infection (UTI) and decreased mobility. Patients who may benefit from urodynamic studies should be identified and referred. Several therapeutic modalities are available to treat lower urinary tract dysfunction in elderly women. These include behavioral therapy, pharmacological treatment, surgery and non-specific supportive treatments. Education for patients and caregivers is critical for the success of most therapies.

EPIDEMIOLOGY

Thomas et al[4] investigated the prevalence of incontinence in the community by conducting both postal and interview surveys. They defined incontinence as involuntary leakage twice or more per month and demonstrated an increase in incontinence of all types with age (Fig. 30.2), with a prevalence of 10–20% in women over 60 years. A similarly

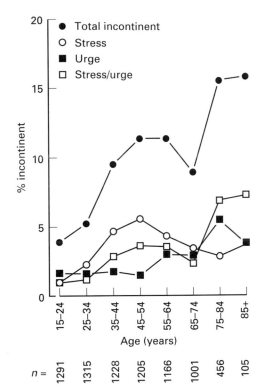

Fig. 30.2 Prevalence of stress, urge and mixed incontinence in women by age. (From Thomas TM, Plymat KR, Blannin J, Meade TW 1980. Prevalence of urinary incontinence. Br Med J 281: 1243–1245, with permission.)

significant number of incontinent elderly women in the community has been confirmed in other studies.[5,6] Dramatically increased levels of incontinence are present in elderly hospitalized or institutionalized women. Between 22% and 47% of elderly hospitalized women were found to be incontinent by Milne and colleagues,[7] and Burton[8] estimates of incontinence in up to 70% of patients in extended care facilities.

The role of estrogen deficiency in the increased prevalence of lower urinary tract symptoms in postmenopausal women remains unclear. Certainly, estrogen receptors have been identified in the human bladder, trigone and urethra,[9] as well as in pelvic floor muscles.[10] A Swedish study[11] of more than 900 women aged 61 years indicated that 29% complained of incontinence and 70% of these related the onset of their symptoms to the menopause. However, it is difficult to separate the influence of aging from that of the menopause. A study we conducted,[12] comparing lower urinary tract symptoms in two groups of postmenopausal women, one group having been on continuous hormone replacement therapy (HRT) and the other not, suggested that except for nocturia, estrogen deficiency does not seem to be an important factor in the pathogenesis of urinary symptoms in postmenopausal women.

CAUSES OF URINARY INCONTINENCE

A multitude of factors, physical, social and environmental, predispose to the increased prevalence of lower urinary tract dysfunction in the elderly. Some of the effects of aging on the lower urinary tract may be listed as follows:

1. Urethra
   a. Decreased collagen content
   b. Decreased epithelial vascularity
   c. Thin epithelium
   d. Decreased anatomic support
2. Bladder
   a. Decreased capacity
   b. Impaired bladder emptying
   c. Increased incidence of asymptomatic bacteriurea
   d. Increased incidence of UTIs
   e. Thin urothelium with impaired bacterial resistance
   f. Increased incidence of trabeculation.

The diagnosis and treatment of urinary incontinence in elderly women is aided by classification into either transient or established incontinence.[13] Transient incontinence is important as this group is generally more amenable to therapeutic intervention. Common causes may be indicated as follows:

- UTI
- confusional states
- fecal impaction
- estrogen deficiency
- restricted mobility
- depression
- drug therapy.

Urinary tract infection can tip the balance between continence and incontinence and should always be excluded. Any acute illness, such as pneumonia, or hospitalization can disrupt normal continence behavior patterns. The patient's motivation to be dry is important and may be decreased by affective disorders such as depression or confusional states. Drug therapy which may result in transient incontinence includes the use of anticholinergics, α-adrenergic blockers, sedatives and diuretics. Antihistamines and tricyclic antidepressants can cause detrusor relaxation, leading to retention with overflow incontinence. Prazosin, an α-adrenergic blocker, may decrease the urethral closure pressure resulting in stress incontinence. Rapidly acting diuretics may result in a patient being unable to reach the toilet in time. Certainly the causes of transient incontinence should be sought and treated before more complex investigations are carried out.

The causes of established incontinence may be listed as follows:

- genuine stress incontinence
- detrusor instability
- mixed genuine stress incontinence and detrusor instability
- retention with overflow
- urethral diverticula
- fistulae.

However it is most often due to detrusor instability (DI), genuine stress incontinence (GSI) or a combination. The prevalence of both of these conditions is increased in the elderly.[4] Other causes include urinary retention with overflow, which is more common in the elderly, and occasionally fistulae and urethral diverticula.

A common description of incontinence in both elderly men and women is of urinary leakage with no warning. This appears to be unrelated to bladder volume. It is suggested[14] that the origin of this involuntary detrusor contraction is at the suprapontine level, as opposed to the mid-brain level which is the presumed level of origin of un-inhibited detrusor activity in younger women. As the involuntary detrusor contraction is not perceived until it is actually in progress, it would appear to be independent of the cortical control of the bladder and may not be due to lack of cortical inhibition of bladder function. There may also be a perception sensory deficit associated with urge incontinence in older people which may alter the facilitatory–inhibitory balance of the central nervous system control of micturition. This would result in a failure of the normal unconscious inhibition of the bladder.

Stress incontinence, as well as urge incontinence, is different in older women. In the elderly, GSI has more of an intrinsic urethral dysfunction component than is the case in younger women, in whom an anatomical defect, hypermobility or poor pressure transmission are usually responsible. In many cases both components are present and this fact will affect the choice of surgery, if it is required, and subsequent success rates.

INVESTIGATION

The clinical history is important, although it must be kept in mind that symptoms of lower urinary tract dysfunction are not an accurate indicator of the underlying pathology.[15] However, the history does indicate those aspects which concern the patient most and their severity. Hilton & Stanton[16] assessed 100 elderly women and found that the complaint of stress incontinence was not restricted to urethral sphincter incompetence in older patients, and was present in half of all those referred. Urge incontinence was a common and non-specific complaint and urinary frequency was present in two-thirds of patients (Table 30.1).

A kind and sympathetic approach is essential, as elderly women often find it difficult and embarrassing discussing such subjects. Communication may also be difficult due to confusion or senility and information from relatives or nursing staff may be required. The history should determine the type of incontinence, the frequency and amount, associated symptoms and conditions as well as the presence of any precipitating factors. Enquiry should be made regarding neurological and psychological symptoms in addition to past surgical history. Current medications should be reviewed and the patient's social and environmental conditions assessed.

The physical examination should include pelvic inspection for signs of estrogen deficiency, and assessment for bladder distension, genital

Table 30.1   Percentage incidences of symptoms related to urodynamic diagnosis

Diagnosis	Stress incontinence	Urgency	Urge incontinence	Enuresis	Frequency	Nocturia	Strain in void	Poor stream	Incomplete emptying
Detrusor instability (n = 29)	33	84	80	46	68	52	0	9	4
Detrusor instability and urethral sphincter incompetence (n = 10)	43	100	71	60	67	67	0	38	38
Urethral sphincter incompetence (n = 30)	63	70	57	30	67	50	10	30	33
Voiding difficulty (n = 14)	77	58	58	62	62	38	43	72	33
No abnormality detected (n = 12)	20	90	90	0	70	50	10	20	20
Miscellaneous (n = 5)	33	33	33	50	40	60	0	25	0
All patients (n = 100)	49	76	68	39	65	51	10	30	23

From Hilton and Stanton 1981.[16] Reproduced by permission of *British Medical Journal*

Table 30.2   Abbreviated mental test score

1. Age
2. Time (to nearest hour)
3. Address for recall at end of test – this should be repeated by patient to ensure it has been heard correctly: 42 West Street.
4. Year
5. Name of hospital
6. Recognition of two persons (doctor, nurse, etc.)
7. Date of birth (day and month sufficient)
8. Year of First World War
9. Name of present monarch
10. Count backwards 20–1
3B. Recall of address

Dementia score = 10

From Hodkinson 1972.[17] Reproduced by permission of *Age and Ageing*

prolapse, stress incontinence or a fistula. Special attention is paid to any evidence of neurological deficit. Anal sphincter tone and perianal pinprick sensation assess S2,3,4 outflow. Rectal examination excludes fecal impaction. In elderly women, this clinical examination should be supplemented by a simple dementia survey and assessment of the woman's mobility. An example of a dementia survey is the Northwick Park Abbreviated Mental Test,[17] in which the patient answers a series of questions asked by the clinician (Table 30.2). Less than 9 out of 10 indicates significant mental deficiency. A mobility score is easily determined and is a useful indicator of how easily the patient can get to the toilet (Table 30.3).

A urinary diary is helpful in patient assessment although it may need to be completed by family or nursing staff if the woman is infirm. It indicates daily fluid intake and output, with urinary volumes voided and episodes of incontinence. The diary gives a baseline for the assessment of therapeutic regimens and aids behavior modification programs.

Table 30.3 Mobility score

1. Mobile
2. Walks with stick or frame
3. Confined to chair, but can stand
4. Cannot stand, but in chair
5. Bedbound

Mobility score = 5

Controversy exists about how far to pursue urinary evaluation in the elderly, and in particular the role of urodynamics. Certainly, urodynamic studies are not indicated in all elderly women with lower urinary tract symptoms and conservative therapy may initially be appropriate in many. However, as in younger patients, the clinical diagnosis of the

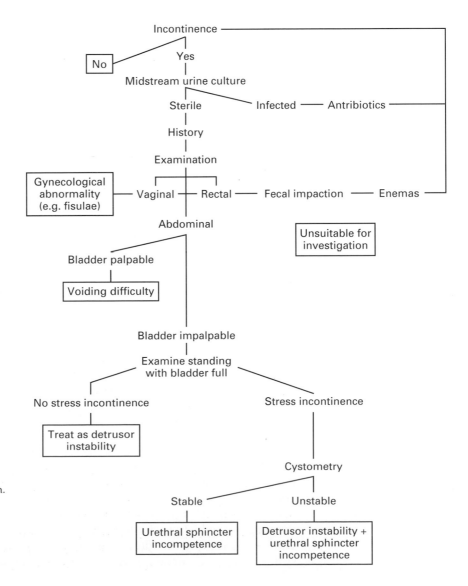

Fig. 30.3 Algorithm for assessment of urinary continence in elderly women. Hilton P, Stanton S L 1981. Algorithmic method for assessing urinary incontinence in elderly women. Br Med J 282: 940–942, with permission.)

cause of incontinence on the basis of symptoms alone is unreliable.[18] Hilton & Stanton[16] have suggested that approximately 60% of elderly women can be given a diagnosis and treated without resort to formal urodynamic testing. An algorithmic approach was recommended for the assessment of the elderly incontinent woman (Fig. 30.3). Following exclusion and treatment of those with UTIs, fecal impaction and voiding difficulties, those with clinically evident stress incontinence have cystometry performed while the others are treated as detrusor instability.

Hilton & Stanton[16] believed that patients with demonstrable stress incontinence should have DI excluded by urodynamic studies in order to determine accurately who will benefit from surgery. Urodynamic studies should also be undertaken when conservative management has failed, when voiding difficulties are present, and when previous incontinence surgery has failed. Some authors[19] suggest the use of a simplified form of cystometry which can be performed at the bedside in all incontinent women. The bladder is filled in increments of 50 ml using a bulb syringe, observing for fluid back-up in the syringe as an indicator of detrusor overactivity. However, this method will give erroneous results in a proportion of cases.

Specific tests

Urodynamic studies in the elderly generally take more time to complete than in younger women and a greater degree of nursing input is required. Therefore, the investigations performed need to be tailored to the individual, her symptoms, her degree of fragility and the information expected from each test.

The urine should be tested in all symptomatic women to exclude infection. The prevalence of UTI increases with age from 1% in healthy young women to 20% in women over 70 years.[20,21,22] Significantly higher rates occur in debilitated and institutionalized patients.[20,21] The relationship between urinary infections and incontinence remains unclear. Whereas an acute UTI can certainly precipitate incontinence, the treatment of asymptomatic infections does not improve incontinence[23] and may even encourage the emergence of resistant bacterial strains.

The measurement of urinary flow rates is a simple urodynamic test. Flow rates generally fall with age (Fig. 30.4) and are often less than 10 ml/s in women over 75 years.[24] Voiding flow rates are dependent on bladder volume,[25] and bladder capacities are lower amongst the elderly.[2] The lower flow rates may be partly related to the decreased bladder capacities but are also secondary to the reduction in detrusor shortening velocity which occurs with advancing age.[24]

Assessment of urinary residual is required and can be achieved either by catheterization or by ultrasound. The latter is less invasive and does not increase the risk of an acute UTI. However, catherization gives a good specimen of urine on which to exclude current infection. More than one assessment of residual volume is required to gain an accurate estimate on which to base management. The post-micturition urine volume is elevated in elderly women (Fig. 30.5), particularly if they are suffering from dementia, cerebrovascular disease, multiple sclerosis or

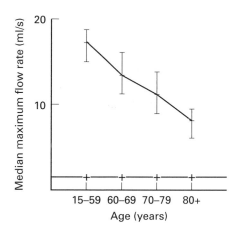

Fig. 30.4 Median maximum flow rate in women by age group with 95% confidence intervals. (From Malone-Lee JG 1989, with permission.)

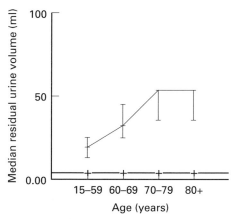

Fig. 30.5 Median residual urine volume in women by age group with 95% confidence intervals. (From Malone-Lee JG 1989, with permission.)

diabetes. The median residual urine volume in women over 75 years is approximately 50 ml, compared with approximately 20 ml in those under 75 years.[26]

Filling cystometry will identify women with DI or low bladder compliance and give an estimate of bladder capacity. However, Malone-Lee questions the value of the filling phase of urodynamics when 75–85% of elderly women over 75 years with lower urinary tract symptoms will be diagnosed as having an unstable bladder.[24] He also suggests that with regard to contractility, the elderly bladder is able to provide the isometric component of a detrusor contraction (change in pressure but no change in length) but is less adept at isotonic detrusor activity (change in length but no change in pressure).[26] The high frequency of DI in the elderly is reflected in higher maximum filling pressures and higher end filling pressures.

In assessment of the voiding phase of urodynamic studies in the elderly, it is helpful to use plots of the detrusor pressure against the voiding flow rate throughout micturition.[26] These graphs are computer-generated and the typical pattern seen in a younger woman is shown in Fig. 30.6. A different pattern often seen in elderly women is shown in Fig. 30.7. In this graph, micturition starts at a higher pressure, probably

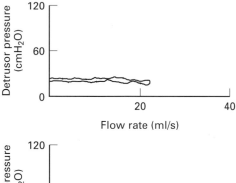

Fig. 30.6 The relationship between detrusor pressure and flow rate in a normal woman. (From Malone-Lee JG 1991, with permission)

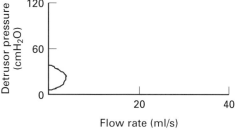

Fig. 30.7 Plot of detrusor pressure against voiding flow rate indicating the delayed sphincter opening and poorly sustained detrusor contraction which commonly occurs in elderly women

reflecting a delay in sphincter opening. Detrusor pressure then decays once micturition begins, due either to detrusor fatigue, reduced detrusor shortening velocity or neurological control being unable to maintain the detrusor contraction. Common urodynamic findings in elderly women are shown below:

- decreased flow rate
- elevated urinary residual
- delayed first desire to void
- decreased bladder capacity
- higher filling pressures
- reduced speed of detrusor contractions
- decreased urethral closure pressure
- impaired pressure transmission to proximal urethra
- lower voiding pressures
- high incidence of DI.

THERAPY

General as well as specific therapeutic measures are of particular importance in the management of lower urinary tract dysfunction in the elderly. These general measures may be listed as follows:

1. Treat any UTI present.
2. Treat constipation.
3. Maximize mobility.
4. Improve toilet access.
5. Assess medications.
6. Rationalize fluid intake.
7. Ensure regular toileting.

Acute UTI should be treated, as should constipation. A decrease in mobility often precipitates incontinence, so this should be addressed and toilet access also improved. The provision of a bedside commode may be of great assistance. Advice regarding fluid intake is given and drug therapy reviewed to ensure that all medications are appropriate and unwanted side effects minimized. This particularly relates to diuretic therapy, which can unnecessarily exacerbate urinary symptoms. Regular toileting (e.g. 2-hourly) can dramatically improve continence, while expert and dedicated nursing care is invaluable.

Specific therapeutic measures include pelvic floor physiotherapy, bladder retraining, electrical stimulation, drug therapy, surgery and catheterization. The decision on the most appropriate management regimen is often not easy and depends on a number of factors including the complexity and severity of the bladder dysfunction, the mental and functional status of the patient, and the family and social support that is available.

Genuine stress incontinence

Pelvic floor denervation is an important etiological factor in the genesis of GSI, and denervation increases with aging. A denervated pelvic floor gives poor urethral support resulting in impairment of pressure transmission to the proximal urethra.[28] There is also a progressive fall in the number of functioning motor units in urethral and pelvic floor skeletal muscle after 60 years of age, resulting in impairment of the urethral closure mechanism.[29]

Genuine stress incontinence is common in the elderly. The management is complicated by the fact that GSI in this age group often coexists with DI and/or voiding difficulties. Certainly, conservative modalities of therapy should initially be tried for the elderly woman with GSI. This should also include treatment of chronic bronchitis and asthma, reduction of smoking and improving bowel habit by attention to diet. Although weight loss makes surgery easier there is little evidence that it improves urinary symptoms, per se. Pelvic floor exercises (PFE) can strengthen pelvic floor muscles and reduce the symptom of stress incontinence,[30,31] but are only effective when the woman can actively participate in the program. Elderly women often have difficulty learning the technique and their poor compliance frequently leads to disappointing results. Initial biofeedback therapy, with a perineometer, can be of assistance in the use of PFE in the elderly.

Electrical stimulation can be used alone or as an adjunct to PFE. It has been shown to cause muscle hypertrophy and enhance reinnervation. Although it has been used for many years with good success,[32] studies of its efficacy in elderly women are lacking. Like PFE, functional electrical stimulation requires a co-operative patient. Short-term transvaginal electrical stimulation may be the most effective form of treatment and improvement within 6 weeks is expected. Maintenance therapy is required for most patients. Pelvic floor exercises and interferential therapy is probably a suitable combination therapy for elderly women. During electrical stimulation the sensation of a pelvic floor contraction is perceived and may aid in training patients how to do PFE. This form of therapy may not be appropriate for all elderly women as some have difficulty using a vaginal electrode because of arthritic changes in their hands or vaginal atrophy.

The lower urinary tract is known to be estrogen-sensitive and estrogens may be used as an adjunct to treatment of GSI in the elderly. Symptomatic benefits in postmenopausal stress incontinence have been described.[33] Although slight increases in urethral pressure and functional urethral length have been shown, it is likely that most benefit is obtained from improvement in the pressure transmission to the proximal urethra.[34,35] There are few good studies showing objective improvement in stress incontinent women treated with estrogen therapy. However, a significant decrease in urine loss with oral estriol 4 mg/d has been described.[36] Similar improvement could not be shown using oral piperazine estrone sulphate[37] or oral conjugate estrogen.[38]

α-Adrenergic agonists, such as phenylpropanolamine (PPA), have been found to be of some benefit in stress incontinence. Hypertension and ischemic heart disease are contraindications to this form of therapy. The combination of an α-adrenergic agonist and estrogen therapy has been examined in a number of studies. Subjective and objective improvement was seen using vaginal estrogen cream and PPA 50 mg twice daily.[38] Also, in a placebo-controlled trial,[36] patients preferred combined estriol and PPA to either drug alone. Estrogen therapy improves the discomfort of atrophic vaginitis and is likely to aid wound healing when given prior to surgery.

Surgery for genuine stress incontinence

Surgery is indicated in the elderly woman with GSI if it is severe or conservative management has failed, and should not be withheld on the basis of age alone. Severe incontinence, of whatever cause, may defeat a woman's ability to remain independent. With modern anesthetic techniques most are able to tolerate a surgical procedure although the recovery period is usually longer. It remains unclear which is the most appropriate procedure in the elderly. There is less morbidity with the endoscopic needle procedures such as the Stamey and Raz operations, but a better and more prolonged result may be achieved by a colposuspension. Pelvic relaxation is common in these women, and where it is the predominant complaint, an anterior colporrhaphy with buttressing of the bladder neck may be the most appropriate procedure. The periurethral injection of GAX collagen (glutaraldehyde cross-linked bovine collagen) may have a role in the management of some elderly women with GSI. It is associated with minimal morbidity and can be inserted under local anesthesia if required. The use of periurethral collagen is most efficacious in type III stress incontinence but repeat injections are often necessary. Data on which to base firm conclusions as to the best operation for the over 75s are deficient. Postoperative complications are more common in these women, particularly urinary retention. Those at particular risk of developing voiding difficulties following surgery should be identified if possible, as intermittent self-catheterization can be difficult to sustain in the elderly.

Postoperative management includes early mobilization, chest physiotherapy and suprapubic bladder drainage. If the peritoneal cavity is entered, the cul de sac should be obliterated by plication of the uterosacral ligaments or by the Moschowitz procedure. Surgery for incontinence in elderly women has a reported 3- to 5-year cure rate of 90%.[39] Stanton & Cardozo,[40] using the Burch colposuspension in elderly women, reported an objective cure rate of 74% which compares favourably with the rate of 86% for all ages.[41]

Detrusor instability

As in the younger woman, the management of DI in the elderly is based on bladder retraining,[42] drug therapy or a combination of the two. Bladder retraining, which has been shown to decrease incontinence in older women,[43] is not suitable for demented or immobile women. Drug therapy which may be beneficial includes in particular oxybutynin,[44] imipramine[45] and propantheline bromide. The latter two are often used in combination. Anticholinergic side effects are to be expected with these medications. The most common of these are dry mouth, blurred vision, esophageal reflux and constipation. Imipramine in particular can cause confusion and may also be associated with postural instability, so therapy should be instituted gradually and low doses prescribed initially, especially in the frail elderly.

Propantheline is the traditional anticholinergic medication and is used in a variable dosage from 15 mg twice daily up to 30 mg three times a day. Imipramine, which is generally well tolerated in the elderly, is commenced at a dose of 10–20 mg at night, and is particularly helpful for nocturia. It can be combined with probanthine with synergistic effect. Oxybutynin is probably the most efficacious of these medications and is therefore drug of first choice. An initial dose of 2.5 mg twice a day is appropriate as the half-life is increased in the elderly.[26] A high urinary residual should be excluded before starting oxybutynin as it may exacerbate voiding difficulties and lead to urinary retention.

If anticholinergic therapy is being considered, then the presence of visual symptoms or a history of glaucoma should be sought, as glaucoma is a contraindication to such therapy. Where nocturia is a significant problem, and has not responded to simpler therapy, night-time urine production can be decreased by intranasal desmopressin (DDAVP), a vasopressin analog.[46] This therapy is contraindicated in those with heart failure. Functional electrical stimulation can be tried as an alternative therapeutic modality, although studies in the elderly are lacking. A 6-week course is initially indicated and up to 50% have significant improvement.[47]

Combined genuine stress incontinence and detrusor instability

The combination of GSI and DI is common in the elderly. An initial accurate diagnosis is essential. A careful history helps determine the relative severity of the patient's symptoms, enabling the physician to concentrate on the problem and select the treatment most likely to be beneficial to the woman. Where symptoms of both conditions are significant, initial emphasis on controlling the DI will minimize the need for surgery in many women.[48] Treatment of the individual conditions is as suggested above. Imipramine has the advantage of a dual action. It reduces bladder contractility as well as acting on urethral smooth muscle by its α-adrenergic activity, possibly improving stress incontinence. Functional electrical stimulation can have a beneficial effect on both conditions, although it may be necessary to alter the frequency settings at certain intervals. Despite treatment of the DI and conservative management of the GSI, some women will still require surgery. In a number of these the DI will also be cured by the surgery, but most will require continuing therapy for their DI.

Voiding difficulties

Voiding difficulties are more common in the elderly. They often coexist with DI or GSI and complicate their management as the treatment of both of these conditions can exacerbate voiding problems. Urodynamic assessment is required to differentiate between outflow obstruction and poor detrusor function, the latter being much more common. Voiding difficulties may result in chronic retention and overflow incontinence. This can be diagnosed by history, examination and measurement of urinary residual (usually more than 400 ml in these cases). Some of the many causes of overflow incontinence may be listed as follows:

- drug effects
  —anticholinergics
  —sedatives, narcotics
- overdistension following surgery
- aging effects on nerve supply
- diabetes mellitus
- fecal impaction
- confusional state
- acute illness/immobility
- multiple sclerosis
- pelvic mass
- detrusor–sphincter dyssynergia.

Urinary residuals of 150–200 ml may cause recurrent UTIs and exacerbate symptoms of frequency, urgency and nocturia.

Once reversible causes have been eliminated, the management of retention and voiding difficulties is either pharmacotherapy, surgery or catheterization. The decision on which to employ depends on urodynamic assessment with pressure/flow studies and urethral pressure profilometry. Drug therapy is aimed at either increasing detrusor activity with cholinergics such as bethanecol (10–50 mg three times a day) or prostaglandins, or decreasing urethral resistance with α-adrenergic agonists (e.g. prazosin 0.5–2 mg twice daily) or skeletal muscle relaxant (e.g. diazepam 5–15 mg twice daily). Clean intermittent self-catheterization can be learnt by most elderly female patients, although a moderate degree of manual dexterity and mental clarity is required. Antibiotic pro phylaxis is not usually required and asymptomatic bacteriuria should not be treated. Those who cannot master self-catheterization can often be improved by urethrotomy.[49] This should only be undertaken when the maximum urethral closure pressure has been demonstrated to be high, otherwise incontinence may result.

Urinary tract infections

The incidence of UTIs is high in the elderly and is the most common cause of acute bacterial sepsis in those over 65 years. The prevalence of bacteriuria also rises with age from less than 5% in those under 50 years of age to more than 20% in those women over 65 years. The likely causes for the higher prevalence of bacteriuria are impaired bladder emptying and a fall in natural host defences. The normal hypoestrogenic state of the elderly woman is probably also a factor. It leads to an increased vaginal pH and subsequent alteration in vaginal flora which predisposes to UTIs. Those women who develop sepsis secondary to a UTI usually have a compounding factor such as voiding difficulties, catheterization or intercurrent disease. Recurrent as well as sporadic infections are a problem in the elderly. It is estimated that some 13% of women over 60 years suffer from recurrent lower urinary tract infections[50] and this prevalence is higher in nursing homes.

The organisms responsible for bacteriuria and UTIs in the elderly are usually Gram-negative bacilli, with *Escherichia coli* being the most commonly isolated. Clean midstream specimens are often difficult to achieve in the elderly and have a false positive rate of 17%.[50] Better specimens can be obtained from a catheter or by suprapubic aspirate. Hospitalization and indwelling catheters increase the incidence of infection with *Proteus*, *Klebsiella*, *Pseudomonas* and *enterococci*. The presence of bacteria on a urine microscopy specimen is abnormal. If leucocytes are also present then infection is likely. Culture and sensitivities should be obtained so that appropriate treatment can be instituted. Asymptomatic bacteriuria in the elderly does not require treatment.

Acute bacterial cystitis does require therapy, and effectiveness of antibiotic treatment should be checked by repeating the urine culture following completion of the course. Pyelonephritis can develop insidiously in elderly women and many will not display the classical signs of loin tenderness and fever. Prophylaxis should be considered for those with recurrent UTIs. There is recent evidence that estrogen therapy in elderly women, by lowering the vaginal pH and decreasing colonization of the vagina by fecal organisms, may reduce the number of infections in those with recurrent UTIs.[52] This beneficial prospect requires further assessment. Vaginal estriol cream is recommended for this indication.

Estrogens and lower urinary tract dysfunction

The various parts of the lower urinary tract, including bladder, trigone and urethra, have estrogen receptors[9] and are estrogen-sensitive. However, the role of postmenopausal estrogen deficiency in the increased incidence of lower urinary tract symptoms in elderly women is unclear. Atrophic changes do develop in the lower urinary tract of many women and it would be surprising if this did not result in symptoms in at least some. Certainly, estrogen therapy improves many urinary symptoms in postmenopausal women, including urinary frequency, urgency, urge incontinence, nocturia and dysuria.[53,54]

Unfortunately, there have been insufficient good studies assessing estrogen therapy in incontinent postmenopausal women. Although there appears to be some subjective improvement in stress incontinence with estrogen therapy, the data showing objective benefit are limited. The results of studies assessing combined estrogens and α-adrenergics are encouraging and this therapy should be considered in mild cases of GSI and where surgery is inappropriate. Estrogen supplementation definitely improves the quality of life of many postmenopausal women, and therefore makes them better able to cope with their other disabilities.

It is probable that the main role of estrogens in the management of postmenopausal urinary dysfunction is as an adjunct to other methods of treatment such as surgery, physiotherapy or drugs. As there are generally minimal risks and side effects to estrogen replacement therapy, and there are significant long-term benefits, the use of estrogens should probably be tried in most postmenopausal women with lower urinary tract dysfunction as improvement in symptoms will occur in many.

Estrogen deficiency and hormone replacement therapy

Estrogen deficiency is the hallmark of the postmenopausal years. The lack of estrogens can affect many different tissues, and symptoms may therefore be of different types. Symptoms may be acute, as with those of vasomotor instability, including hot flushes and night sweats. The onset of other symptoms may be slower and more gradual due to the longer term deprivation of estrogen, as in urogenital atrophy.

The vagina contains estrogen receptors and is sensitive to changes in systemic concentrations of estrogen. Falling estradiol levels after the menopause lead to reduced vascularity of the tissue, along with a decrease in the glycogen content of the cells. This in turn leads to a fall in lactobacilli content and an increase in pH, encouraging the growth of certain bacteria including coliforms and streptococci. A decrease in estrogen levels also results in atrophy of the vaginal epithelium with more parabasal and fewer superficial cells seen on vaginal cytology. Associated symptoms include vaginal dryness, soreness and dyspareunia. Replacement of estrogen, even in small amounts, is effective in reversing vaginal atrophy and increasing vaginal lubrication.

The major long-term consequences of the menopause are osteoporosis and cardiovascular disease. The rate of bone loss increases in the years immediately following the menopause. This is mainly due to a disturbance in the balance between bone resorption and formation, with an overall increase in resorption. Although there is a gradual age-related decline in bone density, the most important factor in postmenopausal osteoporosis is loss of the protective effect of estrogen. Postmenopausal bone loss particularly affects the distal radius, the neck of the femur and the vertebral bodies. It leads to an increase in fractures at these sites, classically with minimal trauma. Estrogen use plays a crucial role in preventing postmenopausal osteoporosis and the associated risk of fractures. Hormone replacement therapy will arrest the further development of osteoporotic bone loss, even in those women with significant disease.

Arterial disease is currently the leading cause of death in post-menopausal women in developed countries. Estrogen replacement therapy has been demonstrated to reduce the risk of coronary heart disease[55] and stroke[56] by over 50%. Although the precise mechanism remains unclear, there appears to be a direct beneficial effect of estrogen on vessel walls as well as an improvement in lipid profiles.

At present there is no clear evidence that estrogen therapy increases the risk of developing breast cancer. The only absolute contraindications to HRT are the presence of hormonally dependent cancers (breast, endometrium), active gall-bladder or liver disease, active thromboembolic disease and undiagnosed vaginal bleeding.

All types of estrogen therapy will relieve symptoms of the menopause when adequate serum levels of estrogen are attained. However, the metabolic effects of estrogen may be influenced by the route of administration. Urogenital atrophic changes in elderly women can be reversed using vaginal estrogen creams. Initial treatment is with one applicator of cream each night for 2–4 weeks, followed by a maintenance level of the same dose 2–3 times a week. As systemic absorption can occur, there is the potential risk of endometrial hyperplasia following continuous vaginal estrogen therapy. Therefore in non-hysterectomized women, therapy should be either intermittent (such as 3 out of every 4 weeks), or combined with progestogens if used continuously.

Estrogen therapy can also be administered orally, transdermally or via a subcutaneous implant. Estradiol given orally is subject to metabolism in the gut wall and liver, requiring the use of higher doses to achieve therapeutic plasma levels. An advantage of this method is the associated elevation of the protective HDL-cholesterol. Transdermal and implant therapy avoid the first-pass hepatic effect and more closely mimic the premenopausal environment.

Catheterization, pads and pants

In general, long-term indwelling urethral catheters should be avoided if at all possible. Catheter use increases bladder irritability and the incidence of UTIs and stone formation. The use of pads and pants, in conjunction with protective creams for the vulva and perineum, is usually preferable when continence has not improved in response to other therapies. It is vital that reversible causes of incontinence should be excluded before pads and catheters are used as a primary management tool for incontinence. There has been marked improvement in incontinence pad design over the past decade and continence advisors should be able to give appropriate advice on the most suitable products as the quality varies considerably. The elderly usually have a lower fluid intake and less urine output than the young, making them eminently suitable for management with modern incontinence pads (see Ch. 44). The availability of a continence advisory service is of great benefit in the management of urinary dysfunction in this population. They can be of considerable assistance in the diagnosis, assessment and management of lower urinary tract dysfunction.

Chronic catheterization may be required for:

- Management or prevention of decubitus ulcers or other skin wounds
- Overflow incontinence
- Women with pain on movement making linen changes difficult
- Those in whom the benefits of dryness outweigh the risks of catheterization.

Chronic catheterization may be by either a urethral or a suprapubic catheter. Urethral catheters are easier to insert as they do not require special expertise or a full bladder. Catheter leg bags should be changed and cleaned twice a day. Catheters should always be fixed in two places to prevent inadvertent removal or kinking. They should probably be changed monthly. Chronic suprapubic catheters are usually wide (18F) to prevent obstruction with mucus. They can usually be replaced without difficulty once the fistula tract matures. However, the use of clean intermittent catheterization is generally a preferable option to long-term urethral catheterization and progress towards a catheter-free state should be attempted.

CONCLUSION

Industrialized countries are rapidly becoming aging societies and much of the practice of urogynecology in the future will involve the investigation and treatment of older women. Urinary dysfunction and incontinence increase with age but are not inevitable accompaniments of the aging process. Both women in general and the medical community need to understand this. All elderly women with urinary problems deserve assessment and appropriate investigation including urodynamic studies where indicated. The complexity of incontinence in older women is generally greater than in young women. Stress and urge incontinence often coexist in the elderly patient and the pathophysiology of both of these may be different from that in younger women. Management decisions depend on many factors, including general health status and mental and functional status. Older women and their families are demanding a higher quality of life than was previously expected. This translates into greater challenges for medical and nursing staff. Good results are more difficult to achieve than in the younger population but are attainable in many women and should be pursued.

REFERENCES

1 Williams ME, Pannill FC. Urinary incontinence in the elderly: physiology, pathophysiology, diagnosis and treatment. Ann Intern Med 1982; 97(6) 895–907.

2 American Urogynecologic Society Quarterly Report, vol 10, no 3. July 1992.

3 Hu TW. Economic impact of urinary incontinence. Clin Geriatr Med 1986; 1: 673–680.

4 Thomas TM, Plymat KR, Blannin J, Meade TW. Prevalence of urinary incontinence. Brit Med J 1980; 281: 1243–1245.

5 Yarnell JWG, St Leger AS. The prevalence, severity and factors associated with urinary incontinence in a random sample of the elderly. Age and Ageing 1979; 8: 81–85.

6 Brocklehurst JC, Fry J, Griffiths LL, Kalton G. Dysuria in old age. J Am Geri Soc 1971; 19: 582–585.

7 Milne JS, Williamson J, Maule MM, Wallace ET. Urinary symptoms in older women. Modern Geriatrics. 1972; 2: 198–212.

8 Burton JR. Managing urinary incontinence – a common geriatric problem. Geriatrics 1984; 39: 46–62.

9 Iosif CS, Batra SC, Ek A, Astedt B. Estrogen receptors in the human female lower urinary tract. Am J Obs Gynae 1981; 141: 817–820.

10 Ingleman-Sundberg A, Rosen J, Gustafsson SA, Caristrom K. Cytosol estrogen receptors in the urogenital tissues in stress incontinent women. Acta Obstet Gynecol Scand 1981; 60: 585–586.

11 Iosif CS, Bekassy Z. Prevalence of genito-urinary symptoms in the late menopause. Acta Obstet Gynec Scand 1984; 63: 257–260.

12 Benness C, Abbott D, Cardozo L, Savvas M, Studd J. Lower urinary tract dysfunction in postmenopausal women – the role of estrogen deficiency. Neurourol Urodyn 1991; 10: 315–316.

13 Resnick NM, Yalla SV. Management of urinary incontinence in the elderly. N Engl J Med 1985; 313: 800–805.

14 O'Donnell. Geriatric issues in female incontinence. In: Walters M, Karram M (eds) Clinical urogynaecology. Mosby, 1993, pp 409–402.

15 Cantor TJ, Bates CP. A comparative study of symptoms and objective urodynamic findings in 214 incontinent women. Br J Obstet Gynaecol 1980; 87: 889–892.

16 Hilton P, Stanton SL. Algorithmic method of assessing urinary incontinence in elderly women. Br Med J 1981; 282: 940–942.

17 Hodkinson HM. Evaluation of a mental test score for assessment of mental impairment in the elderly. Age and Ageing 1972; 1: 233–238.

18 Sand PK, Hill RC, Ostergard DR. Incontinence history as a predictor of detrusor instability. Obstet Gynecol 1988; 71: 257.

19 Bent AE. Geriatric urogynecology. In: Ostergard D, Bent A (eds) Urogynecology and urodynamics – theory and practice. 3rd edn. Williams & Wilkins. 1991, pp 518–531.

20 Bentzen A, Veilsgaard R. Asymptomatic bacteriuria in elderly subjects. Dan Med Bull 1980; 27: 101–105.

21 Dontas AS, Kasviki-Charvati P, Papanawiotou PC, Marketos SG. Bacteriuria and survival in old age. New Eng J Med 1981; 304: 939–943.

22 Nicolle LE, Bjorson J, Harding GKM, Macdonell JA. Bacteriuria in elderly institutionalised men. N Engl J Med. 1983; 309: 1420–1425.

23 Fossberg E, Sander S, Beisland HO. Urinary incontinence in the elderly. A pilot study. Scand J Urol Nephrol 1981; 60: 51–53.

24 Malone-Lee JG. New data on on urodynamics in the symptomatic elderly. Neurourol Urodyn 1990; 9: 409–410.

25 Siroky MB, Olsson CA, Krane RJ. The flow rate nomogram 1. Development. J Urol 1979; 122: 665–668.

26 Malone-Lee JG. Bladder dysfunction in the elderly. In: Recent advances in obstetrics and gynaecology. Edinburgh: Churchill Livingstone, pp 209–221.

27 Griffiths DJ, Urodynamics – medical physics handbooks. Bristol: Adam Hilger, 1980.

28 Smith ARB, Hosker GL, Warrell DW. The role of partial denervation of the pelvic floor in the etiology of genito-urinary prolapse and stress incontinence of urine: a neurophysiological study. Br J Obstet Gynecol 1989; 96: 24–28.

29 McComas AJ. Neuromuscular function and disorders. London: Butterworths, 1977.

30 Burns PA, Pranikoff K, Nochajski T, Desotelle P, Horwood MK. Treatment of stress incontinence with pelvic floor exercises and biofeedback. J Am Geriatr Soc 1990; 38: 341–344.

31 Ferguson KL, McKey PL, Bishop KR, Kloen P, Verheul JB, Dougherty MC. Stress urinary incontinence: effect of pelvic floor exercise. Obstet Gynecol 1990; 75(4): 671–675.

32 Plevnik S, Janez J, Vrtacnik P, Trsinar B, Vodusek D. Short-term electrical stimulation: home treatment for urinary incontinence. World J Urol 1986; 4: 24.

33 Slunsky R. Complex conservative therapy of urinary incontinence in elderly women with ubreticology oesmoil and gymnastic exercises. Wien Klin Wochenschr 1973; 85: 759–762.

34 Rud T. Urethral pressure profile in continent women from childhood to old age. Acta Obstet Gynecol Scand 1980; 59: 331–335.

35 Hilton P. Urethral pressure measurement by microtransducer: observations on the methodology. The pathophysiology of genuine stress incontinence and the effects of its treatment in the female. Doctoral Thesis. University of Newcastle, 1981.

36 Walter S, Kjaergaard B, Lose G et al. Stress urinary incontinence in postmenopausal women treated with oral estrogen (estriol) and an alpha-adrenoreceptor stimulating agent (phenylpropanolamine) A randomised double-blind placebo-controlled study. Int Urogyn J 1990; 2: 74–79.

37 Wilson PD, Faragher B, Butler B et al. Treatment with oral piperazine estrone sulphate for genuine stress incontinence in postmenopausal women. Br J Obstet Gynaecol 1987; 94: 568–574.

38 Hilton P, Tweddell AL, Mayne C. Oral and intravaginal estrogens alone and in combination with alpha-adrenergic stimulation in genuine stress incontinence. Int Urogyn J 1990; 2: 80–86.

39 Gillon G, Stanton SL. Longterm followup of surgery for stress incontinence in elderly women. Br J Urol 1984; 56: 478–481.

40 Stanton SL, Cardozo LD. Surgical treatment of incontinence in elderly women. Surg Gynecol Obstet 1980; 150: 555–557.

41 Stanton SL, Cardozo LD. Results of colposuspension operation for incontinence and prolapse. Br J Obstet Gynecol 1979; 86: 693–697.

42 Frewen WK. A reassessment of bladder training in detrusor dysfunction in the female. Br J Urol 1982; 54: 372–373.

43 Burton JR, Pearce KL, Burgio KL, Engel BT, Whitehead WE. Behavioural training for urinary incontinence in elderly ambulatory patients. J Am Geriatr Soc 1988; 36: 693–698.

44 Koyanagi T, Maru A, Taniguchi K et al. Clinical evaluation of oxybutynin hydrochloride tablets for the treatment of neurogenic bladder and unstable bladder. A parallel double-blind controlled study with placebo. Nishinihon J Urol 1986; 48: 1052–1072.

45 Castleden CM, George CF, Renwick AG, Asher MJ. Imipramine – a possible alternative to current therapy for urinary incontinence in the elderly. J Urol 1981; 125: 318–320.

46 Hilton P, Stanton SL. The use of desmopressin for nocturia in the female. Br J Urol 1982; 54: 252–255.

47 Fossberg E, Sorensen S, Ruutu M et al. Maximal electrical stimulation in the treatment of unstable detrusor and urge incontinence. Eur Urol 1990; 18: 120–124.

48 Karram MM, Bhatia NN. Management of coexistent stress and urge incontinence. Obstet Gynecol 1989; 73(1): 4–7.

49 Moolgoaker AS, Ardran GM, Smith JC, Stallworthy JA. The diagnosis and management of urinary incontinence in the female. J Obs Gyn Brit Commonwealth 1972; 79: 481–487.

50 Iosif CS, Bekassey Z. Prevalence of genitourinary symptoms in the late menopause. Acta Obstet Gynecol Scand. 1984: 63: 257–260.

51 Ouslander JG. Lower urinary tract disorders in the elderly female. In: Raz S (ed) Female urology. Philadelphia: Saunders, 1983: 308–325.

52 Brandberg A, Mellstrom D, Samsioe G. Low dose estriol treatment in elderly women with urogenital infections. Acta Obstet Gynaecol Scand 1987; (Suppl 140): 33–38.

53 Walter S, Wolf H, Barlebo H, Jensen HK. Urinary incontinence in postmenopausal women treated with estrogens. Urologia Int 1978; 33: 135–143.

54 Samsioe G, Jansson I, Mellstrom D, Svanborg A. Occurrence, nature and treatment of urinary incontinence in a 70 year old female population. Maturitas 1985; 7: 335–342.

31 Neurological disorders

INTRODUCTION

This chapter deals with the effect of neurological lesions at different sites, and resulting disturbances of continence and voiding in women who have overt neurological disorders. It also deals in part with an interesting group of problems presented by women who have disorders of voiding or continence, without good clinical evidence of a neurological disorder or structural urological cause. In some members of this latter group, a putative neurological disorder can be identified on investigation. However, the essential difference between the two groups is that in the first the urogynecological problems presented are primarily those of functional diagnosis and symptom management; there is already a relevant neurological diagnosis. In the second, there is a need for both diagnosis and management.

This distinction, important though it may be, has led to the adoption of some terminologies which distinguish between 'neurological' and 'idiopathic' disorders in a way which may not be conducive to understanding of the underlying pathophysiology. For example, detrusor contractions seen during filling urodynamics in a patient with a known neurological lesion are termed 'detrusor hyperreflexia'. The same response seen as an idiopathic phenomenon is termed 'detrusor instability.'[1] The implication may be taken that while in the first case the fault is in the innervation, in the second case the fault is in the detrusor itself. There is no evidence to support such a distinction.

This chapter will not deal with the relevant basic sciences (Section 1), nor give details of the available methods of investigation (Section 2), special treatments (Section 6) or nursing aspects (Section 7). It will deal with the effect of lesions at different levels of the neuraxis, and with a selection of important and typical neurological disorders, and the localized neurological disorders of pelvic function, some of which can be diagnosed by appropriate neurophysiological testing. It will deal briefly with the appropriate planning of investigations in these patient groups.

Neuro-physiology

The basic levels of neural control of continence and voiding as they apply in disease are shown in a simplified form in Fig. 31.1, in which the main components represented are the cerebral, pontine, segmental and peripheral mechanisms and their interconnections, and the connections

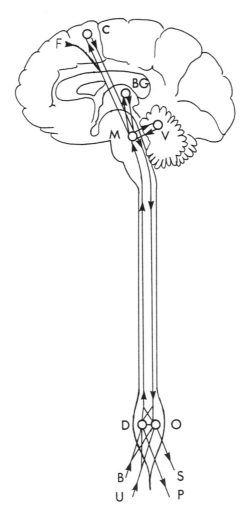

Fig. 31.1 Principal spinal and supraspinal pathways involved in the control of micturition. Afferent pathways are shown on the left, efferent on the right. D, detrusor nucleus; O, Onuf's sphincteromotor nucleus; M, pontine micturition centre; V, cerebellar vermis; BG, basal ganglia connections; C, sensorimotor cortex; F, frontal micturition-regulating areas; B, afferent pathways from bladder wall; U, afferent pathways from urethra; S, somatic sacral outflow to sphincters and pelvic floor; P, parasympathetic sacral outflow.

to the basal ganglia and cerebellum. In the functional model represented here, the basic organization of urinary voiding resembles a switch.[2] This switching function is organized in the pontine micturition centre of Barrington. Most of the time the system is switched to a 'fill' mode, in which the detrusor is inhibited, the bladder neck is closed and striated sphincter tone is maintained. Whether the bladder accommodates entirely passively, or whether there is an active (probably adrenergic) accommodation reflex in this phase in women, is uncertain, but there is good evidence for it in several animal species.[2,3] When voiding is desired and socially convenient, the function switches in a co-ordinated fashion. The striated sphincter relaxes first, and then the bladder neck opens and the detrusor contracts. The detrusor contraction is maintained until the bladder is empty. Several influences converge on the pontine micturition center to promote voiding: proprioceptive impulses from the bladder wall detect stretch and signal fullness; 'exteroceptive' impulses from the urethra detect flow and signal that voiding is in progress; and impulses from the frontal lobes initiate voluntary voiding.

The cerebral influence on the pontine micturition center is normally inhibitory, and dominates in that fullness alone (within normal capacity) does not initiate detrusor contractions. Even during voiding, the active detrusor can be switched off. In this case, however, voiding is interrupted initially by sphincter contraction, following which the detrusor contraction dies away and urine is 'milked back' into the bladder by closure of the proximal urethra and bladder neck. The initial sphincter closure achieves rapid cessation of micturition (usually because some emergency has arisen during micturition), and it also removes the reflex stimulus to continued voiding which arises from urethral flow. Voluntary sphincter closure is doubtless cortical in origin; a fast corticospinal pathway to the sphincters has been demonstrated.[4]

Other central pathways

The pontine micturition center is also anatomically linked by reciprocal pathways with the basal ganglia and the cerebellum. Animal experiments suggest that the cerebellum and basal ganglia may have an inhibitory effect on the pontine micturition center,[5] and this fits in with the clinical observation that patients with Parkinson's disease may exhibit detrusor hyperreflexia. Patients with pure cerebellar lesions do not typically complain of any voiding disorder, but they may show urodynamic abnormalities.[6] However, the functional significance of the connections to the basal ganglia and cerebellum remain unclear.

Lesions and symptoms

The specific disorder experienced by an individual, therefore, may indicate where the control system has been damaged, thus reflecting the site of the lesion, but not necessarily its pathology. However, both the site and distribution of lesions is often characteristic for a particular disease, in which case the constellation of symptoms may also be characteristic. Of course, many neurological illnesses affect the nervous system at more than one level. In that case, the clinical problems are often mixed. Multiple sclerosis, for example, is considered in this chapter among brain disorders, but could just as well have been included among the spinal cord diseases. At all levels of the central nervous system, the control of micturition is bilateral, so that unilateral central lesions do not usually have a severe or permanent effect. For example, patients with hemiplegic stroke may suffer a transient phase of incontinence, but this typically resolves in those patients who do well otherwise.[7] This does not necessarily apply to peripheral lesions, or where function is already compromised, so that for example a complete, but unilateral, pudendal nerve lesion can have a permanent and devastating effect on urinary continence in a woman with pre-existing borderline stress incontinence.

Investigation

Details of methods of investigation are given in Section 2. Only a few general points will be made here. In patients with established neurological disorders and bladder disturbance, investigation is not required to help in making the primary diagnosis, but it does have to serve several purposes. First, it has to exclude any unrelated structural cause, such as urethral stricture or ligamentous laxity. Secondly, it must establish the pathophysiological basis of the dysfunction, so as to guide the choice of treatment. Thirdly, it must search for urinary complications of neurological illness, such as renal or bladder stone, hydronephrosis, ureteric reflux or bladder trabeculation and diverticula. Both structural and functional investigations may therefore be required.

Urodynamics testing will detect detrusor hyperreflexia or hypotonia. However, in order to discover whether detrusor–sphincter dyssynergia or uninhibited urethral relaxations are present, cystometry should be combined with videocystourethrography.

Patients with spinal cord lesions require particular attention, because they commonly develop serious upper tract complications. Their initial assessment usually includes intravenous pyelogram (IVP) or ultrasound urodynamics with video, and cystoscopy. They should be followed up with regular ultrasound assessments to exclude stone, hydronephrosis and excess residual volume, and with regular renal function tests and urine culture.

Patients who are severely immobile as a result of neurological disease, or who have an indwelling catheter, are also liable to develop urolithiasis. This is caused by a negative calcium balance and by alkaline, infected urine. Urinary acidification (e.g. with ascorbic acid) may help.

BRAIN DISORDERS

In terms of the model in Fig. 31.1, cerebral dysfunction will impair efficient voluntary control over the pontine micturition center. In infancy, before the cerebral pathways are fully developed, the micturition center functions autonomously, resulting in efficient reflex urinary voiding (enuresis). In childhood (and often in normal old age) there is a reduced ability to inhibit voiding when the bladder becomes full, and a reduced ability to initiate voiding when the bladder is only partly filled. It should be noted that the cerebral mechanism involved in inhibiting reflex voiding when the bladder is full is not a function of 'will', or even awareness. Will, as ordinarily understood, is absent during sleep. However, whilst an infant voids during sleep when the bladder becomes full, a normal adult does not. Adult enuresis is dealt with later.

Diffuse and localized cerebral disease

In diffuse cerebral disorders such as Alzheimer's disease, and in localized bilateral disorders affecting connections to the frontal lobes, such as hydrocephalus, a pattern similar to the infantile is seen, with regression towards reflex voiding. Other diffuse and localized causes of cerebral lesions which may result in this type of disorder may be listed as follows:

1. Congenital
   a. Cerebral palsy
   b. Cerebral dysgeneses
   c. Craniocervical malformations

d. Syringobulbia
2. Space occupying and neoplastic
   a. Primary tumor (intrinsic or extrinsic)
   b. Secondary tumor
   c. Edema
   d. Hydrocephalus
   e. Extradural, subdural or intracerebral hematoma
3. Traumatic
   a. Closed head injury
   b. Penetrating brain injury
4. Vascular
   a. Cerebrovascular stroke
   b. Aneurysms and AV malformations
   c. Subarachnoid hemorrhage
5. Inflammatory
   a. Encephalitis
   b. Meningitis
   c. Multiple sclerosis (acute phase)
   d. AIDS encephalopathy
6. Degenerative
   a. Alzheimer's disease
   b. Huntington's disease
   c. Creutzfeldt-Jakob disease
   d. Multiple system atrophy
   e. Multiple sclerosis (chronic phase)
   f. Parkinson's disease
7. Functional
   a. Major epilepsy.

When the disorder is diffuse, there is often a concomitant loss of social inhibition and embarrassment at inappropriate voiding. However, when the lesion is localized (particularly involving the superomedial part of the frontal lobes and the corpus callosum), control may be lost but social awareness preserved. This dissociation, like continence during sleep, suggests that tonic cerebral inhibition of the micturition center is separate from the will.

Head injury

Severe or moderate closed head injury may cause diffuse white matter degeneration, intraparenchymal hemorrhages, infarcts and localized cerebral contusions.[8] The resulting specific voiding disorders must be distinguished from changes in voiding behavior resulting from cognitive impairment, spasticity, immobility, loss of communication, challenging behavior patterns, depression and loss of motivational drive. This distinction can be made by urodynamic testing.[9] The common abnormal findings in head injury are uninhibited detrusor contraction, uninhibited sphincter relaxations, difficulty in initiating voiding and detrusor hypotonia. Detrusor–sphincter dyssynergia is relatively uncommon and, when it does occur, is associated with diffuse bilateral brain damage. The abnormalities have been shown to be significant, and urinary infections to be common,[9] even in patients who had never been catheterized.

Stroke

Incontinence of urine is common in the early stages following stroke,[7] and is usually associated with frontal or capsular lesions.[10] Recovery usually occurs in 4–12 weeks, though it may occur as late as a year.[11] Failure to recover continence is associated with extensive or bilateral lesions and a poor prognosis.[7,12] However, care should be taken to ascertain whether stress or urge incontinence may have been present before the stroke. Recovery of continence is a good predictor of a recovery sufficient for early return home. Urodynamic testing shows that incontinence following stroke is associated with detrusor hyperreflexia or uninhibited urethral relaxation; detrusor–sphincter dyssynergia is uncommon. Depending on the site of the lesion, many stroke patients with loss of cortical inhibition of the detrusor reflex do nevertheless retain voluntary sphincter closure, probably via the direct corticospinal pathway.[4] Retention of urine in stroke patients is common and is associated with an increased probability of urinary infection.

Multiple sclerosis

In multiple sclerosis the plaques of demyelination are scattered in the white matter of the brain and spinal cord, with sites of predilection where flexion or pulsation occurs, such as the periventricular region, the optic nerves and the cervical cord. Because of this scatter, the longest pathways are the most heavily damaged, so disturbance of micturition is a prominent feature. Occasionally, urinary incontinence or retention is the initial presenting feature of multiple sclerosis. Much more commonly, the presence and severity of disturbances of urinary function parallel the level of disability, particularly in the legs, as a consequence of the pyramidal tract, propriospinal, cerebellar and sensory lesions,[13] which can be determined both clinically and electrophysiologically.[14] Most patients with disabling multiple sclerosis have disorders of voiding or continence, or both, and most have uninhibited bladders.[15] Dyssynergia is common, and has been correlated closely with the presence of up-going plantar responses. In a recent magnetic resonance imaging study, a correlation was found between severe urinary dysfunction and the presence of midbrain lesions.[16] For reasons which are unclear, patients with multiple sclerosis who have incomplete or dyssynergic voiding seem to be at lesser risk of upper tract damage than patients with spinal paraplegia who have similar urodynamic abnormalities.[17] In patients with mild reflex incontinence the symptoms may be controlled with anticholinergic drugs, such as oxybutynin. If incontinence is more severe, and if voiding difficulty is also present, patients can be taught intermittent self-catheterization, which may need to be combined with anticholinergic treatment. If the hands are too weak or ataxic to self-catheterize, the management choices are between intermittent catheterization by the attendant, indwelling urethral or suprapubic catheter, urinary diversion or protective pads and pants.

Parkinson's disease

Urinary urgency is common in Parkinson's disease. The problems caused may be exacerbated by slowness in reaching the toilet, due to the associated rigidity, bradykinesia and postural instability. Correspondingly, detrusor hyperreflexia is often found to be present on urodynamic testing.[18] Rigidity and tremor of the pelvic floor and sphincters have been found,[19] but the relationship with the symptoms is not clear. Many women with Parkinson's disease have symptoms suggesting stress incontinence, but while some do have genuine stress incontinence, most have detrusor hyperreflexia, and a few have an atonic bladder with overflow. Urodynamic testing is therefore essential[20] in order to make an accurate functional diagnosis, because there is no set of findings that is specific for Parkinson's disease.

Huntington's disease

In this late onset progressive autosomal dominant familial dementing illness, incontinence is a common late feature. Urodynamic studies show either detrusor hyperreflexia or normal results.[21] Sometimes there are choreiform contractions of the abdomen or pelvic floor, which are present during filling and inhibited during voiding.

Alzheimer's disease

There has been little or no work on the mechanisms of the incontinence which is a common late feature of Alzheimer's disease, but clinically the urgency and enuresis due to loss of cortical control of voiding are often exacerbated by confusion, disorientation and urinary infection.

Cerebral palsy

Children with cerebral palsy are commonly late in gaining control, and may have persisting enuresis; on urodynamic testing, detrusor hyperreflexia is frequently found to be present.[22] As they progress into adulthood, poor voiding and chronic retention become more common. Poor voiding was shown in one study[23] to be attributable to pelvic floor spasticity, rather than a true detrusor–sphincter dyssynergia. However, evidence of sphincter denervation in addition is not uncommon.

SPINAL CORD DISORDERS

Pathophysiology

Ascending and descending impulses relating to bladder and urethral sensory and motor functions run in the long tracts of the cord (Fig. 31.2). Proprioceptive impulses from the bladder wall run in the posterior column, while exteroceptive impulses from the urethra run in the spinothalamic tract. The motor pathways are bilateral, and roughly equatorial in position in the cord. Bilateral cord lesions therefore disrupt the regulation of the filling and voiding states which is normally controlled by the pontine micturition center.

The most important causes of spinal cord lesions that can disturb micturition are as follows:

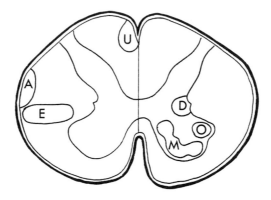

Fig. 31.2 Spinal long tracts (left) and conus medullaris nuclei (right), concerned in micturition. All of them are in reality bilateral. Left: A, approximate location of bladder afferent pathway; U, urethral afferent pathway; E, micturition motor pathway. Right: D, detrusor motoneurone colony in intermediolateral column; O, Onuf's nucleus of sphincter motoneurones; M, motoneurones to extrinsic muscles of the pelvic floor.

1. Congenital
   a. Spinabifida and myelodysplasia
   b. Progressive kyphoscoliosis
   c. Tethered cord
2. Space occupying and neoplastic
   a. Primary tumors (intrinsic or extrinsic)
   b. Secondary tumors (usually bony)
   c. Extradural abscess
   d. Malignant meningitis
3. Traumatic
   a. Closed injury
   b. Penetrating injury
4. Vascular
   a. Angioma or arteriovenous malformation
   b. Anterior spinal artery occlusion
   c. Artery of Adamkiewicz occlusion
   d. Aortic dissection
5. Inflammatory
   a. Multiple sclerosis (acute phase)
   b. Transverse myelitis
   c. Paraneoplastic myelitis
   d. Zoster myelitis
   e. Syphilitic myelitis
   f. AIDS myelopathy
6. Degenerative
   a. Cervical spondylosis
   b. Prolapsed thoracic disk
   c. Syringomyelia
   d. Multiple sclerosis (chronic phase).

Following an acute cord lesion there is a period of 'spinal shock' during which segmental reflex function is reduced. In humans it may be several weeks before segmentally organized reflex detrusor contractions recover, although sphincter tone may reappear in only a few hours.

In patients with stable incomplete lesions, the ability to initiate micturition may be lost. In some patients with a complete cord lesion the detrusor may remain permanently atonic.[24] However, loss of inhibition ('detrusor hyperreflexia') is much more commonly encountered, both for complete and incomplete lesions.

In patients with complete lesions, suprasegmental control is lost; all that remain are the peripheral intrinsic and spinal segmental mechanisms. These function in a way that is variable, and sometimes damaging to the upper urinary tract.

Segmentally organized reflex voiding can be provoked by bladder fullness, either alone or in combination with external stimuli. However, it is inefficient, and differs from pontine reflex voiding in the following ways. First, the detrusor may be activated before the bladder has reached full capacity. This can be interpreted as a loss of descending inhibition. Secondly, detrusor contraction is often associated with striated sphincter activation, which may be phasic or tonic (detrusor–sphincter dyssynergia). This reflects loss of the reciprocal innervation of detrusor and sphincter, which is normally organized suprasegmentally by the pontine center. Less commonly there is a failure of bladder neck opening. Thirdly, detrusor contraction is often poorly sustained. This reflects loss of detrusor facilitation which again is normally a suprasegmental function. Thus, once some urine is passed, the stretch signal from the sensory endings in the bladder urothelium wanes, while the reflex by which urine distending the urethra maintains detrusor contraction[25] is ineffective at segmental level. Lastly, uninhibited sphincter relaxations can occur, unassociated with detrusor contraction but resulting in incontinence.

These faults, if left untreated, may commonly lead to serious consequences. Poor or incomplete voiding will predispose to urinary infection. High pressure or dyssynergic voiding may cause detrusor hypertrophy, trabeculation and the formation of sacs or diverticula, which further increase residual volume. High voiding pressure and changes in the bladder wall lead to ureteric reflux, with hydronephrosis, renal damage and upward transmission of infection.

Autonomic dysreflexia

Spinal cord lesions above a neurological level of about T6 leave a substantial part of the sympathetic outflow, particularly the splanchnic outflow, disconnected from the brain but functionally connected to the isolated distal segments of the spinal cord. Some states of the cord can then result in a massive vasoconstriction, mediated by sympathetic pathways, causing uncontrolled paroxysmal hypertension. This response, called autonomic dysreflexia, can be precipitated by pain impulses entering the cord below the lesion, or by signals from a distended bladder or bowel, uterine contraction or orgasm. Headache, above-lesion flushing and below-lesion piloerection and sweating are the early symptoms of an attack. It may require emergency treatment of the hypertension, and removal of the offending stimulus.

Paraplegia

In the United Kingdom, the incidence of traumatic paraplegia in women is about 1/250 000 per year (225 per year), and the prevalence is less than the prevalence of paraplegia in multiple sclerosis; the reverse is true in men, who suffer less multiple sclerosis but are more liable to be injured in accidents. Other medical causes of paraplegia are much less common. Closed injury resulting in traumatic paraplegia most commonly occurs at mid-thoracic or low cervical level.

Managing the bladder in paraplegia – 'simple' methods

The aims of bladder management in paraplegia are to preserve the integrity of the upper tracts and renal function,[26] to avoid infection and lower tract damage and to achieve continence. During the acute period of spinal shock the patient may require an indwelling catheter to monitor fluid balance. When the patient becomes medically stable, a choice of bladder management technique has to be made, as between intermittent clean catheterization,[27] chronic suprapubic catheter,[28] long-term urethral catheter or reflex voiding. The best initial choice depends on the clinical circumstances.

Intermittent self-catheterization (ISC) is often very satisfactory, and is used by more paraplegics than any other single method. It achieves complete emptying without requiring surgery or an indwelling device. It is applicable to patients with a high outflow resistance or sphincter dyssynergia. It is difficult for patients with a cervical lesion and impaired hand function to self-catheterize, but assistive devices are available, or the carer can learn to do it. If the bladder is hyperactive, ISC can be combined with anticholinergic treatment, intravesical atropine, oxybutynin or capsaicin, or occasionally a bladder augmentation.

Reflex voiding is often combined with manual expression. A reflex detrusor contraction is provoked when the bladder is sufficiently full. The most effective stimulus varies; common methods include pressing or tapping the lower abdomen, straining or anal stretch. As a result of the sources of segmental reflex voiding inefficiency, detailed above, reflex training for micturition may give unsatisfactory results, even in the best hands. Reflex incontinence is common, and is a serious problem for paraplegic women, for whom wearable urine-collecting devices are less than satisfactory. Upper urinary tract damage associated with ureteric reflux caused by high filling and voiding pressure is a danger, though less so than it is for men, who are more likely to have a severe functional outflow obstruction. Incomplete reflex voiding results in a liability to recurrent urinary tract infection. When infection causes inflammation of the bladder, hyperreflexia of detrusor and sphincter is further exaggerated, so reflex incontinence is made worse. The detrusor reflex may be hypoactive, poorly sustained or difficult to provoke.[24] If outflow resistance is low, then adding manual expression may result in success, although it has been associated with upper tract dilatation.[29] If outflow resistance is high with striated sphincter spasticity, then reflex voiding, like expression, is an unsuitable method of management. However, bladder neck smooth muscle dyssynergia may sometimes be treated with an α-adrenergic blocker such as prazosin. Reflex voiding may be accompanied by dyssynergic sphincter contractions; these cannot be controlled except by sphincterotomy or deafferentation. Sphincterotomy is unsuitable for paraplegic women, because it results in intractable stress incontinence. Deafferentation will abolish reflex voiding, and is not used alone. Alternatively, the voiding reflex may be hyperactive, or triggered at the wrong time by bladder fullness, cough or trunk movement. In this case, titrated anticholinergic treatment using oxybutynin or propantheline may be successful. Intravesical capsaicin has also been described. In all paraplegic patients who are using reflex voiding it is essential to monitor regularly for upper tract dilatation and deteriorating renal function.

Chronic urethral catheterization is used much less frequently than in the past as a long-term method of bladder management in active patients. Permanent bacteriuria is almost universal. Serious disadvantages such as ascending infection, pyelonephritis and progressive urethral dilatation with leakage past the catheter are common. Septicemia is commonly associated with a catheter change, which may have to be covered by intravenous antibiotics.

Surgical methods

Surgical treatment must be considered if none of the simple methods is satisfactory. Here the choice depends on the problem. If the problem is a small, high-pressure, refluxing or persistently hyperactive bladder, then the choice is between urinary diversion, bladder augmentation or sacral root stimulation with deafferentation. If the problem is incontinence due to sphincter weakness, then the choice is between a suprapubic catheter, continent urinary diversion or artificial sphincter.

Chronic suprapubic catheterization is occasionally used where the urethra is dilated and incompetent, or severely damaged and requiring closure.[30]

Urinary diversion to an ileal loop with stoma restores perineal dryness, but has been shown often to be associated with renal deterioration in the long term. The bag can be eliminated by using a continent stoma,[31] which the patient or attendant must learn to catheterize.

Bladder augmentation using a segment of detubularized cecum or sigmoid colon can reduce intravesical pressure and restore continence when combined with intermittent self-catheterization.[32]

Sacral anterior root stimulation (SARSI) is usually combined with sacral deafferentation, so as to cure reflex incontinence, loss of detrusor compliance and detrusor–sphincter dyssynergia. Poor voiding and/or reflex incontinence in paraplegia is the main indication for SARSI.[33] The patient is rendered continent, and voids by stimulation (Fig. 31.3). Stimulation is applied in bursts of a few seconds, separated by a few seconds' gap. During the gaps, detrusor pressure rises, urethral pressure falls and

Fig. 31.3 Sacral anterior root stimulator (SARSI) equipment. The driving box (A), which is kept in a pocket or handbag, is battery-driven. It is connected by a cable (B) to the transmitter block (C), which is held over the implanted 'radio' receiver when voiding is required. The receiver has 3 channels (S2,3,4), and is of similar form to the transmitter. The receiver is connected by implanted cables to electrodes on the sacral anterior (motor) roots. About once a week, the driving box is recharged overnight, using the charger (D).

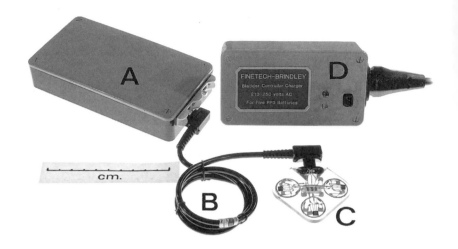

voiding occurs (Fig. 31.4). Stimulus parameters are adjusted during cystometry so as to optimize voiding pressure to the physiological range and minimize residual volume. Any preoperative ureteric reflux is usually improved or cured.[34]

Artificial sphincter is indicated mainly in patients with severe sphincter incompetence, often with lower motor lesions. The bladder must be low-pressure, without reflux. Pressure necrosis, and infection requiring removal, are more common in paraplegia than in the non-paraplegic population.[35] If voiding is poor, the artificial sphincter may be combined with intermittent self-catheterization.

DISORDERS OF SPINAL ROOTS, NERVES AND GANGLIA

Cauda equina

The gross neuroanatomy of the lower urinary tract (Fig. 31.5) has been well described.[2,36] The relevant roots for the somatic and parasympathetic outflow are S2–4, which intradurally form part of the cauda equina. The innervation of the rhabdosphincter originates in Onuf's nucleus in the conus medullaris, and passes mainly in the S3 anterior roots and the pudendal nerves. The parasympathetic efferent supply originates in the intermediolateral cell column in the S2–4 segments (mainly S3), with its preganglionic myelinated fibers passing in the anterior roots, which it leaves to form the pelvic nerves, shortly after exiting the dura. The sympathetic innervation of the pelvis is derived from the inter-mediolateral cell column at T11–L2. It also separates from the somatic motor roots after exiting the dura, and passes to the lumbar sympathetic (paravertebral) ganglia, where many axons synapse, and form the superior hypogastric plexus anterior to the aorta. In the pelvis, the pelvic nerves and superior hypogastric plexus merge to form the inferior hypogastric

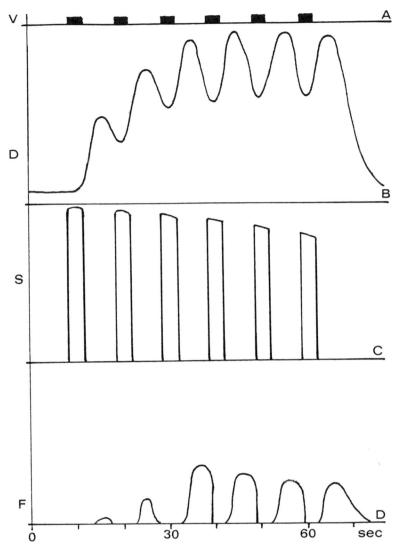

Fig. 31.4   Voiding using the sacral anterior root stimulator (SARSI) device. A. Bursts of stimulation pulses (V) are delivered to the motor roots. Each burst lasts 2–5 s, with gaps of 4–10 s between bursts. The optimum burst and gap lengths depend on the speed of detrusor contraction and relaxation, which varies between individuals. B. The response of detrusor pressure (D), which shows a latency of several seconds in its response to each stimulus burst. The stimulus parameters are adjusted during postoperative urodynamics testing, so that the peak voiding pressure is in the normal range (not more than 80 cmH$_2$O for women). C. The response of sphincter pressure (S) to the same pattern of stimulation; the somatic motor fibers to the rhabdosphincter lie in the same roots as the fibers to detrusor. The latency of contraction and relaxation of the closing muscles is relatively very short (almost instantaneous, on this time scale). Consequently, the urethral pressure is usually well above detrusor pressure *during* stimulation bursts; but it is always well below detrusor pressure *between* stimulation bursts. D. The pattern of voiding. Voiding flow (F) occurs during the gaps, when detrusor pressure is high and outflow resistance is low. In this diagram, detrusor pressure never exceeds the outflow closure pressure during a burst, so there is never any flow during a burst. This is true of a majority of patients. In some patients (including some who have not had sphincter surgery) it does not hold, and a reduced flow continues even during the bursts

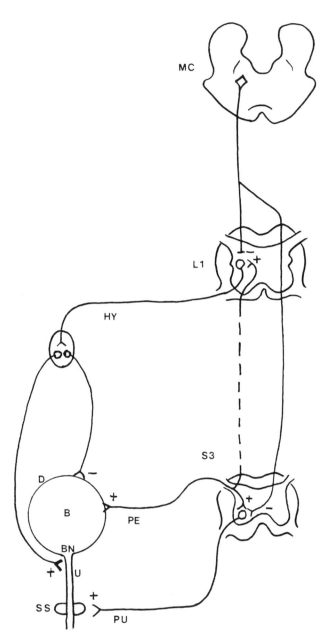

Fig. 31.5 The peripheral motor, sensory and reflex pathways involved in the storage and voiding of urine, showing some excitatory and inhibitory actions. The dashed pathway is presumptive in humans. MC, micturition center; L1, first lumbar segment; S3, third sacral segment; HY, hypogastric nerves; PE, pelvic nerves; PU, pudendal nerves; SS, striated sphincter; U, urethra; B, bladder; D, detrusor; BN, bladder neck

plexus, which innervates the pelvic organs. The parasympathetic ganglia are in the effector organ walls, with short unmyelinated postganglionic fibers. As noted earlier, it is not certain how important the lumbar sympathetic is in the control of the bladder. It is probably active in accommodating to filling, modulating parasympathetic ganglion transmission to the detrusor and maintaining bladder neck closure.[2,3]

The common causes of peripheral autonomic lesions are as follows:

1. Congenital
    a. Sacral agenesis
    b. Tethered cord syndrome with root traction
    c. Myelodysplasia involving cauda equina
    d. Familial dysautonomia (Riley-Day)
    e. Hereditary sensory motor neuropathies
2. Space-occupying and neoplastic
    a. Tumours of cauda equina
    b. Malignant meningeal infiltration
    c. Pelvic carcinomatosis or lymphoma
    d. Neurofibromatosis
3. Traumatic
    a. Lumbar spinal injury
    b. Radical pelvic surgery
    c. Abdominal aortic surgery
4. Vascular
    a. Angioma or arteriovenous malformation of cauda equina
    b. Radicular artery occlusion
5. Inflammatory
    a. Guillain-Barré neuropathy
    b. Zoster neuropathy
    c. Spinal arachnoiditis
    d. Tabes dorsalis
    e. AIDS polyradiculitis
    f. Autoimmune neuropathies
    g. Paraneoplastic neuropathy
6. Degenerative
    a. Central lumbar disk prolapse
    b. Lumbar spinal stenosis
    c. Progressive autonomic failure (Shy-Drager)
    d. Multiple system atrophy
    e. Acute or subacute pandysautonomia
7. Toxic and metabolic
    a. Diabetes mellitus
    b. Alcoholic neuropathy
    c. Vitamin B^1 or B^{12} deficiency
    d. Hypothyroidism
    e. Porphyria
    f. Amyloid neuropathy
    g. Dopamine β-hydroxylase deficiency
    h. Sympathetic or parasympathetic blocking drugs.

Compressive lesions of the cauda equina, such as central lumbar disk protrusions, affect somatic and parasympathetic, motor and sensory, fibers together. Only the sympathetic innervation escapes. Acute lesions are associated with radicular or girdle pain, acute urinary retention, perineal sensory loss and a pattern of leg weakness and sensory loss which depends on the level of the lesion. Long-standing or progressive lesions are associated with an atonic bladder of abnormally large capacity and sphincter weakness. This combination may allow urinary voiding by abdominal compression. Associated features include wasting of gluteal and calf muscles and loss of ankle reflexes.

Pelvic and pudendal nerves

Lesions of the pelvic nerves may be due to local disease or surgery, or may be a feature of a more widespread autonomic neuropathy. Local diseases are most commonly malignant infiltrations in the pelvis, such as lymphomas or carcinomas (e.g. of the rectum, cervix or uterus). Surgical damage usually occurs in the course of radical pelvic surgery such as abdominoperineal resection, proctocolectomy or radical hysterectomy.

The pelvic (parasympathetic) and hypogastric (sympathetic) nerves lie more medially, adjacent to the rectum, and the pudendal nerves more laterally in the pelvis. It is therefore not surprising that pelvic nerve injury (causing an atonic bladder), or superior hypogastric plexus injury (causing loss of smooth muscle tone in the bladder neck) occur more commonly than pudendal nerve injury (causing sensory loss and striated sphincter weakness). Lesions may be complete or incomplete, and accurate postoperative diagnosis of an iatrogenic incontinence or voiding difficulty requires a full urodynamic assessment. Incomplete or unilateral ablative or traction injuries of the pelvic or hypogastric nerves are often followed by recovery, which may take 6–12 months.

Clinical and urodynamic features in pelvic neuropathies

Interruption of the parasympathetic (S2–4) innervation of the detrusor causes poor voiding, while interruption of the pudendal innervation of the sphincters and pelvic floor results in incontinence.[37] The bulbocavernous reflex is lost. If S1 is involved, the ankle jerk is diminished or lost as well. Sensory mapping gives a good indication of the extent of the lesion. Patients may void successfully by abdominal straining or compression, because of the low outflow resistance. Urodynamic testing shows a low filling pressure, large capacity and loss of detrusor-initiated voiding. The denervated detrusor shows increased sensitivity to bethanechol. Subtracted pressure recording shows that voiding is achieved by abdominal straining. Electrophysiologically, the sphincters show denervation changes and sacral evoked responses are delayed or absent. If the main problem is retention, treatment with intermittent self-catheterization is usually successful. If incontinence is severe, women may require an artificial sphincter or a urinary diversion. In patients whose pelvic neuropathy is iatrogenic and follows major pelvic surgery, such as abdominoperineal resection or radical hysterectomy, the autonomic lesion is variable and often recovers, provided that the pudendal nerves are preserved.

AUTONOMIC FAILURE

There are many peripheral causes of autonomic dysfunction and these have been listed on p. 493. However, the causes of autonomic failure per se can be classified into system degenerations and peripheral neuropathies with autonomic involvement. The most prominent of the system degenerations are the degenerative disorders such as the Shy-Drager syndrome[38] of progressive autonomic failure, and multiple system atrophy (MSA).[39] Whether MSA, with prominent central nervous system involvement, and the Shy-Drager syndrome, with mainly peripheral autonomic system degeneration, are separate diseases or the two ends of a spectrum of disorders is controversial. In the second group are those causes of peripheral neuropathy which attack the autonomic nerves, of which diabetes mellitus is much the most common. Alcoholic neuropathy is just as common, but causes significant autonomic neuropathy less often. In both types of autonomic failure, bladder symptoms are common. In men they are usually preceded by impotence, but in women difficulty voiding, poor stream and incomplete voiding are often the first symptoms to present. In this discussion the MSA–Shy–Drager spectrum is taken as representing the central autonomic neuropathies, and diabetes mellitus the peripheral group.

Multiple system atrophy

Disturbances of micturition often develop together with the motor and systemic features, such as parkinsonism, ataxia or postural hypotension. Nocturia is prominent, probably as a result of polyuria caused by recumbent hypertension. In the central degenerations, stress and urge incontinence is attributable to loss of neurones in Onuf's nucleus, as part of the disease. The changes of partial denervation can be seen on sphincter electromyography (EMG),[40] and this can help in the distinction between Parkinson's disease and MSA, which often presents with parkinsonian features. Urodynamics testing typically shows a selection from the following: reduced compliance and an open bladder neck (sympathetic failure); detrusor hyperreflexia (striato-nigral degeneration); increased residual volume (parasympathetic failure); and reduced urethral sphincter pressure (degeneration of Onuf's nucleus). The clinical and urodynamic picture thus depends on the extent and distribution of the lesions. Intermittent self-catheterization may be taught if the residual is >100 ml. Desmopressin nasal spray may help in treating excessive nocturia, and also improve morning postural hypotension.[41]

Diabetes mellitus

In diabetes, symptomatic autonomic failure is more common in those who are insulin-dependent than in those who are not, and mild failure is much more common than severe.[42] However, it may be progressive, with the development of a large atonic bladder with associated loss of bladder sensation. Patients often present with recurrent urinary tract infections, due to retention with glycosuria. Urodynamics testing typically shows a low-pressure bladder of increased capacity, with poor voiding pressure, reduced flow rate and increased residual volume. Less commonly there is detrusor instability, loss of compliance or stress incontinence. Management may be by teaching regular bladder drill to encourage complete voiding, or by teaching clean intermittent self-catheterization.

OCCULT NEUROLOGICAL DISORDERS

Detrusor instability

The most common urogynecological 'occult neurological disorder' is urge incontinence due to detrusor instability, and this is so common that it is dealt with in its own right in Section 4, and a full account is not included here. This is a urodynamic diagnosis, the defining abnormality being active detrusor contraction(s), usually greater than 15 cmH$_2$O, occurring at a volume of <300 ml.[1] Other urodynamic abnormalities, such as loss of detrusor compliance, or uninhibited urethral relaxations, may also be present. The diagnosis also requires the exclusion of urological causes of urgency such as outflow obstruction, infection or urethral trauma. By definition, there are no abnormal clinical neurological signs. There are no diagnostic abnormalities in pelvic electrophysiology. In these circumstances, neurological investigation is not likely to be fruitful, unless the symptoms are particularly severe and of sudden onset. It is often associated with anxiety and depression, and it is difficult to disentangle cause and effect. Treatment options include anticholinergic smooth muscle relaxant drugs such as oxybutynin or propantheline, bladder drill and biofeedback.[43] Detrusor instability and some forms of adult enuresis may be parts of a spectrum, rather than separate disorders.

Adult enuresis

Enuresis may be defined as a habitual involuntary voiding act which occurs after early childhood in the absence of any relevant structural or neurological disorder.[44] As such, it may be nocturnal (night-time only) or diurnal (day and night). It usually resolves during childhood, but may persist into adult life. Adult enuresis seldom arises de novo, but it can be primary or secondary; thus secondary enuresis is the recurrence of enuresis after childhood enuresis has been broken by a late gain of continence, usually at about puberty.[45] The relapse usually occurs in the second, third or fourth decade. Primary nocturnal enuresis sometimes converts to nocturia in adult life, and it is often accompanied by persisting diurnal urgency.[46]

Although there are by definition no relevant structural or neurological lesions, there are functional disturbances which suggest that adult enuresis may not be a single disorder. Filling cystometry may be completely normal, or it may show uninhibited detrusor contractions, either on a normotonic or hypertonic background, resembling the findings in detrusor instability. Cystometric capacity is reduced only in enuretics with uninhibited detrusor contractions.[45] This group of enuretic women also have sphincter hypertrophy, which is believed to be secondary. A few seem to have uninhibited sphincter relaxations as a primary disorder. Treatment methods include behavior modification, scheduled voiding, imipramine and anticholinergic drugs.[47]

Sphincter hypertonia

Urinary retention may occur in women (Table 31.1) with or without known neurological disease, as a temporary phenomenon following childbirth or abdominal, particularly anorectal, surgery. It may also follow

Table 31.1   Causes of retention and poor voiding in women

Overtly neurological	
Frontal lobe lesions (very rarely)	
Pontine lesions	Internuclear ophthalmoplegia may be associated
Suprasacral spinal cord lesions	Spinal shock phase
	Detrusor–sphincter dyssynergia
Conus lesions	
Cauda equinal lesions	Lumbar disk
	Ankylosing spondylitis
	Tumor
	Viral polyradiculitides
Multiple system atrophy	
Pelvic autonomic neuropathy	Guillain–Barré syndrome
	Diabetes mellitus
	Pelvic surgery
Occult neurological	
Urethral sphincter hypotonia	
Bladder neck dyssynergia	
Overdistension injury	
Smooth myopathy	
Anticholinergic drugs	

epidural anesthesia, anticholinergic drug treatment, impacted constipation or an episode of acute retention. In one survey, the incidence of presentation to casualty of women in acute retention was 7/100 000 per year.[48] If there is no obvious explanation, or if poor voiding persists, there should be a gynecological examination to exclude a pelvic tumor, and cystoscopy should be done to exclude urethral stricture, cyst, stone, tumor and caruncle.

After the cystoscopically identifiable causes have been eliminated, there remains a group of mostly young women who present with recurrent retention without any obvious antecedent cause or cystoscopic structural abnormality. Because of the lack of associated features, it has often been supposed that the retention was of psychological or hysterical cause.[49] This was an unsatisfactory explanation, because there were usually no associated signs of psychological disturbance. It has been shown by Fowler and co-workers, and recently independently confirmed, that there is in fact a localized EMG abnormality which is confined to the urethral sphincter in these women, and which is associated with a failure of sphincter relaxation.[50,51] The EMG abnormality is a complex repetitive discharge (CRD) of low jitter occurring with decelerating bursts (DB) suggesting ephaptic transmission between muscle fibers in the sphincter. Treatment remains difficult. There is a suggestion that the condition may have a hormonal basis, because these patients have a higher than expected rate of polycystic ovaries, and of previous problems such as menstrual irregularity, acne or hirsutism. However, hormonal approaches to treatment have not so far proved effective; nor have botulinum toxin injections into the sphincter.[52] Sphincterotomy may result in incontinence. Intermittent self-catheterization may be successful, but may be painful because of the tight sphincter. In some women who have been shown to have the typical picture of DB and CRD, the episodes of retention have been precipitated by childbirth, surgery or anticholinergic drug treatment, suggesting that the disorder may remain compensated and subclinical until unmasked by an intercurrent event.

The condition should be distinguished from two others. First, there is pseudo detrusor–sphincter dyssynergia,[53] in which the sphincter EMG is normal and the sphincter spasm is either psychogenic or occurring in response to painful conditions of the urethra. Secondly, there is bladder neck dyssynergia, in which the bladder neck fails to open during attempted voiding. However, this condition, though not uncommon in paraplegic women, rarely presents as an idiopathic problem in women, though it is quite a common cause of idiopathic functional obstruction in young men. Treatment is with α_1-adrenergic blockers such as prazosin.

SUMMARY

The clinical pattern of disturbances of continence and voiding is a poor predictor of the underlying pathophysiological mechanisms. Patients with established neurological disease involving urinary complaints therefore require investigation of their lower urinary tract function before they can be treated rationally. Coincidental structural disorders and complications must also be excluded. There is a group of urinary disorders which have characteristics suggesting a neurological basis, but in which there is no independent clinical evidence of a neurological lesion. These disorders are diagnosed following the appropriate investigations of lower urinary tract function. Investigation in these patients is necessary in order to make the primary diagnosis.

REFERENCES

1 Bates CP, Bradley WE, Glen ES et al. Fourth report on the standardisation of terminology of lower urinary tract function. Terminology related to neuromuscular dysfunction of lower urinary tract. Brit J Urol 1981; 53: 333–335.
2 De Groat WC, Booth AM, Yoshimura N. Neurophysiology of micturition and its modification in animal models of human disease. In: Maggi VA (ed) The autonomic nervous system, vol 3: Nervous control of the urogenital system. London: Harwood Academic, 1993: pp 227–290.
3 Edvardson P. Nervous control of the urinary bladder in cats. 1. The collecting phase. Acta Physiol Scand 1993; 72: 157–171.
4 Merton PA, Hill DK, Morton HB, Marsden CD. Scope of a technique for electrical stimulation of human brain, spinal cord and muscle. Lancet 1982; 2: 597–600.
5 Bhatia NN, Bradley WE. Neuroanatomy and physiology: innervation of the urinary tract. In: Raz S (ed) Female urology. Philadelphia: Saunders, 1983.
6 Leach GE, Farsali AA, Kark P, Raz S. Urodynamic manifestations of cerebellar ataxia. J Urol 1982; 128: 348–350.
7 Wade DT, Hewer RL. Outlook after an acute stroke: urinary incontinence and loss of consciousness compared in 532 patients. Quart J Med 1985; 56: 601–608.
8 Strich SJ. Shearing of nerve fibres as a cause of brain damage due to head injury: a pathological study of 20 cases. Lancet 1961; 2: 443–448.
9 Kalisky Z, Morrison PD, Meyers CA, van Laufen A. Medical problems encountered during rehabilitation of patients with head injury. Arch Phys Med Rehabil 1985; 66: 25–29.
10 Khan Z, Herlanu J, Young WC, Melman A, Leiter E. Predictive correlation of urodynamic dysfunction and brain injury after cerebrovascular accident. J Urol 1981; 126: 86–88.

11 Brocklehurst JC, Andrews K, Richards B, Laycock PJ. Incidence and correlation of incontinence in stroke patients. J Amer Geriat Soc 1985; 33: 540–542.

12 Garrett VE, Scott JA, Costich J, Aubrey DL, Gross J. Bladder emptying assessment in stroke patients. Arch Phys Med Rehabil 1989; 70: 41–43.

13 Awad SA, Gajewski JB, Sogbein SK, Murray TJ, Field CA. Relationship between neurological and urological states in patients with multiple sclerosis. J Urol 1984; 132: 499–502.

14 Eardley I, Nagendran K, Lecky B, Chapple CR, Kirby RS, Fowler CJ. Neurophysiology of the striated urethral sphincter in multiple sclerosis. Brit J Urol 1991; 68: 81–88.

15 Goldstein I, Siroky MB, Sax DS, Krane RJ. Neurourologic abnormalities in multiple sclerosis. J Urol 1982; 128: 541–545.

16 Grasso MG, Pozzilli C, Anzini A, Salvetti M, Bastianello S, Fieschi C. Relationship between bladder dysfunction and brain MRI in multiple sclerosis. Funct Neurol 1991; 6: 289–292.

17 Petersen T, Pedersen E. Neurourodynamic evaluation of voiding dysfunction in multiple sclerosis. Acta Neurol Scand 1984; 69: 402–411.

18 Berger Y, Blaivas JG, DeLaRocha ER, Salines JM. Urodynamic findings in Parkinson's disease. J Urol 1987; 138: 836–838.

19 Galloway NT. Urethral sphincter abnormalities in Parkinsonism. Br J Urol 1983; 55: 691–693.

20 Khan Z, Starer P, Bhola A. Urinary incontinence in female Parkinson disease patients. Pitfalls of diagnosis. Urology 1989; 33: 486–489.

21 Wheeler JS, Sax DS, Krane RJ, Siroky MB. Vesico-urethral functions in Huntington's chorea. Brit J Urol 1985; 57: 63–66.

22 Decter RM, Bauer SB, Khoshbin S et al. Urodynamic assessment of children with cerebral palsy. J Urol 1987; 138: 1110–1112.

23 Mayo ME. Lower urinary tract dysfunction in cerebral palsy. J Urol 1992; 147: 419–420.

24 Light JK, Faganel J, Beric A. Detrusor areflexia in suprasacral spinal cord injuries. J Urol 1985; 134: 295–297.

25 Barrington FJF. The relation of the hindbrain to micturition. Brain 1921; 44: 23–53.

26 Tribe C. Renal failure in paraplegia. London: Pitman, 1969.

27 Guttman L, Frankel H. The value of intermittent catheterisation in the early management of traumatic paraplegia and tetraplegia. Paraplegia 1966; 4: 63–70.

28 Grundy D, Fellows G, Gillett A, Nuseibeh I, Silver J. A comparison of a fine bore suprapubic and an intermittent urethral catheterisation regime after spinal cord injury. Paraplegia 1983; 21: 227–232.

29 Smith P, Cook J, Rhine J. Manual expression of the bladder following spinal injury. Paraplegia 1972; 9: 213–218.

30 Hulecki S, Hackler R. Closure of the bladder neck in spinal cord injury patients with urethral sphincteric incompetence and irreparable urethral pathological conditions. J Urol 1984; 131: 1119–1121.

31 Bennett J, Gray M, Green B, Foote J. Continent diversion and bladder augmentation in spinal cord-injured patients. Semin Urol 1992; 10: 121–132.

32 Sidi A, Becher E, Reddy P, Dykstra D. Augmentation enterocystoplasty for the management of voiding dysfunction in spinal cord injury patients. J Urol 1990; 143: 83–85.

33 Brindley GS, Polkey CE, Rushton DN, Cardozo LD. Sacral anterior root stimulators for bladder control in paraplegia: the first 50 cases. J Neurol Neurosurg Psychiat 1986; 49: 1104–1114.

34 Brindley GS, Rushton DN. Long-term follow-up of patients with sacral anterior root stimulator implants. Paraplegia 1990; 28: 469–475.

35 Light JK, Scott FB. Use of the artificial urinary sphincter in spinal cord injury patients. J Urol 1983; 130: 1127–1129.

36 De Groat WC. Neurophysiology of the pelvic organs. In: Rushton DN (ed) Handbook of neuro-urology. New York: Marcel Dekker, 1994.

37 Kirby RS, Fowler CJ, Gilpin SA, Gosling JA, Milroy EJG, Turner-Warwick RT. Bladder muscle biopsy and urethral sphincter EMG in patients with peripheral nerve injury to the bladder. J R Soc Med 1985; 79: 270–273.

38 Shy GM, Drager GA. A neurological syndrome associated with orthostatic hypotension. Arch Neurol Chicago 1960; 2: 511–527.

39 Oppenheimer DR, Graham JG. Orthostatic hypotension and nicotine sensitivity in a case of multiple system atrophy. J Neurol Neurosurg Psychiat 1969; 32: 28–34.

40 Eardley I, Quinn NP, Fowler CJ et al. The value of urethral sphincter electromyography in the differential diagnosis of parkinsonism. Brit J Urol 1989; 64: 360–362.

41 Lees AJ. The treatment of multiple system atrophy. In: Bannister R, Mathias CJ (eds)

Autonomic failure: a textbook of clinical disorders of the autonomic nervous system, 3rd edn. Oxford: Oxford University Press, 1992: pp 646–656.

42 Watkins PJ, Grenfell A, Edmonds M. Diabetic complications of non-insulin dependent diabetes. Diabetic Med 1984; 4: 293–296.

43 Cardozo L. Biofeedback methods. In: Krane RJ, Siroky MB. Clinical neuro-urology, 2nd edn, Boston: Little, Brown, 1991: pp 511–522.

44 Miller A. Adult enuresis. Brit J Urol 1966; 38: 697–699.

45 Torrens MJ, Collins CD. The urodynamic assessment of adult enuresis. Brit J Urol 1975; 47: 433–440.

46 Yeates WK. Bladder function: increased frequency and nocturnal incontinence. In: Bladder control and enuresis. Clinics in developmental medicine. 1966; 49: 151–155.

47 Kunin SA, Limbert DJ, Platzker ACG, McGinley J. The efficacy of imipramine in the management of enuresis. J Urol 1970; 104: 612–615.

48 Klarsov P, Andersen JT, Asmussen CF et al. Acute urinary retention in women: a prospective study of 18 consecutive cases. Scand J Urol Nephrol 1987; 21: 29–31.

49 Montague DK, Jones LR. Psychogenic urinary retention. Urology 1979; 13: 30–35.

50 Fowler CJ, Kirby RS, Harrison MJG. Decelerating bursts and complex repetitive discharges in the striated muscle of the urethral sphincter associated with urinary retention in women. J Neuro Neurosurg Psychiat 1985; 48: 1004–1009.

51 Webb RJ, Fawcett PRW, Neal DE. Electromyographic abnormalities in the urethral and anal sphincters of women with idiopathic retention of urine. Brit J Urol 1992; 70: 22–25.

52 Fowler CJ, Betts CD, Christmas TJ, Swash M, Fowler CG. Botulinum toxin in the treatment of chronic urinary retention in women. Brit J Urol 1992; 70: 387–389.

53 Raz S, Smith RB. External sphincter spasticity syndrome in female patients. J Urol 1976; 115: 443–446.

RECOMMENDED FURTHER READING

Krane RJ, Siroky MB (eds). Clinical neuro-urology, 2nd edn. Boston: Little, Brown, 1991.
Rushton DN (ed). Handbook of neuro-urology. New York: Marcel Dekker, 1994.

32

Sex and the bladder

INTRODUCTION

In women the lower urinary and genital tracts are embryologically and anatomically closely related. Both originate from the primitive urogenital sinus, and in the adult woman, the urethra and bladder base lie immediately ventral to the anterior vaginal wall. Disorders of the lower urinary and genital tracts are therefore commonly associated and it is not surprising that sexual activity may cause urinary symptoms and that lower urinary tract dysfunction may lead to sexual problems.

Sexual dysfunction in women with lower urinary tract dysfunction can arise by one of several mechanisms. The presence of urinary symptoms, or the reaction of either partner to them, can cause sexual difficulties where none previously existed. Secondly, a pre-existing but often unacknowledged sexual problem may be blamed, either consciously or subconsciously, on the presence of urinary symptoms. Thirdly, urinary symptoms may be the presenting feature of an underlying sexual conflict and a means of bringing that conflict to the fore.

Sexual intercourse, especially if associated with the use of a contraceptive diaphragm, may result in cystitis or urethritis. Urinary tract infection is also common in the elderly, when vaginal atrophy secondary to estrogen deficiency results in both dyspareunia and an increased risk of ascending bacterial infection. Similarly, the successful or unsuccessful surgical management of genuine stress incontinence (GSI) may lead to dyspareunia and subsequent sexual difficulty.

Incontinence appliances (particularly pads, pants and catheters) are important for the management of symptoms in many women, particularly those with neurological bladder urinary dysfunction. The appropriate choice of pads and catheterization technique is important for the subsequent sexual fulfilment of the patient.

Irrespective of the causal mechanism it is necessary to investigate, treat or exclude disorders of the lower urinary tract prior to re-establishing satisfactory sexual relations. Adequate support and an understanding of and informative approach to the woman and her partner are often of paramount importance to the resumption of a normal sex life.

CAUSES OF LOWER URINARY TRACT DYSFUNCTION

There are three major symptom complexes of bladder and urethral function: urinary incontinence; irritative bladder symptoms (urgency, urge incontinence, frequency, nocturia and dysuria); and voiding difficulties (straining to void, incomplete emptying, poor flow, hesitancy). Each can have an adverse effect on normal sexual activity. The major causes of urinary incontinence are as follows:

- genuine stress incontinence
- detrusor instability (detrusor hyperreflexia)
- overfow incontinence
- fistula
- urethral diverticulum
- temporary (e.g. urinary tract infection, drugs, fecal impaction)
- functional (e.g. immobility)
- congenital.

URINARY INCONTINENCE

Urinary incontinence (UI) is the involuntary loss of urine that is a social or hygienic problem and objectively demonstrable.[1] A recent national survey has shown that at least 14% of women are incontinent of urine.[2] Research has focused largely on the accurate diagnosis, mechanisms and treatment of incontinence, without adequate measures to assess the impact of this devastating condition or its clinical management on women's lives. Little has been done to study the way in which help is offered or indeed sought, and it is not surprising to find that women often wait for over 4 years before seeking medical assistance for this socially unacceptable condition.[3]

Stress incontinence is the commenest symptom with which women present. It is a symptom, or a sign, but not a diagnosis. Genuine stress incontinence is a diagnosis made by urodynamic assessment to confirm urinary leakage per urethram due to an increase in intra-abdominal pressure, in the absence of detrusor activity. It is the most common cause of urinary incontinence in women, accounting for about 50% of cases. Stress incontinence is most commonly caused by coughing or sneezing, but in severe cases occurs with only minimal activity such as walking. It occurs mainly in parous women and is exacerbated by lifting, straining and constipation.

The most common mechanism of GSI is thought to be urethral hypermobility due to pelvic floor weakness, which decreases passive abdominal pressure transmission to the proximal urethra. There is histological[4] and electromyographic[5] evidence that denervation of the pelvic muscles and damage to the urethra as a result of parturition are important in the etiology of this condition.

Detrusor instability (DI) is the second most common cause of incontinence, accounting for 20–40% of referrals for urodynamic investigation

The incidence increases with age and DI is the most common cause of urinary incontinence in the elderly.[6] The condition is termed 'detrusor hyperreflexia' if there is overt neurologial pathology.

An unstable bladder is one which contracts involuntarily, either spontaneously or on provocation, during the filling phase of cystometry whilst the patient is attempting to inhibit micturition. Urodynamic assessment is required for diagnosis. Women usually present with multiple symptoms, most commonly urgency, urge incontinence, frequency and nocturia.

The common causes of frequency and urgency of micturition may be listed as follows:

1. Gynecological/urological
a. Urinary tract infection
b. Detrusor instability
c. Inflammation (e.g. interstitial cystitis)
d. Fibrosis (radiation)
e. Atrophy (menopause)
f. Intravesical lesion (e.g. calculus)
g. Urethral pathology (e.g. urethral syndrome)
h. External pressure (e.g. pelvic mass, fibroids)
i. Pregnancy
2. Medical/psychological
a. Drugs (e.g. diuretics)
b. Diabetes
c. Neurological disease (e.g. multiple sclerosis)
d. Excessive fluid intake
e. Habit.

The pathophysiology of DI is poorly understood, and an underlying cause for the condition is rarely found. In the majority of cases therefore the term 'idiopathic detrusor instability' is used. Detrusor instability and urethral sphincter incompetence (GSI) can occur together, and DI can arise de novo following surgery for stress incontinence.

Sensory urgency is diagnosed when there are intense irritative bladder symptoms in the absence of unstable detrusor contractions. Patients have a reduced functional bladder capacity, daytime frequency, nocturia and sometimes incontinence. It may be caused by inflammatory conditions of the bladder or urethra (e.g. interstitial cystitis, atrophic urethritis), and can be diagnosed by cystoscopy and bladder biopsy.

URINARY INCONTINENCE AND SEXUAL PROBLEMS

Although by definition UI is a social or hygienic problem, the condition has far wider reaching implications for the quality of life of sufferers, affecting not only their social life but also their work and home-life. The majority of women are embarrassed and often ashamed of their condition and recent studies have shown that UI can result in a deterioration in women's interpersonal relationships.[7]

There are many other reasons why UI and sexual dysfunction are associated. Lack of libido and diminished self-esteem due to a fear of leakage are major factors; however, urinary leakage during penetration, or at orgasm, as well as dyspareunia secondary to urine dermatitis or incontinence surgery, play a major role.

Over 50% of sexually active incontinent women suffer sexual dysfunction as a result of their urinary symptoms,[8] and 1 in 4 are incontinent during sexual intercourse.[9,10,11] Women with GSI commonly leak on penetration, whereas those with DI are more likely to be incontinent at orgasm.[11] There are, however, neither anatomical nor urodynamic factors capable of predicting those with or without associated coital leakage.[9,10]

Although incontinence during intercourse is important in the development of sexual dysfunction many women complain of sexual difficulties attributable to their urinary symptoms but not of coital incontinence itself. Patients with DI tend to suffer greater sexual dysfunction, although women with GSI are more likely to suffer coital incontinence, the latter increasing with worsening severity of GSI as determined by videourodynamic investigation.

Norton & Stanton[12] have shown that women with DI have no greater psychiatric morbidity than other incontinent women, although women with DI suffer greater psychological distress as a result of their urinary symptoms. Perhaps due to the unpredictable nature of their symptoms women with DI are more anxious than those with GSI, and it is likely that they fear the unforeseeable and often uncontrollable leakage with orgasm and are therefore more apprehensive about sexual contact. An interesting finding by Norton & Stanton[12] was that women with DI experience greater obstetric complications during parturition and it is possible that this too could lead to greater sexual difficulties post partum. Often women with DI and sensory urgency, may complain of bladder and urethral pain at the time of or shortly after intercourse, and this too may be a major factor in their sexual difficulty.

An interesting group of patients are those with both urinary symptoms and resulting sexual difficulties, but in whom the findings of urodynamic investigations are normal. A recent study has shown that over 50% complain of coital incontinence and 27% of sexual dysfunction as result.[7] These women have been shown by Norton & Stanton[12] to have similar psychiatric morbidity to psychiatric out-patients. In the absence of a urodynamic diagnosis it is often difficult to determine the cause of either of these problems and the commencement of empirical treatment without a sound diagnosis does not appear to improve their condition in the majority of cases.

The adverse reactions to urinary incontinence can often become incorporated into the lifestyle and personality of patients, and it is not surprising to find that women with urinary incontinence have a depressed mood similar to other patients suffering long-standing distressing conditions.[13]

Most cases of sexual dysfunction become worse over time due to the development of performance anxiety, where the goal of sexuality is no longer enjoyment but 'getting it right'. Such factors, described by Master

& Johnson[14] as 'spectating', are important in perpetuating sexual difficulty, and if these are corrected the problem itself may resolve.

Recently, Darling et al[15] have reported a possible homologous female prostate gland, originally referred to as the Grafenberg spot,[16] that may be involved in a sudden spurt of fluid being released at the time of orgasm. Of respondents to an anonymous questionnaire distributed to over 2000 women in the USA and Canada, 40% experienced ejaculation of fluid at the time of orgasm. It is possible that these women are in fact describing coital incontinence, but are neither embarrassed nor disturbed by its occurrence, or construe it as ejaculate, rather than admit to incontinence.

It is likely that a number of factors contribute to the sexual dysfunction of women who are incontinent of urine, and that the psychological consequences of this distressing condition are as important, if not more so, than coital incontinence itself. Long-standing urinary symptoms and sexual difficulty are, however, a source of appreciable morbidity and once established can become incorporated into an individual's lifestyle and personality. This may have major implications for management in these women, as the successful treatment of lower urinary tract symptoms may not necessarily improve their sexual dysfunction.

INCONTINENCE SURGERY AND SEXUAL DYSFUNCTION

The majority of studies evaluating the outcome of incontinence surgery do so in terms of objective urodynamic investigation and urinary symptom questionnaires. Improvement in quality of life is usually ignored. This limited approach to the audit of treatment efficacy clearly fails to recognize the true aims of surgical intervention. For women with sexual difficulty the type of surgery and the subsequent risks of dyspareunia are important considerations when planning operations or auditing treatment efficacy.

Few recent studies have addressed the effect of incontinence surgery on sexual function, despite the fact that urinary incontinence and sexual dysfunction are so closely related.

In a prospective study by Haase & Skibsted,[17] 13 out of 55 women experienced an improvement in their sexual life, 35 out of 55 no change, and 5 out of 55 a deterioration. Improvement was found to result from a cure of coital incontinence, and deterioration from dyspareunia secondary to a posterior repair of the vagina. The authors found that provided women were adequately counseled preoperatively, postoperative sexual difficulty was not a problem.

In a retrospective study, Francis & Jeffcoate[18] examined and interviewed 140 patients at least 2 years after anterior and posterior colpoperineorrhaphy, plus either vaginal hysterectomy or amputation of the cervix. They found that 52 patients virtually ceased coitus whilst 18 suffered considerable discomfort whenever it was attempted. The authors concluded that posterior colpoperineorrhaphy should be avoided if possible, especially in combination with anterior colporrhaphy.

The only study to have examined the effect of Burch colposuspension alone on sexual function has shown that it does not lead to significant dyspareunia despite altering the vaginal profile.[17] Two other studies have addressed the same issue and found that 8% (3/36)[19] and 17% (7/39)[20] of women complained of postoperative dyspareunia, although in the latter series no attempt was made to exclude the effects of previous vaginal surgery.

Little interest has focused on the sexual function of women undergoing major reconstructive lower urinary tract surgery. A study by Nordstrom & Nyman[21] examined the sexual function of 26 women following ileal conduit diversion for either bladder cancer or refractory incontinence. Five of the 6 women undergoing cystectomy who were sexually active before the operation reported a decrease or cessation of sexual activity postoperatively. The main problems were a lack of sexual desire, dyspareunia and vaginal dryness, although one woman reported an inability to experience orgasm after surgery. Compared to women with bladder cancer those undergoing surgery for other indications were more likely to have an active sexual life after urostomy. Seven females in this group, of whom 4 were sexually active preoperatively, increased their sexual activity after the operation primarily because it removed the need to wear incontinence pads or indwelling catheters.

CATHETERS

The most common indications for catheterization are acute and chronic retention, the need for postoperative bladder drainage, neuropathy of the bladder and intractable urinary incontinence.

An indwelling urethral or suprapubic catheter is the most commonly used method. Long-term urethral catheterization has the drawback of discomfort, urethral trauma and a high incidence of symptomatic urinary tract infection by contamination from the perineal flora. Suprapubic catheterization is often more comfortable, particularly in patients who are sexually active,[22] and the lower density of bacteria on the anterior abdominal wall results in fewer significant urinary tract infections.

Clean intermittent catheterization, performed by the patient or carer should be considered for women with a neuropathic or hypotonic bladder associated with voiding difficulties and urinary retention. It can also be used for postoperative voiding difficulty and retention. This technique is of particular benefit to women who remain sexually active.[22]

URINARY TRACT INFECTION AND SEXUAL INTERCOURSE

It is widely recognized that urinary tract infection is one of the most commonly encountered infectious diseases in medical practice and a frequent cause of general practitioner consultations. It is characterized by a significant bacterial colonization of the bladder (greater than 10^5 cfu/ml),[23] and is marked by the symptoms of dysuria, frequency and urgency of micturition. Estimates suggest that 20% of women will experience urinary tract infection symptoms in any year and that half of these will seek medical help.[24]

These overall figures mask the fact that the number of urinary tract infections is not evenly distributed amongst sufferers, and there appears to be a small number of women for whom recurrent urinary tract infections account for an unusually large number of reported cases. Mabeck[25] estimated that one-sixth of sufferers account for 70% of recurrences.

Several behavioral factors have been shown to enhance the risk of recurrent urinary tract infections. These include deferred voiding after sexual intercourse,[26,27] frequency of intercourse,[28] low fluid intake[29] and deferred voiding after the initial urge to micturate.[30]

Many women have an urge to void urine during or immediately after sexual activity.[31] A rigid perineum and nulliparity often result in post-coital dysuria known as 'honeymoon cystitis'. This is commonly followed by urinary tract infection. Organisms are massaged into the bladder and urethra during intercourse and if they are not voided out soon after, they multiply and cause infection. Some women are particularly sensitive to postcoital urinary tract infection and this may be related to voiding difficulty following intercourse due to a relatively high intraurethral pressure. Contraceptive diaphragms may further reduce urinary flow and research has shown that the risk of referral to hospital for urinary tract infection was two to three times higher amongst diaphragm users than among well-matched controls.[32] Spermicidal cream can often result in vaginal irritation, as can the use of spermicidal lubricated condoms. Hypoallergenic spermicidal cream and the use of 'allergy' condoms will usually resolve this problem.

Acute urethritis may also be due to infections with organisms such as *Chlamydia*, which although difficult to isolate respond well to a 14-to 21-day course of doxycyline.

Simple preventative measures can be taken to reduce the risk of post-coital urinary tract infection, namely the avoidance of contraceptive diaphragms, the use of a vaginal lubricant, change of coital technique, close attention to perineal hygiene and postcoital voiding. Estrogens can be used in postmenopausal women, in whom urinary tract infections are often associated with urogenital atrophy. If these simple measures are unsuccessful antibiotic prophylaxis can be taken to cover coitus, and a fluid preload taken before intercourse will encourage postcoital voiding. Culture of a midstream urine sample and appropriate antibiotic treatment is advocated if symptoms persist.

SEXUAL DYSFUNCTION AND ESTROGEN DEFICIENCY

Estrogen deficiency following the menopause results in generalized urogenital atrophy. Elderly women are therefore at risk of dyspareunia, vaginal irritation, pruritus, pain and symptoms of urgency, frequency, dysuria and urinary incontinence. Estrogen deficiency is also an important etiological factor in the pathogenesis of recurrent urinary tract infections.

A study of the age-related frequency of sexual intercourse has shown that among 46- to 50-year-olds, 86% were sexually active, among those aged 56–60, 58%; and among 61- to 65-year-olds, 39%. There was an average sexual frequency of once per week for the age group 45–60.[33]

Urogenital atrophy is a common manifestation of estrogen deficiency and is characterized by vaginal dryness and a thinning and reduced elasticity of the vaginal and urethral epithelium. An increase in vaginal pH promotes an alteration in the normal vaginal flora. Decreased numbers of lactobacilli and increased colonization by pathogenic fecal flora result in an increased incidence of urinary tract infection.

Dyspareunia is a common result of genital atrophy, although few women (even amongst those attending a menopause clinic) complain of vaginal symptoms unless specifically asked.[34] Vaginal dryness is, however, the cause of significant sexual dysfunction and results in a decrease in orgasmic experience and reduced coital enjoyment.[34]

Unfortunately, urogenital atrophy is a late manifestation of the menopause and consequently often underdiagnosed and undertreated. Many women fear the side effects of systemic estrogen therapy and few wish to resume menstrual loss with combined estrogen-progestogen cyclical hormone replacement therapy.

Although various lubricants are available to remedy vaginal dryness[35] their effect is short-lived, and they confer none of the additional benefits available from estrogen replacement therapy. Despite earlier fears, recent research has shown that continuous unopposed low-dose estrogen replacement therapy can be administered topically without significant risk of endometrial stimulation.[36,37] Topical vaginal estrogen can be administered as low-dose estradiol[37,38] or estriol,[39,40] avoiding the enterohepatic circulation and at doses low enough to cause minimal systemic side effects whilst adequately relieving urogenital atrophy and symptoms of frequency and urgency of micturition. Topical low-dose therapy also reduces vaginal pH and has been shown to decrease symptoms of frequency and dysuria and provide prophylaxis against recurrent urinary tract infections whilst encouraging recolonization of the vagina by lactobacilli.

Topical estrogen can be administered as a cream, pessary[40] or tablet [38] or via an impregnated sustained release intravaginal ring.[41] The latter have been shown to be acceptable to patients and do not result in dyspareunia.

The value of estrogen replacement therapy as a treatment of urinary incontinence is controversial and to date there is little substantial evidence to conclude that estrogen replacement therapy alone is of value in the treatment of this condition.

CONCLUSION

The female genital and urinary systems exists in close anatomical and functional proximity, disorders of one resulting in dysfunction of the other. The investigation and management of lower urinary tract disorders must take this important relationship into consideration, as neither can be viewed in isolation.

REFERENCES

1 Bates P, Bradley WE, Glen E. Standardisation of terminology of lower urinary tract function. J Urol, 1979; 121: 551–554.
2 Health Survey Questionnaire: Market and Opinion Research International (MORI), 1990. 95 Southwark Street, London SE1 OHX.
3 Kelleher CJ, Cardozo LD, Wise BG, Cutner A. The impact of urinary incontinence on sexual function. Neurourol Urodyn 1992; 11(4): 359–360.
4 Gilpin SA, Gosling JA, Smith ARB, Warrell DW. The pathogenesis of genitourinary prolapse and stress incontinence of urine. A histological and histochemical study. Br J Obstet Gynaecol 1989: 96: 15–23.
5 Smith ARB, Hosker GL, Warrell DW. The role of partial denervation of the pelvic floor in the aetiology of genitourinary prolapse and genuine stress incontinence of urine. A neurophysiological study. Br J Obstet Gynaecol 1989; 96: 24–28.
6 Ouslander JG, Hepps K, Raz S, Su HL. Genitourinary dysfunction in an elderly outpatient population. J Am Ger Soc 1986; 34: 507–514.
7 Kelleher CJ, Cardozo LD, Khullar V, Wise BG, Cutner A. The impact of urinary incontinence on sexual function. J Sexual Health.
8 Sutherst JR. Sexual dysfunction and urinary incontinence. B J Obstet Gynaecol 1979; 86: 387–388.
9 Thiede HA, Thiede FK. A glance at the urodynamic database. J Reprod Medicine 1990; 35 (10): 925–931.
10 Korda A, Cooper M, Hunter P. Coital urinary incontinence in an Australian population. Asia Oceania J Obstetrics and Gynaecology 1989; 15(4): 313–315.
11 Hilton P. Urinary incontinence during sexual intercourse: a common but rarely volunteered symptom. B J Obstet Gynaecol 1988; 95: 377–381.
12 Norton KRW, Bhat AV, Stanton SL. Psychiatric aspects of urinary incontinence in women attending an outpatient urodynamic clinic. BMJ 1990; 301: 271–272.
13 Macaulay AJ, Stern RS, Holmes DM, Stanton SL. Micturition and the mind: psychological factors in the aetiology and treatment of urinary symptoms in women. BMJ 1987; 1 294: 540–543.
14 Masters WH, Johnson VE. Human sexual inadequacy. London: Churchill Livingstone, 1970.
15 Darling CA, Davidson JK Sr, Conway Welch C. Female ejaculation: perceived origins. The Grafenberg spot/area and sexual responsiveness. Archives of Sexual Behaviour 1990; 19(1): 29–47.
16 Grafenberg E. The role of the urethra in female orgasm. Int J Sexology 1950; 3: 145–148.
17 Haase P, Skibsted L. Influence of operations for stress incontinence and/or genital decensus on sexual life. Acta Obstet Gynaecol Scand 1988; 67: 659–661.
18 Francis WJA, Jeffcoate TNA. Dyspareunia following vaginal operations. J Obstet Gynaecol Br Commonwealth. 1961; 68: 1–10.
19 Walter S, Olsen KP, Frimodt-Moller C, Hald T, Hedjorn S. Urinary incontinence in women treated with colposuspension. Ugeskr Laeger 1975; 2979.
20 Kamper AL, Tikjob G, Bay Nielsen A. Kolposuspension A. M. Burch. Ugeskr Laeger 1982; 144: 1921.
21 Nordstrom GM, Hyman CR. Male and female sexual function and activity following ileal conduit urinary diversion. Br J Urol 1992; 70(1): 33–39.
22 Roe BH, Brocklehurst JC. Study of patients with indwelling catheters. J Adv Nursing 1987; 12: 713–719.
23 Kass EH. Bacteriuria and the diagnosis of infections of the urinary tract. Arch Int Med 1957; 100: 709–714.
24 Sanford JP. Urinary tract symptoms and infections. Ann Rev Med 1975; 26: 485–498.
25 Mabeck CE. Treatment of uncomplicated urinary tract infection in non pregnant women. Postgrad Med J 1972; 48: 69–75.
26 Strom BL, Collins M, West SL. Sexual activity, contraceptive use, and other risk factors for symptomatic and asymptomatic bacteriuria. Ann Intern Med 1987; 107: 816–823.
27 Fihn SD. Behavioural aspects of urinary tract infection. Urology 1988; 32: 16–18.

28 Foxman B, Frerichs RR. Epidemiology of urinary tract infection 1. Diaphragm use and sexual intercourse. Am J Public Health 1985; 75: 1308–1313.

29 Ervine C, Komaroff AL, Pass TM. Behavioural factors and urinary tract infection. JAMA 1980; 243: 330–331.

30 Adatto K, Doebele KG, Galland L. Behavioural factors and urinary tract infection. JAMA 1979; 241: 2525–2526.

31 Cardozo L. Sex and the bladder. Leading article. BMJ 1988; 296, 6622: 587–588.

32 Gillespie L. The diaphragm, an accomplice in recurrent urinary tract infections. Urology 1984; 254: 240–245.

33 Pfeiffer E, Verwoerdt A, Davis GC. Sexual behaviour in middle life. Am J Psychiatry 1972; 128: 1262–1267.

34 Channon LD, Ballinger SE. Some aspects of sexuality and vaginal symptoms during menopause and their relation to depression. Br J Med Psychol 1986; 59: 173–180.

35 Riley AJ. Vaginal dryness and dyspareunia. J Sex Health 1992; 2(8): 7–9.

36 Mattsson LA, Cullberg G, Eriksson O, Knutsson F. Vaginal administration of low dose oestradiol–effects on the endometrium and vaginal cytology. Maturitas 1989; 11: 217–222.

37 Mettler L, Olsen PG. Longterm treatment of atrophic vaginitis with low dose oestradiol vaginal tablets. Maturitas 1991; 14: 23–31.

38 Erikson PS, Rasmussen H. Low dose 17Beta oestradiol vaginal tablets in the treatment of atrophic vaginitis: a double blind placebo controlled study. Eur J Obstet Gynaecol Reprod Biol 1992; 44: 137–144.

39 Iosif CS. Effects of protracted administration of oestriol on the lower genitourinary tract in postmenopausal women. Arch Gynaecol Obstet, 1992; 251: 115–120.

40 Kirkengen AL, Andersen P, Gjersoe E, Johannessen GR, Johnsen N, Bodd E. Oestriol in the prophylactic treatment of recurrent urinary tract infections in postmenopausal women. Scand J Prim Health Care 1992; 210: 139–142.

41 Smith P, Heimer G, Lindskog M, Ulmsten U. Oestradiol releasing vaginal ring for treatment of postmenopausal urogenital atrophy. Maturitas 1993; 16: 145–154.

33 Psychiatric aspects of urinary incontinence

INTRODUCTION

The prevalence of psychiatric disorders amongst non-psychiatric patients is high,[1,2,3] and underreporting of psychological distress is common in the general population[4]. As psychological problems and lower urinary tract dysfunction[5] are both common, it is not unusual for them to coexist. An association of psychological and urinary problems has long been recognized, although at present it is unclear whether this relationship is coincidental or causal.

Urinary symptoms may accompany or be the initial presentation of overt psychiatric illness, and psychological symptoms may result from distressing urinary problems. It is important to recognize patients with psychological problems, as they seldom respond adequately to conventional treatment of lower urinary tract dysfunction.

Patients with established psychiatric disease pose both a diagnostic and therapeutic challenge. Dilemmas focus on the reliability of urinary symptoms, the practicality of conventional urodynamic techniques, the choice of treatment and patient compliance. Although seemingly of secondary importance to severe psychiatric illness, urinary incontinence may be a preventable and unnecessary additional handicap to the psychiatric patient and her carers. Irrespective of the underlying cause there are few women for whom incontinence cannot be treated, and all incontinent patients whether they be of sound mind or otherwise should be appropriately investigated and offered sensible and practical advice.

Although psychological factors may be associated with all causes of lower urinary tract dysfunction they are particularly commonly reported amongst women with detrusor instability, sensory urgency, urethral syndrome and voiding difficulties. Psychological problems have also been implicated in the etiology of recurrent urinary tract infections and childhood nocturinal enuresis.

Undoubtedly, severe urinary symptoms are the cause of significant psychological morbidity, and therefore anxiety, depression and other psychiatric symptoms may well be associated with incontinence in general rather than specific diseases of the lower urinary tract.

PSYCHOLOGICAL MORBIDITY IN UROGYNECOLOGY

Delayed presentation of urinary symptoms

Cross-sectional surveys of patients in primary health care have shown that over a quarter demonstrate psychological morbidity, ranging from frank psychiatric illness in a minority to subtle but often disabling forms of demoralization and depression in others. Such patients utilize far more than their proportionate share of health care resources. They seek and receive treatment for their mental ill-health under the guise of many different somatic complaints, including urinary symptoms. Often underlying psychological problems are unrecognized or become mislabelled by doctors.

Urinary symptoms are the source of considerable morbidity which can become incorporated into the lifestyle and personality of patients. Unfortunately, the assessment and treatment of urinary incontinence are often delayed, compounding psychological distress yet further.[6]

Delay may result from a failure to recognize urinary symptoms as a significant health problem, from lack of information regarding the availability of effective treatment, or more commonly from embarrassment and reluctance to admit to urinary incontinence. Norton et al[6] studied 201 incontinent women and found that a third delayed presentation for 1–5 years and a quarter for more than 5 years after their urinary symptoms became troublesome. More than half said that their urinary symptoms affected their work-life, and reported feeling odd and different from other people. It has been shown that psychological morbidity is a consequence of any long-standing distressing condition, and in this respect urinary incontinence sufferers are no exception.[3,7]

PSYCHOLOGICAL FACTORS AND INVESTIGATION OF URINARY PROBLEMS

The International Continence Society standardization of terminology of lower urinary tract dysfunction has provided a universally recognized classification of lower urinary tract dysfunction.[8] Genuine stress incontinence is characterized by stress urinary leakage due to urethral sphincter incompetence in the absence of detrusor instability. Surgical[9] and conservative[10] treatments have been shown to be highly effective in the management of this condition, and treatment failures, although not always avoidable, can usually be explained on the basis of urodynamic findings.

In many cases of detrusor instability, sensory urgency, voiding difficulty and urethral syndrome, the underlying pathology is poorly understood and response to treatment may be inadequate.[11] Additionally, urodynamic investigations are not always able to diagnose the cause of urinary symptoms, and whilst this may reflect a lack of sensitivity of the investigations themselves,[12] it may also represent the absence of organic pathology.

It is tempting to speculate that any disease which lacks an identifiable structural abnormality and proves difficult to treat is largely of psychosomatic origin. If this were so it would be understandable that such conditions would not necessarily respond to drug therapy any better than to placebo, and would be more suitably managed by behavioral means of psychotherapy. Interestingly, the treatment of detrusor instability does include behavioral modification, biofeedback and psychotherapy, which are traditionally the tools of clinical psychologists and psychiatrists.

A correlation between the degree of neuroticism and response to specific treatments has, however, not been clearly shown,[13,14,15] and no association has been demonstrated between placebo response and psychoneuroticism in controlled clinical trials.[16] Additionally, Moore et al[17] failed to show any difference in the ability of women with different levels of psychoneuroticism to perform 'one shot biofeedback' and exercise cortical control of micturition.

Women who complain of significant urinary symptoms but for whom the findings of all investigations are normal present a particular management problem. Characteristically, these women have long-standing severe symptoms which have usually been previously investigated. In the absence of a diagnosis, response to empirical treatment is often suboptimal. Although it is poor clinical practice to label any long-standing condition which is difficult to identify and treat as psychosomatic, significant psychiatric morbidity has been identified amongst these women. Norton et al[18] have shown by psychological questioning that such women have profound psychiatric morbidity within the range expected of psychiatric out-patients and many have a previous psychiatric history. We have been unable to reproduce their results.

It is conceivable that psychological factors contribute to the severity if not the cause of urinary symptoms, and intervention studies[19] suggest that these factors play at least a maintaining role.

It is also possible that their psychological disorder is secondary to long-standing severe symptoms and the failure of extensive and often unpleasant investigations to reach a diagnosis. It may be for this reason that we have been unable to reproduce the results of Norton et al,[18] as ambulatory urodynamics form part of our urodynamic assessment and were not used in their study. Additionally, no mention was made in their study of cystoscopy being performed on women in their study in whom the findings of cystometry were negative, nor were any of the women given a diagnosis of sensory urgency.

Irrespective of their cause, urinary symptoms often result in significant psychological and emotional distress. It is partly for this reason that research interest has focused on the identification of psychiatric illness amongst incontinence sufferers, rather than a search for incontinence amongst known psychiatric patients.

PSYCHIATRIC ASPECTS OF URINARY INCONTINENCE

Detrusor instability and sensory urgency

Straub et al[20] found that symptoms of urinary frequency and urinary retention correlated with variations in emotional state and life situation. They found that unstable detrusor contractions could be provoked by emotional stress in the laboratory setting, and reinforced and perpetuated by a stressful work and social environment. Voiding difficulties and urinary retention in the absence of anatomical or neurological causes were also related to stressful life events.

Jeffcoate & Francis[21] found that 61% of 246 women with urge incontinence appeared obsessional or depressed. Frewen[22] postulated that urge incontinence developed as a result of psychic trauma, but provided little evidence to substantiate this view. Crisp & Sutherst[23] found that 15 patients with detrusor instability were more neurotic on Eysenck Personality Inventory testing[24] than 42 patients with genuine stress incontinence, and these results agreed with a study of depression and life events by Pierson et al.[25] Using the Psychosocial Adjustment to Illness Scale, we have shown that women with sensory urgency and detrusor instability suffer greater psychological impairment as a result of their urinary symptoms than other incontinent women.[26]

Macauley et al[27] showed than all women with urinary symptoms were more anxious and depressed than continent women of a similar age on three different self-rating scales: the Spielberger State/Trait Anxiety Inventory,[28] the Wakefield Depression Scale[29] and the Crown–Crisp Experiential Index (CCEI).[30] Patients with genuine stress incontinence were no more anxious than general medical in-patients, whereas women with sensory urgency or detrusor instability were significantly more so (p <0.05). Levels of hysteria were higher for incontinent patients than continent controls, and higher for women with detrusor instability and sensory urgency than women with genuine stress incontinence. Roughly one-quarter of their patients felt that life was not worth living because of their urinary symptoms. These patients were found to be as anxious, depressed and phobic as psychiatric in-patients, but the authors were unable to conclude whether an abnormal mental state generated the urinary symptoms or vice versa.

In contrast, Norton et al[18] found that women with detrusor instability had no greater psychiatric morbidity than other incontinent women. Unfortunately, the small number of patients in their study, and the significantly different duration of urinary symptoms between the groups, may have contributed to their conclusions. Additionally, women with detrusor instability scored lower on subjective incontinence severity scales and social impairment scales than women with other diagnoses, which is at conflict with other studies.[31]

It is possible that the limited number of women with detrusor instability (33) in their study may not truly reflect this group as a whole; however, Morrison et al[32] reached similar conclusions and found no difference in the Eysenck Personality Inventory scores of patients with detrusor instability and 50 other incontinent patients. Unfortunately, almost one-third of the women entering this study were excluded from the overall results due to high scores on the lie subscale of the test!

Using the Hospital Anxiety and Depression (HAD) scale,[33] Kelleher et al[34] have shown that women with detrusor instability have significantly higher levels of anxiety and depression than women with genuine stress incontinence, although no significant differences were seen between these two diagnoses using the CCEI. When the suggested cut-off scores of the HAD for probable anxiety and depression were analyzed, no significant differences in clinically recognizable psychopathology were seen between the two diagnostic groups.

A potential bias in reported levels of neuroticism between these two diagnoses may well be attributable to the nature of irritative bladder symptoms. Because of the wording of questions in the HAD, particularly those relating to anxiety, it is highly likely that women with detrusor instability will achieve higher scores than women with symptoms solely of stress incontinence.

The difference in psychiatric morbidity between women with detrusor instability and sensory urgency and other incontinent women may be explained by a number of factors. It is feasible that severe psychological morbidity amongst incontinence sufferers is a reflection of the severity and duration of their urinary symptoms, but it is also possible that the converse is true, and that severe and refractory urinary symptoms are the manifestation of underlying psychological morbidity.

A number of studies have investigated this relationship by correlating objective and subjective assessments of the severity of urinary symptoms with the results of psychological status questionnaires.

Subjective quality of life assessments have shown that women with detrusor instability and sensory urgency suffer greater quality of life impairment as a result of their urinary symptoms than women with other urodynamic diagnosis.[31,35,36] Perhaps the unpredictability and severity of their urinary leakage imparts greater emotional, social and sexual restrictions than in the case of other diagnoses, and hence greater quality of life impairment.

If psychological morbidity was a manifestation of the subjective severity of incontinence it would be understandable that detrusor instability and sensory urgency would impart greater distress. Using the Nottingham Health Profile and the CCEI, we have shown a significant correlation between the scores obtained on quality of life and psychological status questionnaires for women with all forms of lower urinary tract dysfunction.[26] Similarly, Macauley et al[27] recorded greater psychological morbidity in women with detrusor instability and sensory urgency, but irrespective of the urodynamic diagnosis patients with the most severe disease (judged by a self-rating scale) were the most abnormal on psychological function testing.

Moore et al[37] studied 109 women with detrusor instability using the CCEI and both objective and subjective measures of the severity of urinary incontinence. They showed that the severity of psychological impairment correlated significantly with the severity of urinary symptoms and objective measures of the amount of urinary leakage. Although psychological morbidity appears to be most common amongst women with detrusor instability and sensory urgency, research suggests that this is by virtue of the greater subjective severity of these conditions. Unfortunately, by whatever mechanism the two are related, psychological factors may be a major impairment to the successful treatment of affected women, and although no causal link has been proven, psychological factors are likely to play a maintaining role in the natural history of these conditions.

Urethral syndrome

The urethral syndrome is characterized by frequency of micturition, urgency, dysuria and often urethral, back and abdominal pain, in the absence of infection, anatomical abnormalities or frank urological disease.

The role of psychological and personality factors in the etiology of this condition has received scant attention. Carson et al[38] used the Minnesota Multiphasic Personality Inventory (MMPI)[39] to assess 56 women with the urethral syndrome. They found that scores on the hypochondriasis, hysteria and schizophrenia scales of the questionnaire were high, and similar to those found in patients suffering from classical 'conversion hysteria'. Symptoms referred to the back, head, abdomen or bladder often reflected periods of stress or tension, and were used to escape from painful or stressful situations.

The symptoms of urethral syndrome may not necessarily reflect the presence of organic disease, but a psychophysiological process whereby women focus on lower urinary tract symptoms. This may explain the common failure of conventional treatments and a need to concentrate on the psychological difficulties of these patients.

Psychogenic urinary retention

Female urinary retention in the absence of anatomical, physiological, neurological, infective or other causes is difficult to explain and consequently often poorly treated. Approximately 60 years ago Braasch & Thompson[40] described the role of transurethral resection in females for the correction of sphincteric 'ectasia' on one basis of the largely esoteric diagnoses of 'female prostate', 'bladder neck polyps' or 'mucosal proliferation'. This treatment proved unsuccessful and fraught with complications.

Williams & Johnson[41] and Chapman[42] published detailed individual psychiatric case studies of women with urinary retention due to emotional factors. These included rape, incest and in one case self-punishment for a patient's hostility towards her mother. When urinary retention is encountered it is uncommon to recognize the possible psychogenic aspect of this presentation.

Larson et al[43] examined 25 cases of female urinary retention, in all of which the findings of intravenous urography, cystourethroscopy and neurological assessment were normal. Many of the women had previously undergone unsuccessful 'transurethral resection'. Documented urinary retention was found in all the patients, although the residual urine volume varied significantly between investigations. The women all had a high incidence of previous surgical procedures, mainly gynecological or gastrointestinal surgery, and complained of a variety of other somatic complaints including low back pain, headaches and vague gastro-intestinal symptoms. Although all denied the possibility that emotional factors could be implicated in their presenting complaint, assessment using the MMPI showed 17 of the women to be neurotic and 8 to be psychotic. Twelve of the neurotic group were given a diagnosis of conversion hysteria and 3 of neurotic depression. Five of the 8 psychotic patients were diagnosed as schizophrenic and the remaining 3 as psychotic depressives.

It is apparent, therefore, that for a small subgroup of women psychological or emotional factors are a cause of their urinary retention. Their denial of psychological symptoms is typical of the hysteroid personality, and often makes subsequent psychiatric management difficult. Many of these patients prefer to have extensive investigations and invasive management than admit to psychiatric disease. Conservative management by catheterization and urological investigation is usually necessary and allows time for a thorough assessment of the psychological state of the patient.

Nocturnal enuresis

It is generally accepted that nocturnal enuresis affects 15–20% of 5-year-old children. Of these cases, approximately 15% resolve spontaneously each year. The incidence of enuresis is higher amongst boys than girls, and genetic factors appear to be particularly important.[44] Two types of enuresis have been described: type 1 (primary) enuresis, where the child has never been dry at night; and type 2 (secondary), where the child has been dry for a period of at least 6 months and has started to bed-wet again. Secondary enuresis accounts for about 10–15% of cases. Aboulker & Chertok[45] stated that enuresis was essentially a psychogenic disorder, and Kolvin & Taunch[46] found that the association between enuresis and psychiatric disturbance was particularly common in children with secondary enuresis. Moffat[47] found that enuretics actively seeking medical help differed psychologically from other enuretic children, and suggested that these children were under greater stress and consequently had more behavioral symptoms.

In an 8-year longitudinal study of 1265 children, Fergussen et al[48] showed a lack of correlation between psychosocial problems and nocturnal enuresis. Unrelated to enuresis were a broad range of psychosocial factors, including social and economic background, adverse family events and changes in residence. Additionally, no differences were found in achieving nocturnal continence in children with or without psychosocial problems.

Ditman & Blinn[49] showed that enuresis occurred in any stage of sleep, but most often during light sleep. They felt that light sleep and 'physiological wakefulness' represented a dissociative reaction, and should be managed by psychotherapy. Broughton[50] found that enuresis started in deep sleep with signs of arousal, followed by a lightening of sleep and micturition. Schiff[51] concluded similarly that enuresis sufferers have a maturational defect in their sleep/arousal system, and Ritvo et al[52] classified enuretics into two types on this basis: an arousal and a non-arousal pattern. They also found that patients with arousal prior to enuresis had increased evidence of neuroticism and a negative family history for enuresis, whereas minimal evidence of psychological disturbance or maladjustment was seen in the group showing non-arousal enuresis.

Although psychological factors may be important in the etiology and maintenance of nocturnal enuresis the results of studies are conflicting, and no firm causal link has been clearly demonstrated. Nature appears to cure most children, but when medical intervention takes place psychosocial factors do not appear greatly to influence its success.

Psychological factors in recurrent urinary tract infection

Sanford[53] estimated that 20% of women experience symptoms of a urinary tract infection each year, and half of these seek medical help. This figure masks the fact that the number of presentations is not evenly distributed amongst sufferers and many women present with recurrent symptoms. Mabeck[54] estimated that one-sixth of sufferers account for 70% of recurrences. Behavioral factors have been shown to be important in the etiology of recurrent infections[55] (see Ch. 32), although psychological and personality factors may also be of significance.[56,57]

Hunt & Waller[57] used Foxman & Frerichs' 'Inventory of Habits,[58,59] the Eysenck Personality Inventory and the Maudsley Obsessive-Compulsive Inventory[60] to assess behavioral, psychological and personality variables of recurrent urinary tract infection sufferers and a control group of patients with other infections. They found that urinary track infection sufferers were significantly more obsessive, neurotic and introverted than controls, and a higher number of urinary tract infections over the previous year was associated with a more neurotic personality type. They concluded that psychological factors are important in determining which patients develop recurrent urinary tract infections and how often infections occur. Intervention studies[40] suggest that psychological factors have at least a maintaining role, and where physical factors are insufficient to account for the presence or severity of symptoms, psychological factors should also be assessed. It is recognized that some women complain of 'recurrent cystitis', particularly when under stress, although bacteriological investigations are often negative.

Stress incontinence

Chronic urinary symptoms have a detrimental effect on the psychological function of women, and psychological problems may be a normal response to such symptoms. Macauley et al[27] showed that patients with genuine stress incontinence were more anxious than the general population, but were no different from other patients with chronic illness.

Obrink et al[61] used the Eysenck Personality Inventory to show that patients receiving surgical treatment for genuine stress incontinence who were both subjectively and objectively cured had an improvement in neurotic and depressive symptoms. Those subjectively but not objectively cured were similarly improved, whereas those objectively but not subjectively cured remained both neurotic and depressed.

Rosenweig et al[62] also studied the effect of incontinence surgery on the psychological status of genuine stress incontinence sufferers. Sixty-three women without prior psychological histories were evaluated before and after incontinence surgery. An assessment was made of nervousness, depression, tension, sleep disturbance, appetite, somatic weakness and headaches. Patients who were objectively and/or subjectively cured reported a statistically significant improvement in psychological status. Those for whom surgery was unsuccessful did not report a significant change in their psychological status. Sleep disturbance and tension were most commonly affected by treatment, improving significantly with successful treatment and deteriorating with its failure. Subjective treatment failure resulted in a statistically significant increase in depressive symptoms.

Treatment of stress incontinence may be instrumental in improving psychological dysfunction. Subjective failure but objective success of incontinence surgery may indicate the presence of underlying psychological problems. Such patients may derive secondary gains from their urinary symptoms and the apparent failure of surgical treatment perhaps warrants formal assessment of their psychological status. Conversely, these findings may indicate that patients' expectations of treatment and a successful surgical outcome do not necessarily parallel the views of the doctor or the results of objective clinical tests.

PSYCHIATRIC ASPECTS OF THE TREATMENT OF URINARY SYMPTOMS

From this review of the literature it would appear that long-standing urinary symptoms are the source of appreciable psychological morbidity, which itself may be important in the maintenance and severity of lower urinary tract dysfunction. Although there is insufficient evidence to conclude that urinary incontinence is the result of underlying psychological morbidity, psychological factors may be important in the etiology of detrusor instability, sensory urgency, recurrent urinary tract infection and unexplained urinary retention.

Of the various causes of lower urinary tract dysfunction, detrusor instability has been most extensively investigated. The results of studies do, however, conflict and this appears to be related to the method by which psychological morbidity is assessed. If detrusor instability were primarily the result of psychological disturbance, the more severely neurotic patients would be more difficult to treat by conventional means. This does not appear to be the case.[13,14,15,17]

Moore et al[16] used the CCEI to assess women completing a double-blind placebo-controlled crossover trial of oxybutynin for the treatment of detrusor instability. Although the CCEI was only completed after treatment, and therefore improvement in CCEI scores could not be assessed, the scores of poor responders to treatment were significantly higher than those of good responders.

We have recently shown that women with a good subjective response to treatment of both detrusor instability and genuine stress incontinence have lower HAD scores[63] and CCEI scores[34] before treatment than poor responders. This would suggest that psychological factors are important for the prediction of treatment successes and failures, although it would also appear that high scores reflect more severe urinary symptoms, which would undoubtedly be more difficult to treat!

In the absence of a readily identifiable cause for detrusor instability and in view of poor results of pharmacological therapy,[11] it is understandable that behavioral therapy, biofeedback and psychotherapy have all been used for its treatment. Frewen[64] offered women with detrusor instability an in-patient treatment package consisting of a urinary diary, bladder retraining, anxiolytic and anticholinergic medication and supportive care, and achieved a cure rate of 82.5%.

There have been numerous studies demonstrating the value of bladder retraining, behavioral therapy and biofeedback for the treatment of detrusor instability.[64–69] Millard & Oldenberg[14] reported a short-term improvement rate of 70% following bladder retraining and biofeedback, although by 18 months 5–10% had relapsed. Although the authors found considerable psychopathology amongst their patients prior to treatment, this improved substantially following successful therapy.

Oldenberg et al[70] assessed 53 women with detrusor instability using two psychological profile questionnaires, the SCL 90 and the Locus of Control of Behavior. Following bladder retraining with or without biofeedback there was substantial improvement in psychological profile scores at 18-month follow-up. This improvement occurred largely irrespective of the response to treatment, and therapists were unable to predict on the basis of psychological profile scores for which patients treatment would succeed.

Hafner et al[13] used the Eysenck Personality Inventory to assess the results of psychotherapy in patients with detrusor instability. They found that 50% of the most neurotic but only 11% of the least neurotic patients benefited from psychotherapy. The authors felt that the least neurotic subjects actually denied their neuroticism although scores on the lie scale of the test did not appear to substantiate this view.

Macauley et al[27] used a number of self-rating scales to assess the psychiatric profile of patients with detrusor instability or sensory urgency before and after treatment. Following assessment women were randomly allocated to receive either psychotherapy, bladder retraining or medication (propantheline 15 mg three times daily) for 3 months. Nocturia, urgency and incontinence improved with psychotherapy, although frequency was unaltered. There were no appreciable changes in psychological ratings following psychotherapy, although the authors felt that this resulted from increased self-awareness and introspection masking any potential benefit. Bladder retraining decreased the detrusor pressure rise during filling cystometry and the first sensation of desire to void, and was associated with a significant improvement in patients' psychoneurotic profile. None of the women treated with propantheline showed significant cystometric improvement, although the dose of propantheline used in the study was probably too low to have been effective.

Undoubtedly, there is a large placebo response to the treatment of irritative bladder symptoms.[71] Although there are numerous placebo-controlled trials in the literature suggesting that active drugs are superior to placebo for the treatment of detrusor instability, many studies are inconclusive. One study even suggested that placebo was the drug of choice, improving symptoms in 75% of patients.[72]

Whilst the placebo response in psychosomatic conditions is often believed to be high, Moore et al[16] found no association in the treatment of detrusor instability between psychoneuroticism and good response to placebo. This would cast doubt on the suggestion that idiopathic detrusor instability is largely a psychosomatic disorder.

URINARY INCONTINENCE AND ESTABLISHED PSYCHIATRIC ILLNESS

Whilst considerable research interest has focused on the psychological correlates of urinary problems amongst seemingly normal women, there is little literature concerning those with established psychiatric illness. In addition to the usual causes of female urinary incontinence encountered in normal populations additional causes of incontinence may be encountered more frequently amongst women with established psychiatric illness. These may be listed as follows:

- drugs, e.g. lithium, antidepressive drugs, anxiolytics, antipsychotics
- motivational/behavioral/personality disorders
- mental retardation/dementia
- poor hygiene
- bowel problems, e.g. constipation.

Motivational, behavioral and personality disorders may all prevent or limit normal toileting, and mental retardation or dementia are often associated with poor hygiene, abnormal bowel function and urinary incontinence.

Many of the drugs used for the management of psychiatric disorders have potent effects on bladder function. Lithium may result in excessive thirst, polydipsia and increased diuresis, and antidepressives and antipsychotics possess potent anticholinergic effects which may result in voiding difficulties, urinary retention with overflow and recurrent urinary tract infections. Anxiolytics and sedatives may decrease awareness of the need to pass urine, resulting in enuresis and overflow incontinence.

A thorough clinical history, mental state examination and functional assessment are therefore mandatory when assessing lower urinary tract dysfunction in these patients. Treatment should always be carefully planned and tailored to the individual needs and functional requirements of the incontinent psychiatric patient.

A recent move towards community psychiatric care has resulted in the closure of many psychiatric in-patient units and placed additional workloads on already overstretched community services. The importance of continued assessment of the needs of incontinent psychiatric patients should, however, not be underemphasized and appropriate management should be tailored to changes in their mental state and physical requirements. There are few women for whom incontinence cannot be improved by the provision of suitable treatment.

Advances in neuroscience and brain imaging have further improved the investigation of urinary problems affecting psychiatric patients. Bonney et al[73] have recently shown an increased incidence of detrusor instability and urinary incontinence in patients with chronic schizophrenia compared to patients with other psychiatric disorders. Positron emission tomography scanning of the brain has suggested the presence of neuroanatomical lesions to account for this finding and more detailed studies are eagerly awaited.

CONCLUSION

The association between psychological and urinary problems is complex but it is possible to draw several conclusions:

1. Long-standing distressing urinary symptoms are the source of considerable psychological morbidity, and the severity of urinary symptoms and leakage are major determinants of the degree of psychological impairment.
2. Women with greater psychological morbidity often respond worse to treatment, although this may be a reflection of the greater severity of their disease.
3. The treatment of urinary problems improves psychological distress and failure of adequate diagnosis or treatment may intensify psychological symptoms.
4. Assessment of incontinent psychiatric patients should include a detailed clinical history, mental state and functional assessment, and a psychiatric illness should not restrict the appropriate management of their urinary symptoms.

At present there is insufficient conclusive evidence to substantiate a primary psychological cause for lower urinary tract dysfunction, although psychological factors may be important in the etiology of unexplained urinary retention and urethral syndrome and some cases of detrusor instability and sensory urgency.

REFERENCES

1 Shepherd M, Davis B, Culpan RH. Psychiatric illness in a general hospital. Acta Psychiatr Scand 1960; 35: 518–525.
2 Maguire GP, Julier DL, Hawton KE, Bancroft JHL. Psychiatric morbidity and referral on two general medical wards. Br Med J 1974: 1; 268–270.
3 Moffic HS, Paykel ES. Depression in medical inpatients. Br J Psychiatry 1975: 126; 346–353.
4 Veit CT, Ware JE. The structure of psychological distress and wellbeing in general populations. J Cons and Clin Psychology 1983; 51 (5): 730–742.
5 Health Survey Questionnaire: Market and Opinion Research International (MORI), 1990; 95 Southwark Street, London SE1 OHX.
6 Norton PA, MacDonald LD, Sedgewick PM, Stanton SL. Distress and delay associated with urinary incontinence frequency and urgency in women. Br Med J 1988; 297: 187.
7 Stewart AL, Greenfield S, Hays RD et al. Functional status and well-being of patients with chronic conditions: results from the medical outcomes study. JAMA 1989; 262 (7): 907–913.

8 Abrams P, Blaivas JG, Stanton SL, Anderson JT. The standardisation of terminology of lower urinary tract function. Scand J Urol Nephrol 1988; Suppl 114: 5–19.

9 Jarvis GJ. Surgery for genuine stress incontinence. Br J Obstet Gynaecol 1994; 101 (5): 371–374.

10 Kelleher CJ, Cardozo LD. Treatment options in urinary incontinence. Rev Contemp Pharmacother 1994; 5: 163–177.

11 Brading AF, Turner WH. The unstable bladder: towards a common mechanism. Br J Urol 1994; 73: 3–8.

12 Webb RJ. Griffiths CJ, Neal DE. Ambulatory monitoring in neuropathic bladder dysfunction. Neurourol Urodyn 1991; 10 (4): 419–420.

13 Hafner RJ, Stanton SL, Guy J. A psychiatric study of women with urgency and urgency incontinence. Br J Urol 1977; 49: 211–214.

14 Millard RJ, Oldenberg BF. The symptomatic, urodynamic and psychodynamic results of bladder re-education programmes. J Urol 1983; 130: 715.

15 Ferrie BG, Smith JS, Logan D et al. Experience with bladder training in 65 patients. Br J Urol 1984; 56: 482–484.

16 Moore KH, Sutherst JR. Response to treatment of detrusor instability in relation to psychoneurotic status. Br J Urol 1990; 65 (5): 486–490.

17 Moore KH, Richmond DH, Sutherst JR, Manasse P. One shot biofeedback in relation to psychoneurotic status and treatment response in detrusor instability. Neurourol Urodyn 1992; 11(4): 365–366.

18 Norton KRW, Bhat AV, Stanton SL. Psychiatric aspects of urinary incontinence in women attending an outpatient urodynamic clinic. Br Med J 1990; 301: 271–272.

19 Lumsden L, Hyner GC. Effect of educational intervention on the rate of recurrent urinary tract infections in selected female outpatients. Women Health 1985; 10: 79–86.

20 Straub LR, Ripley HS, Wolf S. Disturbance of bladder function associated with emotional states. JAMA 1949; 141: 1139–1143.

21 Jeffcoate TNA, Francis VJA. Urgency incontinence in the female. Am J Obstet Gynaecol 1966; 94: 604–608.

22 Frewen WK. An objective assessment of the unstable bladder of psychosomatic origin. Br J Urol 1978; 50: 246.

23 Crisp A, Sutherst J. Psychological factors in women with urinary incontinence. Proceedings of the International Urodynamics and Continence Society 1983; 1: 174–176.

24 Eysenck HJ, Eysenck SBG. Manual of the Eysenck Personality Inventory. London: Hodder & Soughton, 1978.

25 Pierson CA, Meyer CB, Ostergard DR. Vesical instability, a stress related entity. Proc Int Cont Soc 176–177.

26 Kelleher CJ, Khullar V, Cardozo LD. Psychoneuroticism and quality of life in healthy incontinent women. Neurourol Urodyn 1993; 12(4): 393–394.

27 Macauley AJ, Stern RS, Holmes DM, Stanton SL. Micturition and the mind: psychological factors in the aetiology and treatment of urinary symptoms in women. Br Med J 1987; 294: 540.

28 Spielberger CD, Gorsuch RL, Lushene RE. The stait-trait anxiety inventory. Palo Alto: Consulting Psychologists' Press, 1970.

29 Snaith RP, Ahmed SN, Mehta S, Hamilton M. Assessment of the severity of primary depressive illness (Wakefield Self-assessment Depression Inventory) Psychol Med 1974; 1: 143–149.

30 Crown S, Crisp AH. Manual of the Crown–Crisp Experiental Index. London: Hodder & Stoughton, 1979.

31. Wyman JF, Harkins SW, Fantl JA. Psychosocial impact of urinary incontinence in the community dwelling population. J Am Geriatric Soc 1990; 38: 282.

32 Morrison LM, Eadie AS, McAlister ES, Taylor GJ, Rowan D. Personality testing in 226 patients with urinary incontinence. Br J Urol 1986; 58: 387–389.

33 Zigmond AS, Snaith RP. The Hospital Anxiety and Depression scale. Acta Psychiatr Scand 1983; 67: 361–370.

34 Kelleher CJ. The impact or urinary incontinence on the quality of life of women. MD thesis, University of London, 1995.

35 Hunskaar S, Vinsnes A. The quality of life in women with urinary incontinence as measured by the sickness impact profile. JAGS 1991; 39: 378–382.

36 Grimby A, Milstrom I, Molander U, Wiklund I, Ekelund P. The influence of urinary incontinence on the quality of life of women. Age and Ageing 1993; 22: 82–89.

37 Moore KH, Richmond DH, Sutherst JR, Manasse P. Is severe wetness associated with severe madness in detrusor instability? Neurourol Urodyn 1992; 11 (4): 460–461.

38 Carson CC, Osbourne D, Segura JW. Psychologic characteristics of patients with female urethral syndrome. J Clin Psychol 1974; 35: 312–313.

39 Swenson WM, Pearson JS, Osborne D. An MMPI source book. Basic item, scale, and pattern data on 50,000 medical patients. Minneapolis: University of Minnesota Press, 1973.

40 Braasch WF, Thompson GJ. Treatment of atonic bladder. Surg Gynec Obstet 1935; 61: 379–384.

41 Williams GE, Johnson AM. Recurrent urinary retention due to emotional factors. Report of case. Psychosom Med 1956; 18: 77–80.

42 Chapman AH. Psychogenic urinary retention in women. Psychosom Med 1959; 21: 119–122.

43 Larson JW, Swenson WM, Utz DC, Steinhilber RM. Psychogenic urinary retention in women JAMA 1963; 184 (9): 697–700.

44 Bakwin H. The genetics of enuresis. In: Kolvin I, MacKeith RC, Meadow SR (eds) Bladder control and enuresis. London: William Heinemann, pp 73–77.

45 Aboulker P, Chertok L. Emotional factors in stress incontinence. Psychosom Med 1962; 24: 507.

46 Kolvin I, Taunch J. A dual theory of nocturnal enuresis. In: Kolvin I, MacKeith RC, Meadow SR (eds) Bladder control and enuresis: London: William Heinemann, pp 156–172.

47 Moffat MEK. Nocturnal enuresis. Psychologic implications of treatment and non-treatment'. J Paediatrics 1989; 114 (Suppl): 697–704.

48 Fergussen DM, Horwood LJ, Shannon FT. Factors related to the age of attainment of nocturnal bladder control; an eight year longitudinal study. Paediatrics 1986; 78: 884–890.

49 Ditman L, Blinn LA. Sleep levels in enuresis. Am J Psychiatry 1955; 111: 931.

50 Broughton RJ. Sleep disorders: disorders of arousal. Enuresis, somnambulism, and nightmares in confusional states of arousal, not in dreaming sleep. Science 1968; 159: 1070.

51 Schiff SK. The EEG, eye movements and dreaming in adult enuresis. J Nerv Ment Dis 1965; 140: 397–404.

52 Ritvo ER, Ornitz EM, Gottleib F et al. Arousal and non arousal enuretic events. Am J Psychiatry 1969; 126: 115–122.

53 Sanford JP. Urinary tract symptoms and infections. Ann Rev Med 1975; 26: 485–498.

54 Mabeck CE. Treatment of uncomplicated urinary tract infection in non pregnant women. Postgrad Med J 1972; 48: 69–75.

55 Adatto K, Doebele KG, Galland L et al. Behavioural factors and urinary tract infection. JAMA 1979; 241: 2525–2526.

56 Rees DLP, Farhoumand N. Psychiatric aspects of recurrent cystitis in women. Br J Urol 1977; 49: 651–658.

57 Hunt JC, Waller G. Psychological factors in recurrent uncomplicated urinary tract infection. Br J Urol 1992; 69: 460–464.

58 Foxman B, Frerichs RR. Epidemiology of urinary tract infection. Diaphragm use and sexual intercourse. Am J Public Health 1985a; 75: 1308–1313.

59 Foxman B, Frerichs RR. Epidemiology of urinary tract infection. 2. Diet, clothing and urination habits. Am J Public Health 1985b; 75: 1314–1317.

60 Rachman SJ, Hodgson RJ. Obsessions and compulsions. New Jersey: Prentice Hall, 1980.

61 Obrink A, Fedor-Freyberg P, Hjelmkvist M. Mental factors influencing recurrence of stress incontinence. Acta Obstet Gynaecol Scand 1979; 58: 91.

62 Rosenweig BA, Hischke D, Thomas S, Nelson A L, Bhatia N N. Stress incontinence in women. Psychological status before and after treatment. J Reprod Med 1991; 36, 12, 835–838.

63 Kelleher CJ, Cardozo LD, Khullar V, Salvatore S, Hill S. Anticholinergic therapy: the need for continued surveillance. Neurourol Urodyn 1994: 13(4): 432–433.

64 Frewen WK. A reassessment of bladder training in detrusor dysfunction in the female. Br J Urol 1982; 54: 372.

65 Frewen WK. Urgency incontinence (review of 100 cases). J Obstet Gynaecol Br Commonw 1972; 79: 77–79.

66 Cardozo LD, Abrams PD, Stanton SL, Feneley RC. Idiopathic bladder instability treated with biofeedback. Br J Urol 1978; 50: 521.

67 Burgio KL, Whitehead WE, Engel BT. Urinary incontinence in the elderly. Bladder sphincter feedback and toilet skills training. Ann Intern Med 1985; 103: 507–515.

68 Holmes DM, Plevnik S, Stanton SL. Bladder neck electrical conductivity in the treatment of detrusor instability with biofeedback. Br J Obstet Gynaecol 1989; 96: 821–826.

69 Jarvis GJ. A controlled trial of bladder drill and drug therapy in the management of detrusor instability. Br J Urol 1983; 53: 565–566.

70 Oldenberg B, Millard RJ. Predictors of outcome following a bladder retraining programme. J Psychosom Res 1986; 30: 691.
71 Carter R, Aitchison MA. Placebo responses in the treatment of urge incontinence. International Urogynaecology Journal 1993; 4: 229–231.
72 Meyhoff HH, Gerstenberg TC, Nordling J. Placebo– the drug of choice in female motor urge incontinence. Br J Urol 1983; 55: 34–37.
73 Bonney W, Gupta S, Arndt S, Anderson K, Hunter DR. Neurophysiological correlates of bladder dysfunction in schizophrenia. Neurourol Urodyn 1993; 12 (4): 347–348.
74 Macauley AJ, Stern RS, Stanton SL. Psychological aspects of 211 female patients attending a urodynamic unit. J Psychosom Res 1991; 35 (1): 1–10.

34

Urinary tract involvement by benign and malignant gynecological disease

INTRODUCTION

The urinary and genital tracts have a common embryological origin and throughout life the lower urinary tract and the genital organs lie in close proximity within the confines of the female pelvis. Thus disorders of the genital tract may affect the ureters, bladder or urethra. Symptoms usually arise either due to direct invasion and involvement of the lower urinary tract as part of the disease process or, more commonly, by a mass effect produced by an enlarging pelvic tumor.

This chapter is devoted to the effect which benign or malignant gynecological disease has on the lower urinary tract. The following problems will be considered:

1. Gynecological cancer
2. Fibroids
3. Adnexal disease
   a. Pelvic inflammatory disease
   b. Benign ovarian disease
4. Endometriosis
5. The effect of 'simple' hysterectomy.

Any of these conditions may give rise to lower urinary tract dysfunction, so it is important to consider the possibility of a gynecological cause when investigating urinary symptoms, as treatment of the underlying gynecological disorder may cure the urinary symptoms. In addition, gynecological pathology is often treated surgically. In order to minimize the risks of intraoperative trauma or postoperative complications the surgeon (gynecologist or urologist) must be aware of the possibility of lower urinary tract involvement prior to operative intervention.

GYNECOLOGICAL CANCER

Gynecological cancer accounts for approximately 25% of all female cancers. As the mean female life-expectancy continues to rise, gynecologists may expect to see an increase in the incidence of genital cancer as many of the tumors are more common in old age.

Urinary dysfunction can occur either secondary to the malignancy or more commonly as a consequence of treatment involving surgery, radiotherapy and/or chemotherapy. Usually the primary disease is responsible for the symptoms, although metastatic disease may occasionally be the cause. Involvement of the lower urinary tract greatly reduces the chances of successful treatment and is therefore an important component in the staging of genital tract tumors.

Carcinoma of the cervix

Despite the advent of the Papanicolaou smear and routine screening of all sexually active women, cervical cancer continues to kill approximately 2500 young women each year in the UK. It also produces significant urological morbidity both due to the disease itself and the sequelae of treatment.

Carcinoma of the cervix spreads chiefly in two ways: by direct extension into surrounding tissues, and via the lymphatics to the regional lymph nodes. Blood-borne metastases do occur but are usually found in either very advanced or anaplastic tumors.

The disease may spread by direct extension superiorly, in the stroma and stromal lymphatics, to the uterine canal and myometrium. Extension inferiorly involves the vaginal fornices and from there the disease can spread to the rest of the vagina, whence it extends to involve the bladder and urethra anteriorly or the rectum posteriorly. There may also be unilateral or bilateral extension into the parametrium, towards the pelvic side wall which may cause unilateral or bilateral ureteric involvement.

Tumor dissemination within the lymphatic network appears to be quite orderly (Fig. 34.1). The first nodes to be involved are the parametrial nodes, situated at the intersection of the uterine artery and the ureter. From here spread occurs to involve the following, usually in order: obturator nodes, surrounding the obturator vessels and nerves (Fig. 34.2); the

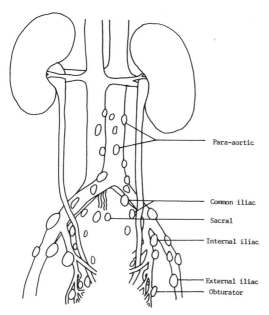

Para-aortic

Common iliac

Sacral

Internal iliac

External iliac
Obturator

Fig. 34.1 The lymphatic drainage of the female pelvis

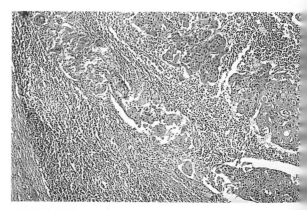

Fig. 34.2 An obturator lymph node involved by metastatic carcinoma of the cervix

internal and external iliac nodes; the common iliac nodes; and finally the para-aortic nodes. The ureter may become obstructed by enlarged lymph nodes as it enters the true pelvis at the bifurcation of the common iliac vessels over the sacroiliac joint, or during its course along the pelvic side wall and in the base of the broad ligament.

The incidence and prognostic significance of urinary tract involvement in cervical carcinoma is dependent on whether the tumor is primary or recurrent.

Primary cervical cancer

The most common single cause of death in women with carcinoma of the cervix is urinary obstruction, which is responsible in at least 50% of cases.[1] The ureter usually becomes obstructed at the urterovesical junction. This is caused by extrinsic compression rather than invasion of the ureter, which is rare.[2] This compression may be caused by the tumor itself or by metastatic deposits in pelvic lymph nodes[3] (Fig. 34.3A and B).

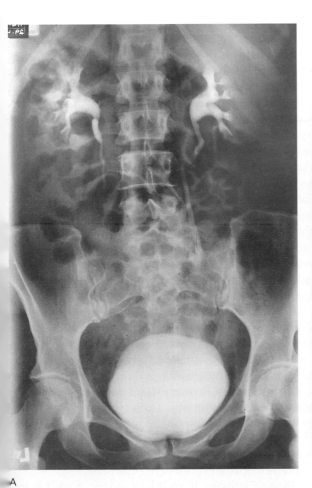
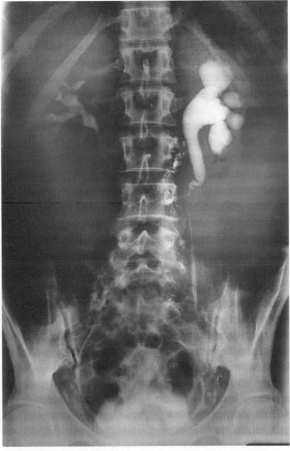

A   B

Fig. 34.3 Normal intravenous urography (IVU) performed as part of the staging procedure in a woman with carcinoma of the cervix. (stage IB on clinical criteria) (**A**). An IVU 1 year after Wertheim's hysterectomy in the same woman, when she presented with a history of loin pain and hypertension (**B**). This now shows obstructive changes in the left kidney due to enlarged lymph nodes at the mid-ureter, later confirmed at postmortem

In a large study performed in 1950, Aldridge et al studied 458 patients of which 334 had intravenous urography (IVU) performed prior to treatment. Of the patients tested 219 were found to have a normal IVU, while 115 (34.5%) had abnormalities thought to be related to the carcinoma. In the group with an abnormal IVU the overall survival rate was only 16%, compared to 62% in the group with a normal IVU.[4] Since then many authors have studied the incidence and prognostic significance of urinary tract involvement by invasive cervical cancer.[5,6,7,8] In these studies, involving a total of 3593 patients, the incidence of urinary tract involvement in all stages of disease was found to vary between 19.1% and 34.5%, with an overall incidence of 23.2%.

The 5-year survival rates for patients with or without ureteric obstruction were compared to illustrate the prognostic significance of this finding. In patients without ureteric obstruction the survival rates were found to vary between 22% and 62% with an overall average of 50%. In patients with ureteric obstruction the survival rates varied between 8.8% and 24% with an average of 14%.

Ureteral obstruction has therefore been shown to be of grave prognostic significance, and this has resulted in placing patients with this finding into an advanced stage group (IIIB). It is therefore essential that the urinary tract be evaluated preoperatively in all women with cervical cancer. This may require an IVU although abdominal ultrasound or computerized tomographic scanning may also be used as alternatives.

Carcinoma of the cervix involving the bladder is uncommon and places the patient in the stage IV group of the disease. The presence of bullous edema or a growth bulging into the bladder does not allow allocation of a case to stage IV unless bladder invasion is proved by histological examination of a biopsy. The vast majority of these patients are incurable as they already have distant metastases, but even in those patients considered for treatment the overall 5-year survival rate is only about 11%.[9]

In patients who are allocated to the stage IV group because of bladder invasion alone, the 5-year survival rate following treatment with anterior pelvic exenteration and/or radiotherapy is about 30%. However, this group represents less than 2% of all stage IV carcinomas of the cervix.[9]

Recurrent cervical carcinoma

The diagnosis of recurrent cervical carcinoma is often difficult and may be made on IVU which shows lower urinary tract involvement. The reason for this is that following treatment it may be difficult to distinguish between recurrent disease, radiotherapy reaction and postoperative scarring or adhesions. Unfortunately, urinary tract involvement again carries a grave prognosis. In patients with obstructive uropathy there are no survivors at 5 years compared to about 40% overall 5-year survival for recurrent disease.[10,11] Bladder involvement has also been shown to decrease the 5-year survival rate[12] and is related to the incidence of lymph node metastasis, thereby further influencing the prognosis.

Because of the signficance of urinary tract involvement, both for the treatment and subsequent prognosis of carcinoma of the cervix, routine assessment of urinary tract involvement should be carried out in all cases of invasive cervical carcinoma.

The importance of an abnormal IVU and cystoscopy have already been discussed, and these remain the standard for the assessment of urinary tract involvement. More recently, computerized axial tomography (CT) and nuclear magnetic resonance imaging techniques (NMRI) have been employed.

Computerized tomographic scanning has been quite extensively studied but unfortunately the results are not very encouraging, particularly as there is still difficulty in assessing parametrial involvement (Fig. 34.4).

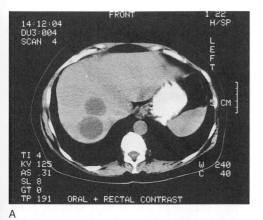

A

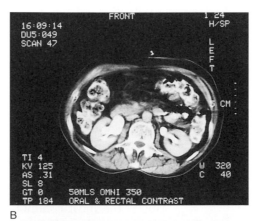

B

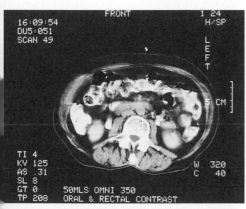

C

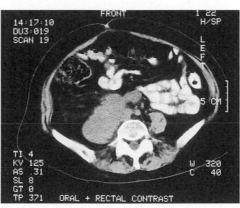

D

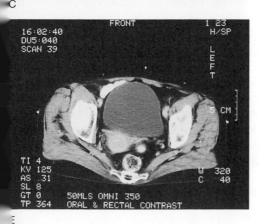

E

Fig. 34.4 Computerized axial tomography of the abdomen and pelvis in advanced cervical carcinoma (stage IV). Metastatic lymph node deposits within the liver (**A**). Right-sided hydronephrosis (**B**) and hydroureter (**C**). Grossly enlarged para-aortic lymph nodes (**D**). The cervix shows bilateral parametrial involvement (R>L) not extending to the pelvic side wall (**E**), also note the loss of a clear border between the cervix and the bladder anteriorly

However, it may demonstrate loss of the periureteral fat plane, due to parametrial involvement before hydronephrosis is present.[13] Involvement of the bladder is characterized by nodular indentations along the posterior bladder wall or intraluminal tumor mass. An earlier sign is loss of the posterior perivesical fat plane; however, it may still prove difficult to distinguish between bladder invasion and external compression.

Reports on the use of NMRI have been encouraging. They have shown that NMRI findings correlate better with the surgical pathology than either clinical evaluation or CT scanning.[14] This test has not yet been fully evaluated with respect to lower urinary tract involvement but it is to be hoped that it will yield good results in the future.

The majority of women with urinary tract involvement by cervical cancer do not have urinary symptoms. Ureteric obstruction may cause flank pain, fever or evidence of renal failure but often causes no symptoms if unilateral. If the bladder is compressed there may be symptoms of urgency and frequency and direct invasion into the bladder may cause hematuria, or in advanced disease there may be symptoms due to a urinary fistula or urethral obstruction.

Endometrial carcinoma

This is the most common malignant tumor of the female genital tract, comprising about 15% of all malignant tumors in women. It is preceded by endometrial hyperplasia in some women, and usually starts in the fundus of the uterus.

Depending on the degree of differentiation of the tumor (grades I–III), there is a greater propensity for the tumor to infiltrate the myometrium, starting at the endometrial surface and extending through the myometrium to the serosal surface and on to involve adjacent organs. Invasion is seen in approximately 5% of well-differentiated tumors (grade I), as compared to 30% of poorly differentiated tumors (grade III).

The presence of myometrial invasion is directly related to the incidence of pelvic lymph node metastases and has a negative impact on survival.[15] Another factor influencing metastatic dissemination is the stage of the tumor. The tumor may extend to the isthmus and rarely to the vagina (5%). When this occurs the tumor is usually noted in the suburethral region.

The lower urinary tract is not involved as commonly as in cervical carcinoma; this can be accounted for by the greater distance between the uterine fundus and the bladder and ureters, and is also because uterine carcinoma does not extend beyond the confines of the uterus as rapidly as does a cervical lesion. Carcinoma involving the isthmus of the uterus may spread laterally into the parametrium and in advanced cases as far as the pelvic side wall. When such invasion occurs the ureter may become compressed, leading to hydronephrosis. The ureter may also become compressed or displaced by metastatic inguinal or para-aortic lymph nodes.

Bladder involvement by endometrial carcinoma is rare and usually only occurs in advanced disease.

Where the tumor has spread on to the anterior vaginal wall the urethra is not uncommonly involved, leading to outflow obstruction; this is usually suspected on clinical grounds and may be confirmed by urethroscopy.

Vaginal and vulval carcinoma

Vulval carcinoma accounts for approximately 5% of all genital cancers and vaginal cancer is even rarer. In both tumors lower urinary tract involvement occurs in advanced disease. Urinary symptoms may occur, but patients will usually present prior to this with other symptoms such as a mass causing discharge or pain or bleeding.

Urinary tract complications following the treatment of gynecological cancer

Urological problems developed in 28% of women treated for carcinoma of the cervix, in a retrospective study of 1161 cases of carcinoma of the cervix presenting to the Royal Marsden over a 20-year period. Of these 7% had major complications, of which 43% had no evidence of active disease.[16] These complications result from surgery and radiotherapy either alone or used in combination or from recurrent disease.

Surgery

Surgery for early-stage carcinoma of the cervix has a 5-year cure rate of over 85% in selected populations, the mainstay of surgical management being the Wertheim's hysterectomy.[17]

Ureterovaginal and vesicovaginal fistulae have, in the past,[18] been the most important urological complications of radical hysterectomy, but now that their postoperative incidence has been reduced to less than 1% in most centers[19,20] they have been superseded in importance by disorders of micturition.

About 50% of patients will develop some form of urinary abnormality following surgery,[21] although for most of them this presents only minor difficulties. The frequency of urinary incontinence has been found to vary between 11% and 28%,[22,23] being severe in at least 5% of patients. It is thought to occur partly due to damage of the nerve supply to the bladder and urethra. This damage may occur when the cardinal and uterosacral ligaments are divided and may relate to the radicality of the surgery performed,[23] although this has been questioned.[24] Seski & Diokno[25] suggest that postoperative edema, hematoma and scar formation may be contributing factors but that partial parasympathetic denervation leading to detrusor hypotonia together with decreased sensation are the fundamental problem. If postoperative bladder care is inadequate then asymptomatic overdistension of the bladder may occur, leading to decompensation and permanent voiding difficulties, which does not seem to be affected by radiotherapy.[21]

Appropriate postoperative bladder care will expedite the return to normal function,[26,27] and takes the form of continuous bladder drainage, preferably suprapubic, for at least 8 days postoperatively or until normal voiding function returns. If necessary this can be replaced by clean intermittent self-catheterization in the medium term until the resumption of normal voiding.

Radical vulvectomy is the primary treatment option for vulval carcinoma. Unfortunately, the tumor is often situated close to the urethra, which may need to be partially removed in order to obtain adequate excision margins. Misdirection or spraying of the urinary stream is the most common complaint and is found in 17%[28] to 65%.[29]

Genuine stress incontinence may also occur and it is thought that this is due to urethral rather than bladder compromise. Reid et al[29] in a study of 21 women, pre- and postoperatively, showed that the distal urethral pressure is reduced following surgery and that there was also a reduction in urethral length, although this was not significant.

Currently, there is a trend towards less radical vulvectomy with individualization of patient care, and it is suggested that this will lead to fewer urinary complications.[30]

Radiotherapy

Because of the anatomical position of the cervix it is inevitable that both the ureter and the bladder may be damaged by radiotherapy given for cervical or uterine malignancy. The degree of damage is dose-dependent and can thus be reduced by careful placement of the radioactive source. Symptoms are acute or chronic. Acute symptoms are usually irritative: frequency, urgency, cystitis and hematuria, whilst chronic symptoms are related to decreased bladder compliance and a decreased bladder capacity. Urinary tract infection is often concurrent in women suffering from radiation trauma. Women should therefore be screened for this and given appropriate treatment.

Unfortunately, conventional therapy in the form of anticholinergic medication is often ineffective and as a last resort a urinary diversion or augmentation cystoplasty may be required.

Urinary fistulae occur in less than 5% of women following radiotherapy and are related to tumor recurrence in 50%[31] (Fig. 34.5). Treatment is usually conservative with long-term bladder drainage and antibiotics. Some fistulae will resolve with this treatment, although primary repair or more usually urinary diversion may be required.

FIBROIDS

Fibroids are not only the most common tumor of the genital tract but are in fact the most common tumor in the human body (Fig. 34.6). They are present at necropsy in approximately 20% of all women and are more common during the reproductive years. They commonly arise from the smooth muscle of the uterus but may rarely occur anywhere within the genital tract, including the bladder.[32] Although they are known to be hormone-sensitive their exact etiology remains uncertain.

Macroscopically the appearance is of a firm, round tumor with a smooth surface situated in the uterine wall. In this position they are called intramural, although they may also be subserous, submucous or intraligamentary. Subserous fibroids may become pedunculated, and submucous fibroids polypoidal. Rarely pedunculated fibroids may become adherent to other structures, gain a second blood supply and lose their

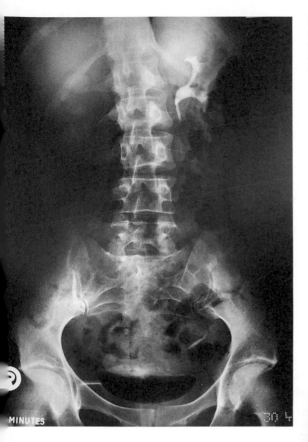

Fig. 34.5 Intravenous urography showing delayed excretion and hydronephrosis of the right kidney and the presence of air in the bladder from a rectovesical fistula, in a 43-year-old woman following treatment of stage IIB cervical carcinoma with radiotherapy

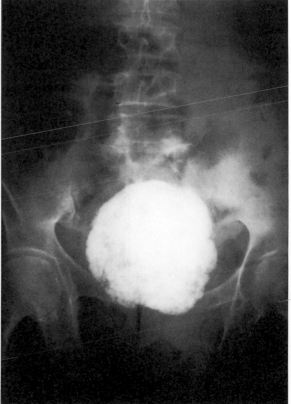

g. 34.6 Plain abdominal X-ray showing calcified uterine ɔroids

original uterine attachment and are then called 'parasitic'. When such a parasitic leiomyoma occurs in relation to the ureter then ureteral obstruction may occur.[33]

Fibroids normally have a smooth surface and are mobile, but they can become fixed in position if associated with other pelvic pathology such as pelvic inflammatory disease or endometriosis.

Enlargement of uterine fibroids within the pelvis causes compression of adjacent organs. The urinary bladder is particularly susceptible to this as it is closely approximated to the front of the uterus (Fig. 34.7). Usually this compression causes distortion of the bladder, giving rise to the symptom of urinary frequency (Fig. 34.8). Less commonly, the bladder may become lifted by low-lying fibroids and the urethra may be distorted or obstructed leading to symptoms of voiding difficulty, poor stream and incomplete emptying, or even acute urinary retention.

The incidence of urinary complications is related to the size, position and mobility of the tumor. Fibroids which are small rarely cause problems and usually present as an incidental finding; however, not all urinary symptoms are related to the size of the fibroids. Langer et al[34] showed that a 55% reduction in the size of large fibroids, induced by luteinizing hormone releasing hormone analogs, reduced the symptoms of diurnal frequency, nocturia and urinary urgency but did not affect symptoms of urge or stress incontinence. Occasionally, they become large enough to fill the whole of the abdominal cavity. Even in such cases it is unusual for the ureters to be significantly obstructed. This is because

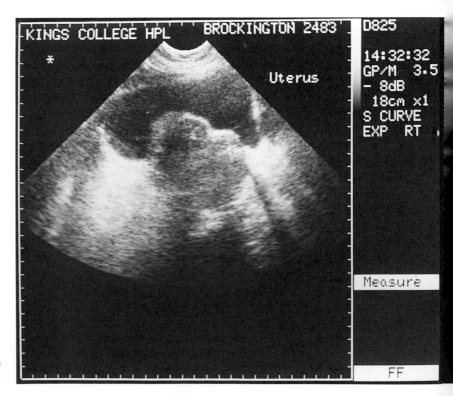

Fig. 34.7 Ultrasound scan of pelvis showing a large fibroid uterus causing compression of the urinary bladder

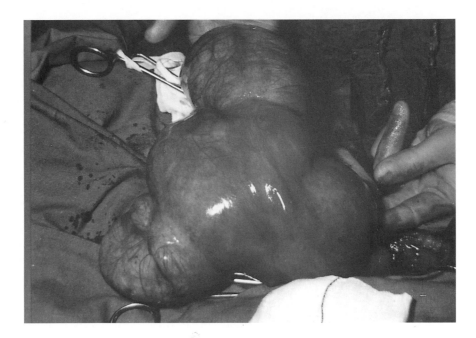

Fig. 34.8 Fibroid uterus at hysterectomy, causing symptoms of urinary frequency and urgency

fibroids are usually mobile irrespective of their size, and as they are firm they do not mold well to the shape of the pelvis. The extraperitoneal position of the ureter also protects it from external compression.

Ureteral obstruction usually occurs at the level of the pelvic brim and is more common on the right side than the left. This is thought to be because of the difference in the anatomy of the two sides, especially the protection afforded to the left ureter by the sigmoid colon.

In all reported series ureteral compression is more common in tumors large enough to be palpable above the pelvic brim.[35,36,37] In these studies some degree of ureteral obstruction, in the presence of large fibroids (above the pelvic brim), was found in between 66.6% and 72.5% of cases. More recently these figures have been disputed; Buchsbaum & Brady[38] found significant ureteral obstruction in only 9 of 598 patients with fibroids of all sizes.

The position of the fibroids is also important. Intraligamentary fibroids, situated between the leaves of the broad ligament, are relatively fixed, and because of their position, enlargement is more likely to cause ureteral displacement and obstruction.[36]

When fibroids are found in association with other pelvic pathology which causes fibrosis and adhesions, such as pelvic inflammatory disease or endometriosis, they become relatively fixed and are thus more likely to cause ureteral obstruction.[37]

The ureteral obstruction and dilatation produced by uterine fibroids does not usually lead to permanent renal damage and once the pelvic mass has been removed the radiographic changes rapidly revert to normal. Care should be taken, especially when removing intraligamentous tumors, not to damage the lower urinary tract as the course of the ureter may be greatly deviated from its normal position. A preoperative IVU is advisable in selected cases.

ADNEXAL DISEASE

Pelvic inflammatory disease

Pelvic inflammatory disease (PID) is an extremely common gynecological problem and is responsible for a large proportion of all admissions to acute gynecological wards. It is particularly common in developing countries, but its incidence in the Western world has increased dramatically over the last two decades.

The term 'pelvic inflammatory disease' is in many ways unsatisfactory, as it covers all inflammatory disorders of the genital tract irrespective of their etiology or severity.

Gonococcal infection is considered to initiate most cases of primary ascending infection,[39] and may precede infection by other oganisms. Infection starts in the lower genital tract and if untreated ascends to involve the fallopian tubes. The epithelium is damaged and cilial motility is lost leading to a build-up of inflammatory exudate (pus).

Initially, the fimbrial end of the tube remains patent and pus may enter the peritoneal cavity. Here it causes severe inflammation and becomes walled off by bowel, ovary and omentum to form a tubo-ovarian abscess. If the fimbrial end of the tube becomes sealed off, then pus accumulates within the fallopian tube to form a pyosalpinx.

During its course through the pelvis the ureter lies in contact with the peritoneum of the pouch of Douglas and then travels forwards and medially, in the loose areolar tissue of the parametrium, into the bladder. It is therefore situated in a prime site for involvement by the inflammatory process of PID. Acute inflammation of the ureter may lead to impaired peristalsis and urinary stasis;[37] this may be exacerbated by some bacterial toxins which cause paralysis and atony of the ureter. Inflammation of the ureter may resolve on antibiotic therapy or may lead to permanent stricture formation.

Pelvic abscesses are fixed to the pelvic peritoneum by adhesions caused by the acute inflammatory process, therefore one would expect ureteric obstruction to be a common sequel to an enlarging pelvic abscess. However, the incidence of this complication varies widely in the available reports. While it is widely accepted that urinary tract obstruction does not occur even in extensive pelvic infection, whereas Long & Montgomery[37] found dilatation of the upper urinary tract in 49.9%, and an abnormal delay in drainage in a further 9%, of patients with extensive PID.

Pelvic abscesses, especially those secondary to surgery or the intrauterine contraceptive device, may rarely drain into the bladder by the formation of a fistula. This is characterized by the passage of thick purulent material in the urine, with a simultaneous reduction in size of the pelvic mass and a reduction in the severity of symptoms.[40,41] Spontaneous closure of the fistula occurred in the 3 cases described, on appropriate antibiotic therapy, once the abscess had drained.

Ovarian neoplasia

Ovarian neoplasia exerts a very similar effect on the lower urinary tract to that of fibroids. It is rare to find direct invasion into the bladder even in advanced stages of malignant ovarian tumors (Fig. 34.9). They usually

A

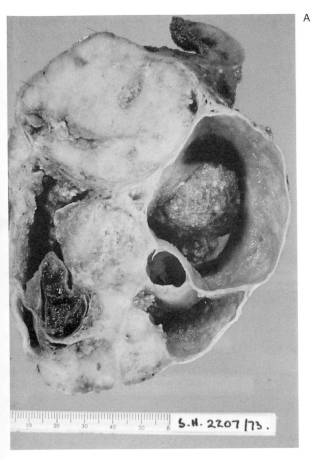

B

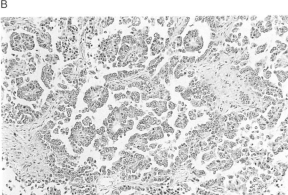

Fig. 34.9 Serous cystadenocarcinoma of the ovary. Pathological specimen removed from a 57-year-old woman who presented in acute urinary retention (**A**), and the microscopic appearance of this tumor (**B**); note the large number of mitotic figures and nuclear pleomorphism

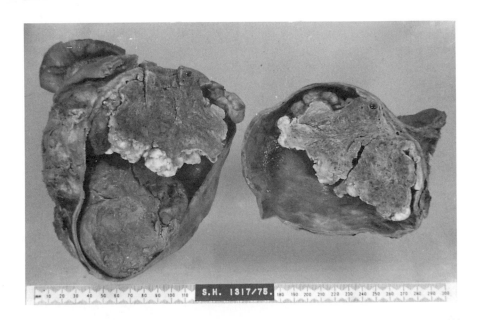

Fig. 34.10 Malignant teratoma of the ovary. This caused both symptoms of frequency and urgency and was found to be displacing the left ureter on a preoperative intravenous urogram (Fig. 34.11)

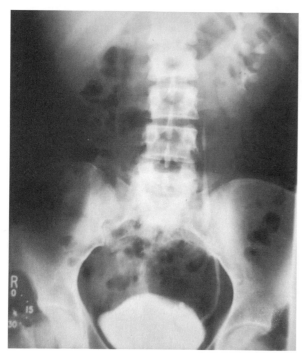

Fig. 34.11   Preoperative intravenous urogram in a woman with a malignant teratoma showing lateral displacement of the left ureter

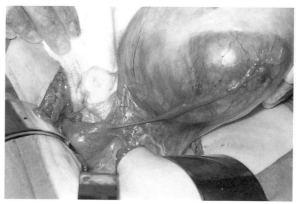

Fig. 34.12   Intraoperative picture of a large cystic ovarian neoplasm

alter lower urinary tract function by a direct pressure effect either on the bladder or the ureters (Figs. 34.10 and 11). Ureteric obstruction is more likely to occur in ovarian tumors because they tend to be cystic and mould to the contours of the pelvis more readily than do leiomyomata (Fig. 34.12). The incidence of ureteric obstruction by large ovarian neoplasms has been reported at between 40% and 81.8%.[35] It has been found to be slightly more common in malignant (69.2%) than benign (57.8%) tumors.

The site of ureteric obstruction is probably related to the size, consistency and shape of the tumor and usually occurs at the pelvic brim, on the side from which the tumor originates.[37] Malignant ovarian tumors may, by metastasis to regional lymph nodes, lead to further displacement and obstruction of the ureters. This is particularly likely to occur when the common iliac lymph nodes become enlarged. After removal of the neoplasm ureteric function, as observed by radiological studies, rapidly returns to normal in most cases.[42]

Paraovarian cysts

These are cystic dilatations of the vestigial remnants of the wolffian duct and occur between the fallopian tube and the ovary. Their effect on the lower urinary tract is similar to that of ovarian cysts. Because of their position in relation to the distal ureter they may cause ureteric obstruction and a hydroureter but usually only when they become very large.

Ovarian remnant syndrome

The ovarian remnant syndrome is the condition in which remnants of ovarian cortex, left in situ after surgical removal of the ovaries, become functional and/or cystic, giving rise to pain with or without a pelvic mass.

It occurs following 'difficult' oophorectomy in conditions such as endometriosis and PID, when the ovary is embedded in dense adhesions.[43] The presenting symptoms are persistent pelvic pain and pressure, as well as deep dyspareunia. The diagnosis is confirmed by surgery and pathological studies which demonstrate the presence of ovarian tissue where there should be none.

The ovarian remnant is usually a complex of corpus luteum cysts and dense fibrous tissue. It is situated on the lateral pelvic side wall and may obstruct the ureter at this site. Several reports of this condition involving the ureter have been published.[44,45,46,47] Treatment consists of surgical removal of the ovarian remnant and surrounding fibrous tissue. In order to avoid surgical trauma to the ureter during the procedure it must be identified and mobilized. This is best performed by the placement of an indwelling retrograde ureteral catheter prior to the operation.[48]

ENDOMETRIOSIS

Endometriosis is an extremely common gynecological disease, most often seen in the late reproductive years in nulliparous women of high social class. In this condition tissue similar to normal endometrium is found in sites other than the lining of the uterine cavity (Fig. 34.13). Numerous theories have been suggested to account for this phenomenon and it seems that no one theory will explain all forms of the disease. The three most commonly accepted are: the theory of implantation via retro-

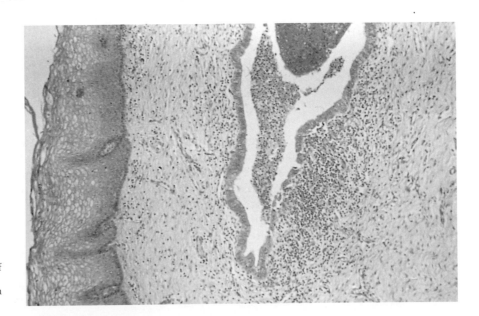

Fig. 34.13 Endometriosis of the cervix showing both endometrial-type epithelium and stroma

grade menstruation, the coelomic metaplasia theory and the lymphatic and vascular dissemination theory.

The true incidence of urinary complications with endometriosis is not known as not all sufferers are fully urologically investigated, but a study of 720 patients by Ball & Platt[49] found that 34 had major urological complications. These findings and those of other authors[50] would suggest that it is important to consider urinary tract involvement in all cases of severe endometriosis.

It most commonly involves the urinary bladder, followed by the ureters.[51] The urethra is very rarely involved, but occasionally a nodule may be seen at the urethral meatus which increases in size at the time of menstruation.

The bladder may be involved on its epithelial or serosal surface; commonly a serosal deposit infiltrates and involves the full thickness of the bladder, thus forming an endometrioma which is visible on the epithelial surface.

Urinary symptoms tend to be cyclical. Frequency, urgency, dysuria, suprapubic pain or 'bladder irritation' are reported in approximately 80% of patients, and hematuria in about 30%. The symptoms may be aggravated in the second half of the cycle and during menstruation.[52]

The severity of the symptoms is related more to the size of the lesion, which may exceed 8 cm, than to its location. A lesion near the relatively fixed trigone is not disturbed much by bladder filling and emptying, and therefore produces less pain than a lesion in the relatively mobile fundus.

In about half the cases a bladder mass can be palpated, but it is unusual for the bladder to be the only site of endometriosis and bimanual examination may reveal a retroverted uterus fixed in the pouch of Douglas, involvement of the uterosacral ligaments and cysts on the ovaries adherent to the broad ligament or pelvic side wall.[53]

If endometriosis of the bladder is suspected then a cystoscopic examination is mandatory. The findings vary with the size and location of the lesion: a subepithelial lesion may only be seen as bullous edema, whereas an epithelial lesion will be seen as a bluish nodule, if the epithelium is intact, or as an ulcer if it is breached. The ectopic endometrium causes an inflammatory reaction in the surrounding tissue, marked by reddening, congestion and edema.[49] A biopsy should be taken under direct vision to differentiate the lesion from a primary neoplasm or metastatic disease in the bladder from other pelvic organs.

The management may be conservative or surgical, depending on such factors as the severity of the disease, age or the desire for future pregnancies. Surgical therapy still seems to offer the best results[54] and involves excision of the endometrioma (partial cystectomy) combined with a total abdominal hysterectomy and bilateral salpingo-oophorectomy. If the patient wishes to have more children a more conservative approach is indicated. Nehzat & Nehzat[55] report the use of laparoscopic segmental bladder resection rather than open surgery, whilst various non-surgical treatments such as continuous progestogens, the combined oral contraceptive pill, danazol and ablation of the ovaries by irradiation have been tried with some degree of success.[49,56]

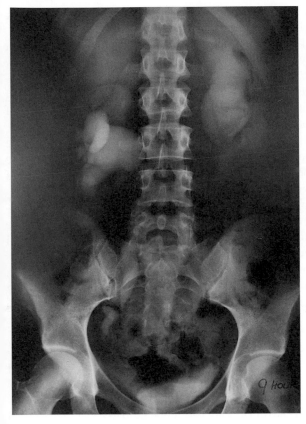
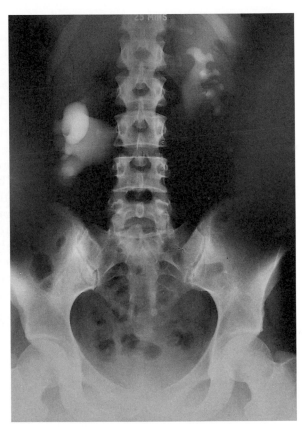

A   B

Fig. 34.14 Intravenous urogram (IVU) in a 31-year-woman with a 7-year history of endometriosis previously treated by a total abdominal hysterectomy and bilateral salpingo-oophorectomy. The IVU (**A**) shows gross bilateral hydronephrosis and hydroureter with obstruction of both lower ureters. At surgery both ureters were mobilized and the left ureter reimplanted into the bladder. A repeat IVU (**B**) 1 month later shows great improvement on the left but none of the right, which was subsequently also reimplanted into the bladder

Ureteral involvement by endometriosis is a well-known but very uncommon finding, to date approximately 100 cases having been reported in the literature. Endometriosis involving the ureter is not a completely benign condition: about 25% of kidneys are lost when endometriosis obstructs the ureter.[50,54,57] Obstruction may occur when there is extensive endometriosis (Fig. 34.14A), but can also complicate relatively minimal disease particularly when it involves the uterosacral ligaments.[54]

The ureter may be involved in two ways, extrinsic or intrinsic. In extrinsic involvement the ureter becomes compressed by endometriosis originating at another site, e.g. the broad ligament or ovary. Intrinsic involvement implies that there is endometriosis within the ureteral wall itself, usually in the muscularis, causing significant narrowing of the lumen. This is much rarer than extrinsic involvement.

Urinary symptoms are caused either by hemorrhage or ureteric obstruction, which leads to hydroureter, hydronephrosis and in time obstructive nephropathy. In most instances ureteral obstruction occurs insidiously with few symptoms and may progress relatively asymptomatically to cause renal failure.[58] Symptoms such as loin pain, oliguria and hematuria may be cyclical or may mimic ureterolithiasis,[59] especially when they are caused by an endometriotic ureteral nodule. More commonly, however, the symptoms are caused by ureteral compression or stricture, and are steadily progressive mimicking urological problems following obstructive disease from other causes.

As with the bladder, it is uncommon for the ureter alone to be involved by endometriosis, although this has been reported,[60] and therefore clinical examination will usually reveal the cause of the obstruction.

Cystoscopy is normally unrewarding, although bleeding from the terminal ureter may be seen if performed during menstruation. The passage of ureteral catheters is not particularly helpful when performed as a single examination, but if performed at different times during the menstrual cycle may reveal varying degrees of obstruction. Intravenous urography, too, may show obstruction of the ureter but again may have to be performed at different times in the cycle if the obstruction is partial.

The investigations above are often unrewarding and it may be impossible to differentiate between endometriosis and other lesions giving rise to ureteric obstruction, such as gynecological or retroperitoneal malignancy, inflammatory stricture of PID; even at laparotomy frozen section may be required in order to make the correct diagnosis.

Extrinsic endometriosis involving the ureter is managed by surgical removal of the endometriosis, thereby releasing the ureter from the constricting mass (Fig. 34.14). A portion of the ureter only will need to be removed if there is intrinsic involvement of the ureteric wall by an endometrioma. More radical surgery for the endometriosis, particularly bilateral salpingo-oophorectomy seems to improve the long-term prognosis.[50,61]

Conservative measures are the same as for bladder endometriosis and when used as a first-line treatment may relieve ureteric obstruction, as long as this is not caused by a secondary inflammatory stricture.[56] They should be considered in all cases following surgical treatment.

'SIMPLE HYSTERECTOMY'

Hanley[62] in an anecdotal report suggested an association between urinary symptoms and total hysterectomy. In his report of many years of clinical experience he comments that they are more common following total rather than subtotal hysterectomy, though he freely admits that this feeling is not based on any prospective, comparative or controlled study. In addition, no attempt was made to obtain a record of preoperative urinary symptoms in women undergoing hysterectomy, nor did he give any analysis of the indications for the operation. Nevertheless, it has been widely accepted that hysterectomy may cause debilitating bladder symptoms.

However, a large proportion of hysterectomies are performed in perimenopausal women in whom there is a high prevalence of lower urinary tract dysfunction. Thus a number of prospective studies have been performed in which pre and postoperative urinary symptoms have been evaluated. Jequier[63] studied urinary symptoms preoperatively and at 6 weeks and 6 months postoperatively in 104 women undergoing total abdominal hysterectomy. She found that 62% were symptomatic preoperatively and 50% postoperatively, with frequency and urgency of micturition being the commonest symptoms.

More recently studies have been performed comparing pre and postoperative urodynamic data and urinary symptoms. Parys et al[64] in a study of 42 women found a significant increase in urinary symptoms after hysterectomy and a new urodynamic abnormality in 14 women. Genuine stress incontinence was found in 5, detrusor instability in 2 and urethral obstruction in 3. In addition, they found a significant increase in sacral reflex latencies postoperatively, suggesting a possible neurological cause for these.

Griffith-Jones et al,[65] however, failed to show any increase in urinary symptoms after hysterectomy. In an elegant study they compared urinary symptoms before and after hysterectomy with symptoms prior to and following dilatation and curettage. No urinary symptom was found more commonly after hysterectomy than after curettage.

In summary, urinary symptoms are often reported as having occurred since hysterectomy but in many instances the symptoms predate the operation. It is true, however, that some women may develop problems de novo. There is no evidence to suggest that subtotal hysterectomy should be performed in preference to total hysterectomy, but as surgeons gynecologists must be wary of the possibility of causing urinary symptoms and exercise caution in their bladder dissection.

Trauma to the bladder or ureters may also occur during bladder dissection, securing of the uterine pedicles and uterosacral ligaments and vaginal cuff closure. It is not the remit of this chapter to discuss this in detail, although there has recently been renewed interest in this complication, particularly as it appears to occur relatively commonly during the 'learning curve' associated with minimal access surgery and laparoscopically assisted vaginal hysterectomy.[66]

CONCLUSIONS

Gynecological pathology is common, and for the most part benign disorders are easy to treat without producing significant morbidity. However, it is often stated that gynecologists are not sufficiently aware of the possibility of damage to the lower urinary tract, especially during surgery for endometriosis or cervical cancer and more recently during minimal access surgery.

Similarly, urologists who are used to dealing with urinary tract disease may not always consider the possibility of underlying gynecological pathology. It is therefore imperative that those who operate in the pelvis and who treat women with lower urinary tract dysfunction should be familiar with both systems, and consider the problem as a whole rather than dealing with their own specialty in isolation.

The lower urinary tract may be involved by gynecological disease or may be damaged during treatment. The pelvis is therefore a multi-disciplinary area and must be considered as such during diagnosis and treatment of benign or malignant gynecological disorders.

REFERENCES

1 Henriksen E. The lymphatic spread of carcinoma of the cervix and of the body of the uterus. Am J Obstet Gynecol 1949; 58: 924–927.
2 van Nagell JR Jr, Donaldson ES, Wood EG et al. The significance of vascular invasion and lymphocytic infiltration in invasive carcinoma of the cervix. Cancer 1978: 41: 228–234.
3 van Nagell JR Jr, Donaldson ES, Gay ER. Urinary tract involvement by invasive cancer. In: Buchsbaum HJ, Schmidt (eds) Gynecologic and obstetric urology, 3rd edn. Philadelphia: WB Saunders, 1982.
4 Aldridge CW, Mason JT. Ureteral obstruction in carcinoma of the cervix. Am J Obstet Gynecol 1950: 60: 1272–1280.
5 Burns BC, Everett HS, Brack CB. Value of urologic study in the management of carcinoma of the cervix. Am J Obstet Gynecol 1960: 80: 997–1004.
6 Barber HRK, Roberts S, Brunschwig A. Prognostic significance of preoperative non-visualising kidney in patients receiving pelvic exenteration. Cancer 1963: 16: 1614–1615.
7 Kottmeier HL. Surgical and radiation treatment of carcinoma of the uterine cervix. Acta Obstet Gynecol Scand 1964: 43 (Suppl 12): 1.
8 Bosch A, Frias Z, de Valda GG. Prognostic significance of ureteral obstruction in carcinoma of the cervix uteri. Acta Radiol 1973: 12: 47–50.
9 Million RR, Rutledge F, Fletcher GH. Stage IV carcinoma of the cervix with bladder invasion. Am J Obstet Gynecol 1972: 113: 239–246.
10 Halpin TF, Frick HC III, Munell EW. Critical points of failure in the therapy of cancer of the cervix; a reappraisal. Am J Obstet Gynecol 1972: 114: 755–758.
11 Van Dyke AH, van Nagell JR Jr. The prognostic significance of ureteral obstruction in patients with recurrent carcinoma of the cervix uteri. Surg Gynecol Obstet 1975: 141: 371–373.
12 Spratt JS, Butcher HR Jr, Bricker EM. Exenterative surgery of the pelvis. Philadelphia: WB Saunders, 1973: p 49.
13 Vick CW, Walsh JW, Wheelock JB et al. CT of the normal and abnormal parametria in cervical cancer. Am J Roentg 1984: 143: 597–603.
14 Rubens D, Thornbury JR, Angel C et al. Comparison of clinical, MR, and pathological staging. Am J Roentg 1988: 150: 135–138.
15 Creasman WT, Boronow RC, Morrow CP et al. Adenocarcinoma of the endometrium: its metastatic lymph node potential. Gynecol Oncol 1976: 4: 239–243.
16 Jones CR, Woodhouse CRJ, Hendry WF. Urological problems following treatment of carcinoma of the cervix. Br J Urol 1984: 56: 609–613.
17 Wertheim E. The extended abdominal operation for carcinoma uteri. Am J Obstet Gynecol 1912: 66: 169–173.
18 Meigs JV. Radical hysterectomy with bilateral lymph node dissections. A report of 100 women operated on five or more years ago. Am J Obstet Gynecol 1957: 62: 854–858.
19 Lerner HM, Jones HW, Hill EC. Radical surgery for the treatment of early invasive cervical carcinoma (stage IB): review of 15 yrs experience. Obstet Gynecol 1980: 56: 413–418.
20 Larson DM, Malone JM, Copeland LJ et al. Ureteral assessment after radical hysterectomy. Obstet Gynecol 1987: 69: 612–614.
21 Kadar N, Saliba N, Nelson JH. The frequency, causes and prevention of severe urinary dysfunction after radical hysterectomy. Br J Obstet Gynecol 1983: 90: 858–863.
22 Lewington W. Disturbances of micturition following Wertheim hysterectomy. J Obstet Gynecol Br Emp 1956: 63: 861–864.
23 Forney JP. The effect of radical hysterectomy on bladder physiology. Am J Obstet Gynecol 1980: 138: 374–382.
24 Photopulos GJ, Vander Zwaag R. Class II hysterectomy shows less morbidity and good treatment efficacy compared to class III. Gynecol Oncol 1991: 40: 21–25.
25 Seski JC, Diokno AC. Bladder dysfunction after radical abdominal hysterectomy. Am J Obstet Gynecol 1977: 128: 643–648.
26 Green TH, Meigs JV, Ulfelder H et al. Urological complications of radical Wertheim hysterectomy: incidence, etiology, management and prevention. Obstet Gynecol 1962: 20: 293–312.

27 Glahn BE. The neurogenic factor in vesical dysfunction following radical hysterectomy for carcinoma of the cervix. Scand J Urol Nephrol 1970: 4: 107–111.

28 Culame RJ. Pelvic relaxation as a complication of the radical vulvectomy. Obstet Gynecol 1980: 55: 716–718.

29 Reid GC, DeLancy JOL, Hopkins MP et al. Urinary incontinence following radical vulvectomy. Obstet Gynecol 1990: 75: 852–854.

30 Burke TW, Stringer A, Gerhenson DM et al. Radical wide excision and selective inguinal node dissection for squamous cell carcinoma of the vulva. Gynecol Oncol 1990: 38: 328–331.

31 Cushing RM, Tovell HMM, Liegner LM. Major urological complications following radium and x-ray therapy for cervical carcinoma of the cervix. Am J Obstet Gynecol 1969: 101: 750–754.

32 Knoll LD, Segura JW, Scheithauer BW. Leiomyoma of the bladder. J Urol 1986: 136: 906–908.

33 Zaiton MM. Retroperitoneal parasitic leiomyoma causing unilateral ureteral obstruction. J Urol 1986: 135: 130–131.

34 Langer Z, Golan A, Neuman M et al. The effect of large uterine fibroids on urinary bladder function and symptoms. Am J Obstet Gynecol 1990: 163: 1139–1141.

35 Kretschmer HL, Kanter AE. The effect of certain gynecological lesions on the upper urinary tract. J Am Med Assoc 1937: 14: 1097–2003.

36 Chamberlin GW, Pain FL. Urinary tract changes with benign pelvic tumors. Radiol 1944: 42: 117–120.

37 Long JP, Montgomery JB. The incidence of ureteral obstruction in benign and malignant gynecologic lesions. Am J Obstet Gynecol 1950: 59: 552–562.

38 Buchsbaum HJ, Brady PS. Urinary tract involvement by benign and malignant gynecological disease. In: Buchsbaum HJ, Schmidt (eds) Gynecological and obstetric urology, 3rd Philadelphia: WB Saunders, pp 489–503.

39 Esenbach DA, Holmes KK. Acute pelvic inflammatory disease: current topics of pathogenesis, aetiology and management. Clin Obstet Gynecol 1975: 18: 35–36.

40 Altman LC. Ovarian abscess and vaginal fistula. Obstet Gynecol 1972: 40: 321–322.

41 London AM, Burkman RT. Tuboovarian abscess with associated rupture and fistula formation into the urinary bladder: report of two cases. Am J Obstet Gynecol 1979: 135: 1113–1134.

42 Morrison JK. The ureter and hysterectomy. Including the effects of certain gynecological conditions on the urinary tract. J Obstet Gynecol Brit Emp 1960: 67: 66–72.

43 Symmonds RE, Pettit PDM. Ovarian remnant syndrome. Obstet Gynecol 1979: 54: 174–177.

44 Kaufman JJ. Unusual causes of extrinsic ureteral obstruction, part II. J Urol 1962: 87: 328–332.

45 Horowitz MI, Elguezabal A. Obstruction of the ureter by a recent corpus luteum located in the retroperitoneum: report of two cases. J Urol 1966: 95: 706–710.

46 Major FJ. Retained ovarian remnant causing ureteral obstruction. Obstet Gynecol 1968: 32: 748–750.

47 Scully RE, Galdabini JJ, McNeely BV. Case records of the Massachusetts General Hospital. Case 48–1979. New Eng J Med 1979: 301: 1228–1232.

48 Berek JS, Darney PD, Lopkin C et al. Avoiding ureteral damage in pelvic surgery for ovarian remnant syndrome. Am J Obstet Gynecol 1979: 15: 221–222.

49 Ball TL, Platt MA. Urological complications of endometriosis. Am J Obstet Gynecol 1962: 84: 1516–1521.

50 Kerr WS. Endometriosis involving the urinary tract. Clin Obstet Gynecol 1966: 9: 331–335.

51 Abeshouse BS, Abeshouse G. Endometriosis of the urinary tract: a review of the literature. J Int Col Surg 1960: 83: 100–102.

52 Aldridge KW, Burns JR, Singh B. Vesical endometriosis: a review and two case reports. J Urol 1985: 134: 539–541.

53 Kane C, Drouin P. Am J Obstet Gynecol 1985: 151(2): 207–211.

54 Moore JG, Hibbard LT, Growden WA et al. Urinary tract endometriosis: enigmas in diagnosis and management. Am J Obstet Gynecol 1979: 134(2): 162–172.

55 Nehzat CR, Nehzat FR. Laparoscopic segmental bladder resection for endometriosis: a report of two cases. Obstet Gynecol 1993: 81: 882–884.

56 Lavelle KJ, Melman AW, Cleary RE. Ureteral obstruction owing to endometriosis: reversal with synthetic progestin. J Urol 1976: 116: 665–666.

57 Stanley KE Jr, Utz DC, Dockerty MB. Clinically significant endometriosis of the urinary tract. Surg Gynecol Obstet 1965: 120: 491–493.

58 Gourdie RW, Rogers CN. Bilateral ureteric obstruction due to endometriosis presenting

with cyclical hypertension and cyclical oliguria. Br J Urol 1986: 58: 224.

59 Traub YM, Fischelovitch J, Neri A et al. Endometriosis mimicking ureterolithiasis. Br J Urol 1976: 48: 27–30.

60 Bulkley GJ, Carrow LA, Estensen RD. Endometriosis of the ureter. J Urol 1965: 93: 139–143.

61 Langmade CF. Pelvic endometriosis and ureteral obstruction. Am J Obstet Gynecol 1975: 122(4): 463–469.

62 Hanley HG. The late urological complications of total hysterectomy. Br J Urol 1969: 41: 682–684.

63 Jequier AM. Urinary symptoms and total hysterectomy. Br J Urol 1976: 48: 437–441.

64 Parys BT, Haylen BT, Hutton JL, Parsons KF. The effects of simple hysterectomy on vesicourethral function. Br J Urol 1989: 64: 594–599.

65 Griffith-Jones MD, Jarvis GJ, McNamara HM. Adverse urinary symptoms after total abdominal hysterectomy – fact or fiction? Br J Urol 1991: 67: 295–297.

66 Kadar N, Lemmerling L. Urinary tract injuries during laparoscopically assisted hysterectomy: causes and prevention. Am J Obstet Gynecol 1994: 170: 47–48.

Section 6 Urological Aspects

35 Surgery of the female bladder (lower urinary tract)

This chapter will cover endoscopic and open surgical procedures on the female bladder. It has been written from a urological perspective and although safe practice demands some urological training, it would not be unreasonable for an experienced gynecologist to include these procedures in his or her repertoire. The only exception is the endoscopic resection of a bladder tumor, which it is reasonable to perform for a small papillary lesion but can be very difficult in those larger than 3 cm, since it may lead to a dangerous bladder perforation that potentially converts a superficial cancer into an invasive one. It is also recommended that a more detailed operative text be consulted before undertaking a cystoplasty or cystectomy and suggestions for further reading are given at the end of the chapter.

The following topics will be covered:

1. Bougies and catheters
2. Endoscopic procedures
   a. Transurethral resection
   b. Litholapaxy
3. Open procedures
   a. Cystoplasty
   b. Cystectomy.

Cystoscopy is covered in detail in Ch. 12.

URETHRAL BOUGIES/DILATORS

These instruments are made of metal or silk and are solid with no lumen. There are three types, the most common of which is the metal bougie. This is of a short, straight design when used for the female urethra. The bougie à boule has an olive-shaped tip with graduation marks at 1-cm intervals in order to measure the depth of a possible stenosis. The filiform bougie is the slimmest bougie and is semi-rigid. The tip has a screw to which special metal bougies or catheters can be attached so that gradual and contiguous dilatation can take place. This latter bougie system is particularly useful when there is only a pinhole meatus present.

Metal bougies are employed to dilate the urethra in cases of urethral stenosis (which is uncommon in women), or where the introduction of a large-caliber transurethral instrument would produce unnecessary trauma without prior dilatation. There is no place in modern urological surgery for an empirical urethral dilatation in the absence of true stenosis. This procedure used to be carried out frequently for a variety of functional bladder disorders that were rarely investigated with complete urodynamics.

There are two measurement systems to denote the sizes not only of bougies but also of catheters and endoscopes. The term 'size' refers to the outer circumference. The French system is the most commonly employed standard and is expressed as 1F, 2F etc. up to 30F or as Ch1, Ch2 etc. up to Ch30. The diameter of a circle (cross-section) approximates to the circumference divided by 3 (π) and so '1 French' represents a diameter of one-third of a millimeter and every subsequent unit represents an increment of the same value. The diameter can therefore be calculated by dividing the F value by 3 mm. It is generally possible to insert instruments up to 24F into the normal female urethra. Instruments larger than this should be inserted only after gentle and gradual dilatation to 1 or 2F larger than the instrument itself.

CATHETERS

In general, catheters are instruments with an internal lumen constructed of flexible rubber, synthetic materials, silk or metal. They are employed for a variety of purposes in the field of urology including the drainage of urine, washing the bladder and instillation of contrast medium and therapeutic agents. Various catheters have differently designed tips, apertures and methods of opening the aperture (Fig. 35.1). The most common catheters are now described.

The Nelaton catheter is a semi-rigid catheter with a rounded tip. Nelaton catheters employ the English standard in which 1 represents 1.5 mm and every subsequent unit represents increments of 0.5 mm. The aperture is located close to the tip but because there is only one aperture, it can be obstructed by compression from the mucosa. This is not self-retaining

Types of catheter

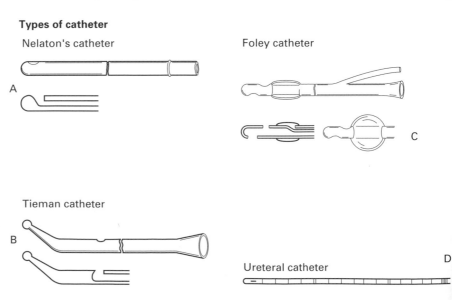

Nelaton's catheter

A

Tieman catheter

B

Foley catheter

C

Ureteral catheter

D

Fig. 35.1 Urethral catheter tips. **A** Nelaton; **B** Tieman; **C** Foley; **D** Ureteral

but is very useful for in-out catheterization. The Tieman catheter is slightly less flexible and has an angled olive-shaped tip. This is useful in male patients who have an obstructing prostate but it can also be useful in a female patient where there is a tight urethral stenosis. The balloon or Foley catheter is the most commonly used urethral catheter. There is a balloon extending for several centimeters from the tip which can be inflated by liquids or air, after insertion, to keep it in place. It is often used as an indwelling catheter. The balloons vary in volume but rarely is it necessary to inflate a balloon more than 5 ml. Any greater volume will create a sump of urine between the aperture and bladder base which negates some of the purpose of an indwelling catheter. Foley catheters are available in a wide variety of sizes (6–30F) and all are now 'siliconized'. The addition of silicone has reduced the incidence of periurethral inflammation and stricture formation and they can be left in situ safely for 3 months.

Although there are specially designed sets for suprapubic bladder catheterization, these are usually an unnecessary luxury and indeed many of these specially designed catheters are of a very small caliber and can become obstructed with blood clots or mucus. It is now possible to obtain either a disposable or non-disposable trocar and peel-away cannula introducer (Fig. 35.2) for a standard 12–16F Foley catheter that can be used suprapubically. This can be easily inserted with local anesthetic. Blind suprapubic catheterization should only be carried out when either urethral catheterization has failed or there is urethral pathology. Suprapubic catheterization can be dangerous if one does not have any information concerning the supposedly full bladder beneath. It is not unknown for a suprapubic catheter to be inserted into either dilated bowel or a bladder tumor with disastrous results. A simple ultrasound examination should ideally take place before suprapubic catheterization, or the bladder should be filled with at least 300 ml of saline via a urethral catheter.

ENDOSCOPIC PROCEDURES

Endoscope design

There can be few areas of surgery in which endoscopic techniques have made such a great impact as urology. In the early days of surgery, open operations on the bladder were frequently complicated by sepsis and urinary fistulae, whether performed via a transabdominal or transperineal approach.

Just over 100 years ago, bladder calculi were common in Western Europe and often treated by a transperineal lithotomy, a procedure which was performed rapidly (within 2 min) but was associated with an average hospital stay of 30 days and a 30% mortality. The greatest single advance which changed this type of surgery was the introduction of a transurethral lithotrite and subsequently an endoscopic version. The in-patient stay dropped to 10 days and the mortality to 2%. This was the impetus behind the creation of St Peter's Hospital for 'stone', which has gone on to become one of the greatest urological institutions in the

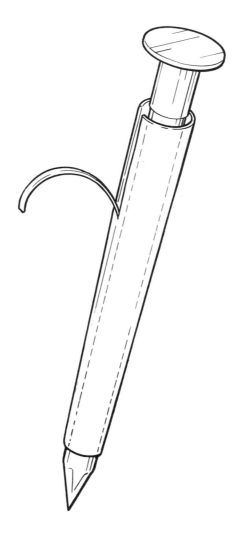

Fig. 35.2 A 'peel away' trocar and cannula allows easy access for a suprapubic standard 2-way Foley catheter

world. Although crude tube-like instruments were used many centuries ago, the first modern cystoscope was made by Nietze in 1879. This instrument had distal illumination by a platinum wire, a lens system and an instrument channel. It was improved further with the invention of the Edison bulb in 1891, which replaced the rather cumbersome platinum wire light source. Although many changes took place during the nineteenth century, the next major milestones occurred in the 1950s. These were the introduction, by Hopkins, of a rod-lens system which improved the view enormously and also the introduction of fiber optics by the same eminent scientist. The efficient light-transmitting fiber optics enabled the introduction of better light source leads and then, when more refined, to their visual use in a fiber optic flexible telescope.

Transurethral resection

The resectoscope mechanism within a sheath, usually 2–3F larger than a cystoscope, is a routine instrument employed by the urologist to remove prostatic tissue. The same instrument is used to remove superficial bladder tumors, and more recently endometrium. It requires a safe technique that comes only with great experience so only small fingernail-sized bladder lesions should be tackled by the inexperienced resectionist. In the case of the large tumor, it is preferable to take biopsies of the tumor and tumor base and a random mucosal biopsy and leave the definitive therapy to someone more experienced.

The aim of resecting a small lesion, which in Western Europe is usually a papillary transitional cell carcinoma (95%; 4% are squamous cell tumors and 1% are adenocarcinomas), is to remove the lesion together with the underlying muscle layer. This ensures not only complete removal but also histological assessment of invasion. A post-resection bimanual examination should then reveal no palpable residual lesion. Even small, well-differentiated tumors can recur and the patient should be referred postoperatively to a urologist for follow-up. Recurrences can occur up to 20 years later and progress to invasive disease in 5%. Follow-up will be tailored to the size, histological grade, multiplicity, time to first recurrence and dysplasia.

Transurethral litholopaxy

This is one of the earliest minimally invasive urological techniques but is more safely achieved when carried out with an optical lithotrite. Bladder stones are much less common in Western Europe now than they were in the nineteenth century, and are usually only seen in neuropathic bladders or after long-term catheterization. The optical lithotrite is easy to use but remember to lift the grasped stone clear of the bladder mucosae to avoid damage to an already edematous and inflamed bladder wall.

The fragments are washed out through the sheath. The presence of stones and their subsequent crushing prevent ideal inspection of the whole bladder mucosae. A second look, say flexible cystoscopy, will be required at least 2 weeks later in order to exclude any mucosal lesion. Squamous metaplasia and sometimes frank carcinoma are associated with the presence of stones.

OPEN PROCEDURES

Cystoplasty

This term covers a variety of procedures ranging from a simple transection to a complete substitution. Interestingly, until only recently a subtotal augmentation was thought to be the most radical that one could do in a female. However, recent communications from the United States and France suggest that a complete substitution can be anastomosed on to a neurologically intact female urethra with excellent functional continence. Many urologists working in this field await the follow-up of a published series.

A transection cystoplasty is a procedure used to treat the unstable bladder when all more conservative options have failed or cannot be tolerated. It can be regarded as a less invasive alternative to an augmentation cystoplasty when there is no need to increase bladder capacity. It has been attempted both transurethrally and laparoscopically with varying degrees of success (personal communication).

An open surgical simple bladder transection should be approached extraperitoneally via a Pfannenstiel incision. The transection can be effected in a longitudinal, transverse or complete horizontal direction. After complete division of the serosa and mucosa, the wall is sutured back together again with a single layer of 2-0 Vicryl or PDS. (One observation for the successful trend in bladder reconstruction is that single continuous lines of the newer absorbable sutures are quite safe in bladder surgery if protected by a catheter). One advantage of the longitudinal incision is that no lateral dissection and division of the superior vesicle pedicles is required. A urethral catheter is left to drain the bladder for 7 days.

The varying results of this procedure reflect our ignorance of the exact pathophysiology of each individual patient with recalcitrant instability and therefore a sometimes poor selection of patients. The purpose of this procedure is often described as an interruption of surrounding autonomic nerve fibers but this has never been convincingly shown histologically and the most likely mechanism of action is to produce a disruption of smooth muscle syncytial conductivity and strength of contractions. It does work spectacularly well sometimes.

The 'clam' cystoplasty is the most commonly performed augmentation cystoplasty in Great Britain. It was first described by Bramble[1] and is a relatively simple technique using detubularized ileum that produces lower compliance than when the cecum or tubularized large bowel is utilized. It is indicated for bladder instability again when conservative management fails. Those sceptical of a simple bladder transection will go immediately to this operation but such an augmentation cystoplasty is associated with a greater morbidity because of the need for bowel reconstruction. The name 'clam' has been given because the bladder is opened transversely like a clam and a pedicled segment of detubularized small bowel is interposed. The twofold objective is both to interrupt contractile pathways and to increase bladder capacity, so increasing compliance. Follow-up urodynamics often shows that unstable contractions do still occur in the filling phase but these do not usually reach significant levels to produce incontinence and also minimize clinical urgency. Unfortunately, because this is also an empirical operation, detrusor activity can be overcompensated and hypotonia during voiding occurs. Approximately 10% of patients will need to intermittently self-catheterize (ISC).[2] However, if the operation was being performed for intractable urge incontinence, then an informed patient will still be pleased with the postoperative result if she is continent, even if ISC is now necessary.

Such a clam cystoplasty is sometimes required in combination with bladder neck surgery when two discrete functional abnormalities coexist. In these cases it is even more difficult to produce a functional voider, but again the main objective is to produce a 'dry' patient and the procedure is done in recognition of the fact that detrusor hyperreflexia or instability gets worse when urethral resistance is increased.

The use of only a small portion of bowel in the urinary tract rarely produces any metabolic disturbances but many patients experience increased mucus production for up to 6 months and there is a very small but definite risk of malignant change over 15–20 years. It is not clear how to follow these patients up but a 2-yearly flexible cystoscopy would be a reasonable suggestion with biopsy of any visible abnormalities at the previous vesicointerstitial junction. This operation is not uncommonly performed on young women and there has always been a concern that pregnancy would produce anatomical problems. This has not been borne out and, in fact, an elective Caesarean section is also quite safe but the surgeon should leave no room for error in his incision.

Cystectomy

This is commonly performed for malignant disease as part of an anterior pelvic exenteration in combination with a radical hysterectomy. The author has seen this performed by a combination of laparoscopic and open vaginal dissection but this technique will require further evaluation before becoming accepted. At present, the safest method is an open technique through a lower midline incision. The midline incision usually facilitates access to bowel mesentery for a subsequent urinary diversion of some sort (see Ch. 36).

Once again the reader is directed to fuller surgical texts, but there is a fundamental technical step that the author suggests is a great aid to a successful cystectomy. This is to begin with an iliac and obturator lymphadenectomy. It is an infrequently practised step in the UK but almost mandatory in the United States and Germany.

Although the majority of oncological surgeons recognize that a lymphadenectomy has no therapeutic value, it is of prognostic significance such that frozen sections may be positive in up to 20% of patients and bring into question subsequent, more complex reconstructive urinary diversions. The patient with only a 6 to 12-month prognosis may not wish for a 25% chance of revision if something like a Mitrofanoff or Kock diversion procedure is carried out.

However, the practical value of a lymphadenectomy, irrespective of what diversion is chosen, is that the surgeon is forced clearly to dissect out the branches of the internal iliac artery. The subsequent cystectomy and hysterectomy can be completed.

The last section refers to the vaginal reconstruction following a cystectomy. An anterior section of vagina should be taken with the bladder. Obviously, the vagina should not then be simply approximated but care must be taken into bringing the distal flap downwards to provide adequate width with an acceptable loss of length. The flap must be brought all the way down to the defect created by excision of the urethra or else a proximal vaginal stricture will occur.

IATROGENIC INJURIES

The majority of injuries to the bladder and ureter can now be managed by a minimally invasive method. In general, any reparation of the urinary tract will heal if urine is diverted away. Large tears of small structures, i.e. ureter or urethra, will also require stenting, which allows re-epithelialization to occur around a predetermined shape, a process that has been shown to take 4–6 weeks. Catheters are rarely left in for this length of time because the need for perfect epithelial healing must be balanced against the dangers of retrograde infections. All bladders being drained by a urethral catheter, even in a closed system, will reveal a bacteriuria within 10–14 days. This is why one usually ignores a positive culture in a catheterized patient unless the patient has a pyrexia or is immunosuppressed.

Bladder perforation

These can be caused during either open or endoscopic surgery. Open repair at the time of operation can accelerate healing but all perforations will heal with a draining catheter eventually. A reasonable working policy would therefore be to repair bladder perforations caused by open surgery and noticed during that surgery but to manage everything else with a simple catheter. Repaired bladders should be drained for 5 days and conservatively treated bladders drained for 10–14 days. Rarely this conservative policy fails and it is because the catheter is not adequately draining the bladder and is actually stenting open the perforation. The patient will probably have an ileus from peritoneal absorption of urine which will produce a classic hyperchloremic acidosis – the serum urea will also be elevated in the presence of a near normal serum creatinine.

Ureteric obstruction

I will mention ureteric obstruction at this juncture because of its occurrence post-hysterectomy. It is suspected from the clinical picture and an intravenous urogram that shows delayed or absent nephrograms and is confirmed by ultrasound. It requires a cystoscopy and retrograde ureterogram to confirm it. The same open-ended 6 or 7F catheter should be used as mentioned above. Olive-tipped catheters are not used now because the larger, soft-nosed, open-tipped catheters (borrowed from the interventional radiologists) can not only produce a good ureterogram but allow passage of a guide wire through them and often up to the kidney. The majority of post-hysterectomy 'cut' or 'ligated' lower ureters are in reality only partially damaged or obstructed and can be managed with a ureteric stent for 6 weeks. This conservative approach produces excellent results and an open reimplantation of the ureter is only indicated in 20% of cases now.

REFERENCES

1 Bramble FJ. The clam cystoplasty. B J Urol 1990; 66: 337–341.
2 Mundy AR, Stephenson TP. Clam ileocystoplasty for the treatment of refractory urge incontinence. B J Urol 1985; 57: 641–646.

FURTHER READING

Rob and Smith's operative surgery (Genitourinary surgery – ed HN Whitfield) 5th edn, Butterworth-Heinemann 1993.

Urinary diversion in the female patient

INTRODUCTION

This simple form of diversion must never be underestimated in terms of its impact in our clinical practice. A 6 or 7 F nephrostomy tube can easily be inserted under ultrasound or X-ray control, producing an immediate effect whilst definitive reconstruction is planned. This chapter will concentrate on those permanent forms of urinary diversion that are utilized in the female patient and the surgical principles involved. The technique of an ileal conduit will be described in detail but the reader who wishes to perform the other procedures described is also encouraged to read a urological atlas of surgery. In the cancer patient, they will be associated with a cystectomy or anterior exenteration. In benign conditions, associated removal of the bladder is not always required but the functionless bladder that is left may produce a pyocystis. This latter problem can be countered by either an initial vesicovaginal fistula (Spence procedure) or a secondary cystectomy. Many of these forms of permanent urinary diversion require a working knowledge of the principles and techniques of bowel surgery and these will be outlined before specific diversion procedures are illustrated. A variety of conditions can lead to an acute obstructive uropathy and the simplest diversion, albeit only temporary, that leads to a restoration of normal renal function is the percutaneous nephrostomy tube insertion.

A distinction also needs to be made between those diversion procedures requiring an external appliance (incontinent) and various continent urinary diversion procedures that have been refined and are now in widespread use. In general terms, a continent type of diversion is a more complicated and extensive procedure, with a significant revision rate in the order of 25%, but the benefits are outstanding. This must be contrasted with the simple incontinent type of diversion such as the ileal conduit, which is relatively straightforward and rarely requires revision. The younger patient with a good prognosis is the best patient for whom to recommend a continent diversion but this is only a general consideration and all options should be discussed with the patient prior to choosing a specific procedure.

A second important practical concept is that the choice of procedure must sometimes be changed during an operation. Any surgeon contemplating urinary diversion should be able to perform a variety of procedures depending on the findings at operation, regardless of what the original plan had been. The safest and simplest fall-back position is usually to select an ileal conduit but one's working knowledge of other procedures and, in particular, the general principles that govern one's choice may provide alternative options that do not require an external collecting appliance if the patient prefers to avoid one.

HISTORY

For the large part of the twentieth century most urinary diversions were performed into the intact intestinal tract because external collecting devices were imperfect and implantations to the skin were felt to place a great burden of care and discomfort on the patient because of incontinence. Thus continent urinary diversion into the intact fecal stream was the standard of the day. Some surgeons advocated in addition either complete or partial diversion of the fecal stream so as to diminish ascending infection. Continent urinary diversion was first reported by Simon.[1] He operated on a patient with bladder exstrophy and performed a ureterorectal anastomosis. However, the earliest attempt to fashion an artificial bladder from bowel was made in a dog by Tizzoni.[2] He created an isolated closed loop of intact ileum and re-established bowel continuity. One month later, he anastomosed ureters into the blind ileal loop and sutured the loop into the bladder neck. The dog survived.

The first clinical use of the small intestine to fashion a continent urinary reservoir was performed by Cuneo in 1911. The high operative mortality (approximately 50%) experienced with this procedure and modifications made over the next 10–20 years led to the temporary abandonment of attempts to create a continent urinary reservoir or conduit separate from the fecal stream. The concept behind all of these procedures was that continence depended upon a functional anal sphincter. Goldenberg[3] employed an ileal segment which was reimplanted into the cecum in an antiperistaltic fashion. The trigone was anastomosed to the distal end. Berg[4] isolated a segment of ileum and anastomosed Roux-en-Y to the rectum. The trigone was anastomosed to the transposed ileal segment at a second procedure. Intervening intestinal segments anastomosed to the fecal stream also resulted in a high operative mortality (approximately 40%).

Thus, in the preantibiotic era, intestinal surgery to reconstruct the urinary tract was extremely hazardous. In an attempt to minimize the mortality and complication rates, procedures were developed to anastomose the ureter directly to the intact colon.

Numerous methods of ureteral implantation were described in the late nineteenth and early twentieth centuries. Many of these procedures which were described as new represented subtle permutations of existing concepts. In general, these various procedures were designed to decrease the risk of peritonitis. Bacterial peritonitis in the preantibiotic era was associated with a high mortality rate and, when accompanied by failed surgical anastomosis, was almost universally fatal. Hinman[5] recognized and described 11 unique surgical principles which evolved into the concept of the perfect ureterointestinal anastomosis. Some of these principles have since been discarded but many form the backbone of the procedures that we perform today.

The introduction of effective antibiotic therapy after World War II resulted in a significant decrease in postoperative mortality. The combination of improved patient survival of major surgery such as a cystectomy and the lack of socially and medically accepted forms of urinary diversion was responsible for the wave of enthusiasm that greeted Bricker's[6] report on his technique for an ileal conduit.

It was in fact Seiffert[7] who reported the construction of an ileal conduit 15 years earlier, but his name is rarely remembered because he lacked an effective means of collecting and storing urine. Bricker utilized Rutzen's bag, which was attached to the anterior abdominal wall with adhesive. It was this breakthrough that facilitated the socially acceptable (in the West) non-fecal urinary diversion. The ease of construction and the low incidence of complications led to the Bricker ileal conduit becoming the urinary diversion of choice.

A growing number of urological surgeons over the last 20 years have not been satisfied with a simple ileal conduit diversion. It is becoming apparent that the lack of any anti-reflux procedure to protect the upper tracts leads ultimately to upper tract dilatation and renal impairment.

This is not in itself a reason to abandon such a reliable technique because the effect may not be seen until 20–25 years postoperatively. But the accumulative response has been to revisit the various types of continent diversion and these have been modified and refined in such a way that they have had an enormous clinical impact. A successful continent diversion leaves the patient with a positive self-image and has been greeted universally by our younger and, in particular, female patients.

GENERAL PRINCIPLES

Bowel preparation

Urological operations in which the bowel is utilized for reconstruction are usually elective and bowel preparation is therefore appropriate. Although the bacterial population in the stomach is relatively low, the remainder of the bowel including jejunum and ileum have high bacterial population counts and therefore require both mechanical and antibiotic preparation. Patients who have intestinal procedures on unprepared bowels have an increased wound infection rate and a higher instance of intraperitoneal abscess formation and anastomotic dehiscence rate when compared with patients who have had a proper bowel preparation prior to surgery. Complications that occur as a result of bacterial contamination are a major cause of morbidity and mortality. The mechanical preparation reduces the amount of feces whereas the antibiotic preparation reduces the bacterial count. Bacterial flora in the bowel consists of aerobic and anaerobic organisms. The bacterial concentration in the jejunum ranges from 10^0 to 10^5, in the distal ileum from 10^5 to 10^7, in the ascending colon from 10^6 to 10^8 and in the descending colon from 10^{10} to 10^{12} organisms per gram of fecal content.

Mechanical bowel preparation

Mechanical bowel preparation reduces the total number of bacteria but not their concentration. The spilling of enteric contents during a procedure is less likely following mechanical preparation of the bowel because there is literally less of it to spill. However, once spilled, the concentration of the inoculum is the same as if the bowel had not been prepared. Conventional bowel preparations often exhaust the patient and are unnecessary. Whole gut irrigation has been found to be no more effective in reducing wound infections and septic complications than conventional preparations. The days of placing a nasogastric tube and infusing 9–12 l of lactated Ringer's solution over a several-hour period are, fortunately for our patients, only of historical interest. A polyethylene glycol electrolyte lavage solution has been shown to be just as effective in preparing the gut for both elective colon and rectal surgery as well as urological surgery in which bowel is utilized. If this is taken by mouth, it is better tolerated if the solution is chilled and the addition of orange juice also makes it a little more palatable. The rectal effluent must be clear and free of particulate matter irrespective what method of mechanical bowel preparation is used, and this is often overlooked if a nurse does not pay particular attention.

Antibiotic bowel preparation

Many surgeons do not now use preoperative oral antibiotic regimens to sterilize the bowel. The marginal improvement in the septic complication rate has to be balanced by the increase in incidence of diarrhea and more rarely pseudonembranous enterocolitis. It is now routine practice to give intravenous antibiotics at the time of induction that cover both aerobes and anaerobes. It remains controversial how long these antibiotics should be continued but the consensus of opinion is to stop after 3 days unless there are any septic complications, by which time specific cultures and sensitivities should be known.

Abdominal pain and diarrhea in the absence of a fever constitute a relatively benign complication of antibiotic overusage which disappears if the antibiotic is stopped. However, there is rarely the danger of overgrowth of *Clostridium difficile* which can produce the potentially dangerous pseudomembranous enterocolitis. Antibiotics can destroy the bacteria that inhibit the growth of *Clostridium difficile* and thereby allow it to flourish. Its growth is associated with the liberation of toxins that produce a diffuse inflammatory response and causes profuse diarrhea. The diagnosis is suggested by the symptomatology and endoscopic findings and is confirmed by the culture of the organism. Since culture takes a prolonged period of time, it is important to identify the toxin through tissue culture techniques. Once it has been diagnosed, the treatment involves the administration of vancomycin and the discontinuation of other antibiotics which the patient is receiving. Rarely, this treatment fails or is given too late and a toxic megacolon occurs that requires a subtotal colectomy as a life-saving procedure. Fortunately, this is very rare.

Intestinal anastomoses

Principles

Irrespective of the type of anastomosis or the methods utilized to perform it, certain fundamental principles must be observed in order to minimize morbidity and mortality from intestinal surgery. Complications in the immediate postoperative period may be related either to the enteroenterostomy or to the segment interposed in the urinary tract. The following principles should be firmly ingrained in the surgeon undertaking the diversion:

1. Ensure adequate exposure.
2. Maintain a good blood supply to the severed ends of the bowel.
3. Prevent local spillage of enteric contents.
4. Maintain an accurate apposition of the serosa to serosa of the two segments of bowel to be anastomosed.
5. Do not tie the sutures so tight that the tissue is strangulated.
6. Realign the mesentery of the two segments of bowel to be joined.

Types of anastomosis

Intestinal anastomoses may be performed with sutures or staples. In general, sutured anastomoses are preferable for intestinal segments which will be exposed to urine because of the possibility of stone formation on staples. A two-layer suture anastomosis is only required when there is a history of local radiotherapy or when the anastomosis is between bowel ends of discrepant diameters. The majority of enterostomies can be performed with a single-layer row of interrupted subserosal sutures. This type of anastomosis is identical for both small and large bowel. It is possible to use 2–0 Vicryl or PDS but the latter requires an extra throw on each knot to ensure that it does not unravel. The subserosal sutures should be placed approximately 3 mm apart and 3 mm form each margin. This type of anastomosis produces extremely good tension, does not leak and allows the vascular mucosa to produce an excellent seal from the very beginning. A single layer of sutures also produces a larger functional diameter for the anastomosis and is associated with an earlier return of normal peristaltic function.

The advantage of a stapled anastomosis is that it can be performed in much less time but this is only probably a saving of 10–15 min. The complication rates in sutured and stapled anastomosis are identical.[8] The one area in urology in which the stapling device is superior is in the ileocolonic end to side anastomosis. This utilizes the circular stapling device and a widely patent anastomosis can be achieved.

Complications

The complications following a bowel anastomosis include leakage of fecal contents, sepsis, wound infections, abdominal abscesses, hemorrhage, anastomotic stenosis, pseudo-obstruction of the colon (Ogilvie's syndrome) and intestinal obstruction. These events increase morbidity and are frequently major contributors to mortality. The complication rates for elective colocolonic and ileocolonic anastomosis performed in prepared bowel are: intestinal leak, 2%; hemorrhage, 1%; stenosis or obstruction, 4%. These complications require reoperations in 1% of patients and may result in death in up to 0.2% of patients.[9]

Ureterointestinal anastomoses

The ureter may be anastomosed to the colon or small bowel in such a manner as to produce a refluxing or non-refluxing anastomosis. Considerable controversy still exists as to whether a non-refluxing anastomosis is desirable in urinary tract reconstruction. Deterioration of the upper tracts is usually a consequence of infection or stones or, less commonly, of obstruction at the ureterointestinal anastomosis.

Because bacteriuria occurs in almost all conduits and because the intestine certainly does not inhibit and may in fact promote bacterial colonization, many have suggested that a non-refluxing anastomosis would minimize the instance of renal deterioration. Unfortunately, it is very difficult to perform a standard non-refluxing anastomosis between the ureter and small bowel because of the difficulty in separating the mucosa from the serosal layers.

Ureteral small bowel anastomoses

A number of ureteral small bowel anastomoses are possible and these are of two basic types, end to side and end to end. The end to side anastomosis may be constructed in a non-refluxing manner but this is often associated with failure. The Bricker anastomosis is a refluxing end to side ureteral small bowel anastomosis that is simple to perform and has a low complication rate.[6] Although originally described for the small bowel, it may be employed in any suitable intestinal segment. The original description involved suturing the adventitia of the ureter with interrupted silk sutures to the serosa of the bowel. The mucosa and serosa were incised and a small mucosal plug removed, and using fine reabsorbable chromic sutures, the full thickness of the ureter was sewn to the mucosa of the bowel. A less cumbersome method of performing this anastomosis is to excise a small button of seromuscular tissue and mucosa, spatulate the ureter for 0.5 cm and suture the full thickness of the ureter to the full thickness of the bowel with 4–0 PDS.

Another frequently employed anastomotic technique is that of Wallace, in which the end of the intestine is sutured to the end of the ureter.[10] This is a refluxing anastomosis. The intestinal segment employed may be either small bowel or colon. There are three basic types of Wallace anastomosis (Fig. 36.1) and these are:

1. The end of one ureter is sutured to the end of the other ureter. This anastomosis is then sutured to the end of the bowel.
2. A Y-anastomosis of the ureters is created, which is sutured to the end of the bowel rather like a pair of trousers.
3. A head to tail uretero-anastomosis is formed (affectionately known as 'the 69 position'), which is then sutured to the end of the bowel.

3–0 chromic catgut or 4–0 PDS should be utilized for each anastomosis. The Wallace anastomosis has the lowest complication rate of any of the ureterointestinal anastomotic techniques. Stricture formation is approximately 3%. All of these types of anastomosis require stenting for a minimum of 7 days and this is usually facilitated by suturing a ureteric catheter or infant feeding tube in place with an absorbable fine catgut suture that will dissolve after 1 week and so allow the stent to be removed percutaneously. A tunneled small bowel anastomosis can be attempted to establish a non-refluxing situation. This requires dissection between the mucosa and serosa which often leads to perforation, and few surgeons use this technique in small bowel. An alternative method for establishing a non-refluxing anastomosis is to employ a nipple mechanism. A 0.5-cm

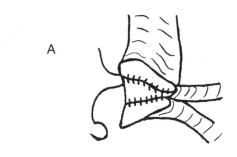

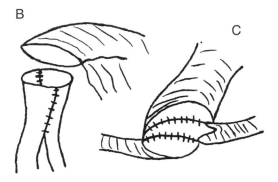

Fig. 36.1 Wallace ureterointestinal anastamosis. Both ureters are spatulated and laid against each other in one of three options. **A** Apex of one ureter is sutured to the apex of the other ureter. **B** 'Trouser' graft arrangement. **C** Head to tail or '69' configuration. The choice of alignment is best indicated by how the ureters lie at the time of reconstruction.

longitudinal incision in the ureter is made and the ureteral wall turned back on itself creating a nipple at least twice as long as its width. The cuff is stabilized at the corners with sutures and then the whole thing is passed through a buttonhole in the small bowel. This latter technique can prevent reflux in up to 50% of patients but it is more prone to stenosis than the routine Wallace non-refluxing technique.

Ureterocolonic anastomoses   The most commonly used technique (Fig. 36.2) is that described by Leadbetter & Clarke.[12] It establishes a non-refluxing ureterocolonic anastomosis by employing a submucosal tunnel. Injection of the submucosal

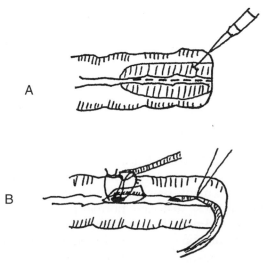

Fig. 36.2 Leadbetter–Clarke ureterointestinal anastomosis. **A** Injection of submucosal tissues assists dissection. **B** Linear incision is made in the taenia. A small button of mucosa is removed, the ureter is spatulated and then sutured to the mucosa with 4–0 CCG. The seromuscular layer is then sutured over the ureter.

tissues facilitates the dissection of the mucosa away from the serosa. A linear incision is made in the taenia and the mucosa away from the serosa. A linear incision is made in the taenia and the mucosa identified. A small button of mucosa is removed. The ureter is spatulated and is then sutured to the mucosa with a 4–0 PDS or Vicryl suture. The seromuscular layer is then sutured over the ureter, being careful not to compromise or occlude the ureter.

The complications reported with this procedure include a leak rate of 2.5%, a deterioration of the upper tracts that varies between 4.3% and 25% and a stricture rate that varies between 8% and 14%.

The transcolonic technique of Goodwin establishes a similar non-refluxing ureterocolonic anastomosis by creating a submucosal tunnel but by working from within the bowel. The bowel must be opened and if it is performed leaving this segment of bowel in continuity with the gastro-intestinal tract, then a non-crushing occlusive clamp is applied just proximal to the point of the anastomosis. The tunnel can be made without incising the roof and then resuturing it with the Goodwin technique.

Complications of ureterointestinal anastomoses

The complications that occur with ureterointestinal anastomoses include leakage, stricture and reflux in those anastomoses that were performed to prevent reflux and pyelonephritis. With respect to stricture formation and leakage, it appears that the Wallace technique has the best results.

Urinary fistulae invariably occur within the first 7–10 days post-operatively, with an incidence of between 3% and 9%. The incidence of leaks is markedly reduced by the use of soft Silastic stents. A leak may cause periureteral fibrosis and scarring with subsequent stricture formation. In general, antirefluxing techniques have a slightly higher incidence of strictures. Some strictures have been reported to develop many years following a procedure and stricture can also occur away from the uretero-intestinal anastomosis. This latter problem may be due to ischemia caused by aggressive dissection of the ureter and angulation of the ureter under the inferior mesenteric artery. Once the stricture has developed, various minimally invasive techniques such as balloon dilatation can be utilized to rectify the situation but there is a success rate of at best 50%. Whilst a conservative form of management is worthwhile in all cases, restenosis should be treated by re-exploration, excision of the stenotic segment and a reanastomosis of the ureter to the bowel.

Acute pyelonephritis occurs both in the early postoperative period and long term. The incidence is approximately 12% in patients who underwent diversion with ileal conduits and 9% in those who underwent diversion with antirefluxing colon conduits. When sepsis is associated with decreasing renal function, the morbidity and mortality are markedly increased. The incidence of renal deterioration itself following a conduit urinary diversion has varied from 10% to 60%. This is perhaps due to the fact that many reports include both renal units that were abnormal as well as those that were normal prior to diversion. The incidence of both sepsis and renal failure is greater than in those with conduits because of contamination from bowel in patients with ureterosigmoidostomies.

Renal function necessary for urinary intestinal diversion

The amount of renal function required effectively to combat the reabsorption of urinary solutes by the intestinal segment and prevent serious metabolic side effects is dependent on the urinary intestinal diversion created, the amount of bowel used and the length of time the urine will be exposed to intestinal mucosa. Thus a greater degree of renal function is necessary for continent diversions that utilize a reservoir than for short conduit diversions. In a patient with a raised serum creatinine level who has been considered for a urinary reservoir or on whom long segments of intestine will be used, a more detailed analysis of renal function is necessary. If the patient has a urine pH of 5.8 or less following an ammonium chloride load and a glomerular filtration rate that exceeds 35 ml/min and minimal protein in the urine then she may be considered fit enough for a more complex procedure.

Metabolic sequelae of urinary intestinal diversions

The metabolic complications include electrolyte abnormalities, altered conscious affective disorders, abnormal drug metabolism, osteomalacia, growth retardation in children, persistent and recurrent infections, formation of renal and reservoir calculi, problems ensuing from the removal of portions of the gut from the intestinal tract and development of urothelial/intestinal cancer. Many of these complications are a consequence of altered solute absorption across the intestinal segment. The factors that influence the amount of solute and type of absorption are the segment of bowel utilized, the surface area of the bowel, the amount of time the urine is exposed to the bowel, the concentration of the solutes in the urine and the renal function and pH of the fluid.

Serum electrolyte complications and the type of electrolyte abnormalities that occur are different depending on the segment of bowel utilized. If stomach is employed, a hypochloraemic metabolic alkalosis may occur. If jejunum is the segment used, hyponatremia, hyperkalemia and metabolic acidosis occur. If the ileum or colon is utilized, a hyperchloremic metabolic acidosis ensues. Other electrolyte abnormalities that have been described include hypokalemia, hypomagnesemia, hypocalcemia, hyperammonemia and elevated blood urea and creatinine levels.

Risk of cancer

The incidence of cancer developing in a patient with a ureterosigmoidostomy varies between 6% and 29%.[12] Generally, a 10–20 year delay occurs before the cancer becomes manifest. Histologically, the tumours include adenocarcinomata, adenomatous polyps, sarcomas and transitional cell carcinomas. Case reports of tumors developing in patients with ileal conduits, colon conduits and bladder augmentation have also more recently been described.[13] The etiological mechanism of the development of these carcinomas is not understood. Whether the tumor arises from transitional or colonic epithelium is unclear.

Adenocarcinomas have been shown to arise from transitional cell epithelium exposed to the fecal stream in the experimental animal. What is puzzling is that if the urothelium is left in contact with the intestinal mucosa even though the diversion is defunctionalized and the area is not bathed in urine, adenocarcinoma may still develop. Other evidence including cell staining techniques suggests that the colon is the primary organ of origin.[14] Whether the urothelium or intestine is the primary site of origin, it seems likely that tumors can arise from both tissues. The highest incidence of cancer occurs when the transitional epithelium is juxtaposed to the colonic epithelium and both are bathed by feces and urine.[15]

SPECIFIC DIVERSION PROCEDURES

Procedures requiring appliances (incontinent)

Cutaneous ureterostomy

Urinary diversion by means of a cutaneous ureterostomy offers the distinct advantage of being able to achieve the goals of the procedure without the need for bowel surgery. Therefore, many of the complications associated with bowel anastomoses can be avoided and one need not be concerned at all about reabsorption of urinary constituents by the bowel mucosa.[16] However, the major disadvantage of a cutaneous ureterostomy relates to the condition of the ureter itself. If a normal caliber ureter is brought to the skin even with a V-flap insertion technique designed to widen the stoma, the incidence of stomal stenosis is considerable.[16] This is because the length of the ureter that must be freed from its blood supply in order to traverse the distance from the retroperitoneum to the anterior abdominal skin necessitates that the ureter be dependent on collateral circulation for its survival, and a stricture often occurs. Also, a reasonable degree of ureteral peristaltic power is required for the ureter to propel urine through the relatively obstructing posterior rectus sheath and rectus muscles. If both ureters are dilated, they can be brought to the anterior abdominal wall as a double-barreled stoma site.

If one ureter is dilated and the other is of normal caliber, the dilated ureter could be brought out as a single-barreled stoma and the normal caliber ureter managed by a proximal transureteroureterostomy. Every attempt should be made to avoid two separate stoma sites.

Conduits

Ileal Urinary diversion by an ileal conduit diverting the urine to a short ileal segment that is directed to the anterior abdominal wall. Urinary diversion by means of an isolated ileal segment has become the most common surgical option in a patient who requires removal of the bladder for malignancy or who lacks functional or anatomical integrity of the urinary bladder. Because the majority of patients with uretero-intestinal urinary diversions suffer from bacteriuria and because bacteriuria in the presence of renal reflux is generally considered to be of adverse prognostic potential, a diversion that provides an antireflux anastomosis is preferred. However, this preference is imposed most often in the young surgical candidate rather than in the more typical older candidate whose bladder must be removed for purposes of cure from malignancy and it is the young patient to whom one normally offers a continent diversion, so the current practice is generally to provide ileal conduits with a safer non-refluxing ureterointestinal anastomosis for the older age group.

The selected stoma site is usually in the right lower quadrant but the ileum may be directed by rotation along its axis to the left lower quadrant if the left ureter is short or there is excessive scarring on the right side of the abdomen. In patients with terminal ileitis, a more proximal piece of bowel should be used (jejunum). There will be a potential for reabsorption of urinary constituents but in the ordinary patient with normal renal function, this should not constitute a clinically significant problem. In the patient with pre-existing damage to renal function, an ileal conduit can tip the balance and great care should be taken to select the shortest portion of bowel that will be capable of diverting the urine in these patients.

The procedure (Fig. 36.3) can be carried out through a low midline or transverse incision. When selecting an appropriate bowel segment for division from bowel continuity, it is helpful to transilluminate the bowel mesentery.

The mesenteric attachments of the isolated conduit should be as broad as possible. Its base should contain at least two major vascular supplies. The length of bowel segment should be equal to the length from the sacral promontory to the anterior abdominal wall plus 5 cm. It should not be taken from the terminal 20 cm of the ileum so that vitamin B12 and bile salt absorption are not disturbed. The mesenteric windows can be created with either a mechanical stapling device or by ligation with 3–0 Vicryl ligatures. After the ileal segment is isolated, it is dropped down caudally to lie below the area of selected ileal reanastomosis. The mesenteric window is closed with interrupted 3–0 Vicryl sutures in this operation (as well as in all procedures where bowel segments are isolated) to avoid postoperative internal herniation of bowel loops. The ileal reanastomosis can be made with either staples or a single layer of interrupted subserosal sutures (see above).

A preliminary cystectomy will have already freed the distal ureters, which should have been intubated with infant feeding tubes and the urine collected in small bags. When a cystectomy is not being performed, the ureters can be left attached to the bladder for convenient drainage until the ileal segment has been completed. One's attention then turns to the ureteroileal anastomosis. A standard end to end Wallace ureteroileal anastomosis is recommended using a continuous 3–0 Vicryl or PDS suture. Just prior to completion of each ureteral anastomosis, the infant feeding tube should be directed up towards each renal pelvis. These are temporarily stabilized using a 4– or 5–0 catgut suture. The stents are then brought out through the ileal segment and on to the anterior abdominal wall. The site of the ureteroileal anastomosis is then brought down towards the sacral promontory and the base is thoroughly retroperitonealized by bringing the excess right-sided retroperitoneum anteriorly to cover it. A suction drain is placed beneath this recreated peritoneal leaflet and then directed through the left lower quadrant. The skin is excised in a circular fashion over the chosen stoma site by pulling up the skin with a Lanes

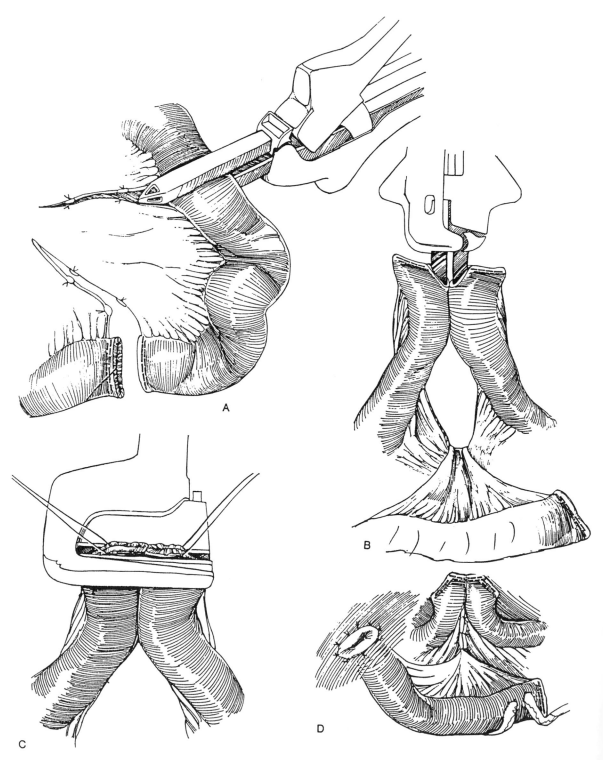

Fig. 36.3A–C   The bowel is transected utilizing a GIA stapler. Bowel continuity is restored by opening the antimesenteric corner of the two ileal ends and sliding the arm of the GIA down each limb. Prior to firing, proper orientation is assured. The opening is closed with a TA-55 stapler. **D** The ileal segment is dropped caudally so as to lie below the area of selected ileoileal anastomosis. The mesneteric trap is closed wth interrupted non-absorbable sutures. (From Hinman F Jr 1989. Atlas of urologic surgery. Philadelphia: WB Saunders, with permission.)

tissue holder. A cruciate incision is made in the fascia. The bowel end and stents are brought up through this hole to the anterior abdominal wall. A 2–0 Vicryl suture is placed between each corner of the fascial incision and attached to the bowel serosa approximately 6 cm from its end.

The terminal bowel segment is then folded back on itself like a rosebud and interrupted 2–0 CCG sutures join the full thickness of the bowel to the skin.

A review of serious complications associated with the ileal conduit urinary diversion has been completed by Benson et al.[17] It is surprising how often a second operation is required for even this the simplest of standard urinary diversions, either in the early postoperative period (15–23%) or more long term (17–23%). The most significant complication resulting from this procedure is related to the intestinal reanastomosis. A postoperative ileus is to be expected but this will normally resolve within 2–3 days. It is always important to remember that when a diversion is undertaken on a patient with a neurological disease such as multiple sclerosis, then the neuropathic bladder will almost always produce a much more prolonged ileus. Any suggestion of mechanical obstruction at the site of bowel reanastomosis can be managed conservatively for a short time but should be re-explored if there is no improvement. A leak from the anastomosis rarely produces generalized peritonitis but can lead to abscess formation. These again can usually be managed conservatively either with antibiotics alone or with percutaneous drainage under ultrasound control. However, in the absence of improvement, exploration is recommended. As many as 5–10% of individuals who undergo an ileal conduit urinary diversion experience bowel complications at some time in the future,[18] and this most often takes the form of intermittent diarrhea. Ureterointestinal stenosis may occur at any time in a patient with any bowel conduit. Any patient with a previous history of urothelial malignancy who develops ureteral obstruction should be thoroughly investigated by means of urinary cytology, imaging and endoscopy of the conduit to rule out any anaplastic cause. The non-malignant stenosis is usually caused by a poor vascular supply sometimes associated with an early urinary leak. Balloon dilatation is associated with a high short-term success, up to 50% of these strictures recur and open reconstruction is then required.

Jejunal

The only indication to use a jejunal segment is when the pelvis has been exposed to radiotherapy and the ileum has suffered visible effects of either a frozen pelvis or partial ischemia. Such findings are unpredictable after radiotherapy. However, in deciding to use the jejunum, which will be away from the site of radiotherapy, one must also take into account that the pelvic portions of the ureters should also be avoided and the ureters should be anastomosed at a point just above the pelvic brim. This should be the sole indication for using jejunum because of the physiological disadvantages. Electrolyte complications from urine absorption are very common and the majority of patients will require salt replacement. These problems can be minimized if the bowel segment chosen is as short as possible. The stoma will have to be positioned somewhere above the umbilicus.

Colonic

Either the sigmoid or the transverse colon can be used. These share the theoretical advantage of allowing a non-refluxing ureterointestinal anastomosis to be formed but the theoretical avoidance of upper urinary tract deterioration that it brings has not always been borne out in clinical series.[19] A tunneled anastomosis cannot be made with a dilated ureter. The transverse colon is chosen when the pelvis has received radiotherapy. Postoperative complications are unexpectedly as few as when using small bowel, with the exception of a slightly higher incidence of ureterointestinal stenosis (13%) as well as a high incidence of parastomal herniation or stomal prolapse (13%), but there is a lower incidence of stomal stenosis when using large bowel.[20]

Continent urinary diversion procedures

Ureterosigmoidostomy

A ureterosigmoidostomy can be regarded as the original continent urinary diversion.[21] Despite the metabolic complications of hyperchloremic acidosis, hypocalcemia, pyelonephritis and development of colonic malignancy, this procedure still has a place when a rapid, simple diversion is required, particularly in a patient with a poor prognosis from an advanced malignancy. The absence of a bowel anastomosis means a rapid recovery and an improved quality of what may turn out to be a shortened remaining lifespan. The patient with established renal impairment is a poor candidate for this operation or indeed any continent diversion. It should also be avoided in patients who have been exposed to pelvic irradiation. Various tests have been proposed to assess sphincter integrity. The most useful are those that require the patient to retain an enema solution of solid and liquefied material for a specified time in the upright and ambulatory position without incontinence. A thin mixture of oatmeal and water serves well for this. The patient should retain 400–500 ml for 1 h in the upright position. However, this operation is often utilized in patients where a more elaborate diversion had been planned and a laparotomy reveals a more extensive disease. In these cases obviously the preoperative assessment of continence would not have been made and, fortunately, the majority of these patients still do well and are continent.

The various techniques of ureterocolostomy have been described earlier in this chapter. The easiest method is to open the sigmoid colon between stay sutures and carry out a tunneled anastomosis. The stents can be brought out of the anus along with a larger defunctioning catheter.

Rectal bladder (Fig. 36.4)

Various innovative surgical techniques have been introduced for separating the fecal and urinary streams while still employing the basic ureterosigmoidostomy principle. The various improvements have been brought together by Kock et al.[22] Their procedure is based on three principles. The first is a non-refluxing ureterorectal anastomosis. Secondly, an augmentation of the rectum is carried out with a detubularized small bowel pedicle to reduce the inherent tone of the rectum and increase its capacity.

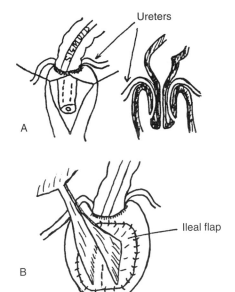

Ureters

Ileal flap

A

B

Fig. 36.4 The Ghoneim augmented rectal bladder. **A** The ureters are anastomosed to the rectum via a submucosal tunnel. An intersusception of sigmoid is made into the rectum and held with four rows of staples. **B** A 20-cm segment of ileum is detubularized and augmented into the rectum

Thirdly, a rectosigmoid intussusception valve is created to prevent retrograde passage of urine into the remaining large bowel and so reduce the risk associated with urine absorption.

Continent catheterizing pouches

Numerous operative techniques (Fig. 36.5) have been developed for continent diversion of urine. A reservoir is created from bowel and this is emptied at intervals by clean self-catheterization through a continent abdominal valve. I will describe five of the more well-known procedures, each of which has its proponents. An expertise in at least one of these needs to be built up together with a working knowledge of the Mitrofanoff[23] principle (Fig. 36.6), which can be applied when revising some of these procedures. It is important that a patient undergoing one of these procedures should have sufficient hand–eye co-ordination to perform clean intermittent catheterization and this is often not the case with quadriplegic patients or those patients with progressive multiple sclerosis. The location of the catheterizing site is usually at the umbilicus or in the lower quadrant of the abdomen through the rectus bulge and below the bikini line in those females who wish to hide this site under either their swimwear or undergarments. The umbilicus is certainly preferred for the individual confined to a wheelchair. A stoma site can usually be covered with gauze or a simple adhesive plaster between catheterizations and this both helps self-image and avoids mucus soiling of clothing which sometimes occurs.

These reservoirs are more complex than the conduit and as such are associated with a more significant morbidity and a higher revision rate. The single most demanding technical feature of each pouch is the construction of a continence mechanism and it is this that often requires revision of surgery, albeit often of a minor nature. It is important to counsel the patient preoperatively with regard to these potential pitfalls

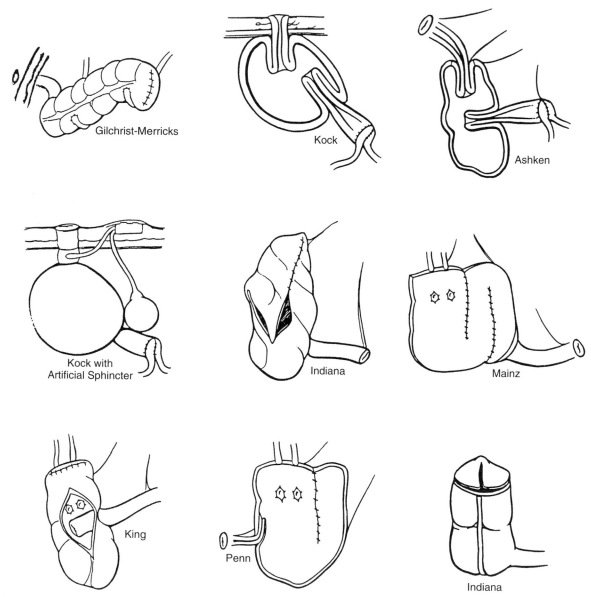

Fig. 36.5   Options for a continent diversion

and many patients who are psychologically fragile may elect to undergo a more simple urinary diversion using a conduit rather than face the increased risk of a second operation.

The frequency of catheterization obviously depends on the capacity of the reservoir (up to 100 ml). The need for catheterization can be fairly accurately assessed by the sensation of discomfort that a patient feels but this can often be minimal in the initial postoperative period and rapid overstretching should be avoided by punctilious emptying, erring on the conservative side. In practice, this usually means between 3 and 5 times a

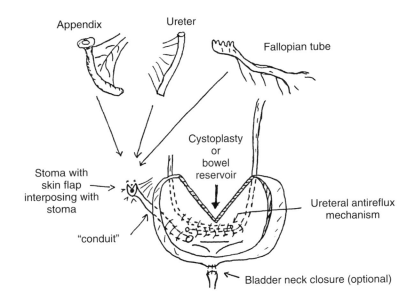

Fig. 36.6 The Mitrofanoff principle. The alternatives are appendicovesicostomy, ureterostomy with transureterureterostomy, fallopian tube conduit, tapered or imbricated ileum, tapered bladder or urethra and appendicocecostomy. A patent bladder neck does provide a pressure valve if the stoma becomes obstructed

day. The reservoirs will usually increase their capacity but not significantly after the first year.

The Kock pouch

This particular procedure described by Kock in 1982 is responsible for reawakening interest in the continent diversion principle which can now be performed much more safely in the era of antibiotics and improved surgical and anesthetic techniques. First 70–80 cm of ileum is isolated and the remaining bowel reanastomosed. A 5-cm segment of proximal ileum and mesentery is sacrificed to provide added mobility to the isolated segment. The middle portion of the ileum is folded in the shape of a 'U' with each limb measuring 20–22 cm in length (see Fig. 36.5). The medial borders of the 'U' are sutured together after detubularization along the antimesenteric border. Nipple valves are created at either end of the segment using a TA55 stapler. Stapling provides the most efficient long-term success of these valves but unfortunately the staples are prone to becoming the nidus for stone formation in up to 10% of patients. This complication can be minimized by removing the distal 6 staples from each cartridge before application to ensure that the tip of the valve is free of staples. The reservoir is completed by folding the U-shaped portion down on itself and completing the anastomosis. The ureters are anastomosed to one nipple valve and this operation is tailor-made for the dilated ureter and will still provide an anti-reflux procedure because of the ileal nipple. The other nipple valve is brought up through the abdominal wall. The Kock pouch has an initial capacity of just over 200 ml but this will increase to over 600 ml after 6 months.

The Mainz pouch The precise operative technique to create the Mainz pouch has been refined so as to utilize the intact ileocecal valve as a means of stabilizing the intussusception.[24] By using large bowel, a tunneled non-refluxing ureterointestinal anastomosis can be performed. The abdominal wall valve is created from an intussusception of the normal but often incompetent ileocecal valve (see Fig. 36.5). Detubularization is again an essential principle that reduces the overall inherent tone of the reservoir. The intussusception valve is secured with metal staples. From a technical point of view this is easier to construct than the Kock pouch, but the use of large bowel produces a reservoir with a slightly higher inherent tone despite detubularization, and this is often a cause of incontinence, particularly at night when the reservoir is full. The Indiana pouch is essentially similar to the Mainz pouch but the ileocecal valve is strengthened by a double row of imbricating sutures rather than being enhanced with internal staple fixations. If offers a more straightforward technique without the problems associated with stone formation on staples, but several patients require revision because the imbricating sutures create a potentially uneven passage for the catheter through the stoma.

The Penn pouch This is the first continent diversion to employ the Mitrofanoff principle, wherein the appendix serves as the continence mechanism to the abdominal wall. The operation is otherwise very similar to the Mainz pouch but in the absence of an appendix or even an appendix of a large caliber then either a fallopian tube or pedicled terminal ureter can be utilized.

Gastric pouches The use of stomach to create a urinary reservoir has both theoretical and practical advantages.[25] Electrolyte reabsorption is minimal even when compared to small bowel. A hyperchloremic acidotic state is virtually impossible given that the gastric mucosa produces a barrier against the absorption of chloride and ammonium and there is also the active secretion of chloride ions in the reverse direction. This makes it the potentially ideal reservoir for individuals with pre-existing renal impairment and it has now been used for many patients, especially finding a place in the pediatric population.

A wedge-shaped segment of stomach in which the greatest width is 7–10 cm is fashioned from the greater curvature taking care not to extend the apex through to the lesser curvature in order to preserve vagal innervation and normal gastric emptying. The pedicle is based on the left gastroepiploic artery. The isolated wedge is refashioned into a spear by folding it back on itself and suturing the edges together. Before pouch closure, one ureter is tunneled into the reservoir in an anti-reflux fashion. The terminal portion of the second ureter is used as a Mitrofanoff valve to the abdominal wall and proximal transureteroureterostomy is performed.

Orthotopic voiding diversions

A reservoir can be constructed based on the techniques for a continent urinary diversion to the abdominal wall but the reservoir instead is anastomosed to the intact urethra. As a technique, it is much simpler than the above-mentioned continent diversion because there is no need for a continent valve at the distal end and the anastomosis with the urethra is quite straightforward. However, continence is dependent on the integrity of the external sphincter and whilst this operation has become quite routine in the male patient following a cystoprostatectomy, the results are very variable in the female patient. The difficulty lies in retaining adequate external sphincter function in women following a cystectomy. The only situation where an orthotopic voiding diversion is reasonable is where a subtotal cystectomy is performed and the diversion is into a subtotal bladder augmentation cystoplasty.

SUMMARY

A urinary diversion can take on a variety of forms. Those utilizing bowel have only been safe in the current antibiotic era but their complexity is unlimited. The ileal conduit is the best compromise for long-term success, has a low incidence of anastomotic stenosis and is relatively easy to perform. The two main indications for a diversion are: (1) following a cystectomy, and (2) following failed incontinence surgery. However, some patients will be suitable for a continent diversion. There are no absolute criteria that should be fulfilled for a patient to undergo a continent diversion but generally it is best that their renal function is normal and that they have the psychological resolution to undergo reoperation when complications occur (25%).

REFERENCES

1 Simon J. Ectropia vesicae (absence of the anterior wall of the bladder and pubic abdominal parietes); operation for directing the orifices of the ureters into the rectum; temporary success; subsequent death; autopsy. Lancet 1852; 2: 568–570.
2 Tizzoni, Foggi. Die Wiederherstellung der Harnblase. Centrabl f Chir 1888; 15: 921–924.
3 Goldenberg T. Ueber die totalextirpation der Harnblase und die Versorgung der Ureteren. Beitr Z Klin Chir 1904; 44: 627–649.
4 Berg J. Ueber die Behandlung der Ectopia vesicae. Nord Med Arki Abt 1907; 1(4):
5 Hinman F, Weyrauch HM Jr. A critical study of the different principles of surgery which have been used in uretero-intestinal implantation. Trans Am Assn GU Surgeons 1936; 29: 15–156.
6 Bricker EM. Bladder substitution after pelvic evisceration. Surg Clin North Am 1950; 30: 1511–1521.
7 Seiffert L. Die 'Darm-siphonblase'. Arch f klin Chir 1935; 183: 569–574.
8 Chassin JL, Rifkind KM, Sussman B et al. The stapled gastrointestinal tract anastomosis: incidence of postoperative complications compared with the sutured anastomoses. Ann Surg 1978; 188: 689–696.
9 Jex RK, van Heerden JA, Wolff BG, Ready RL, Illstrup DM. Gastrointestinal anastomoses. Factors affecting early complications. Ann Surg 1987; 206: 138–141.
10 Wallace DM. Uretero-ileostomy. Br J Urol 1970; 42: 529–534.
11 Leadbetter WF, Clarke BG. Five years' experience with uretero-enterostomy by the 'combined' technique. J Urol 1954; 73: 67–82.
12 Zabbo A, Kay R. Ureterosigmoidostomy and bladder exstrophy: A long-term follow up. J Urol 1986; 136: 396–398.
13 Filmer RB. Malignant tumours arising in bladder augmentation and ileal and colon conduits. Soc Pediatr Urol Newsletter, December 9 1986.
14 Scott McDougal W. Use of intestinal segments in the urinary tract: basic principles. Campbell's urology, 6th edn. New York: Saunders, 1992.
15 Shands C III, McDougal WS, Wright EP. Prevention of cancer at the urothelial enteric anastomotic site. J Urol 1989; 141: 178–181.
16 Chute R, Sallade RL. Bilateral side-to-side cutaneous urethrostomy in the midline for urinary diversion. J Urol 1961; 85: 280–283.
17 Benson MC, Slawin KM, Wechsler MH, Olsson CA. Analysis of continent versus standard urinary diversion. Br J Urol, Submitted 1990.

18 Sullivan JW, Grabstald H, Whitmore WF Jr. Complicatons of ureteileal conduit with radical cystectomy: review of 336 cases. J Urol 1980 124: 797–801.
19 Hill JT, Ransley PG. The colonic conduit: a better method of urinary diversion? Br J Urol 1983; 55: 629–631.
20 Richie JP. Sigmoid conduit urinary diversion. Urol Clin North Am 1986; 13: 225–232.
21 Smith T. An account of an unsuccessful attempt to treat extroversion of the bladder by a new operation. St Barth Hosp Rep 1879; 15: 29–35.
22 Kock NG, Ghoneim MA, Lycke KG, Mahran MR. Urinary diversion to the augmented and valved rectum: preliminary results with a novel surgical procedure. J Urol 1988; 140: 1375–1379.
23 Mitrofanoff P. Cystostomie continente transappendiculaire dans le travail des vessies neurologiques. Chir Pediatr 1980; 21: 297.
24 Thuroff JW, Alken P, Riedmiller H, Jacobi GH, Hohenfellner R. 100 cases of MAINZ pouch: continuing experience and evolution. J Urol 1988; 140: 283–288.
25 Adams MC, Mitchell ME, Rink RC. Gastrocystoplasty: an alternative solution to the problem of urological reconstruction in the severely compromised patient. J Urol 1988; 140: 1152–1156.

Section 7 Additional Aspects

37 Physiotherapy

INTRODUCTION

Genuine stress incontinence (GSI) is a condition defined as the involuntary loss of urine which occurs when the intravesical pressure exceeds the urethral closure pressure, in the absence of detrusor activity.[1] Leakage typically occurs when the urethral sphincter mechanism cannot withstand sudden increases in intravesical pressure generated by exercise, coughing, sneezing, straining or during sexual intercourse. The urethral closure pressure is the product of several factors which together help maintain continence. Elasticity and compliance of the urethra and integrity of the submucosal vascular plexus are important as they help provide a hermetic seal. Urethral smooth muscle, the intrinsic urethral rhabdosphincter and the extrinsic striated muscle of the levator ani are all important in the genesis of urethral closure pressure at rest and during stress episodes. Maintenance of the bladder neck and proximal urethra in an intra-abdominal position is an important factor in the mechanism of continence. In this position, any rise in intra-abdominal pressure will be transmitted equally to the bladder neck and proximal urethra, thus maintaining the positive pressure gradient which normally exists between the urethra and the bladder. Descent of the bladder neck will result in loss of intra-abdominal pressure transmission to the proximal urethra during stress, and incontinence occurs because bladder pressure then exceeds the urethral closure pressure.

The bladder neck and proximal urethra are flanked by the tendineus fasciae pelvis. This is a band of dense connective tissue running from the lower border of the symphysis pubis to the ischial spine. The bladder neck is connected to this structure by the pubovesical muscle, which is a direct continuation of the detrusor, and not ligamentous as previously described.

The vagina is densely adherent to the levator ani muscles, just caudal to the arcus tendineus fasciae pelvis. This attachment is 1 cm long and 0.5 cm wide, and lies in the region of the proximal urethra extending up towards the bladder. Microscopically, connective tissue fibers from the vaginal wall, containing collagen, smooth muscle fibers and abundant elastin, interdigitate with the levator ani muscle. There is no direct connection between the urethra and the levator ani muscles, they are connected only indirectly via the pubovesical muscle. The urethra is closely attached to the vaginal wall and therefore its position and function may be influenced by levator ani contraction.

The connections of the vagina bilaterally to the arcus tendineus fasciae pelvis have been viewed as the ropes supporting a 'hammock' of supporting tissue beneath the urethra.[2] The hammock itself consists of anterior vaginal wall and endopelvic fascia. Raised intra-abdominal pressure acting on the urethra forces it against the supporting layer, resulting in apposition of anterior and posterior urethral walls, increase in intra-urethral pressure and occlusion of the lumen.

Genuine stress incontinence may occur in nulliparous women,[3] but it is more common in multiparous women and may arise following denervation and reinnervation of the pelvic floor which can occur following vaginal delivery.[4] A recent follow-up study of the same patients after subsequent pregnancies suggests that further changes in pelvic floor neurophysiology occur with time, but are not specifically related to parity. The majority of denervation–reinnervation occurs at the first vaginal delivery.[5]

Damage to the supporting structures of the bladder and levator ani muscles leads to the association of GSI and prolapse, although the two conditions can exist independently. Impairment of the function of the urethral sphincter may arise following repeated trauma from surgery, instrumentation or catheterization.

In nulliparous women the etiology of GSI may be different. No concentric needle electromyographic abnormalities were identified in 30 premenopausal nulliparous women with GSI compared to 22 normal controls.[3] It is postulated that abnormalities in the collagen content of the pelvic floor and bladder neck supports predispose to the development of GSI in such women.

Incontinence which results from laxity of the pelvic floor and bladder neck supports may be expected to respond to methods of treatment aimed at strengthening these supporting structures. Traditionally, the treatment of GSI involves bladder neck surgery; however, this is not acceptable or suitable for all women. In cases of mild GSI, women who desire further children and those who are unfit for anesthesia, conservative therapy is preferable.

As yet, however, there is no consensus as to the most effective form of pelvic floor physiotherapy for the treatment of GSI. In 1991 Mantle & Versi conducted a postal questionnaire of all 192 health districts in England.[6] They found the provision of pelvic floor re-education to be heterogeneous, with the use of Kegel exercises and interferential therapy the most commonly offered treatments in 189 out of 192 and 176 out of 192 districts respectively. The use of faradism (103/192) and interrupted direct current (8/192) was much less widespread. A perineometer was used in 50 out of 192 districts as a means of assessing pelvic floor strength prior to therapy or as a means of monitoring treatment outcome. At the time of the survey, vaginal cone therapy was only available in 31 out of 192 districts.

PELVIC FLOOR EXERCISES

Pelvic floor exercises were first described by Arnold Kegel in 1948[7]. He utilized vaginal palpation of the pubococcygeal muscle to enable the

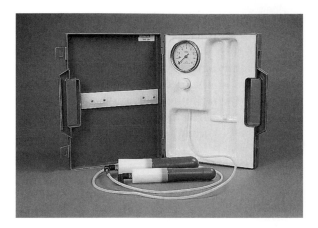

Fig. 37.1 A perineometer

patient to isolate a correct contraction which was then carried out voluntarily at home. He also introduced the perineometer, which consisted of a flexible rubber chamber connected to a manometer. Following insertion into the vagina, the pressure generated by pelvic floor contraction was measured in mmHg. The device also served as a means of biofeedback, demonstrating the presence of a contraction to the patient. A modern perineometer is shown in Fig. 37.1. Kegel stressed the importance of encouragement and supervision in the management of these patients and estimated that restoration of tone and muscle function could be achieved following 20–40 h of progressive muscle resistance exercise, over a period of 20–60 days. His original results were impressive, quoting 64 women with stress incontinence who were made continent for up to 14 months following therapy.[8] In subsequent studies by Kegel and his colleagues[9–15] an overall success rate of 84% in more than 500 patients was reported. More recently, studies[16–30] have confirmed the beneficial effects of pelvic floor exercises in women with GSI. Most of these studies only employed short-term follow-up of weeks to months; however, long-term results indicate that a proportion of women will sustain relief of symptoms for many years following continued pelvic floor re-education.[26,27,30,31]

The rates of cure or improvement quoted in these studies vary. There are differences in study design, inclusion criteria, exercise regimen employed, duration of treatment and means of subjective and objective assessment, which makes direct comparison difficult.

Tapp et al[32] found that the women with GSI most likely to benefit from physiotherapy were premenopausal, with a short duration of symptoms and urodynamic evidence of good urethral function. Older women with more severe incontinence were thought to be more suited to surgical treatment. This finding is supported by Henalla & Hutchins, who found that duration of symptoms was negatively related to treatment outcome.[21]

In contrast, Bo & Larsen[33] used discriminant analysis to classify responders to an intensive program of pelvic floor exercises. Responders were significantly older (48.4 years SD 7.4) than borderline responders (38.3 SD 9.8). Duration of stress incontinence symptoms was greater for responders (12.8 yrs SD 5.7) than borderline responders. Responders had a higher body mass index (23.9 SD 2.4) than borderline responders (21.0 SD 2.3). Pelvic floor muscle strength and objective severity of GSI was significantly greater for responders to pelvic floor re-education. The disparity in the results of these studies may be due to the fact that severity of incontinence was assessed by different means in the studies, and different treatment regimens with different outcome variables were employed. Patient motivation and compliance is another important factor which have led to such contrasting findings in the populations studied. In the short term, the intensity of pelvic floor re-education employed is related to outcome, and continued compliance is vital for long-term benefit to be maintained.

PERINEOMETER/BIOFEEDBACK

The use of a perineometer (Fig. 37.1) to record intravaginal pressure and provide biofeedback during pelvic floor contraction has been investigated by Kegel[7] and subsequently by several authors using different devices.[17,34,35,36] The perineometer may be used as the primary treatment or as a means of facilitating pelvic floor contraction and improving the therapeutic efficacy of Kegel exercises. In a study by Ferguson et al in 1990,[25] however, use of a vaginal balloon perineometer was not associated with any increased benefit in terms of improved pelvic muscle strength or decreased urinary leakage when compared to standard pelvic floor exercises. Laycock & Jerwood have employed a water-filled perineometer to evaluate pelvic muscle strength in women with and without stress incontinence.[37] They recorded the maximum voluntary contraction profile during a pelvic floor contraction held for 10 s. The maximum pressure recorded, the area under the profile and the initial pressure gradient were compared between the two groups. The area under the profile is believed to be a property of slow twitch fibers of the levator ani, the pressure gradient a function of fast twitch fibers, and the maximum pressure a combination of both. Women with reported stress incontinence had lower maximum pressures, smaller areas under the profile and a flatter pressure gradient than their continent counterparts. These differences are insufficient to allow accurate diagnosis of GSI using perineometry, but provide useful information in the planning of a pelvic floor exercise program.

Only recently have perineometry measurements been validated in terms of reproducibility and relationship to bladder volume and timing of the menstrual cycle.[38] If several perineometry readings are taken at one visit, then the first value is significantly greater than the others, which appear to be reproducible. If weekly measurements are taken, then those made at the first two visits are significantly lower than those in subsequent weeks, which tend to become more reproducible. Measurements are affected by bladder volume and should ideally be taken with an empty bladder. No relationship was found between perineometer readings and the timing of the menstrual cycle. There is obviously a learning process in isolating a correct pelvic muscle contraction and no analysis of muscle strength should be made until the third visit. At each visit, the first value should be discarded and the mean of the following three or four contractions used.

Traditional perineometry has been criticized as increases in intra-abdominal pressure as during a Valsalva maneuver may register on the manometer and be misinterpreted as pelvic floor contractions. Surface electromyography electrodes have been developed to circumvent this problem. A vaginal surface electrode placed 3 cm from the introitus will accurately record pelvic floor muscle activity during contraction and provide biofeedback to the patient.[39] In this way erroneous straining or inappropriate muscle contraction may be reduced.

VAGINAL CONE THERAPY

Vaginal cone therapy (Fig. 37.2) provides an alternative means of strengthening pelvic floor musculature which also utilizes the principles of biofeedback. Once the cone is inserted into the vagina, the sensation of it 'falling out' results in pelvic floor contraction in order to retain the cone. It is a simple technique that can easily be performed at home after a few simple instructions. When performing voluntary pelvic floor exercises, women often inadvertently contract the abdominal or gluteal muscles. This is not the case with vaginal cones. When the lightest cone can be retained in the vagina for 20 mins on two separate occasions, the next heaviest weight is employed. The first sets of cones comprised five separate weights ranging from 20 to 100 g.

Cone therapy has been shown to result in subjective and objective improvement or cure in 70% of 30 women treated for 4 weeks.[40] Only 37% of women opted for surgery following the treatment period. Good correlation was found between the increase in cone weight at rest and the objective reduction in urinary leakage on pad testing.

The efficacy of vaginal cone therapy has been compared to inter-ferential therapy in a randomized prospective study.[41] The treatments

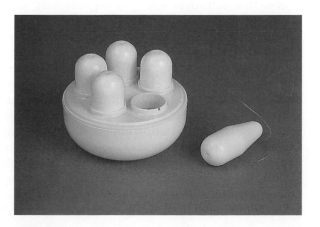

Fig. 37.2 A set of vaginal cones

were found to be equally effective following 1 month's therapy, with subjective improvement in 79% of the cones group and 90% of the interferential group. Objective improvement on pad testing was found in 50% and 76% respectively. Cone therapy necessitated fewer visits to hospital and required less supervision by the physiotherapist. It is interesting to note, however, that both groups of women were taught Kegel exercises which they continued throughout the study period. It is not clear how much this latter intervention contributed to the clinical improvement observed in this study.

Vaginal cone therapy used alone (i.e. without instruction in how to isolate pelvic floor contraction and according to the patient information leaflet accompanying each set of cones) has been compared to standard Kegel exercises.[42] Following a 10-week treatment period, both groups showed significant subjective improvement on a visual analog symptom score. Sixty-two per cent of the pelvic floor exercises group and 74% of the cones group were improved on pad testing. This objective improvement was only significant for the cones group. Difficulty in remembering to carry out the treatment as instructed was a predominant feature in the pelvic floor exercises group but this was not found in the cones group. The presence of significant vaginal atrophy or prolapse was associated with difficulty in cone insertion and reduced compliance with treatment.

Two studies have compared the use of vaginal cones with standard Kegel exercises in the teaching of postnatal exercises.[43,44] Both found that it was easier to teach patients to contract their pelvic floor muscles using cones, and the short-term results in terms of improvement in pelvic muscle strength were superior. Increased compliance with treatment was found for the women treated with cones.

Combination therapy of cones plus Kegel exercises was compared to treatment with cones alone or treatment with maximal electrical stimulation (MES).[45] Following a 12-week treatment period, all three groups were symptomatically improved. The degree of symptomatic improvement, however, was greater for those in the combination treatment group than for those in the cones group or the MES group. A significant reduction in leakage on pad testing was achieved in the cones group and the combination group, but not in the MES group. The degree of objective improvement was significantly greater in the combination therapy group than in the MES group; however, there was no significant difference between the cones group and those treated with cones plus Kegel exercises.

Comparing the two groups that used cones, a greater proportion of women were objectively improved following combination therapy; however, this difference approached but did not reach statistical significance. Similarly, no added effect was found in terms of increase in passive and active cone weight following combination treatment. This suggests that careful instruction on how to contract the pelvic floor muscles by a physiotherapist or continence advisor is not necessary for successful use of vaginal cones, and the practice of performing such contractions regularly throughout the treatment period does not increase efficacy. The use of 'unsupervised' cone therapy should reduce the amount of clinic time required to initiate treatment and enable treatment to be offered by non-specialist practitioners such as the general practitioner or practice nurse.

INTERFERENTIAL THERAPY

Interferential therapy is a form of neuromuscular electrical stimulation which can be applied to the pelvic floor using two electrodes[46] (bipolar or premodulated interferential therapy) or four electrodes[47,48] or via a single vaginal electrode. In clinical studies it has been shown to be an effective primary therapy for GSI with a reported cure rate of around 30%.[46-51] Recently, interferential therapy and pelvic floor re-education using cones plus Kegel exercises were compared.[49,52] Low cure rates of 4.5% and 17.6% respectively were documented with no significant difference between the two methods in terms of subjective or objective improvement. Interferential therapy, however, requires regular attendance at the out-patient clinic, and is time-consuming for the physiotherapist who must supervise each session.

Interferential therapy is employed in the majority of physiotherapy units in the United Kingdom,[6] but the exact techniques employed are heterogeneous. Since its efficacy is no greater than that of Kegel exercises and cone therapy one may question the validity of the providing of such a labor-intensive, and therefore relatively expensive therapy for women with GSI.

INTRAVAGINAL ELECTRICAL STIMULATION

Electrical stimulation was originally proposed to activate the urethral closure mechanism using implantable electrodes by Caldwell in 1963.[53] Such devices were associated with high complication rates due to infection and malfunction of the implanted electrodes, and were superseded by external anal[54] or vaginal stimulators.[55] Regimens using long-term, low-intensity electrical stimulation have a reported success rate of between 37% and 92% in women with stress incontinence.[56,57,58,59,60] Such modalities of treatment have been popular for 15 years in Yugoslavia and Scandinavia, but have gained little recognition in the United Kingdom and the United States.

Intravaginal electrical stimulation is believed to act via stimulation of somatic efferent pathways and not by direct muscle stimulation. It has been shown to restore urethral pressure profile (UPP) measurements following epidural anesthesia, but not after succinylcholine administration, which blocks neuromuscular transmission to striated muscle.[61] Intravaginal electrical stimulation is unlikely to be effective if there is complete denervation of the pelvic floor. In cases of a partial lower motor neurone lesion, the intensity of stimulation required to achieve effective pelvic floor contraction may be so high that it causes pain and possible tissue damage.

There are scant data on the efficacy of short-term MES in the treatment of GSI. Plevnik et al[62] reported the results of short-term maximal electrical stimulation in 310 incontinent patients, 80 of whom had GSI. Twenty-five patients (31%) were cured and a further 13 (16%) improved following 1 month's home treatment. This led to the development of the device shown in Fig. 19.4, which the patient may use at home. More recently, Jonasson et al[63] utilized the same device to treat 17 women with GSI. They reported subjective improvement in 8 patients (47%), with a reduction in leakage on pad testing of >50% in 12 cases (71%). Plevnik found that it was not possible to predict treatment outcome following MES on the basis of the response of UPP measurements to test stimulation. Fall et al[64] found that UPP parameters were not improved in patients who experienced symptomatic relief of stress incontinence following long-term intravaginal electrical stimulation.

We compared short-term MES with cone therapy or a combination of cones plus Kegel exercises in 63 women with GSI.[45] Maximal electrical stimulation did not appear to be an effective treatment for GSI, since subjective improvement was less than for therapy using cones plus pelvic floor exercises, and no significant objective effect was found on pad testing. It was, however, well tolerated by all patients, easy to perform and associated with good patient compliance. In contrast compliance with Kegel exercises is often poor and so combination therapy with home intravaginal electrical stimulation may result in improved uptake of treatment and an overall greater efficacy.

CONCLUSIONS

There is undoubtedly a role for pelvic floor re-education in the treatment of GSI. A proportion of patients will be subjectively and objectively cured and if therapy is continued these benefits may be maintained in the long term. Other women will notice a significant improvement in urinary symptoms such that surgery may be avoided. It is still unclear from studies undertaken which is the most effective form of physiotherapy and which patients are likely to benefit most. Standard methods of patient investigation and pre-treatment evaluation should be employed in all units. Objective measures of outcome should be used wherever possible. At present the number of different pad tests employed in the literature is vast with little evidence of validation.

Whatever method of therapy is employed, supervision by an informed, enthusiastic health professional is essential if good results are to be achieved. Dedicated physiotherapists or continence advisors should be closely incorporated into the team of gynecologists and urologists responsible for the management of women with lower urinary tract dysfunction. The role of pelvic floor exercise programs in the prevention of prolapse and incontinence following childbirth and aging remains to be determined. This is an area of preventative medicine with important implications for women's health which to date has sadly received little attention.

REFERENCES

1 Abrams P, Blaivas JG, Stanton SL, Andersen JT. The standardisation of terminology of lower urinary tract function. Br J Obstet Gynaecol 1990; Suppl 6: 1–16.

2 DeLancey JOL. Three dimensional analysis of urethral support: the 'hammock hypothesis'. Neurourol Urodyn 1992; 11(4): 306–308.

3 Keane DP, Sims TJ, Bailey AJ, Abrams P. Analysis of pelvic floor electromyography and collagen status in pre-menopausal nulliparous females with genuine stress incontinence (GSI). Neurourol Urodyn 1992; 11(4): 308–309.

4 Smith ARB, Hosker GL, Warrell DW. The role of pudendal nerve damage in the aetiology of genuine stress incontinence in women. Br J Obstet Gynaecol 1989; 96: 29–32.

5 Mallett V, Hosker G, Smith ARB, Warrell D. Pelvic floor damage and childbirth: a neurophysiological follow up study. Neurourol Urodyn 1994; 13(4): 357–358.

6 Mantle J, Versi E. Physiotherapy for stress urinary incontinence: a national survey. BMJ 1991; 302: 753–755.

7 Kegel AH. Progressive resistance exercise in the functional restoration of the perineal muscles. Am J Obstet Gynecol 1948; 56: 238–248.

8 Kegel AH. The physiologic treatment of poor tone and function of the genital muscles and of urinary stress incontinence. West J Surg Obstet Gynecol 1949; 57: 527–535.

9 Kegel AH. The nonsurgical treatment of genital relaxation: use of the perineometer as an aid in restoring anatomic and functional structure. Ann West Med Surg 1948; 2: 213–221.

10 Kegel AH, Powell TO. The physiologic treatment of urinary stress incontinence. J Urol 1950; 63: 808–817.

11 Jones EG. The role of active exercise in pelvic muscle physiology. West J Surg Obstet Gynecol 1950; 58: 1–9.

12 Kegel AH. Physiologic therapy for urinary stress incontinence. J Am Med Assoc 1951; 1146: 915–924.

13 Jones EG, Kegel AH. Treatment of urinary stress incontinence, with results in 117 patients treated by active exercise of the pubococcygei. Surg Gynecol Obstet 1952; 94; 179–187.

14 Kegel AH. Sexual functions of the pubococcygeus muscle. West J Surg Obstet Gynecol 1952; 60: 521–528.

15 Kegel AH. Stress incontinence of urine in women: physiologic treatment. J Int Coll Surg 1956; 25: 487–494.

16 Shepherd A, Montgomery E. A pilot study of a pelvic exerciser in women with stress incontinence. J Obstet Gynecol 1983; 3: 201–202.

17 Castleden CM, Duffin HM, Mitchell EP. The effect of physiotherapy on stress incontinence. Age Ageing 1984; 13: 235–237.

18 Sandri SD, Magnaghi C, Fanciullacci F, Zanollo A. Pad controlled results of pelvic floor physiotherapy in female stress incontinence. Proceedings of the 3rd Joint Meeting, International Continence Society 16th Annual Meeting. Boston: Urodynamics Society, pp 233–235.

19 Klarskov P, Belving D, Bischoff N et al. Pelvic floor exercise versus surgery for female urinary stress incontinence. 1986; 41: 129–132.

20 Burgio KL, Robinson JC, Engel BT. The role of biofeedback in Kegel exercise training for stress urinary incontinence. Am J Obstet Gynecol 1986; 154: 58–64.

21 Henalla S, Hutchins CJ. Assessment of the value of physiotherapy in treatment of genuine stress incontinence by a weighed pyridium pad test. Proceedings of the 3rd Joint Meeting, International Continence Society 16th Annual Meeting 1986. Boston: Urodynamics Society, pp 413–415.

22 Benvenuti F, Caputo GM, Bandinelli S, Mayer F, Biagini C, Somavilla A. Reeducative treatment of female genuine stress incontinence. Am J Phys Med 1987; 66(4): 155–168.

23 Wilson PD, Sammarai TAL, Deakin M, Kolbe E, Brown ADG. An objective assessment of physiotherapy for female genuine stress incontinence. Br J Obstet Gynaecol 1987; 94: 575–582.

24 Tschou DCH, Adams C, Varner RE, Denton B. Pelvic floor musculature exercises in treatment of anatomical urinary stress incontinence. Phys Ther 1988; 68: 652–655.

25 Ferguson KL, McKey PL, Bishop KR, Kloen P, Verheul JB, Dougherty MC. Stress urinary incontinence: effect of pelvic muscle exercise. Obstet Gynecol 1990; 75: 671–675.

26 Klarskov P, Nielsen KK, Kromann-Andersen B. Long term results of pelvic floor training and surgery for female genuine stress incontinence. Int Urogynecol J 1991; 2: 132–135.

27 Mouritsen L, Frimodt-Moller C, Moller M. Long term effect of pelvic floor exercises on female urinary incontinence. Br J Urol 1991; 68: 32–37.

28 Cammu H, Van Nylen M, Derde MP. Pelvic physiotherapy in genuine stress incontinence. Urology 1991; 38: 332–337.

29 Hahn I, Sommar S, Fall M. A comparative study of pelvic floor training and electrical stimulation for the treatment of genuine female stress urinary incontinence. Neurourol Urodyn 1991; 10: 545–554.

30 Hahn I, Milsom I, Fall M, Ekelund P. Long term results of pelvic floor training in female stress urinary incontinence. Br J Urol 1993; 72: 421–427.

31 Bo K, Talseth T. Five year follow up of pelvic floor muscle exercise for treatment of stress urinary incontinence. Clinical and urodynamic assessment. Neurourol Urodyn 1994; 13(4): 374–376.

32 Tapp AJS, Hills B, Cardozo L. Who benefits from physiotherapy? Neurourol Urodyn 1988; 7: 259–265.

33 Bo K, Larsen S. Pelvic floor muscle exercise for treatment of female stress urinary incontinence: classification and characterisation of responders. Neurourol Urodyn 1992; 11: 497–507.

34 James ED, Shaldon CS, Niblett PG. Vaginal pressure: its role in urodynamic studies and in re-educating pelvic floor muscles. In: Proceedings of the 14th Annual Meeting of the International Continence Society, 1984; pp 150–151.

35 Gordon H, Logue M. Perineal muscle function after childbirth. Lancet 1985; 2: 123–125.

36 Dougherty MC, Abrams RM, McKey PL. An instrument to assess the dynamic characteristics of the circumvaginal musculature (CVM). Nurs Res 1986; 35: 202–206.

37 Laycock J, Jerwood D. A clinical study of the pelvic floor muscles by perineometry. Neurourol Urodyn 1991; 10(4): 390–391.

38 Wilson PD, Herbison GP, Heer K. Reproducibility of perineometry measurements. Neurourol Urodyn 1991; 10(4): 399–400.

39 Glavind K, Walter S, Nohr S. Biofeedback training of the pelvic floor muscles in the treatment of stress urinary incontinence. Neurourol Urodyn 1990; 9(4): 435–436.

40 Peattie AB, Plevnik S, Stanton SL. Vaginal cones: a conservative method of treating genuine stress incontinence. Br J Obstet Gynaecol 1988; 95: 1049–1053.

41 Olah KS, Bridges N, Denning J, Farrar DJ. The conservative management of patients with symptoms of stress incontinence: a randomised, prospective study comparing weighted vaginal cones and interferential therapy. Am J Obstet Gynecol 1990; 162: 87–92.

42 Haken J, Benness C, Cardozo L, Cutner A. A randomised trial of vaginal cones and pelvic floor exercises in the management of genuine stress incontinence. Neurourol Urodyn 1991; (4): 393–394.

43 Jonasson A, Larsson B, Pschera H. Testing and training of the pelvic floor muscles after childbirth. Acta Obstet Gynecol Scand 1989; 68: 301–306.

44 Norton P, Baker J, Randomised prospective trial of vaginal cones vs Kegel exercises in postpartum primiparous women. Neurourol Urodyn 1990; 9(4): 434–435.

45 Wise BG, Haken J, Cardozo LD, Plevnik S. A comparative study of vaginal cone therapy, cones + Kegel exercises and maximal electrical stimulation in the treatment of female genuine stress incontinence. Neurourol Urodyn 1993; 12(4): 436–437.

46 Laycock J, Green RJ. Interferential therapy in the treatment of incontinence. Physiotherapy 1988; 74: 161–168.

47 Savage B. Interferential therapy. London: Faber and Faber, 1984: pp 94–97.

48 De Domenico. New dimensions in interferential therapy. A theoretical and clinical guide. Lindfield, NSW: Reid Medical, pp 143–151.

49 Dougall DS. The effect of interferential therapy on incontinence and frequency of micturition. Physiotherapy 1985; 71: 135–136.

50 Henalla SM, Hutchins CJ, Castleden C. Conservative management of urethral sphincter incompetence. Neurourol Urodyn 1987; 6: 191–192.

51 Laycock J. Interferential therapy in the treatment of genuine stress incontinence. In: Proceedings of the 18th Annual Meeting of the International Continence Society, 1988: pp 268–269.

52 Laycock J, Jerwood D. Does pre-modulated interferential therapy cure genuine stress incontinence? Physiotherapy 1993; 79(8) 553–560.

53 Caldwell KPS. The electrical control of sphincter incompetence. Lancet 1963; 2: 174–175.

54 Hopkinson BR, Lightwood R. Electrical treatment of incontinence. Br J Surg 1967; 54: 802–805.

55 De Soldenhoff R, McDonnel H. New device for control of female urinary incontinence. Br Med J 1969; 4: 230.

56 Caldwell KPS, Cook PJ, Flack PC. Stress incontinence in females: report on 31 cases treated by electrical implant. J Obstet Gynaecol Br Cwlth 1968; 75: 777–780.

57 Suhel P, Krajl B, Plevnik S. Advances in nonimplantable electrical stimulators for correction of urinary incontinence. TITH Life Sci 1978; 8: 11–16.

58 Fall M. Does electrostimulation cure urinary incontinence? J Urol 1984; 131: 664–667.

59 Eriksen BC, Bergmann S, Mjolnerod OK. Effect of anal electrostimulation with the 'Incontan' device in women with urinary incontinence. Br J Obstet Gynaecol 1987; 94: 147–156.

60 Eriksen BC, Eik-Nes SH. Long-term electrostimulation of the pelvic floor: primary therapy in female stress incontinence? Urol Int 1989; 44: 90–95.

61 Erlandson BE, Fall M, Sundin T. Intravaginal electrical stimulation. Clinical experiments on urethral closure. Scand J Urol Nephrol 1977; (Suppl) 44(3): 31–39.

62 Plevnik S, Janez J, Vrtacnik P, Trasinar B, Vodusek DB. Short term electrical stimulation: home treatment for urinary incontinence. World J Urol 1986; 4: 24–26.

63 Jonasson A, Larsson B, Pschera H, Nylund L. Short-term maximal electrical stimulation – a conservative treatment of urinary incontinence. Gynecol Obstet Invest 1990; 30: 120–123.

64 Fall M, Erlandson BE, Ahlstrom K et al. Contelle: pelvic floor stimulator for female stress-urge incontinence. Urology 1986; 27(3): 282–287.

38

Behavioral therapy

INTRODUCTION

For those of us with small children, behavioral therapy for complete urinary incontinence forms part of everyday life. The success of training relies on the same elements that must be present for behavioral therapy for lower urinary tract dysfunction to succeed. There needs to be normal anatomy, neurology and function of the lower urinary tract. The cognitive state should be such as to perceive the need to void and the mood should encourage motivation for continence. Environmental and functional elements should be adapted to allow and encourage normal voiding.

The National Institute of Health consensus conference[1] concluded that the 'least invasive procedure should be tried first' when treating incontinence and that 'for many types of incontinence, behavioral treatments meet this criterion'. Behavioral therapy is perceived as a low-risk, safe alternative to other therapies with few if any of the side effects. Behavioral therapy, in many instances, may be nurse-based. Successful treatment can be achieved in patients with detrusor instability (DI), genuine stress incontinence (GSI) and detrusor–sphincter dyssynergia. The major disadvantages of behavioral therapy are the requirements for active patient participation and co-operation together with learning and skills that the patient may not possess and, above all, it is time-consuming. The major emphasis in medical schools is still on the surgical correction of incontinence[2] with arguments about different operative approaches reinforcing this. Besides that the specialties to which patients are often referred are surgical in nature (urology and gynecology), with distinct financial advantage to the consultant who operates. In many instances surgery does offer excellent results but it should be remembered that, given the choice, over 50% of women with GSI would elect to have conservative therapy.[2]

Behavioral therapy usually takes the form of operant learning, where behavior leading to favorable consequences is maintained and that with unfavorable results is discarded. To enhance behavioral modification biofeedback is used, where physiological responses are measured and using a display of this measurement the patient learns to change the physiological responses. In many instances several techniques are combined within one treatment regimen.[3] The role of psychological or emotional disturbance in the genesis of lower urinary tract dysfunction has been accepted since Mosso & Pellicani,[4] and in the case of DI this has been particularly developed by Frewen.[5,6] To confirm his theory, Frewen readily identified particular emotional or psychological elements from his patients' histories and he believed successful treatment of the bladder symptoms could be achieved with simple psychomedical measures.[6] The psychosomatic nature of DI has been recognized by many others.[7,8,9,10] However, such a causal relationship must be called into question,[11] as the symptoms of urgency and incontinence have profound effects on psychological and social functioning. Such psychological arguments reinforce the place of behavioral therapy in the treatment of DI. In GSI, where an anatomical defect is proposed as the causative abnormality, behavioral therapy in the form of biofeedback is used as a teaching method in conjunction with pelvic floor physiotherapy where, in many women, voluntary control of the pelvic floor has been lost even during intercourse.

Behavioral therapy by its very nature will not be suitable for all patients within the different diagnostic categories where efficacy has been demonstrated. The patient needs to be ambulant, motivated and cognizant, with intact neurology. Despite this, the behavioral treatment of prompted voiding does show some improvement in the continence of institutionalized non-ambulatory patients.

BIOFEEDBACK

Biofeedback uses the process of operant conditioning of physiological responses. However, simply learning how to inhibit bladder contractions or perform contractions of the pelvic floor is still a long way from using these learnt responses to alter bladder function. Biofeedback, in all instances, is used as a learning technique that is reinforced by training and exercising at home. Wilson in 1948[12] inadvertently discovered that the visual feedback of cystometrogram traces led to symptomatic improvement in half of his patients with urgency or incontinence. Kegel,[13] for stress incontinence, developed his perineometer to help women identify the pubococcygeal muscle. He could then assess the strength of the muscle and use the device to help instruct his patients. Unfortunately, the Kegel perineometer may be influenced by contraction of abdominal muscles alone and is much less commonly used than one might expect considering Kegel's published results. Digital examination of the vagina by the teacher offers a simple alternative but will inevitably be inaccurate and variable and would represent verbal feedback rather than biofeedback.

Cardozo et al[14,15] continued the development of biofeedback in DI using both visual and auditory feedback of detrusor contractions during repeated filling cystometry to teach the patients to inhibit their detrusor contractions. A more complex approach has been proposed which brings together the components of biofeedback used previously both for DI and GSI.[16] Here not only is there a pressure transducer in the bladder but there are simultaneous transducers at the anal sphincter and in the rectum, the latter measuring intra-abdominal pressure. Using this apparatus patients with DI can be taught voluntarily to inhibit detrusor contractions, relax their abdominal muscles and contract their pelvic floors. Patients with stress incontinence may be taught pelvic floor contraction alone without concomitant abdominal muscle contraction. Once these techniques have been taught by biofeedback, reinforcement at home with exercises is encouraged, although the best exercise regimen has still to be developed and tested against others.

Further developments in biofeedback for DI and GSI have included measuring urethral electromyographic activity, bladder neck conductance and the urethral pressure. Success of therapy with biofeedback not only rests with the appropriateness of the treatment but also depends considerably on patient and operator's motivation and the latter's skills. The techniques are time-consuming and require the patient to be ambulatory, cognizant, motivated and living independently.

Biofeedback as a method of treatment is usually combined with other behavioral therapies. The relative efficacy of biofeedback has been tested in a number of small trials. Shepherd et al[17] randomly allocated 22 women with stress incontinence to either pelvic floor exercises or pelvic floor exercises combined with biofeedback using a new kind of perineometer. Those treated with pelvic floor exercises alone showed a 55% rate of cure or improvement, whereas those treated with pelvic floor exercises combined with biofeedback had a 91% rate of cure or improvement. Burgio et al[18] had very similar results in 24 women with stress incontinence with either urethral sphincter biofeedback and pelvic floor exercises (92% cured or improved) or verbal feedback during vaginal palpation and pelvic floor exercises (55% cured or improved). Although these studies imply that biofeedback enhances traditional physiotherapy, other studies have failed to confirm this. Castleden et al[19] in a crossover study compared 2 weeks' physiotherapy with 2 weeks' physiotherapy plus biofeedback and could show no difference in efficacy. This study is open to criticism because of the very short time span for either treatment. Burton et al[20] looked at the role of their complex biofeedback techniques[16] in a mixed elderly population. The study has a number of design deficiencies but they failed to show that the addition of biofeedback improved results.

Eighteen-month follow up of patients treated with biofeedback for urgency or urge incontinence shows a 5–10% rate of relapse over this time in the 70% who were cured by the initial therapy.[21] The most important factor influencing short-term outcome with biofeedback is treatment compliance.[11] This also holds true for long-term outcome but presenting urological symptoms are also correlated with long-term success.[11] Not only does behavioral therapy and biofeedback improve urological symptoms, but measuring psychological functioning over 18 months shows improvement in psychological symptomatology and locus of control which is largely irrespective of the urological response.[11] Psychological factors that are predictive of poor outcome include excessive worry, preoccupation with illness and severe symptoms.

BLADDER RETRAINING

The rationale behind the use of bladder retraining is that voluntary repetitive efforts to suppress and initiate voiding will reinstate central control using the operant learning model where the reward is continence and praise from the trainer. Handley[22] has described four different schedules for bladder retraining. First there is 'prompted voiding', which is popular in institutionalized patients. Here patients are asked at regular intervals if they need to void and are assisted to the toilet. There is probably no long-term learnt benefit from this but there is a reduction in the number of incontinent episodes.[23,24] Secondly, there is 'timed voiding', where a fixed voiding schedule is implemented. This is very easy to organize and remember and is probably good treatment for volume-dependent DI. It is uncertain, however, if any long-term benefit will be achieved. Thirdly, there is 'habit retraining', where the patient is given an initial voiding interval that is modified to fit the habits of the patient. The patient then tries to increase the interval between voids. Finally, there is what we recognize as the widely practised 'bladder drill', when a fixed initial voiding interval is set just short of the natural voiding interval. Using the learnt techniques of abdominal relaxation, levator contraction and the suppression of urgency to inhibit detrusor contractions, the voiding intervals are progressively increased. These are recorded on charts with the final aim of the patient voiding every 3–4 h.

Prompted voiding and timed voiding are most commonly used in institutions. Prompted voiding requires greater commitment from the caring staff and therefore a distinct advantage of this over easily managed timed voiding has to be demonstrated. Burgio et al[23] allocated 41 incontinent elderly residents to different prompted voiding schedules on the basis of their previous incontinence. They were then transferred to a continence research unit. In their prompted voiding schedule a nurse greeted the patient, waited for a self-initiated request for toileting, checked the pad, prompted voiding and assisted the resident to the toilet. The nurse praised the resident if the pad was dry and was mildly disapproving if it was wet. The resident was then informed of the time of the next check. Using such a regimen continence can be improved and this improvement can be seen for up to 3 months after initiation of treatment; however, improvement may not be seen in those most severely incontinent. Prompted voiding intervals of 3 h with improvement of dryness are attainable and this negates some of the disadvantages of the increased nursing workload.

Probably the most important component of bladder drill is not responding to the desire to void by rushing to the toilet but suppressing the urge, remaining still and contracting the pelvic floor until the sensation passes. The evidence suggests that bladder drill is effective for the young, well-motivated woman but less effective in the elderly.[25] In the early 1980s there was a debate about the relative importance of in-patient and out-patient bladder drill. Fantl[26] has outlined an excellent 6-week out-patient bladder drill regimen for patients with DI where the patient is seen on a weekly basis. Patients receive written information and instructions. They are assigned a voiding schedule and inhibit at other times. They are informed that they will have to accept some accidents. Motivation and encouragement are an important part of the clinic visit. The goal for each patient is to be able to void every 3–4 h without urgency or incontinence between these times.

McClish et al[27] attempted to clarify the mechanism by which bladder drill works. They looked at the urodynamic changes before and 6 months after treatment in 108 women (76 GSI, 11 DI, 16 mixed). They found that neither urodynamic variables nor urodynamic diagnoses correlated with the change in the number of incontinent episodes. There was a 50% reduction in incontinent episodes regardless of the change in uro-dynamic diagnosis. They concluded that bladder drill is effective mainly through changes that are undetected by urodynamic techniques and that bladder drill affects behavior rather than laboratory–measured physiology.

DETRUSOR INSTABILITY

Behavioral therapy in many forms, including psychotherapy, behavioral modification and biofeedback, has been used to treat DI. Such treatments may also be combined with pharmacological agents. Frewen[5,6,28,29,30] has published extensively and did a great deal to popularize behavioral therapy in the United Kingdom. Frewen's regimen is commonly in-patient with an average stay of 10 days, although out-patient treatment is entirely acceptable and does not appear to jeopardize the results.[6] Frewen used a combination of bladder drill, anticholinergics, sedatives and simple psychotherapy. With such a regimen cure rates between 82%[28] and 97%[30] are attainable in women with DI. Six-year follow-up shows that those who became dry remain dry, although 34% need some retraining. Not only do the symptoms resolve with such treatment but cure is also associated with a return to normal cystometric findings,[6] although cystometric findings sometimes take longer than symptoms to resolve.

Elder & Stephenson[31] tested the Frewen regimen on 21 patients with a mean age of 45.8 years. Their patients were mixed and had either sensory urgency, DI or low compliance. Of these patients 86% responded, with 52% cured and 33% improved. This group found that only 28% of their patients reverted to stability on cystometric tracing. Low compliance was the cystometric abnormality most likely to revert to normal. Pengelly & Booth[32] had very similar results with the 26 patients who completed their trial. Of these 76% were cured or improved but only 32% had an improvement in cystometry. They found that site of treatment was not an independent variable, although patients were not formally randomized. Failure of therapy in their study was most commonly seen in women with a history of nocturnal enuresis after the age of 10 years, those with a strong isometric detrusor contraction on voiding cystometry and those who failed to show any improvement after the first 2 weeks' treatment.

Fantl et al[28,29] investigated the relative importance of the addition of anticholinergic agents to bladder drill. They found that 78% were cured with bladder drill alone and 83% with bladder drill combined with anticholinergics, and therefore concluded that bladder drill was an important independent variable. Of 8 women who failed with bladder drill alone, only 1 had symptomatic improvement when anticholinergic agents were added.

Cardozo et al,[14,15] using biofeedback as a primary treatment modality, have reported cure rates of 41% in women with DI with a further 40% experiencing some improvement. Burgio et al,[16] with a more complex biofeedback technique, have shown reduction of incontinent episodes by 85% in elderly women with urge incontinence. In a subgroup of patients with sensory urgency there was a 94% reduction in incontinent episodes.[17] Of the 18 women, however, 12 still had some incontinence after treatment. Elderly women do not respond as well as younger women, as Ouslander et al[33] demonstrated (only a 25% reduction in incontinent episodes).

STRESS INCONTINENCE

Despite Kegel[34] reporting a remarkable 90% improvement rate in 455 women with stress incontinence in 1956, it has taken several decades for pelvic floor physiotherapy and biofeedback to compete with surgery as the treatment modality of choice in patients with stress incontinence. Indeed over 50% of women with stress incontinence would prefer conservative therapy.[2] Burgio et al,[16] using a biofeedback technique that resolved the criticism of the effect of abdominal pressure on the Kegel perineometer, have seen an 82% reduction in incontinent episodes in elderly women and Burgio et al[16] and Shepherd[17] have found that biofeedback enhances the efficacy of physiotherapy in stress incontinence by 40%.

Burns et al[35] randomly allocated 123 women with GSI to either pelvic exercises, pelvic floor exercises and biofeedback or control. In this study a vaginal probe was used to measure levator electromyographic activity as the biofeedback. At 3 months the group using the biofeedback plus physiotherapy had 61% fewer losses, whereas the group using physiotherapy alone had a reduction of 54%. Surprisingly, a similar impact was seen regardless of whether the patient had previously undergone incontinence surgery. Of the biofeedback group 23% had a complete cure and of those in the physiotherapy group 16% had a complete cure. The greatest improvement was seen in those women who presented with severe incontinence. The greatest improvement in electromyographic activity was seen in the group using biofeedback. Although not conclusive, this study suggests that biofeedback in combination with physiotherapy may be the non-surgical choice in those with severe incontinence.

DETRUSOR–SPHINCTER DYSSYNERGIA

Biofeedback from the external urethral sphincter[36] or the anal sphincter[37] has been reported to improve continence in patients with detrusor–sphincter dyssynergia.

CONCLUSION

Behavioral therapy either as a primary treatment or in conjunction with other treatments is effective in women with DI or GSI. It is a treatment relatively free from side effects and should form the first line of therapy in motivated, cognizant women with urinary incontinence. It requires considerable time and effort. Therefore facilities should be established, staffed and appropriately funded.

REFERENCES

1 NIH Consensus Conference: urinary incontinence in adults. JAMA 1989; 261: 2685–2696.
2 Richardson PA. Conservative management of urinary incontinence. J Repod Med 1993; 38(1): 659–661.
3 Burgio KL. Behavioral training for stress and urge incontinence in the community. Gerontology 1990; 36 (Suppl): 27–34.
4 Mosso A, Pellicani P. Sur les functions de la vessie. Archives Italiennes de Biologie 1882; 1: 97–128.
5 Frewen WK. Urinary incontinence. Journal of Obstetrics and Gynaecology of the British Commonwealth. 1972; 79: 77–79.
6 Frewen WK. An objective assessment of the unstable bladder of psychosomatic origin. Br J Urol. 1978; 50: 246–249.
7 Smith DR. Psychosomatic cystitis. J Urol 1962; 87: 359.
8 Hafner J, Stanton SL, Guy J. A psychiatric study of women urgency and urgency incontinence. Br J Urol 1977; 49(3): 211–214.
9 Jeffcoate TN, Francis WJ. Urgency incontinence in the female. Am J Obstet Gynecol 1966; 94: 604 618.
10 Cherluk L, Bourguingono O, Guillon F, Aboulker P. Psychosomatic Medicine 1977; 3: 68.
11 Oldenburg B, Millard RJ. Predictors of long term outcome following a bladder retraining programme. J Psychosomatic Research 1986; 30(6): 691–698.
12 Wilson TS. Incontinence of urine in the aged. Lancet 1948; 2: 374–377.
13 Kegel AH. Progressive resistance exercise in the functional restoration of the perineal muscles. Am J Obstet Gynecol 1948; 56: 238–248.
14 Cardozo LD, Abrams PD, Stanton SL et al. Idiopathic bladder instability treated by biofeedback. Br J Urol 1978; 50: 27–30.
16 Burgio KL, Whitehead WE, Engel BT. Urinary incontinence in the elderly: bladder/sphincter biofeedback and toileting skills training. Ann Intern Med 1985; 103: 507–515.
17 Shepherd AM, Montgomery E, Anderson RS. Treatment of genuine stress incontinence with a new perineometer. Physiotherapy 1983; 69: 113.
18 Burgio KL, Robinson JC, Engel BT. The role of biofeedback in Kegel exercise training for stress urinary incontinence. Am J Obstet Gynecol 1986; 154: 58–64.
19 Castleden CM, Duffin NM, Mitchell ED. The effect of physiotherapy on stress incontinence. Age Ageing 1984; 13: 235–237.
20 Burton JR, Pearce KL, Burgio KL et al. Behavioral training for urinary incontinence in elderly ambulatory patients. J Am Geriatr Soc 1988; 36: 693–698.
21 Millard RJ, Oldenburg B. The symptomatic, urodynamic and psychodynamic results of bladder re-education programmes. J Urol 1989; 130: 715–719.
22 Handley EC. Bladder training and related therapies for urinary incontinence in older people. JAMA 1986; 256: 372.

23 Burgio LD, McCormick KA, Scheve AS, Engel BT, Hawkins S, Leahy E. The effects of changing prompted voiding schedules in the treatment of incontinence in nursing home residents. JAGS 1994; 42: 315–320.

24 Creason NS, Grybowski JA, Burgeno S, Whippo C, Yeo S, Richardson B. Prompted voiding therapy for urinary incontinence in aged female nursing home residents. J of Advanced Nursing 1989; 14: 120–126.

25 Sand PK, Brubaker L. Non surgical treatment of detrusor overactivity in post menopausal women. J Repod Med 1990; 35(8): 758–765.

26 Fantl A. Behavioral therapy for detrusor instability of idiopathic etiology.

27 McClisk DK, Fantl JA, Wyman JF, Pisani G, Bump RC. Bladder training in older women with urinary incontinence: relationship between outcome and changes in urodynamic observations. Obstet Gynecol 1991; 77(2): 281–286.

28 Frewen W. Role of bladder training in the treatment of the unstable bladder in the female. Urol Clin North Am 1976; 6: 273.

29 Frewen W. The significance of the psychosomatic factor in urge incontinence. Br J Urol 1984; 56: 330.

30 Frewen WK. A reassessment of bladder training in detrusor dysfunction in the female. Br J Urol 1982; 54: 372.

31 Elder DD, Stephenson TP. An assessment of the Frewen regimen in the treatment of detrusor dysfunction in females. Br J Urol 1980; 52: 467–471.

32 Pengelly AW, Booth CM. A prospective trial of bladder training as treatment of detrusor instability. Br J Urol 1980; 52: 463–466.

33 Ouslander JG, Blaustein J, Conner A et al. Habit training and oxybutynin for incontinence in nursing home patients: a placebo controlled trial. J Am Geriatr Soc 1988; 36: 40.

34 Kegel AH. Stress incontinence in women: physiologic treatment. J Int Coll Surg 1956; 25: 487–499.

35 Burns PA, Pranikoff K, Nochajski TH, Hadley EC, Levy KJ, Org MG. A comparison of effectiveness of biofeedback and pelvic muscle exercise treatment of stress incontinence in older community dwelling women. J Gerontology 1993; 48(4): 167–174.

36 Wear JB, Wear RB, Cleeland C. Biofeedback in urology using urodynamics: preliminary observation. J Urol 1979; 121: 464–468.

37 Maizels M, King LR, Firlit CF. Urodynamic biofeedback: a new approach to treat vesical sphincter dyssynergia. J Urol 1979; 122: 205–209.

Electrical therapy

39

INTRODUCTION

Therapeutic electrical stimulation for lower urinary tract dysfunction is not a new method of treatment. As early as 1895, it was discovered that stimulation of the proximal stump of a transected pudendal nerve resulted in profound inhibition of the detrusor in the cat.[1]

During the 1960s interest in electrical therapy increased to such a degree that by the end of the decade several commercially available products had been evaluated. They were devised to treat patients with stress incontinence who had not benefited from conventional incontinence surgery, which at that time usually meant anterior colporrhaphy.

In 1963 Caldwell[2] presented the results in two patients of a radio-controlled electrode implant inserted into the anal sphincter. One patient with intractable fecal incontinence was treated for 4 months using continuous stimulation. This resulted in continence which persisted even when the stimulation was turned off. A second female patient with urinary incontinence of unspecified cause was similarly cured.

Alexander & Rowan[3] showed that sustained stimulation of the levator ani muscles, using electrodes in close proximity to the pudendal nerves, prevented escape of urine from the bladder in dogs. Following this, they reported a series of 14 patients treated using a radio implant similar to that of Caldwell[4]. The platinum electrodes were inserted transperineally and attached using non-absorbable sutures to the periosteum of the ischium. The exact position was chosen following test stimulation to locate the point of maximal perineal contraction. Leads from the electrodes were tunnelled subcutaneously to the receiver stimulator which was positioned deep to the anterior rectus sheath or subcutaneously in fat patients. Of the 14 patients treated, 10 were women and 4 were men. Eight women with stress incontinence, 5 of whom had undergone an anterior repair on one or more occasion, were treated using the device. Four cases were deemed successful with 2 women cured of their incontinence, whilst no improvement was seen in 4 cases. Six patients with detrusor hyperreflexia were also treated and in 5 cases significant symptomatic improvement was achieved. Surgical complications included inflammation at the site of the receiver stimulator (7 cases) and ulceration of the implant through the abdominal wall (4 cases). They proposed that the mode of action of the stimulator was by increased urethral intraluminal pressure during stimulation. They noted, however, that results were better in patients with 'precipitancy' incontinence rather than stress incontinence and suggested that pelvic floor stimulation resulted in inhibition of the detrusor.

Due to the high complication rate associated with implanted stimulators, external devices were developed. Initially, they were proposed for the treatment of stress incontinence. Alexander & Rowan adapted a Portex ring pessary using two stainless steel wire electrodes.[5] The two coils of ten turns each were wound on to the pessary at an angle of 60–70° to each other. A flexible cable from the pessary was connected to an external stimulator. The pessary was inserted with the electrodes anteriorly and continuous stimulation applied except during micturition. One case was reported of a patient with stress incontinence in whom the pessary alone did not improve symptoms. Following 3 months' electrical stimulation substantial symptomatic improvement was reported.

In a similar way, the Hodge pessary was adapted. Contrary to the case with the ring pessary the electrodes could not be dislodged by rotation, or the wires broken by repeated distorsion of the ring. In one study, 79 patients with urethral sphincter weakness were treated using this device. Twenty-seven cases (33%) were reported as successful.[6]

The vaginal 'Continator' was produced by Vitalograph Ltd in 1969. This consisted of a vaginal pessary, similar in size to a sanitary tampon, connected to an external pulse generator. Twenty-eight women with stress incontinence in combination with varying degrees of cystocele, rectocele and uterine prolapse were treated for 2–3 months using continuous daytime stimulation. Twenty-three were judged to be cured or controlled by the device up to 2 years after commencing therapy.[7]

An external device using an anal electrode was deviced by Hopkinson & Lightwood[8]. Of 9 female patients treated, a successful outcome was achieved in 3 cases.

An automatic electrical stimulator containing a battery inside the vaginal plug electrode was designed by Suhel[9]. The device was automatically turned on when the electrodes touched the vaginal walls and stopped when removed and dried. A similar device has been developed and evaluated by Eriksen et al[10] using chronic anal electrical stimulation for the treatment of stress incontinence, urge incontinence and mixed incontinence. Stimulation was carried out for between 6 and 20 hs/day for 3–36 months (mean 8.8 months). Of 121 patients who entered the study, 23 (19%) did not complete 3 months' therapy and were excluded. Overall 50% became continent and were able to discontinue treatment, 12% needed continuous stimulation to remain continent, 29% were symptomatically improved, and 9% showed no therapeutic effect. Continence was achieved in 64% with stress incontinence, 65% with detrusor instability and 53% with mixed incontinence.

The different electrical parameters employed, the number of patients treated and the reported success rates of these early stimulators are shown in Table 39.1.

All the studies mentioned so far used continuous stimulation, and the devices were primarily designed to treat stress incontinence. Although moderate success rates were obtained in such cases, women with urge incontinence benefited more.

Table 39.1 Stimulation parameters, type of device and success rates of early studies of electrical stimulation for the treatment of urinary incontinence

Author	Freq. (Hz)	Pulse width (mS)	Device	No. of pts. (Treatment)	Success (%)
Caldwell 1963[2]	25–200	0.1–1.0	Implant	2	100
Alexander & Rowan 1968[4]	20	1	Implant	14	GSI 50 DI 83
Alexander & Rowan 1968[5]	20	1	Electronic ring pessary	1	100
Hopkinson & Lightwood 1967	200	1	Anal plug	9	33
DeSoldenhoff & McDonnel 1969[7]	120	0.2	Vaginal electrode	28	82
Doyle et al 1974[6]	200	1	Electronic Hodge pessary	79	33
Suhel 1976[9]	0.5–60	0.2–3.0	Automatic vaginal electrode	Not stated	80

More recently, greater attention has been paid to the effects of electrical stimulation on detrusor inhibition. Inhibition of the detrusor on vaginal or anal dilatation was originally observed in the cat.[11] The same phenomenon was shown to occur in humans following mechanical stimulation of the perineum. Pin-prick stimulation,[12] penile squeeze[13] and anal dilatation[14] all produce similar effects. DeGroat & Ryall[15] demonstrated that such physical stimulation evoked inhibitory postsynaptic potentials and inhibition of discharges in parasympathetic neurones due to a spinal reflex with a somatic (pudendal) afferent limb.

Pompeius[16] concluded that anal stimulation resulted in detrusor inhibition due to a sacral spinal reflex with its afferent pathway in the pudendal nerves and its efferent pathway in the pelvic nerves.

In an experiment using anesthetized cats, anal stimulation at high intravesical pressure resulted in bladder inhibition via a pudendal to pelvic nerve reflex. Electrical stimulation of the proximal end of the pudendal nerve at low bladder pressures induced bladder relaxation via a pudendal to hypogastric nerve reflex[17]. These same reflex pathways were shown to be activated by intravaginal electrical stimulation in cats.[18]

Lindstrom et al[19] were able to record directly from the hypogastric and pelvic nerves during intravaginal electrical stimulation in anesthetized cats. During electrical stimulation, a long-lasting reflex discharge with a latency of 35–50 ms was recorded in the hypogastric nerve. This effect was found to be frequency-dependent with a maximal response at 5 Hz. When bladder pressure was elevated, intravaginal electrical stimulation resulted in abolition of the spontaneous efferent activity in the pelvic nerves. This latter effect was maximal at 5–10 Hz.

The role of the sympathetic nervous system in the control of the human bladder is disputed and so it is more likely that the pudendal to pelvic reflex is the most important pathway responsible for detrusor inhibition following electrical stimulation in man.

Godec et al[20] were the first to use the principles of bladder inhibition clinically. They employed acute maximal electrical stimulation using an anal plug electrode in 40 patients with detrusor hyperreflexia. Treatment was administered on one occasion and only repeated if required. During stimulation 31/40 (78%) showed reduced or absent hyperreflexia. The degree of inhibition was greater than that achieved by manual anal stimulation. An increase in anal pressure during electrical stimulation was found to be a useful prognostic indicator of likely success of chronic electrical stimulation. Those with a poor sphincter response and severe denervation of the pelvic floor were deemed unsuitable for chronic electrical stimulation. An intact or at least partially intact reflex arc appears to be necessary for successful treatment with electrical stimulation. The beneficial effect of acute stimulation in this paper was seen to continue after cessation of therapy, the so-called carry-over effect. This phenomenon was first described by Moore & Schofield,[21] who treated 18 patients with stress incontinence due to pelvic floor weakness using acute maximal perineal stimulation. Ten out of the 18 were completely or partially cured of their symptoms, giving an efficacy comparable to that of chronic stimulation. This important discovery has led several authors to investigate the efficacy of short-term repetitive stimulation as opposed to the chronic continuous stimulation that was employed in earlier studies.

It has been shown that mechanical anal stimulation and vaginal and anal electrical stimulation activate the same pelvic reflex mechanisms which lead to detrusor inhibition. It was originally believed that pelvic floor contraction was an essential part of this mechanism; however, stimulation of non-muscular pudendal nerve afferents has been shown to evoke the same response. Stimulation of the dorsal nerve of the penis was found to have a beneficial effect in 10 of 22 patients.[22] Of 10 patients with detrusor instability, 7 were found to be stable during penile electrical stimulation. Penile or clitoral stimulation using surface electrodes at a stimulus intensity up to 3.5 times the threshold for eliciting the bulbocavernous reflex was found to improve cystometric capacity in 10 patients with suprasacral spinal cord injuries and objectively demonstrable detrusor hyperreflexia.[23] Even electrical stimulation of the common peroneal and posterior tibial nerve has been reported to induce bladder inhibition in a study of 15 patients[24]

Direct stimulation of the pudendal nerve was reported in a pilot study of 3 patients with detrusor hyperreflexia.[25] Satisfactory inhibition of the detrusor was achieved using a stimulus intensity much lower than that required for intravaginal or anal stimulation. It was suggested that the high stimulus intensity necessary for the latter methods was a result of suboptimal stimulus delivery through anal and vaginal electrodes. Ohlsson et al[26] reported 2 cases in which combined intravaginal and intra-anal maximal electrical stimulation (MES) was found to be of no benefit. Direct pudendal nerve stimulation, however, produced a decrease in urinary frequency and an increase in bladder capacity in both cases. It appears that direct pudendal nerve stimulation is a more sensitive and specific means of evoking detrusor inhibition.

The electrical parameters employed in different stimulators are not uniform. The most important parameter appears to be the frequency of the stimulus applied. Fall et al[18] established that a frequency of 5–10 Hz produced the most marked detrusor inhibition in cats, whilst between 20 and 50 Hz was optimal for sphincter closure. In clinical trials, however, stimulation at 5 Hz was found to be less well tolerated and 10 Hz has been suggested as the optimal frequency for bladder inhibition.[19] Vereeken et al[27], however, found no difference in the degree of bladder inhibition upon stimulation with frequencies of 5, 10 or 20 Hz.

The stimulus intensity required depends on the diameter of the afferent nerves involved and the distance from the stimulating electrode. Intravaginal or intra-anal electrical stimulation activates mechanoreceptors supplied with low-threshold myelinated afferents. The threshold for reflex activation is close to the perception threshold in man. Maximal bladder inhibition is achieved at an intensity of stimulation two to three times the threshold intensity; however, such levels are painful. The maximum tolerated level is usually 1.5–2 times the perception threshold.[28] For practical purposes the stimulators used clinically, including those termed 'maximal,' utilize suboptimal stimulus intensity.

Short square wave pulses are most efficient in terms of nerve stimulation. This minimizes the charge transfer required to achieve depolarization of pudendal afferents. A pulse duration of 0.2 ms has been found to be optimal for exciting both sensory and motor nerves in the perineal region[29] This is less than the commonly employed pulse duration of 1 ms, which delivers three times the charge and energy per pulse. Regulated current (constant current) charge balanced biphasic stimulation has been shown to minimize electrochemical processes at the metal-tissue interface, and minimizes tissue injury and electrode corrosion. The stimulation parameters produced by this device are shown in Table 39.2.

Several studies have reported results in women with detrusor instability and genuine stress incontinence following electrical stimulation using the Conmax stimulator. The original work on short-term home electrical stimulation by Plevnik et al[30] was carried out using this device Fig. 19.4. Three hundred and ten unselected men and women with urinary incontinence of differing etiologies were treated with the device either at home or in the clinic. Daily stimulation for 20 min was carried out for 30 days. Outcome was assessed subjectively by questioning on frequency and severity of incontinence following treatment. Overall 56% were cured

Table 39.2 Stimulation parameters of the Conmax intravaginal electrical stimulator

Device	Conmax
Electrodes	Intravaginal/intra-anal
Stimulus configuration	Biphasic, charge balanced, continuous
Pulse amplitude	0–90 mA
Pulse duration	0.75 ms
Pulse frequency	20 Hz
Maximum charge per pulse	67.5 mcC
Maximum current density	6 mcA/mm2
Maximum average charge density	0.3 mcC/mm2
Treatment duration	20 min/day (automatic switch off)

Table 39.3 Success rate by diagnosis for short-term maximal electrical stimulation

Diagnosis	Cured	Improved	Failed
Genuine stress incontinence (GSI)	25	13	42
Detrusor instability (DI)	20	15	32
Mixed (GSI + DI)	14	10	27
Detrusor hyperreflexia	13	10	12
Post-prostatectomy (USI)	3	1	8
Post-prostatectomy (DI)	6	2	4
Enuresis	19	23	11
Total	100 (32%)	74 (24%)	136 (44%)

or improved following therapy. The breakdown of outcome by diagnosis is shown in Table 39.3.

More recently, Jonasson et al[31] treated 17 women with genuine stress incontinence and 20 with detrusor instability using the Conmax stimulator for a period of 12 weeks. Eight out of the 17 women with genuine stress incontinence were subjectively improved, and a significant reduction in leakage on pad testing was seen in 12 cases. In the detrusor instability group, 14 out of the 20 women noticed symptomatic improvement, with 19 showing decreased leakage on pad testing.

Intravaginal MES has been compared to standard conservative treatments for both genuine stress incontinence and detrusor instability.[32] For women with genuine stress incontinence MES was found to be less effective, in terms of symptomatic improvement, than vaginal cone therapy in combination with Kegel exercises. Following a 10-week treatment period with MES, no significant reduction in urinary leakage on pad testing was observed.[33]

Maximal electrical stimulation was compared to oxybutynin in a prospective, randomized study of 60 women with idiopathic detrusor instability or detrusor hyperreflexia[32]. Oxybutynin therapy resulted in greater subjective and objective improvement, but was associated with significant side effects and a high rate of discontinuation of therapy. Following MES therapy, 18% of women were converted to a stable bladder while 60% showed improvement in volume at first sensation to void or cystometric capacity. Seventy-five per cent of women showed a reduced maximum detrusor pressure during cystometry following MES therapy. Intravaginal MES was almost universally acceptable and therefore provides a useful alternative treatment for those women who do not tolerate or benefit from anticholinergic therapy.

Transcutaneous electrical nerve stimulation over the S3 dermatome has been reported effectively to stabilize the detrusor during acute stimulation in women with idiopathic detrusor instability.[34] It may provide an alternative home electrical therapy to MES for the treatment of detrusor instability.

Functional electrical neuromodulation using surgically implanted sacral foramen electrodes has been employed for both detrusor instability and chronic urinary retention. In selected cases S3 stimulation may result in improvement in the symptoms associated with detrusor instability, although objective urodynamic changes following treatment were minimal.[35]

Nine patients with 'idiopathic' chronic urinary retention, associated with abnormal myotonic-like activity of the pelvic floor, inappropriately high urethral pressure profiles and inability to initiate a detrusor contraction during cystometry were treated using a permanent sacral foramen electrode. S3 stimulation was employed and the patients were able to void after deactivation of the continuous stimulation.[36] As with all implantable electrodes, problems with infection, migration of the electrodes and mechanical failure are common complications.

Electrical stimulation of sacral anterior nerve roots, usually combined with division of posterior sacral nerve roots, provides an effective method of managing the bladder of some patients with suprasacral spinal cord injury.[37] Sacral deafferentation produces an areflexic bladder capable of storing large volumes of urine at low pressure. This contributes to continence and protects the upper tracts. It also serves to abolish detrusor-sphincter dyssynergia and autonomic dysreflexia. Electrical stimulation of anterior roots results in detrusor contraction but also in contraction of the urethral rhabdosphincter. In between bursts of stimulation, the urethral sphincter relaxes rapidly whilst the detrusor contraction persists, resulting in bladder emptying leaving small residual volumes of urine. Urinary infection and bacteriuria are reduced, vesicoureteric reflux may be improved, and long-term results over 15 years suggest that technical problems are uncommon and the nerve roots are not damaged by chronic electrical stimulation.[38]

CONCLUSIONS

At present, electrical therapy cannot be advocated as first-line therapy for either detrusor instability or genuine stress incontinence. Alternative treatments are available for both conditions with greater efficacy. Maximal electrical stimulation should be offered to women who cannot tolerate the side effects of anticholinergic medication, but the results are unpredictable. From clinical experience, those patients with detrusor hyperreflexia respond less favorably than women with idiopathic detrusor instability, possibly due to loss of integrity of the necessary reflex pathways. Sacral deafferentation and anterior root stimulation are reserved for selected cases of suprasacral spinal cord injury.

In the conservative management of genuine stress incontinence, MES is less effective than conventional Kegel exercises in combination with vaginal cones, and other modalities of electrical therapy confer no added benefit.

Functional electromodulation is an invasive procedure which has yet to be fully evaluated. It should be reserved only for patients with intractable symptoms in whom conventional management for detrusor hyperreflexia or idiopathic retention has failed.

REFERENCES

1 Griffiths J. Observations on the urinary bladder and urethra. Part 2. The nerves. Part 3. Physiological Journal of Anatomy and Physiology 1895; 29(61): 254.

2 Caldwell KPS. The electrical control of sphincter incompetence. Lancet 1963; 2: 174–175.

3 Alexander S, Rowan D. Closure of the urinary sphincter mechanism in anaesthetised dogs by means of electrical stimulation of the perineal muscles. Br J Surg 1966; 53: 1053–1056.

4 Alexander S, Rowan D. Electrical control of urinary incontinence by radio implant. (A report of fourteen patients). Br J Surg 1968; 55(5): 358–364.

5 Alexander S, Rowan D. An electric pessary for stress incontinence. Lancet 1968; 1: 7–28.

6 Doyle PT, Edwards LE, Harrison NW, Malvern J, Stanton SL. Treatment of urinary incontinence by external stimulating devices. Urol Int 1974; 29: 450–457.

7 De Soldenhoff R, McDonnel H. New device for control of female urinary incontinence. Br Med J 1969; 4: 230.

8 Hopkinson BR, Lightwood R. Electrical treatment of incontinence. Br J Surg 1967; 54: 802–805.

9 Suhel P. Adjustable nonimplantable electrical stimulators for correction of urinary incontinence. Urol Int 1976; 31: 115–123.

10 Eriksen BC, Bergmann S, Mjolnerod OK. Effect of anal electrostimulation with the 'Incontan' device in women with urinary incontinence. Br J Obstet Gynaecol 1987; 94: 147–156.

11 Langworthy OR, Hesser FH. Reflex vesical contraction in the cat after transection of the spinal cord in the lower lumbar region. Bulletin of the Johns Hopkins Hospital 1937; 60: 204–214.

12 Parker MM, Rose DK. Inhibition of the bladder. Arch Surg 1937; 34: 828–838.

13 Kondo A, Otani T, Takita T. Suppression of bladder instability by penile squeeze. Br J Urol 1982; 54: 360–362.

14 Kock NG, Pompeius R. Inhibition of vesical motor activity induced by anal stimulation. Acta Chir Scand 1963; 126: 244–250.

15 De Groat WC, Ryall RW. Reflexes to sacral parasympathetic neurones concerned with micturition in the cat. J Physiol (Lond) 1969; 200: 87–108.

16 Pompeius R. Detrusor inhibition induced from anal region in man. Göteborg: Elanders Boktyckeri, 1966.

17 Sundin T, Carlsson CA, Knock NG. Detrusor inhibition induced from mechanical stimulation of the anal region and from electrical stimulation of pudendal nerve afferents. Invest Urol 1974; 11(5): 374–378.

18 Fall M, Erlandson BE, Carlsson CA, Lindstrom S. The effect of intravaginal electrical stimulation on the feline urethra and bladder. Neurological mechanisms. Scand J Urol Nephrol 1977; Suppl 44(2): 19–30.

19 Lindstrom S, Fall M, Carlsson CA, Erlandson BE. The neurophysiological basis of bladder inhibition in response to intravaginal electrical stimulation. J Urol 1983; 129: 405–410.

20 Godec C, Cass AS, Ayala GF. Bladder inhibition with functional electrical stimulation. Urology 1975; 6(6): 663–666.

21 Moore T, Schofield PF. Treatment of stress incontinence by maximum perineal stimulation. Br Med J 1967; 3: 150.

22 Nakamura M, Sakurai T. Bladder inhibition by penile electrical stimulation. Br J Urol 1984; 56: 413–415.

23 Vodusek DB, Light JK, Libby J. Detrusor inhibition induced by stimulation of pudendal nerve afferents. Neurourol Urodyn 1986; 5: 381–389.

24 McGuire EJ, Shi-Chun Z, Horwinski ER, Lytton B. Treatment of motor and sensory detrusor instability by electrical stimulation. J Urol 1983; 129: 78–79.

25 Vodusek DB, Plevnik S, Vrtacnik P, Janez J. Detrusor inhibition on selective pudendal nerve stimulation in the perineum. Neurourol Urodyn 1988; 6: 389–393.

26 Ohlsson BL, Fall M, Frankenberg-Sommar S. Effects of external and direct pudendal nerve maximal electrical stimulation in the treatment of the uninhibited overactive bladder. Br J Urol 1989; 64: 374–380.

27 Vereecken R, Das J, Grisaf P. Electrical sphincter stimulation in the treatment of detrusor hyperreflexia of paraplegics. Neurourol Urodyn 1984; 3: 145–154.

28 Ohlsson BL. Effects of some different pulse parameters on the perception of intravaginal and intra-anal electrical stimulation. Med Biol Eng Comput 1988; 26: 503–505.

29 Plevnik S, Janez J, Vrtacnik P. Optimization of pulse duration for electrical stimulation in treatment of urinary incontinence. World J Urol 1986; 4: 22–23.

30 Plevnik S, Janez J, Vrtacnik P, Trasinar B, Vodusek DB. Short term electrical stimulation: home treatment for urinary incontinence. World J Urol 1986; 4: 24–26.

31 Jonasson A, Larsson B, Pschera H, Nylund L. Short-term maximal electrical stimulation – a conservative treatment of urinary incontinence. Gynecol Obstet Invest 1990; 30: 120–123.

32 Wise BG. A clinical evaluation of maximal electrical stimulation in the management of female lower urinary tract dysfunction. MD Thesis, University of London, 1996.

33 Wise BG, Haken J, Cardozo LD, Plevnik S. A comparative study of vaginal cones, cones plus Kegel exercises and maximal electrical stimulation in the treatment of female genuine stress incontinence. Neurourol Urodyn 1993; 12(4): 436–437.

34 Webb RJ, Powell PH. Transcutaneous electrical nerve stimulation in patients with idiopathic detrusor instability. Neurourol Urodyn 1992; 11(4): 327–328.

35 Thon WF. Functional electrical neuromodulation of voiding dysfunction using foramen electrodes: results of the European Study Group. Neurourol Urodyn 1992; 11(4): 325–327.

36 Thon WF, Grunewald V, Hofner K, Kramer AEJL, Jonas U. Sacral spinal nerve neuromodulation for the treatment of idiopathic chronic urinary retention. Neurourol Urodyn 1993; 12(4): 385–386.

37 Brindley G, Polkey C, Rushton D, Cardozo L. Sacral anterior root stimulators for bladder control in paraplegia: the first 50 cases. J. Neurol Neurosurg Psychiatry 1986; 49: 1104–1114.

38 VanKerrebroeck P. World wide experience with the Finetech-Brindley sacral anterior root stimulator. Neurourol Urodyn 1993; 12: 497–503.

40

Acupuncture and the bladder

INTRODUCTION

The medical profession has remained suspicious of acupuncture since its introduction into Western Europe in the seventeenth century. This suspicion is founded firstly on disbelief that the insertion of acupuncture needles can exert any more than a powerful placebo effect, and secondly on the reluctance to accept the traditional philosophical theories of the yin and yang into modern medical doctrine. Over the years doubt has slowly dissipated as scientific evidence to support the neurophysiological basis of acupuncture has accumulated.

Acupuncture is of proven value for the relief of musculoskeletal, neurological and visceral disorders and is commonly used in pain clinics. Despite its use for hundreds of years in China to treat many other conditions, including lower urinary tract dysfunction, it has rarely been used for these indications in the West. Neurogenic bladder dysfunction is, however, included in the World Health Organization list of indications for acupuncture.[1]

Acupuncture has many potential benefits, such as the relative absence of side effects, a high degree of patient compliance and the limited expense of acupuncture needles. Unfortunately, at present an appropriate placebo for use in acupuncture studies is unavailable and therefore trials are largely uncontrolled. The use of acupuncture for the management of bladder symptoms, although promising, awaits further clinical evaluation.

Ancient Chinese theory

About 200 years before the Christian era, the basic tenets of Chinese medicine were recorded in a classic work the *Huang Di Nei Jing*, the Yellow Emperor's textbook of physical medicine.[2] Ancient Chinese doctors saw man in a constant equilibrium of 'qi' (vital energy), and 'yin and yang' (forces of opposite polarity), their imbalance resulting in many different pathological processes. The yin and yang give rise to the flow of qi which accumulates in the organs and flows in channels or meridians between them. According to traditional Chinese theory, most illnesses are rooted in the flow of qi, which may be either excessive, deficient or stagnant. It is possible to exert a direct effect on the channels and organs and thus in turn on bodily functions by needling specific acupuncture points.

It is partly a failure by traditional acupuncturists to relinquish this ancient Chinese theory in favor of modern scientific principles that has resulted in widespread suspicion of acupuncture treatment.

Mechanism of action of acupuncture

Originally acupuncture was considered to be a form of hypnosis or suggestion,[3] but experiments on animals, which are neither easily hypnotized nor open to suggestion but do respond to acupuncture, suggest that many other mechanisms of action exist.[4] Double-blind experimental analgesia has shown false suggestion to be worthless for acupuncture analgesia in humans, and this and other physiological studies do not support hypnosis[5] or suggestion as a real mechanism of action of acupuncture. Moreover, acupuncture analgesia is effective even under anesthesia.[6]

Recently, a more scientific understanding of acupuncture has evolved, resulting primarily from the ability to detect and assay neurohumeral transmitter substances. The observation of a delay in acupuncture-induced analgesia, and the persistent effect after the cessation of needling, suggested the release of a humeral mediator. The Research Group of Acupuncture Anaesthesia[7] reported that the transfer of cerebrospinal fluid from rabbits receiving acupuncture resulted in analgesia in recipient animals. Clement Jones et al[8] have since shown an increase in the activity of opiate-like substances in the brain and cerebrospinal fluid of animals and man during and following acupuncture needling.

These endogenous peptides with opiate-like analgesic effects are broadly classified as opioids and include the endorphins, dynorphins and enkephalins. It is thought that the effect of acupuncture analgesia is mediated partly via the release of these endogenous opioids.

The stimulation of peripheral nerve fibers by acupuncture needles results in the activation of three major centers: the spinal cord, midbrain and hypothalamus/pituitary. By complex mechanisms, this results in the blockade of afferent painful stimuli at these three levels and involves the release of enkephalin, dynorphin, γ-aminobutyric acid (GABA), serotonin and many other inhibitory neurohumeral transmitter substances.[9]

Clement Jones et al[8,10] have shown that electroacupuncture significantly increases the level of β-endorphin measured in the lumbar cerebrospinal fluid of humans. Whereas electroacupuncture in heroin addicts led to a significant increase in cerebrospinal fluid levels of metenkephalin with little increase in the level of β-endorphin, the reverse was found for a group of chronic pain patients receiving similar treatment. The difference seen in these two studies may reflect the different conditions being treated or the fact that different stimulation frequencies were used to elicit the differential response.

Research has shown that naloxone, an opiate and opioid antagonist, reduces the analgesic effect of acupuncture by a competitive blockade of the effects of endogenous opioids.[11,12] 5-Hydroxytryptamine (serotonin) also plays a role in the analgesic effect of acupuncture, and the tryptophan hydroxylase inhibitor parachlorophenylalanine, which decreases concentrations of 5-hydroxytryptamine (serotonin) in the brain, reduces the analgesic effect of high-frequency electroacupuncture.[13] Acupuncture also has widespread visceral autonomic effects mediated by the release of cholecystokinin (CCK), noradrenaline, vasoactive intestinal peptide (VIP) and other substances.[1]

It is evident that although the mechanisms of action are complex, acupuncture has a sound neuropharmacological and physiological basis which has yet to be completely determined.

METHODS OF ACUPUNCTURE TREATMENT

Acupuncture is traditionally performed by the insertion of needles into the skin or muscle to stimulate high-threshold sensory nerve afferents (small A delta and C fibers). Modern acupuncture needles are sterile and disposable to avoid the risk of infection. Traditional acupuncture points have strict anatomical landmarks and a full description of these points can be found in an acupuncture atlas.[1] Many modern acupuncturists use trigger points, tender points and segmental points in addition to a number of empirically chosen traditional needling sites.

Traditionally, in order to achieve adequate nervous stimulation the acupuncture needles were stimulated (rotated, jiggled or moved in and out) to elicit 'de qi', a deep acting aching sensation associated with numbness or tingling around the needle site. The value of de qi has recently been challenged and minimal stimulation acupuncture, using smaller-gauge needles with no attempt to elicit de qi, appears to be equally effective for many conditions and more comfortable for the patient (Filshie, personal communication).

As a substitution for vigorous manual stimulation electroacupuncture was developed. This involves the electrical stimulation of needles by a battery-powered stimulator. In modern practice usually 4–8 needles are stimulated simultaneously. Pulses of electricity are applied to the needles in order to stimulate nerves with a pulse width from 0.1 to 0.5 ms duration.

More modern stimulators use biphasic pulses in order to reduce polarization of the needles due to electrolysis. Polarization is a nuisance as it raises the resistance of the needle over time thus reducing the intensity of stimulation, and also occasionally causing the needle to break off in the tissues. The wide margin of error for needle placement is a major advantage of electroacupuncture, particularly for the less experienced acupuncturist.

Transcutaneous electrical nerve stimulation (TENS) is a method of nerve stimulation without the use of needles. Small, flexible electrode pads are attached to the skin over the stimulation point (one pair of electrodes for each stimulator channel). The current/voltage is turned up until the nerves under the skin are activated transcutaneously. Higher currents/voltages are required than for electroacupuncture because the current density is less with pads than with needles. Good contact of the electrode with the underlying skin is of paramount importance to the success of TENS. It is easy to use, requiring even less precision of pad placement than for electroacupuncture needling, and is particularly helpful when patients have a fear of needles.

Conventional TENS, developed in the early 1970s as a result of the Gate theory of pain,[14] works by stimulating large-diameter (A beta) afferent nerves in the same dermatome as the site of pain. This is thought to result in the release of GABA, an inhibitory neurotransmitter substance, and cause presynaptic inhibition of adjacent pain fibers (small-diameter A delta and C fibers) at a spinal level. Analgesia starts within milliseconds of TENS stimulation and may last for up to 10 min after the machine is turned off.

'Acupuncture-like TENS' differs from conventional TENS in the use of low-frequency high-intensity stimulation at acupuncture points to excite small-diameter A delta and C fibers. This results in a longer-lasting effect, possibly because of the substantial release of endorphins, and consequently needs to be administered as little as twice a week.

Neurohumeral transmitters and the lower urinary tract

The effects of opiate premedication and inhalational anesthetic agents on urodynamic parameters have been studied on humans under general anesthesia.[15] Opiate analgesic drugs decrease detrusor pressure and bladder sensation and increase bladder capacity and urethral closure pressure. The use of epidural and intraspinal opiates for postoperative analgesia may be a cause of postoperative urinary retention partly by these mechanisms. These effects might be predicted from the effect of opiates and the opiate antagonist naloxone on the sphincter of Oddi and other smooth muscle sphincters.[16]

The effects of opioids on the lower urinary tract have also been studied both in vitro and in vivo. Enkephalinergic nerves have been demonstrated in smooth muscle of the lower urinary tract and in ganglia of the bladder.[17,18,19]

Klarskov[20] studied the in vitro effects of enkephalins on human detrusor muscle obtained from cystotomy specimens of the dome and trigone of the bladder. Both methionine enkephalin and leucine enkephalin significantly inhibited electrically evoked detrusor muscle contractions, although no effect was seen on contractions elicited pharmacologically with carbachol, PG F2α and substance P, suggesting a presynaptic inhibitory effect of enkephalins on the bladder.

Opioids have been shown to depress bladder motility following intrathecal administration in cats[18,21] and intracerebrovascular injection in rats.[22] Opioid antagonism with naloxone enhances detrusor activity in cats,[23] rats[22] and humans,[24,25] suggesting the role of enkephalinergic bladder control.

Murray & Feneley[25] performed cystometry on 20 patients aged 30–62 before and after intravenous administration of naloxone. Subtracted detrusor pressure increased and bladder compliance and capacity decreased following the administration of naloxone. Peak flow pressure also increased, and in female patients this was associated with a significant decrease in the maximum urethral closure pressure (MUCP). Three patients developed worsening of detrusor instability following the administration of naloxone, although there was no mention of worsening of stress incontinence. These results show that endogenous opioids exert an effect in the control of lower urinary tract function and that this is one likely site of action of acupuncture for the treatment of lower urinary tract dysfunction.

ACUPUNCTURE AND LOWER URINARY TRACT DYSFUNCTION

The mechanisms of action of acupuncture suggest a possible role in the treatment of detrusor instability. Acupuncture has also been used to treat nocturnal enuresis. It is unlikely that acupuncture has a significant clinical effect in patients with genuine stress incontinence despite evidence to suggest that it may increase urethral closure pressure.

Unfortunately, there are no suitably controlled trials of acupuncture treatment due to the absence of a credible acupuncture placebo. Various studies have attempted to use acupuncture needling at different sites as a control treatment. As neither the best needle sites nor the optimum duration of treatment have been fully assessed, the treatment effect of this control cannot be considered negligible. Only one study has compared the efficacy of acupuncture to that of conventional anticholinergic medication for the treatment of irritative bladder symptoms, but this too can be criticized for failing to recognize the significant placebo effect of both treatment arms of the study.[26] Although acupuncture appears to be of benefit to patients with detrusor instability and nocturnal enuresis, large controlled trials are awaited.

Two publications[27,28] have reported the successful management of nocturnal enuresis with acupuncture. Although the studies were uncontrolled and the assessment of treatment was symptomatic only, cure rates of 82% and 70% respectively were achieved.

Pigne et al[29] performed acupuncture using traditional steel needles on 16 women with detrusor instability. Acupuncture needling was performed twice weekly for 5 weeks at acupuncture points bladder 65, 64, 28, 23 and at spleen 6, 9 and conception 3 (Figs. 40.1–40.3). Urge incontinence and urinary frequency were subjectively improved following treatment, and cystometry showed a significant improvement in the first desire to void, bladder capacity and bladder compliance.

Philp et al[30] performed acupuncture on 20 patients with irritative bladder symptoms (frequency, nocturia, urgency and urge incontinence). A frequency/volume chart was completed and urodynamics performed prior to 10–12 weekly acupuncture treatment sessions. Traditional stainless steel acupuncture needles were inserted either at bladder points 23 and 28 plus Du 4, or points Ren 4 and 6 plus spleen 6 (Figs. 40.1–40.3). The needles were manually stimulated to elicit de qi and left in situ for a period of 30 min. Following treatment frequency/volume charting and urodynamic assessment were repeated.

Of the 20 patients 3 had a diagnosis of sensory urgency, 1 man had detrusor instability secondary to locally invasive prostatic carcinoma and

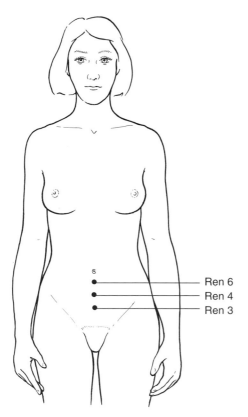

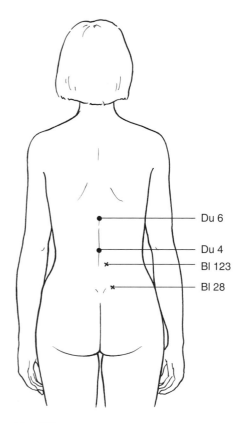

Fig. 40.1   Acupuncture points as referred to in text (Figs 40.1–40.4)

Fig. 40.2

16 patients had idiopathic detrusor instability. Of these 3 were enuretic with no daytime symptoms, and the remainder had diurnal symptoms. The majority of patients had previously received a variety of different medications and most had been prescribed more than one. Prolonged hydrodistension of the bladder had been performed in 7 patients, and in 4 more than once.

None of the patients with sensory urgency noted symptomatic improvement, and all refused cystometry on completion of the study. Short-term symptomatic improvement lasting for 1 week was seen in the man with invasive prostatic cancer.

Of the 3 patients with enuresis, 1 was cured and remained completely dry for at least 9 months. Unfortunately, 2 were unchanged by treatment and refused cystometry. Of the 13 patients with detrusor instability and diurnal symptoms, 10 (77%) noted a significant symptomatic improvement of frequency and nocturia. Urgency was cured in 7 women and although still present in 3 was less troublesome. Urge incontinence resolved in 63% of patients.

Cystometric results were inconsistent with subjective improvement. Detrusor instability was cured in only 1 case, and this woman, who had no symptomatic improvement, was later shown to be clinically depressed.

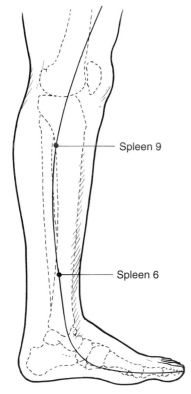

Fig. 40.3

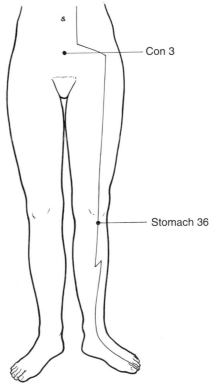

Fig. 40.4

A symptomatic improvement in 66% of patients with detrusor instability and a 77% improvement in those with predominantly daytime symptoms suggest that acupuncture offers a worthwhile treatment, at least as effective as other non-invasive therapies for these patients. Although there was no formal long-term follow-up, symptomatic improvement appeared to last for up to 2 years.

Chang[31] performed urodynamics before, during and after acupuncture at two different acupuncture points (spleen 6 and stomach 36) on women with frequency, urgency and dysuria. Treatment efficacy was assessed by cystometry, urethral sphincter electromyography, urethral pressure profilometry and uroflowmetry.

Urodynamics was performed before, during and after spleen 6 acupuncture on 26 women, and before and after stomach 36 acupuncture on a further 26 women (Figs. 40.1–40.4). The spleen 6 point has been used traditionally for the management of urinary problems, whereas stomach 36, which is traditionally used for the treatment of gastrointestinal disease, was used as a control. Six-centimeter-long acupuncture needles were inserted to a depth of 2–2.5 cm, manually stimulated to elicit de qi, and left in situ for 20 min. Urodynamics was performed 30 min following needling.

Acupuncture at both points resulted in an increased cystometric bladder capacity and time to first sensation of desire to void, although

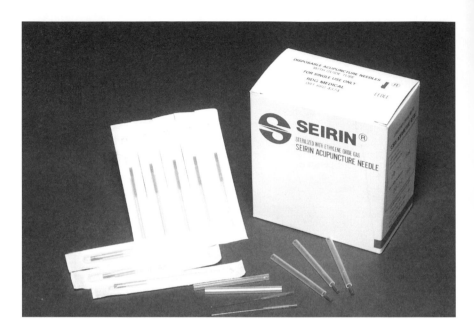

Fig. 40.5

the effect was greater following spleen 6 acupuncture. There were no significant changes in anal sphincter electromyogram after acupuncture at either point, and there were no measurable changes in intravesical pressure during acupuncture at spleen 6. Clinically, 22 (84.6%) women were cured or subjectively improved following acupuncture at the spleen 6 point. Only 6 women (23%) had symptomatic improvement following stomach 36 acupuncture.

The authors were surprised to find that 17 women had an increased cystometric bladder capacity, and were symptom-free after only one acupuncture treatment at the spleen 6 acupuncture point. Cyclical periods of acupuncture were, however, needed to maintain these beneficial effects in 12 patients. A major flaw in this study was the limited number of patients with cystometric abnormalities, only 14 women suffering from detrusor instability.

Gibson et al[32] used infrared low-power laser acupuncture on 28 women with detrusor instability. The patients had been symptomatic from 6 months to 10 years and had previously received various other treatments. Patients were treated twice weekly for 5 weeks using laser acupuncture applied bilaterally for 1 min at the same points used by Pigne[29] (Figs. 40.1–40.3).

Laser acupuncture compared favorably with previous results using both conventional and electroacupuncture. Urgency, frequency and nocturia were significantly improved, and time to first desire to void, bladder capacity and detrusor compliance increased significantly following treatment. Overall 50% of women were completely cured and 25% improved.

We have recently evaluated minimal stimulation acupuncture for the treatment of urgency, urge incontinence, frequency and nocturia in women with idiopathic low compliance.[26] Thirty-nine women aged between 18 and 75 years were included in the study and randomly allocated to receive either acupuncture or oxybutynin (5 mg twice daily) for 6 weeks. All patients completed a detailed urinary symptom questionnaire, a symptom visual analog scale and a urinary diary prior to videourodynamic investigations. These were repeated at the end of the study and the side effects of treatment were also assessed.

Acupuncture was performed by a single experienced acupuncturist, using 36-gauge 3-cm-long disposable needles and a minimal stimulation technique. Fifteen needles were inserted at each of the 6 weekly visits and left in situ a few millimeters below the skin without further stimulation for 10 min. The acupuncture points used were bilateral spleen 6 and stomach 36, conception 3 or 4, bladder 23 and 28. Two further paravertebral segmental lumbar points and four sacral segmental points were employed for their possible autonomic effects. (Figs. 40.1–40.4).

Symptoms of urgency, frequency and nocturia were significantly improved by both treatments and a maximal response was seen following 6 weeks of acupuncture needling. There was no significant improvement in urge incontinence for either group.

Acupuncture resulted in very few side effects although they were common with oxybutynin, all patients experiencing some degree of dryness of the mouth, and over 50% headaches, dizziness, gastrointestinal upset and transient visual impairment, resulting in withdrawal from the study by 3 women.

Both acupuncture and oxybutynin increased the time to first sensation of desire to void and bladder capacity during the filling phase of cystometry. The detrusor pressure rise on filling was decreased for both treatment groups. There were no statistically significant subjective or objective differences between the efficacy of the two treatments. Three months following treatment, 12 patients in the acupuncture group and 7 in the oxybutynin group remained subjectively improved.

In 1984 Lin et al[33] reported an increase in urethral pressure in response to acupuncture in 4 of 8 dogs. Kubista et al[34] studied the effect of electroacupuncture on the urethral pressure profile of humans and found an increase in the MUCP in 17 out of 20 women. Chang[31] noticed periodic increases in intraurethral pressure in the distal urethra of 20 women during spleen 6 acupuncture. Urethral pressure profiles were also measured in 7 of the 20 patients studied by Philp et al[30] but no consistent changes were seen. It seems unlikely that acupuncture is of value to women with genuine stress incontinence, and all the women studied by Kubista et al[34] later underwent bladder neck surgery.

There has been little research using TENS in the treatment of lower urinary tract dysfunction. Webb & Powell[35] treated 24 patients with detrusor instability using a commercially available TENS unit (Microtens). All patients were evaluated without TENS, with TENS applied to the active S3 dermatome, and as a control with TENS applied to the T12 dermatome. The order of the three treatments was randomized.

Active TENS on the S3 dermatome resulted in stable cystometric findings in 11 patients compared to 1 patient with TENS on T12; TENS on S3 also significantly increased bladder capacity and reduced daytime frequency and urgency. Urge incontinence was significantly improved for all patients and cured in 13 patients following S3 TENS.

Although these results appear impressive, the authors failed to state the optimum duration of treatment or the duration of improvement, and it is unclear whether TENS at T12 is a suitable placebo. Further research would be of value, including the use of 'acupuncture-like TENS', which is known to exert a longer-lasting clinical effect.

CONCLUSION

Acupuncture is potentially a cheap and safe treatment for lower urinary tract dysfunction and has few side effects. Many problems are, however, encountered in trials of acupuncture therapy, not least of which are the lack of a credible acupuncture placebo and the large placebo effect encountered in the treatment of irritative bladder symptoms. Unfortunately, despite convincing evidence of the neurophysiological actions of acupuncture, uncontrolled studies are insufficient to prove categorically a beneficial therapeutic effect.

Studies to date, despite their uncontrolled design, have however shown the potential value of acupuncture and TENS for the management of detrusor instability, idiopathic low compliance and nocturnal enuresis. It would seem at present unwise to disregard acupuncture, but perhaps in the face of doubt to reserve it for patients unresponsive to conventional therapy, or for those patients who request alternative therapy.

REFERENCES

1 Stux G, Pomeranz B (eds) Acupuncture textbook and atlas. Berlin: Springer Verlag, 1987; pp 300–302.
2 Needham J, Gwei-Jen L. Celestial lancets– a history and rationale of acupuncture and moxibustion. Cambridge: Cambridge University Press, 1980.
3 Wall PD. Acupuncture revisited. New Scientist 3 Oct 1974; pp 31–34.
4 Janssens LAA, Rogers PAM, Schoen AM. Acupuncture analgesia: a review. The Veterinary Record 9 April 1988; p. 355–358. In:
Stux G, Pomeranz B (eds) Acupuncture textbook and atlas. Berlin: Springer Verlag, 1987.
5 Goldstein A, Hilgard EF. Failure of the opiate antagonist naloxone to modify hypnotic analgesia. Proceedings of the National Academy of Science (USA) 1975; 72: 2041–2043.
6 Tseng CK, Tay AA, Pace NL, Westenskow DR, Wong KC. Journal of the American Veterinary Medical Association 1981; 178: 502.
7 Research Group of Acupuncture Anaesthesia (Peking). The role of some neurotransmitters of brain in finger acupuncture analgesia. Sci Sin 1974; 17: 112–130.
8 Clement Jones V, McLoughlin L, Tomlin S, Besser G M, Rees L H, Wen H L. Increased beta-endorphin but not met-enkephalin levels in human cerebrospinal fluid after acupuncture for recurrent pain. Lancet 1980; 946–948.
9 Stux G. World Health Organisation list of indications for acupuncture. In: Stux G, Promeranz B. Basics of acupuncture. Berlin: Springer Verlag, 1988: p 241.
10 Clement Jones V, McLoughlin L, Lowry PJ, Besser G M. Acupuncture in heroin addicts: changes in met-enkephalin and beta-endorphin in blood and cerebrospinal fluid. Lancet 1979; 380–382.
11 Chapman CR, Colpitts YM, Benedetti C, Kitaeff R, Gehrig JD. Evoked potential assessment of acupuncture analgesia: attempted reversal with naloxone. Pain 1980; 8: 231–236.
12 Mayer DJ, Price DD, Rafii A. Antagonism of acupuncture analgesia in man by the

narcotic antagonist naloxone. Brain Res 1977; 121: 368–372.

13 Cheng RS, Pomeranz B. Electroacupuncture analgesia could be mediated by at least two pain relieving mechanisms. Endorphin and non endorphin systems. Life Sci 1979; 25: 1957–1962.

14 Melzack R, Wall PD. Pain mechanism: a new theory. Science 1965; 150: 971–979.

15 Doyle PT, Briscoe CE. The effects of drugs and anaesthetic agents on the urinary bladder and sphincter. British J Urology 1976; 48: 329–335.

16 McCammon RL, Veigas OJ, Stoelting RK. Naloxone reversal of choledochoduodenal spasm associated with narcotic administration. Anaesthesiology 1978; 48: 437.

17 Alm P, Alumets J, Hakanson R et al. Enkephalin immunoreactive nerve fibres in the feline genitourinary tract. Histochemistry 1981; 72: 351–355.

18 Booth AM, Ostrowski N, McLinden S, Lowe I, De Groat WC. An analysis of the inhibitory effects of leucine enkephalin on transmission in vesical parasympathetic ganglia of the cat. Society for Neuroscience symposia, 1981. Abstract 7, p 214.

19 Kawatani M, Lowe IP, Booth AM, Backes MG, Erdman S, De Groat WC. The presence of leucine enkephalin in the sacral preganglionic pathway of the urinary bladder of the cat. Neuroscience Letters 1983; 39: 143–148.

20 Klarskov P. Enkephalin inhibits presynaptically the contractility of urinary tract smooth muscle. Br J Urol, 1987; 59: 31–35.

21 Hisamitsu T, Roques BP, De Groat WC. The role of enkephalins in the sacral parasympathetic reflex pathways to the urinary bladder of the cat. Society for Neuroscience Symposia, 1982. Abstract 8, p 227.

22 Dray A, Metsch R, Davis TP. Endorphins and the central inhibition of urinary bladder motility. Peptides 1984; 5: 645–647.

23 Roppolo JR, Booth AM, De Groat WC. The effects of naloxone on the neural control of the urinary bladder of the cat. Brain Research 1983; 264: 355–358.

24 Murray KHA. Effect of naloxone induced opioid blockade on idiopathic detrusor instability. Urology 1983; 22: 329–331.

25 Murray KHA, Feneley RCL. Endorphins – a role in lower urinary tract function? The effect of opioid blockade on the detrusor and urethral sphincter mechanisms. Br J Urol 1982; 54: 638–640.

26 Kelleher CJ, Filshie J, Burton G, Cardozo LD. Acupuncture and the treatment of irritative bladder symptoms in women. Journal of the British Medical Acupuncture Society (In press).

27 Bartocci C, Lucentini M. Acupuncture and micromassage in the treatment of idiopathic night enuresis. Minerva Med 1981; 72: 2237.

28 Song Baozhu, Wang Xiyou. Short term effect in 135 cases of enuresis treated by wrist ankle needling. J Tradit Chin Med 1985; 5: 27–28.

29 Pigne A, De Goursac C, Nyssen C, Barrat J. Acupuncture and unstable bladder. Abstracts 15th Annual meeting of the International Continence Society, 1985, pp 186–187.

30 Philp T, Shah PJR, Worth PHL. Acupuncture in the treatment of bladder instability. Br J Urol 1988; 61: 490–493.

31 Chang PL. Urodynamic studies in acupuncture for women with frequency, urgency and dysuria. J Urol 1988; 140: 563–566.

32 Gibson JS, Pardey J, Neville J. Proceedings of the 18th Annual Meeting of the International Continence Society, 1988, pp 146–147.

33 Lin SN, Lue TF, Chang YP, Schmidt RA, Tanagho EA. Acupuncture and urethral function: an experimental study. J Urol 1984; 131: 382A, Abstract 1113.

34 Kubista E, Altmann P, Kucera H. Electroacupuncture's influence on the closure mechanism of the female urethra in incontinence. Am J Chin Med 1976; 4: 177–181.

35 Webb RJ, Powell PH. Transcutaneous electrical nerve stimulation in patients with idiopathic detrusor instability. Neurourol Urodyn 1992; 11(4): 327–328.

FURTHER READING

Han JS. The neurochemical basis of pain relief by acupuncture. The China Medical Technology Publishing House, China, 1987.

Section 8 Nursing

41

The role of the nurse in urodynamics

INTRODUCTION

Urodynamics is the most widely accepted method for investigation of urinary incontinence in women. With an increased number of referrals and the demands of the service to provide 'quality care', the role of the nurse in this specialty has become increasingly important as part of a multidisciplinary team.

There are no formal training courses in urodynamics for nurses. Most experience is gained 'in-house', and given the diversity of units undertaking investigation of incontinence the standard of experience can vary from that of highly skilled clinical nurse specialists, who carry out their own investigations and can undertake a complex workload, to that of nurses whose primary role is to assist the clinician and chaperon the patient. A recent survey carried out in Manchester[1] has shown that 12% of investigations are carried out solely by nursing staff, and that a combination (of doctor and nurse) conduct 26% of investigations. The study does not differentiate as to which tests were carried out solely by nurses and in conclusion the author states that the study is incomplete. However, it does highlight the fact that there is very little formal training for any staff.

At present nurses in the field have access to current data via scientific meetings (International Continence Society, Association for Continence Advice, British Association of Urological Surgeons), but as such have no separate association in the United Kingdom. The only formal discussion of urodynamic interpretation is found in the English National Board urology course (ENB A46) and, if the tutor has an interest, in the English National Board course 'Introduction to Continence' (ENB 978). Many units now hold their own study days, and with the implementation of the PREP (Post-registration Education and Practice Project) requirements for nurses, this may well prove to be a creditable method of acquiring knowledge in promotion of continence.

CLINICAL SKILLS

It is obvious that nursing input can be of paramount importance to the quality of care provided during urodynamic investigation. Quite often it is difficult for a patient to admit that he or she suffers from urinary incontinence. Having reached the stage where investigations are being carried out, a woman will already have had to talk to her family doctor and probably a consultant urologist or gynecologist in the search for a cure for a problem which will significantly affect her quality of life.[2]

Continence advisors do not usually undertake urodynamic investigations themselves. Many nurses do not appreciate that cystometry provides a simple and accurate way of diagnosing urinary symptoms, and do not include this option in the initial assessment. However, Roper[3] defines information gathered by assessment as including not only interview and observation, but also examination and measurement and tests appropriate to the patient. Duffin[4] describes the assessment process in great detail, and much emphasis is placed upon an individualized approach to the patient. By using urodynamics as a method of assessment within the nursing field, it is possible to offer appropriate management without having to implement an inappropriate course of conservative management.

Patients who have been mismanaged will often become disheartened when they feel their condition is not being treated. For this reason urodynamics can now be used to give objective assessment of a patient's problems.

The urodynamic nurse may cover a variety of roles. The UKCC (United Kingdom Central Council for Nursing, Midwifery and Health Visiting) Code of Conduct[5] and Scope of Professional Practice[6] clearly state that individual nurses are accountable for their own practice. Nurses in urodynamics may be working without the support of a nursing hierarchy structure in a very medically orientated environment, and need to be aware of the changing face of nursing protocol in order to provide quality research-based care at a clinical level and to maintain their own identity.

A highly technical skill is required in order to use and maintain the machinery which is available. This should always be done in accordance with manufacturers' instructions, and a recent publication from the Department of Health[7] provides an introduction to the Medical Devices Directorate and the role of the health care professional in using equipment and devices safely. Close contact with the medical physics department will ensure that all equipment is safely maintained in accordance with health and safety requirements. It is also necessary to be aware of infection control issues, the need for on-going management of the patient, for counseling, and to act as a liaision between the urodynamic unit and the other departments which may have an interest. The urodynamic unit provides ample opportunity for a nurse to initiate her own research projects and to participate in large clinical studies.

The Working for Patient[8] and caring for People[9] white papers, which have resulted in the National Health and Community Care Act, will have an effect on existing and future services. Both white papers make reference to the efficient and effective utilization of resources. If this is the case how can nurses use the facilities available to make sure that incontinent patients have the best advice possible at the time? Continence Advisory Services have often developed as a community service and not with the support of hospitals. Urodynamics, however, is seen as the province of the hospital clinician. It is possible to develop a role as a clinical nurse specialist, where the nurse working with the clinician can provide a much more comprehensive care program for the patients in his or her care. Many hospitals and trusts have set various course standards to which the hospitals will work, for example for catheterization. The nurse in the urodynamics department would be responsible for managing these standards of care.

It is envisaged that the public will become more informed. Professional bodies now offer telephone helpline services and public information services such as National Continence Weeks. The public will now be more aware of what is available to help them with their incontinence problems. However, this puts a certain amount of pressure on services. It is possible for a well-trained urodynamic nurse to run her own clinics in conjunction with another nurse, technician or continence advisor. This can be done with the guidance of the consultant and is more suitable for those groups of patients such as the elderly, the disabled and those with learning difficulties or mental illness, and will enable the nurse to carry out a more in-depth assessment in keeping with their special needs. At present at the King's Urogynaecology Unit we undertake in the region of 200 nurse-led investigations annually.

CARE DURING URODYNAMICS

One of the main advantages of a nurse in urodynamics is that she or he will act as patient's advocate.[6] The nurse should make sure that the patient is provided with as much information prior to the test as possible. Depending on how the particular service operates it should be possible to provide patients with information and simple instructions to which they will be able to relate. The nurse should also be sufficiently skilled to be able to cope with any questions that patients may ask prior to the investigation.

In our particular department the nurse takes a major role in patient care during urodynamics. This does not necessarily mean that the nurse is the only person to pass catheters or carry out the investigation, but it is the nurse's responsibility to ensure that whoever carries out the urodynamics does so in such a way as to procure maximum co-operation from the patient. For example, one would not expect a very elderly patient or a child to have to undergo an excessively invasive investigation when the service can provide a nurse who is trained to look after these groups of patients. Indeed, it is often the nursing assessment which indicates the need for urodynamics or may exclude that patient from the investigation if nothing abnormal is found on assessment.

Once the patient has entered the urodynamic environment it is important to make sure that her needs are met at all times. During the catheterization, it will be reassuring to have a female chaperone present in the room. It is not only ethical but is also more acceptable to the patient, especially if there are ethnic considerations.

Patients are referred for urodynamics from many sources. They can come from geriatricians, urologists, neurologists, gynecologists or pediatricians. After investigation the patient may be referred back to the original referral source. If the patients are referred both for investigation and management it is often the responsibility of the nurse to ensure that there is continuity of that care.

In some situations the urodynamic nurse may take on a patient care load herself where she will undertake conservative methods of management. This care may be instigated at ward level if the urodynamics sister is able to assess the patient prior to investigation. This is especially useful if the woman needs to be taught clean intermittent self-catheterization or if ward staff need advice and instruction on catheter procedures.

In our particular department the nurse specialist is able to use ultrasound scanning equipment. Again there is little formal training and experience is gained 'in-house', but this skill is useful for ascertaining urinary residuals and more recently has been employed to assess bladder wall thickness.[10] It is essential that the nurse in the urodynamics room has an understanding of all the techniques that are used during the investigation.

INFECTION CONTROL

Urinary tract infection following urodynamic investigation is reported as between 1.5% and 4%[11,12,13,14] and in our own department the reported incidence is in the region of 2% (1991 unpublished data). A retrospective study by Hamill et al[15] describes an incidence of 18.7% in a group of 274 men. This incidence was reduced by implementing strict aseptic controls in the urodynamics laboratory and consistently screening for bacteriuria and urinary tract infection prior to urodynamics. Even so, the study still reports a 5% rate of acquired infection. However, the author concludes that this may be due to an all male population in the analysis and the nature of the medical conditions, which include spinal injury. This highlights the importance of pre-urodynamic screening and strict maintenance of equipment and application of aseptic technique. It is the nurse's responsibility to maintain such standards, and in the event of infection implement the appropriate measures.

Patients will often complain of dysuria following urodynamic investigation. In a recent study by Carter,[14] 63% of a total of 310 patients complained of dysuria following urodynamics; however, only 1.9% of the total number of patients investigated were found to have developed a urinary tract infection after the investigation. Simple advice following urodynamics should therefore include increasing fluid intake and ensuring that the bladder is emptied completely on voiding. If symptoms of dysuria persist for more than 48 h the patient should contact the unit or consult her general practitioner.

Of paramount importance to good technique is the need to utilize all the resources available. Disposable equipment needs to be continuously evaluated for patient comfort and morbidity. The nurse is responsible for assessment of available resources and ensuring all equipment is in good condition and plentiful supply. This is especially important with disposables, which need to be stored according to the manufacturers' instructions.

TEACHING

Specialists from many disciplines have an interest in urodynamics. These include specialists, visiting doctors, clinical scientists, physicians, pediatricians and geriatricians. The nurse may therefore find herself teaching at various levels. The art of teaching in a clinical environment is a skilled one. Without isolating the patient from the conversation, the nurse needs to be able to teach the visitors so that they gain as much as possible from the investigation. It is not advantageous to the patient to have too many spectators during a urodynamic investigation. Many women find urodynamics undignified and without proper counseling may indeed find it intimidating to have extra personnel in the laboratory.

The specialist skills required in the urodynamic setting can also be of enormous benefit in educating ward-based staff. The urodynamic nurse can be active in ensuring that all current information regarding incontinence is available for both patients and staff, and can be available to assist in an educational role at a clinical level.

MANAGING THE SERVICE

Urodynamic investigation in tertiary referral centers can be a costly and time-consuming exercise. It is essential that all appointment time be utilized and the best available appointment system be used. Once the contract has been agreed and the patient is accepted for urodynamics, it is vital that she should receive as much information as possible regarding the test before her appointment. The patient should be given accurate instructions on how to get to the unit, and she should be aware that any drugs affecting the bladder should be stopped before the test, unless she is instructed otherwise, and that the bladder should be comfortably full on arrival. It is important that patients who are unable to attend should inform us as quickly as possible. The patient's records are of great importance. It is useful to have any previous notes, including the results of investigations, available at the time of urodynamics, as these may provide information essential to a diagnosis.

THE ROLE OF THE NURSE

The nurse plays an essential role in a urodynamic environment. As this is a new specialty it is very much in the interest of the nurse to develop the role within urodynamics so that the patient will receive the best possible care and the unit will provide a high-quality service.

REFERENCES

1 Kilcoyne GVP, Lord J, Smith J, Warrell D. Urodynamic personnel and training in the UK. ICS Prague Read by Title abstracts, pp 357–356, 1994.
2 Kelleher CJ, Khullar V, Cardozo LD. The impact of urinary incontinence on quality of life. Neurourol Urodyn 1993; 12(4): 388–389.
3 Roper N, Logan W, Tierney A. The elements of nursing, 4th edn. Edinburgh: Churchill Livingstone, 1990.
4 Duffin H. Assessment of urinary incontinence: clinical nursing practice: the promotion and management of continence. Prentice-Hall, 1992.
5 UKCC. Code of Conduct for the Nurse, Midwife and Health Visitor, 1992.
6 UKCC. The Scope of Professional Practice, 1992.
7 Department of Health and the Central Office of Information: Doing No Harm: HSSH JO3–2732NJ: 1994.
8 Department of Health. Working for people. London: HMSO, 1989a.
9 Department of Health. caring for people. London: HMSO, 1989b.
10 Khullar V, Salvatore S, Cardozo L, Hill S, Kelleher C. Ultrasound bladder wall measurement – a non invasive test for detrusor instability. Neurourol Urodyn 1994; 13(4): 461–462.
11 Bergman A, McCarthy T. Antibiotic prophylaxis after instrumentation for urodynamic testing. Br J Urol 1883; 55: 568–569.
12 Powell PH, Lewis P, Shephard A. The morbidity of urodynamic investigation. In: Proceedings of the 11th Annual Meeting of the International Continence Society, Lund, Sweden, 1981, pp 140–141.
13 Walter S, Vejigaard R. Diagnostic catheterisation and bacteriuria in women with urinary incontinence. Br J Urol 1978; 50: 106–108.
14 Carter P, Lewis P, Abrams P. Urodynamic morbidity and dysuria prophylaxis. Br J Urol 1991; 67: 40–41.
15 Hamill J, Wright M, Andres N, Koza M. Urinary tract infection following instrumentation for urodynamics. Infect control Hosp Epidemiol 1989; 10(1): 26–32.

42

The role of the continence advisor

INTRODUCTION

Over the past 20 years attitudes to incontinence have changed as it has been increasingly recognized that incontinence is a symptom that is often curable and can nearly always be better managed. Some of the changes in attitudes can be credited to the emergence of nurse specialists who have a responsibility for promoting continence and developing Continence Advisory Services.[1]

The role of the Continence Advisor has not been formally defined. However, the Association for Continence Advice has issued guidelines which include advice on the level of competence and training required and the resources needed to establish a service.[2]

The scope and extent of Continence Advisory Services differ from one health authority to another. The service may cover a unit, a trust or a number of trusts within a district. The range of the service provided is influenced by the number of Continence Advisors and the unit that funds them.

In 1991 The Department of Health reviewed continence services in the United Kingdom and acknowledged the Continence Advisor as a key feature of all effective local services.[3]

DEVELOPMENT OF THE CONTINENCE ADVISOR'S ROLE

In 1972 the Department of Health and Social Services identified a gap in health services and a need for continence promotion. The Chief Nursing Officer suggested that each health authority should identify a nursing officer who would be able to act as a point of reference on the subject of incontinence.[4]

The first Continence Advisor post was established in the private sector by the Disabled Living Foundation in 1974, offering a nationwide advice service. The increase in the number of Advisors was very slow and most of the original post-holders were solely identified as 'Incontinence' Advisors and worked in urology units, urodynamics clinics and specialist departments of geriatric medicine.

The Association of Continence Advisors was set up in 1980 with six founder members of which only one was in a post entitled 'Incontinence Advisor'. As a result of the work of the original members[5,6] the King's Fund in London set up a working group. This group produced a report which made recommendations on the services required to promote continence and manage incontinence.[7] The report is as relevant today as it was when it was produced in 1982. As a result of the King's Fund recommendations more Continence Advisors were appointed. The development of services, however, was patchy and many Continence Advisors found they were working in isolation with little support and without adequate resources.[8] Their role became identified as that of a clinical specialist who gave advice to patients, carers, health care professionals, organizations and voluntary groups. In 1985 the Association of Continence Advisors produced guidelines on the role of the District Continence Advisor[9] and in 1988 the Department of Health issued a circular recommending that a continence advisor be appointed to all health authorities.[10]

The Department of Health white papers 'Working for Patients' (1989a) and 'Caring for People' (1989b) recommend the efficient, effective utilization of health service resources and quality service provisions. Both of these were seen as integral parts of a continence advisor's role. It was feared that the National Health Services and Community Care Act (1990) would threaten the 'seamless care' offered by continence advisors across hospitals and community boundaries. There has been some evidence that the Continence Advisory Services have been affected.[11] However, in 1993 the National Health Service Management Executive guidance EL(93) 54 underlined the importance of an integrated service.[12] The guidance directed regional authorities to ensure that Continence Services conform to the 'Agenda for Action on Continence Services'. This should ensure multidisciplinary teamwork across trust boundaries with the continence advisors playing a major role. In 1993 there were approximately 380 continence advisors in posts with over 80% of all health authorities having at least one.[13]

THE ROLES AND PRINCIPLE FUNCTIONS OF CONTINENCE ADVISORS

In 1988 the Royal College of Nursing produced a report of the working party investigating the development of specialties within the nursing profession.[14] This report clearly identified the key role of nurse specialists and acknowledged that if standards of care were to be maintained and improved the profession must recognize that specialist nurses mean value for money for patients. The core elements of the specialist role were identified as:

- clinical practice
- teaching
- management
- research.

The Royal College of Nursing Continence Care Forum used a workshop approach to produce a consensus view of the role and principle functions of a Continence Advisor. They also developed the principal functions into four, covering the following core elements:[15]

- to meet the needs of people requiring continence care by direct and indirect clinical practice;
- to educate self and the public and other professionals about all aspects of continence care;
- to provide quality management of a comprehensive Continence Advisory Service;
- to have knowledge of research evidence and to use it in any aspect of continence care.

The Association of Continence Advisors in their guidelines provide a similar breakdown of the Continence Advisor's role but have added a further element; that of liaison[2] (Fig. 42.1).

In 1992 the Department of Health commissioned the Social Policy Research Unit of the University of York to carry out an investigation of the role of the Continence Advisor. Their research, which was published in 1993, attempted to discover the responsibilities, needs, views and problems of Continence Advisors.[16] They concluded that:

1. The role requires a mix of skills.
2. The role offers a career within a speciality and new opportunities to acquire a range of skills that can be carried into other fields.

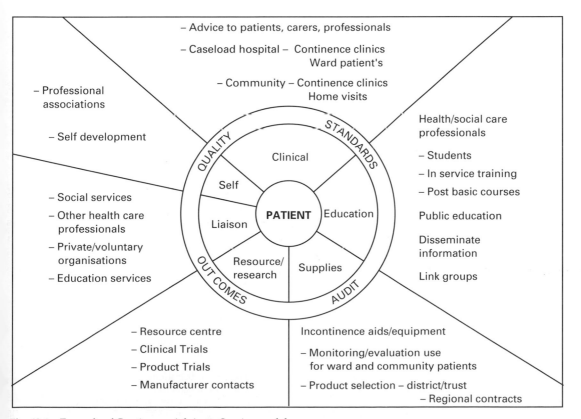

Fig. 42.1   Example of Continence Advisory Service model

3. There is no single model which encompasses continence advisors' practice. It is appropriate to talk in terms of roles of continence advisors.
4. Continence Advisors work across both professional and disciplinary boundaries.
5. Continence Advisors collaborate between health and social care agencies and their positions can provide a model for effective inter-agency collaboration and service integration.

The Social Policy Research Unit research also indicated that of the five main elements of the role, clinical practice, advice, and teaching were the most important, with management and research taking second place (Fig. 42.2). Only 20% of Continence Advisors were actively involved in all five functions, 57% being engaged in four of the five elements.[16]

Clinical practice

The results of the Social Policy Research Unit postal survey of Continence Advisors showed that clinical practice was reported as the most important element of the role. Seventy-two per cent of Continence Advisors carried a personal caseload and 85% were involved in home visits.[3] The Association of Continence Advisors and the Department of Health recommended that Continence Advisors have 'a small caseload'. However, 29% had caseloads of 50 patients and 16% had caseloads of over 100. Sixty-five per cent of patients were seen in clinics (hospitals and community). The research also showed that 82% of Continence Advisors worked closely with urodynamics investigation clinics and 26% were personally involved in urodynamic assessment.

List of conditions thought suitable for management by a nurse continence advisor

Condition	Treatment/management
Stress incontinence	Pelvic floor exercises. Use of cones and insertion devices. Biofeedback–perineometer/electrical stimulation. Dietary advice–psychological support.
Urge incontinence	Bladder retraining. Electrical stimulation. Supervision/advice re drug therapy. Psychological support.
Overflow incontinence	Instruction in voiding techniques. Intermittent catheterization Indwelling catheter/drainage system management. Dietary advice/bowel management. Psychological support.
Functional incontinence	Bladder training. Toileting programs. Advice on environmental and physical functioning. Dietary advice/bowel management. Psychological support.
Passive incontinence	Habit training. Toileting programs. Behavior modification.
Fecal incontinence	Treatment of constipation. Dietary advice/bowel management.

Consideration of suitable aids or equipment to enhance the quality of life of an incontinent patient.

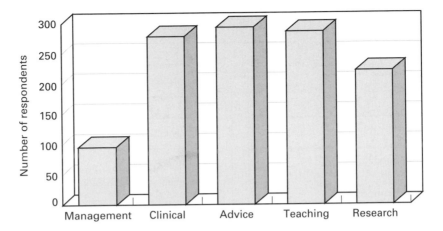

Fig. 42.2 Core functions of the Continence Advisor/clinical nurse specialist role
P. Pogri, G. Palmer – Social Policy Research Unit, The University of York

There is evidence to show that when a nurse specialist is clinically involved as part of a team with close interprofessional liaison this ensures that patients benefit from the most up-to-date clinical practice. By constantly researching and perfecting new methods of practice the Continence Advisor is in an ideal position to be able to affect other health care professionals' practices.[17]

Many continence services have adopted this approach to the dissemination of knowledge.[18] It has been argued that nurse specialists in clinical practice potentially deskill their colleagues. However, deskilling will not occur if the specialist functions as part of a team in an approach to patient care that influences the practice of colleagues. In fact, skills and knowledge are more likely to be gained by using the nurse specialist as a role model. Members of the multidisciplinary team can then use the specialist as a resource to help to meet individual patients' needs as and when required.

Hall et al[18] demonstrated the benefits of having link nurses working closely with the Continence Advisor in clinical practice. These nurses who have additional training in the promotion of continence and management of incontinence are then able to disseminate information and act as a local resource (Fig. 42.3).

The Continence Advisor should be involved with other health and social care professionals in establishing and circulating guidelines for practice, protocols and relevant clinical standards.[19] This should include programs of care indicating a comprehensive range of services available for incontinent patients (Fig. 42.4). These programmes should include performance indicators and targets for clinical audit. Continence advisors should be responsible for acquiring the consent of management concerning the operational policies for clinical continence services.[20]

Protocols for the clinical Continence Advisory Service might include:

- clinics
- home visiting
- access to the service
- referral to other agencies

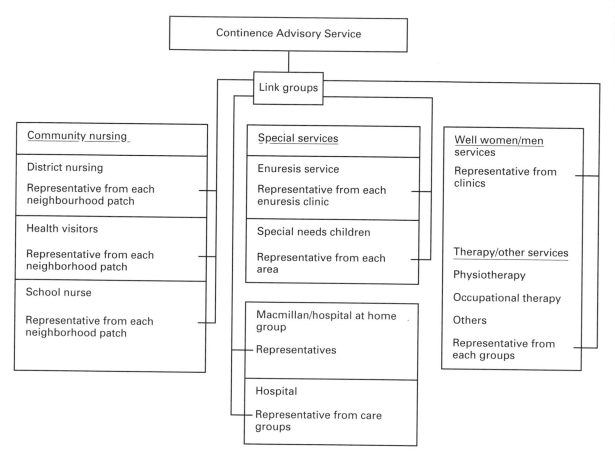

Fig. 42.3   Model of link network

Most Continence Advisors combine the clinical role with that of an advisory role, taking referral for advice from any source and covering any aspect of the service. Some continence advisors will offer a telephone advisory service with an answerphone to take messages when they are not available for direct consultations.

Education

The most important aspect of a specialist role is to educate and help others working in professional practice.[21] Certainly, the success of a continence service is dependent upon the knowledge and attitudes of all carers.[22] A Continence Advisor should, therefore, ensure that there is provision of a comprehensive program of education on the promotion of continence and management of incontinence. This service should be agreed upon with management as part of professional development and continuing education and needs to be regularly evaluated and updated.

The South Thames Continence Advisors in their regional standard for Continence Advisory Services recommended that Health Service Commissioners need to ensure that education is available to the following groups:

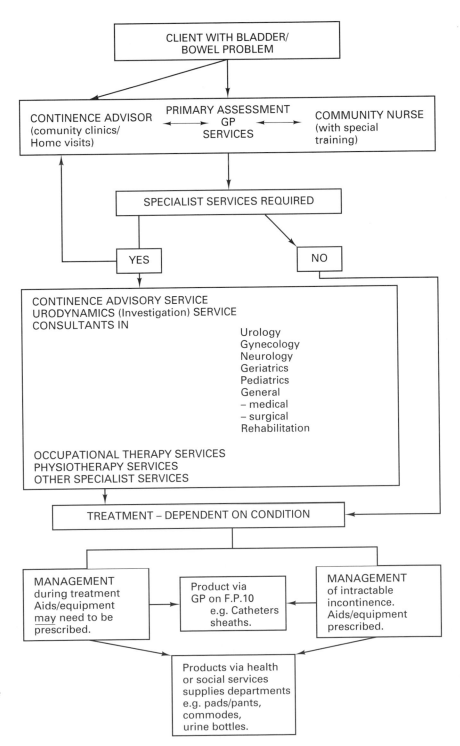

Fig. 42.4 Example of the range of services that may be required for the treatment/management of incontinence

- interested members of the public
- voluntary groups and organizations
- health care staff from all sectors
- carers
- social services staff
- private care facilities
- disability services
- occupational health services.

They also recommended that the Continence Advisory Services should support all health promotion services by supplying current literature on the promotion of continence and be actively involved in national campaigns such as 'National Continence Week'.

Continence advisors are responsible for their own professional development, and when a continence advisor is a nurse, it is now acknowledged that this should be at specialist or advanced nursing practice level.[23]

Resources

Part of the continence advisor's role is to act as a resource for patients and their carers. The services offers:

1. Information on all aspects relating to the promotion of continence and management of incontinence.
2. Information on the range of incontinence products available whether they are available through local health authority providers or by private purchase.
3. Information on the availability of education and training for carers and clients related to the promotion of continence.
4. A resource center with a range of products on view. This should include educational material with leaflets and handouts giving information on continence services available and how to access the service.

Research

It is a vital part of a Continence Advisor's role to be aware of current developments in the promotion of continence and know that their practice is based on research evidence.[24] The specialist can then assist colleagues to improve practice through the application of relevant research and by researching clinical practice on an on-going basis stimulate others to question their practice and develop their knowledge.

Management

The Continence Advisor's management role is increasingly involved with policy decisions, adjudication of tenders and budget holding. Many advisors will be responsible for developing, monitoring and evaluating the systems for the provision of incontinence aids and equipment. They will work closely with supplies and distribution departments to produce information on continence expenditure.

The management of the Continence Service will often be seen within the performance review structure, based on the achievement of the service objectives,[25] the continence advisor offering expertise relevant to the speciaty to all levels of an organization. This should ensure safe and appropriate planning, policies and care delivery, linking technical advice with business decisions.

REFERENCES

1 Wilce F. Spreading the word. Nursing Times 1987; 83: 15, 74.
2 Association of Continence Advisors. Guidance on the role of the continence advisor. London Executive Committee ACA, 1991.
3 Sanderson J. An agenda for action on continence services. (Unpublished report). London: Department of Health, 1991.
4 DHSS. (1977) Standard of Nursing Care. Promotion of continence and management of incontinence, letter C.N.O.SNC 77/1 London: DHSS.
5 Blannin J. Towards a better life. Nursing Mirror 1980; March 20, 31.
6 White H. Setting up an advisory service. Journal of District Nursing 1982; 1 (3): 4–60.
7 King's Fund Centre. Action of incontinence 1983. Report of Working Group, King's Fund Project Paper no 43.
8 Norton C. The development of continence advisors. Nursing for continence. Beconsfield Publishers 297–298.
9 ACA (1985) Guidelines on the role of the District Continence Advisor. London: Association of Continence Advisors.
10 DOH (1988) The development of services for people with physical or sensory disabilities. London: Department of Health, 1988.
11 Potter B. Reform role. Nursing Times 1993; 89, 39 63.
12 DOH Management Executive. Priorities and Planning Guidance 1994-95 E.L.(93)54. London: Department of Health, 1993.
13 ACA 1990 Improving our image. A Public Records pack for the continence advisor. London: Association of Continence Advisors.
14 Royal College of Nursing. Specialties in nursing. London: Ruislip Press, 1988: p 7.
15 Royal College of Nursing. The role of the continence advisor. Continence Care Forum. RCN, London, 1992.
16 Rhodes P, Parker G. The role of continence advisors in England and Wales. Social Policy Research Unit, University of York, 1993.
17 Rooney V. A team for continence. Journal of District Nursing 1994; 2(10): 6–11.
18 Hall C. Advising on continence. Community Outlook. July 1990. 38.43.
19 Standards for Continence Advisory Services (1994). Published by Directorate of Nursing, Quality Programmes. South-East Thames Regional Thames Authority. Thrift House, Bexhill-on-Sea, East Sussex, TN39 3NQ.
20 National Health Services Management Executive (1993). A vision for the future–the nursing, midwifery and health visiting contribution to health and health care. Department of Health, 1993.
21 Castledine G. Continence nurse specialists. British Journal of Nursing 1994: 3(11): 576.
22 Roe B. Setting up a continence advisory service. Clinical nursing practice. Prentice-Hall, 1992, 227.
23 Castledine G. U.K.C.C's standards for education and practice. British Journal of Nursing 1994; 3(5): 233.
24 Briggs A. Report of the Committee on Nursing. London: Her Majesty's Stationery Office, 1992.
25 Roe B. Setting up a Continence Advisory Service. Clinical Nursing Practice. Prentice-Hall, 1992: p 224.

43 Catheters and collecting systems

INTRODUCTION

The use of catheters to enable effective bladder emptying is well established. Catheters are used to relieve anatomical or physiological obstruction of the lower urinary tract, to facilitate postoperative healing and to observe and quantify urine output and appearance.

Reybard[1] was the first to advocate the use of a self-retaining catheter in 1853. Frederick Foley, however, is credited with the production of the first catheter of latex with an integrated balloon and his name is permanently and generically associated with this development.[2] As materials have improved the types of catheter available have developed accordingly: there is now an extensive range of products which health care professionals can draw on for use.[3]

The main use of catheters falls into three groups: the long-term and short-term urethral indwelling catheters, suprapubic catheters and clean intermittent self-catheterization (CISC) catheters.

INDWELLING URETHRAL CATHETERS (FOLEY)

Urethral catheters are used most extensively because it is easy and quick to visualize the urethral orifice and insert a catheter. Each hospital has formulated its own standard of care which relates to the techniques of catheterization. Much debate centers around the catheterization of male patients by nursing staff,[4] but training is now provided and the nurse must use her own accountability in practice.[5] Female catheterization is, however, an accepted nursing procedure and is often used in cases of intractable incontinence.

The female anatomy does not lend itself well to appliances, and a catheter is often seen as the only solution to control of incontinence. The type and size of urethral catheter (Foley) used is often left to the discretion of the nursing staff unless it is being used as a specific postoperative management. In general selection of a catheter is dependent on patient requirements and the length of time it is to remain in situ.[6] Catheters are available in a variety of materials, summarized in Fig. 43.1.

Catheter size

Selection of the appropriate catheter is important. It is usually best to choose a small charrière (12–16) with small balloon size. This

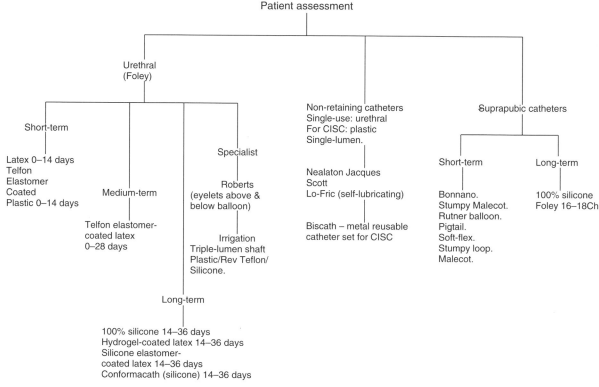

Fig. 43.1 Catheters: duration, type and use

recommendation is based on work carried out by several authors.[7-9] In women catheterized for incontinence, it has been found that a large balloon size is associated with bypassing. Large balloons are designed to be used following prostatectomy to prevent hemorrhage, and should not be used for long-term catheterization. Charrière (Ch), a French term, is used to size the external circumference of the catheter in millimeters, and is equal to about three times the external diameter, although this will vary according to materials.[7] For drainage of a normal bladder, smaller catheters should be used, size 12–16 Ch in an adult. A comparative study by Edwards et al in 1989[8] found that small charrières were suitable to transport the volumes of urine produced by the average human over a 24-h period. In a study of the hydrodynamic properties of 34 different catheters, Ebner 1985[7] concluded that the size 12Ch silicone catheter provided optimal drainage. Large-sized catheters have been associated with the bypassing of urine[9] and pain and discomfort.[10,11] Thus a smaller catheter provides optimal flow with minimal discomfort in long-term catheterized patients.

Catheter length

Catheters are produced in two lengths, male and female. The female catheters are approximately 22 cm long and the male 40 cm, although this may vary to a small degree between manufacturers.[3]

Types of catheter

Plastic or PVC catheters are cheap, stiff and inflexible. They have been found to cause bladder spasm, pain and leakage of urine[12] and are used postoperatively. Coated latex products are more flexible and cheaper but are prone to encrustation and urinary deposits.[12] All latex catheters are manufactured to a British Standard[13] which ensures that they adhere to a recommended level of safety. This follows reports of chemicals leaching out of the catheters, causing urethral adhesions and cytotoxic reactions.[14,15,16] It is now recommended that uncoated latex catheters be avoided because of their mechanical effects. Therefore, coated latex can be used in short-term catheterization (up to a maximum of 14 days) but may absorb body moisture which leads to a reduced internal diameter and therefore reduces drainage of urine.[17]

Teflon-coated latex catheters have a smoother finish. The effect of coating the catheters is to minimize trauma, irritation and encrustation[18] and it makes them suitable for up to 4 weeks' use. Long-term catheters must be suitable for use for 14–36 days: Silicone is an inert material which avoids trauma and causes a lower incidence of urethritis or encrustation. However, as silicone permits gas diffusion, there can be problems associated with balloon deflation.[19] Hydrogel-encapsulated catheters have similar properties to 100% silicone, but when hydrated become smoother, decreasing friction in the urethra.

Studies carried out at Manchester University[20] in 1984 found that the female urethra is not circular, and that a circular catheter therefore tends to distort the urethra. For this reason a catheter with a soft urethral section was described by Brocklhurst et al.[21] The 'Conformacath' was shown in a trial of 52 geriatric patients to be a substantial improvement over the standard Foley. However, studies by Kohl-Ockmore[22] and Pomfret[23] have shown that these catheters do sometimes block and patients experience bypassing. However, this catheter does offer an alternative in women. Further evaluation of this type of catheter is required.

A report by Crow et al[10] has shown that 10–12% of patients admitted to hospital have an indwelling urethral catheter inserted. The same report found that 14% of the patients were catheterized for incontinence and 18% for outlet obstruction or retention. However, now that alternatives such as CISC are available this figure may be reduced. An audit[24] of the use of long-term urethral catheters found that wide variations were found in community nursing management and care was frequently suboptimal.

Catheter management

The care of indwelling Foley catheters is a nursing role. Effective catheter management includes care of the perineal skin and assessing drainage and appearance of the urine. Problems associated with indwelling catheters include blockage, encrustation and urinary tract infection. In the event of catheter blockage bladder washouts or irrigation can be used with self-retaining (Foley) catheters. The introduction of a bladder washout to unblock a catheter[26] or to instill drugs for chemotherapy[25] involves breaking a closed system and this may introduce infection.[27] A study by

Elliot & Gopal-Rao[27] suggested that bladder irrigation further damages the already disrupted urothelium, which increases the predisposition of the bladder to the recurrent infections commonly associated with patients who have indwelling catheters. However, Flack 1993[28] found that the reduction in the incidence of catheter blockage when individual bladder washout regimens with effective solutions are used can increase catheter life and reduce trauma to the patient, and may well be more cost-effective than re-catheterization. Flack also concluded that bladder washouts should not be given to everyone with indwelling catheters; this would support the view taken by Roe[29] that an individual maintenance regimen should be established.

SUPRAPUBIC CATHETERIZATION

Suprapubic catheterization is the insertion of a catheter into the bladder wall just above the symphysis pubis. This may be carried out as a temporary measure following urological or other surgical procedures, or when a patient requires long-term catheterization and is unable to carry out CISC. The only real contraindication to suprapubic catheterization is hematuria of unknown diagnosis, as it is undesirable to place a catheter

Table 43.1

Acute illness	In urinary retention when urethral catheterization fails In acute retention as a primary method of drainage

Intractable incontinence	Following:
	    Failure of CISC
	    Failure to tolerate or manage urethral
	    catheter
	    Pads not sufficient to cope

Gynecological	Following:
	    Colposuspension
	    Stamey needle suspension
	    Vaginal hysterectomy
	    Colporrhaphy
	    Colpoperineorrhaphy
	    Pelvic surgery

Urological	Following:
	    Cecocystoplasty
	    Ileal augmentation
	    Trauma to urethra or bladder
	    Urethral stricture

Anorectal Surgery	Abdominoperineal resection of rectum Proctocolectomy Distal sigmoidocolectomy

Neurogenic bladder	Reflex:
	    Trauma above T12
	    Upper motor neuron
	Mixed:
	    Trauma below T12
	    Lower motor neurone

Cardiothoracic surgery	Open heart Aorta

through a bladder tumor. The types of patient groups using suprapubic catheters are summarized in Table 43.1.

The choice of catheter to insert following surgery will depend on cost, availability and individual preference. Commonly in our department a Bonnano catheter (Fig. 43.2) is inserted following gynecological surgery, although there are many variations which are in current use (Fig. 43.1).

Suprapubic catheters can be inserted using an open or closed technique. Cystotomy into the bladder dome under direct vision at the end of a retropubic procedure is used in the presence of gross hematuria, or when there has been a recent cystotomy. Percutaneous or closed insertion is carried out with the patient in the Trendelenburg position and the bladder filled transurethrally with at least 300 ml of sterile fluid. This is to ensure that no bowel lies between the bladder and anterior abdominal wall. The needle or trocar of the chosen catheter is then inserted, and when drainage through the catheter is visualized the urethral catheter is removed.

Bladder drainage via a suprapubic catheter is beneficial for patients who require long-term management and who are unable to carry out CISC. Barnes et al,[30] in a review of 40 patients with neuropathic bladders, found that suprapubic catheters were well tolerated despite problems of catheter blockage and urinary tract infections.

Long-term catheters need to be changed at least every 8 weeks, and should be 100% silicone Foleys. Care should be taken with reinsertion through the fistula, and in general the first change is carried out by experienced staff in a clinical environment (personal observation). Subsequent catheter changes can be undertaken in the community if required, but a lost catheter should be replaced immediately. A dedicated carer can be trained to reinsert a catheter with close supervision.

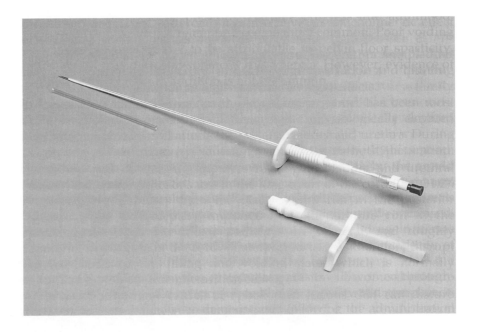

Fig. 43.2 Bonnano catheter

However, failure or delay will result in the need for reinsertion under medical supervision and possible resiting.

In general suprapubic catheterization is seen by patients and nurses as an alternative method of bladder control which is acceptable both from a social and hygienic point of view.

CLEAN INTERMITTENT SELF-CATHETERIZATION

Clean intermittent self-catheterization is a term applied to a method of bladder emptying which enables the patient to control her own bladder, rather than her bladder controlling her life.[33]

The method is simple: the patient is taught to pass a catheter into her urethra and thus effect bladder emptying. This technique has reduced infection hazards and greatly improved the lives of patients with disorders of micturition. However, its success is dependent on the skill of the teacher and the motivation of the patient. Poor technique and lack of understanding on both sides may lead to failure and can be detrimental to a patient's health. Wider[33] has described criteria required to ensure a successful outcome for teaching CISC. A programme for teaching CISC has been recommended by Sheri & Barnes,[34] and can be used for patients in hospital or the community. It is essential that patients taught in a ward environment by hospital-based staff be prepared in the use of CISC in the community. The instructors must therefore have acquired skills to enable the patients to manage their bladders in their own environment. District nurses and continence advisors should then follow up and revise management in the community as necessary.

With the advent of clean intermittent catheterization it has been possible to reduce nursing management of patients with disorders of micturition and establish independence in those who would otherwise be managed with long-term indwelling catheters.

The clean intermittent catheterization technique can be used by both men and women, children and the elderly, in particular those who have neurogenic bladder disorders caused by spinal injury, spina bifida or conditions such as multiple sclerosis. It can be employed by those with hypotonic bladders associated with spinal cord trauma, or neuropathy associated with diabetes, or following overdistension. Obstruction, found more commonly in elderly men and in patients with urethral stricture or stenosis, can be managed with CISC. In our own department women with genuine stress incontinence who have voiding difficulties or persistent urinary residuals on urodynamic investigation are required to learn CISC before any form of surgery is undertaken for their incontinence.

Catheter types

The catheters used for CISC are generally made of PVC. The product types available are described in the Directory of Toileting Aids[3] and shown in Fig. 43.3. Catheters are chosen to meet the requirements of the individual patient. Women may be taught with a male-length (40-cm)

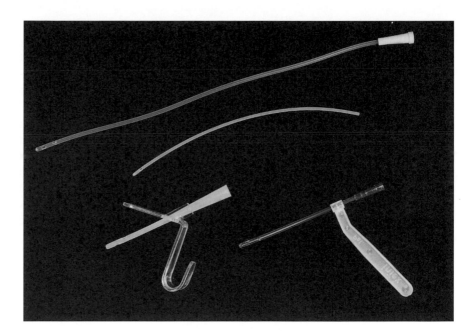

Fig. 43.3 Catheters for clean intermittent self-catheterization catheters

catheter but with developing confidence choose to use the shorter, female-length catheter (22-cm). Most adult women will use a size 10–12Ch. To avoid trauma the eyelets through which the urine will pass should be smooth; it is also essential that the rounded end of the catheter be passed into the urethra. For this reason some catheters designed for CISC have a wide end or funnel, and are useful for those patients with poor eyesight. All catheters should conform to the British Standard for manufacture.[13]

Whilst learning, in a hospital environment, if there is a urinary tract infection or during pregnancy, a new catheter should be used on each occasion. However, in general, if simple care is taken a Nealaton catheter can be used for up to a week. Self-lubricating catheters are available, but are more expensive and can only be used once. This type of catheter has a hydrophilic layer which enables the surface to bind with water, so that the catheter surface is covered by a layer of water on coming into contact with the urethral mucosa. Manufacturers claim this results in less trauma to the urethra and bladder wall when the catheter is inserted. Women do not necessarily need this form of catheter, and care should be taken when prescribing that the type and size of catheter required are made clear. The self-lubricating catheter should be used in accordance with manufacturer instructions. If the patient is not familiar with their use, she may not understand the preparation required and this will result in a traumatized urethra. An overview of the types of catheters available and their use can be seen in Figs. 43.1 and 43.3.

The Biscath system was developed in Birmingham Children's Hospital. It was observed that teenage girls with neurogenic bladders were notoriously bad at caring for their Nealaton catheters, and that therefore as a group they were more susceptible to infection and consequently renal damage (personal communication). The Biscath system was developed to ensure that this group had an acceptable method of bladder management. The system consists of a set of six short metal catheters, in a metal case. These catheters have found success in children and women, perhaps as the fine metal is less traumatic to the urothelium. The initial outlay for this system is expensive. The catheters are sterilized once a day in a domestic oven and have been observed to discolor with use.

Once the technique is established a regimen for undertaking CISC is devised with the patient. The aim is to achieve volumes below 500 ml. Initially, the patient is observed to ensure that there is no bad practice and that catheterization is sufficient to control urinary leakage. Some patients may need to carry out CISC up to six times daily, but constant review will ensure a continuing assessment of the need to catheterize. One of the main worries with a patient newly taught CISC is how he or she will undertake this procedure in a public toilet! Continuing support and use of widely available literature will help to alleviate misconceptions.

DRAINAGE SYSTEMS

Leg bags are designed to be used with long-term or short-term indwelling catheters. The range of products is extensive and current availability and pricing can be found in the Directory of Toileting Aids[3] (Fig. 43.4). The bags are designed to hold varying volumes. In general, bags are available with capacities of 350, 500 and 750 ml for daytime use. Two-litre bags are used for overnight drainage in long-term catheterized individuals. To reduce infection and prevent spillage the overnight bags are connected to the smaller leg bags to avoid disconnection of the system.[35,36]

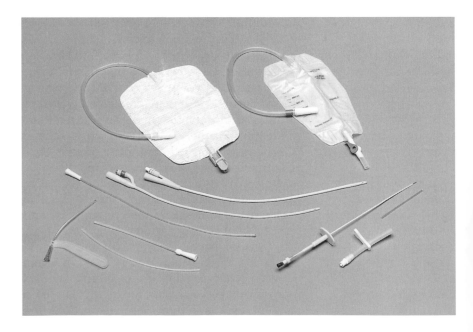

Fig. 43.4 Collecting bags

The types of bags used will depend on the patient assessment. Manual dexterity needs to be taken into consideration when deciding which type of tap should be used. Lifestyle of the patient may dictate where a bag is worn and suitable adaptation may be required.

Some patients find a catheter valve more acceptable. Catheter valves fit into the catheter and can be released at regular intervals to facilitate bladder drainage. In this way the infection risks of using a spigot are avoided. Although there has been little research into this product, it is felt that in the manually dexterous and motivated patient this will promote bladder tone and prevent bladder shrinkage.

Bypassing may also prove to be a problem and education in both nurse and patient is of paramount importance. They should be aware of problems which may be develop, such as urinary infection or blockage.

SUMMARY

Catheterization of an incontinent patient is not a procedure which should be undertaken lightly. If this is the only feasible option after objective investigation, then the catheter of choice should be one which is found by comprehensive assessment to be the most beneficial to that patient.

Care should always be modeled on good research-based practice, as this is the mode whereby quality of life will be maintained.

REFERENCES

1 Reybard JF. Traite pratique des rétrécissements du canal de l'urètre. Paris; Labe, 1853.
2 Zorgniotti AW. Early development of balloon catheter. Urology 1973; 1(1): 75–80.
3 Association of Continence Advisors: Directory of continence and toileting aids. London, 1992.
4 Faber M. New thoughts on male catheterisation. Nursing Times 1986; 64–66.
5 United Kingdom Central Council for Nursing, Midwifery and Health Visiting: Code of Professional Conduct: June 1992.
6 Roper N, Logan W, Tierney A. The elements of nursing, 4th edn. Edinburgh: Churchill Livingstone, 1990.
7 Ebner A, Madersbacher H, Scober F, Marbeger H. Hydrodynamic properties of Foley catheters and its clinical relevance. Proceedings of the 15th Meeting of the International Continence Society, London, 1985: pp 217–218.
8 Edwards LE, Lock R, Powell C, Jones P. Post-catheterisation ureatral strictures: a clinical and experimental study. British Journal of Urology 55: 53–56.
9 Kennedy AP, Brocklhurst JC, Lye MD. Factors related to the problems of long term catheterisation. Journal of Advanced Nursing 1983; 7: 411–417.
10 Crow RA, Chapman RG, Roe B, Wilson JA. A study of patients with an indwelling urethral catheter, and related nursing practice. Nursing Practice Research Unit, University of Surrey, 1986.
11 Roe BH, Chapman RG, Crow RA. A study of the procedures for catheter care recommended by health authorities and schools of nursing. Nursing Practice Unit, University of Surrey, 1987.
12 Blannin J, Hobden J. The catheters of choice. Nursing Times 76: 2092–2093.
13 BSI 1695 (1990). Urological catheters. London: British Standards Institution.
14 Wilksch J, Vernon-Roberts B, Garret R, Smith K. The role of catheter surface morphology and extractable cytotoxic material in tissue reactions to urethral catheters. British Journal of Urology 1983; 125: 48–52.
15 Nacey JN, Tulloch AGS, Ferguson AF. Catheter induced urethritis: a comparison between latex and silicone catheters in a prospective clinical trial. British Journal of Urology 1983; 57: 325–328.

16 Ruutu M, Alfhan O, Anderson LC. Cytotoxicity of latex urinary catheters. British Journal of Urology 1985; 57: 82–87.

17 Ryan-Wooley B. Aids for management incontinence. London: King's Fund, 1987.

18 Blacklock NJ. Catheters and urethral strictures. British Journal of Urology 1986; 58: 475–478.

19 Studer UE. How to fill silicone catheter balloons. Urology 1983; 22: 300–302.

20 Pullman BR, Phillips JI, Hickey DS. Uretral lumen, crosssectional shape: its radiological, determination and relationship to function. British Journal of Urology 1984; 399–407.

21 Brockhurst JC, Hickley DS, Davis I, Kenndy AP, Morris JA. A new urethral catheter. British Medical Journal 1988; 296: 1691–1693.

22 Kohl-Ockmore. Catheter concerns. Nursing Times 1993; Vol 89(2): 34–36.

23 Pomfret I. Conformacath update. Journal of Community Nursing Nov. 1992 14–16.

24 Capewell A, Morris SL. Audit of catheter management provided by district nurses and continence advisors. British Journal of Urology1993; 71: 259–264.

25 Fowler CJ, Beck RO, Betts, Lynn, B, Fowler CG. Intervesical capsaicin for treatment of detrusor hyperreflexia. Neurology and Urodynamics 11(4): 465–466.

26 Slade N, Gillespie W. The urinary tract and catheter infections and other problems. Chichester: wiley, 1985.

27 Elliot TS, Gopal-Rao G. Bladder irrigation. Age and Ageing 1988; 17: 373–378.

28 Flack S. Finding the best solution. Nursing Times 1993; 89(11): 68–74.

29 Roe B. Use of indwelling catheters. clinical nursing practice: the promotion and management of continence. prentice-Hall, 1992.

30 Barnes D, Shaw PJ, Timoney AG, Tsokos N. Management of the neuropathic bladder by suprapubic catheterisation. British Journal of Urology 1993; 72: 169–172.

31 Winder A. Intermittent selfcatheterisation. Nursing Times 1990; 86: 43.

32 Lapides J, Dionka AC, Gould F, Bette S, Lowe BS. Further observations of self catheterisation. American association of Genito Urinary surgeons 67: 15–17.

33 Winder A. Intermittent self catheterisation. Clinical nursing practice: the promotion and management of continence. Prentice-Hall, 1992.

34 Sheri H, Barnes. The development of a comprehensive instructional package for teaching intermittent self catheterisation. Journal Enterostom Ther 1985; 13: 238–241.

35 Kennedy AP. Drainage system on trial. Nursing Mirror 1984; 158(7): 19–20.

36 Roe B, Brocklehurst J. Study of patients with indwelling catheters. Journal of Advanced Nursing 1987; 12: 713–718.

44 Pads and pants

INTRODUCTION

The use of pads and pants for control of incontinence should not be the first line of management. It is essential that the incontinent patient be assessed appropriately so that the best available treatment can be offered in the first instance. However, for some women suffering from incontinence, pads may well be the only practical method of control and they can also be used as a temporary measure while objective investigation is undertaken, or treatment awaited.

Incontinence is not normally a life-threatening condition, but the social stigma associated with it can create enormous pressure for an individual in a society where there are demands for domestic hygiene and cleanliness. To be seen to be incontinent is therefore not acceptable. Many women would rather buy expensive, unsuitable products than seek appropriate help. Incontinence can be an expensive business. Incontinence garments, consisting of an absorbent body-worn pad held in place by special pants or fashioned into a garment, are in common use and are very costly to the health service.[1]

PADS

In the last 10 years the availability of products has increased enormously. In 1974 the Australian Bill Kylie launched an oblong absorbent pad which became the forerunner of the disposable pad industry. In 1983 the Incontinence Action Group published a report which encouraged companies to advertise. In the United Kingdom the consumable industry has developed rapidly since 1970, so it is difficult for even specialist nurses to keep up with the choice available. This is unfortunate, as it is these specialist continence advisors who will normally recommend products for regional use. Furthermore, products are changing all the time so that the results of the limited studies available are often out of date before publication. Thus a review of the literature is disappointing. Few products are assessed in quality trials and most of the current data in the United Kingdom are from one specialist unit.

Current availability of products is documented in the Association of Continence Advisors' Directory of Continence and Toileting Aids.[2] More recently, Philp & Cottenden[3] have produced a comprehensive guide to

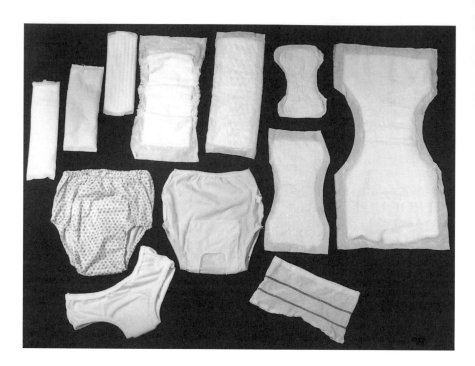

Fig. 44.1 Pads and pants

reusable products available in the United Kingdom. Their article provides information about the products currently in use and the addresses of the companies supplying them.

There are approximately 70 types of reusable pad available today, some of which are shown in Fig. 44.1. Most products are designed for a broad spectrum of users, while others are used for specific groups. In 1992 researchers at St Pancras Hospital, London, published the results of studies they carried out assessing the efficiency, durability and acceptability of these products.[4] In a series of articles they have evaluated the durability of reusables in the light of environmental and consumer benefits.[5,6,7,8,9]

ASSESSMENT

Assessment is a key factor in individualized care. It is defined by Roper[10] as collecting information, reviewing the collected information, identifying the patient's problems and identifying the priority of problems. Before a specific pad and pants system is recommended, a full assessment of the patient's needs will be required to ensure optimal benefit.[11] The assessment and allocation of pads is generally carried out by the continence advisor or district nurse. Important points to consider include:

- the severity of incontinence
- the cause of incontinence (as demonstrated on urodynamics)
- mobility and dexterity
- fluid balance
- concurrent medication
- bowel habits
- provision of toileting facilities
- disposal and laundry facilities
- lifestyle
- occupation
- social activities
- sexual relationships.

These guidelines are not exhaustive and can be adapted to provide individual and on-going care in the presence of changing needs.

PADS

Efforts have been made to produce the most 'user-friendly' pad, but their general purpose and properties remain the same. There is a vast array of pads made from various materials, including wood pulp with or without superabsorbent polymer. Pads are manufactured in numerous shapes and sizes. The most recently developed are those containing super-absorbers. These are a group of polymers capable of absorbing 50 times their own weight under some degree of pressure. Fluff (wood) pulps are cheaper but hold only five times their weight beneath pressures typically found under a seated or supine person.[12] Studies have shown that the performance of the two types of product is not dependent on the quality of absorbency, but also on the shape and how often they are changed.[13] They can therefore be designed for different purposes from double incontinence through to light daytime urinary incontinence. Thus the performance of incontinence pads can be enhanced by design and demand.

The most comprehensive trials of body-worn pads and pants are those published by Journet,[14] Malone-Lee,[15] Faber[16] and more recently Philp.[7] The basic structure of all trials has been to compare different pad and pants systems in groups of incontinent subjects; data were collected by structured interview to assess performance. The pad and pants systems used were compared with regard to their acceptability and efficacy. The studies undertaken concentrated on the performance of the pad, rather than the pants. However, where the pants are an integral part of the garment, it is still the absorbency which carries the most weight when performance is described.

Journet[14] used questionnaires to grade performance of 15 different pad and pants systems (Table 44.1) in 45 handicapped children under the age of 15 years. Each child tested 6 systems for a 1-month period and each product was used by at least 10 children. The results of the trial concluded that no single product was suitable for all handicapped children and that it was vital that a choice should be offered for experimentation.

Table 44.1   Assessment of pads and pants (Journet 1981)[14]

Pads with separate plastic pants	IPS pads and pants	IPS Hospital Supplies Ltd
	Inco roll and drop front pants	Robinsons and Sons Ltd
	Inco roll and pull on pants	Robinsons and Sons Ltd
	Sandra pull-on pads and pants	Henley's Group
	Sandra drop-flat pants and pads	Henley's Group
	Maxi snibb and pads	Molnlycke Ltd
	Feel free pull-on pads and pants	Contenta
	Extra large Readinaps	Robinson and Sons Ltd
	Golden Babe overnight nappies and pants	Smith and Nephew Medical Ltd
Pants with separate textile and pants	Kanga doublet pads and pants	Kanga Hospital Products Ltd
All-in-one nappy	Kanga pads and pants	
	Cosifit	Kanga Hospital Products Ltd
	Peaudouce	Robinsons and Sons Ltd
	Snugglies	Peaudouce (UK) Ltd
		Curity
Plastic-backed pad and stretch net pants	Maxi plus pads and stretch pants	Molnlycke

Table 44.2   Assessment of pads and pants (Malone-Lee et al 1982)[15]

Pads with separate plastic pants	Sandra plastic pads and insert pads	Henley's Group
	Maxi snibb and pads	Molnylcke
Plastic-backed pads and stretch net pants	Comfort insert pads 2245 and 2260 and stretch pants	Ancilla (UK) Ltd
	Tenaform pad and stretch pants	Molnlycke
	Tenaform pad and stretch pants	Molnlycke
	Dandeliner and stretch pants	Smith and Nephew Medical Ltd
Marsupial pads and pants	Kanga lady pants and single pads	Kanga Hospital Products Ltd
	Kanga standard pants and standard pads	Kanga Hospital products Ltd

Malone-Lee et al[15] (Table 44.2) tested 8 different pad and pant systems in 113 subjects. Sixty were community-dwelling and the remainder were resident in Part Three (sheltered) accommodation. They ranged from 30 to 100 years but most subjects were in their 70s and 80s. Of these subjects, 22 had slight incontinence, 51 moderate incontinence and 40 heavy incontinence. The pad systems were trialed for a month each and the subjects or their carers gave their views using structured interviews. The study found that at least 7 of 8 products trialed were the favorite of at least 1 community dweller, but the requirements of those in Part Three accommodation differed from the rest. This underlines the need for individual assessment of incontinent patients with different priorities.

Faber et al[16] used 26 incontinence aid systems (Table 44.3) and 137 testers. The products were divided into three groups depending on the level of incontinence they were designed to deal with. Subjects who had

Table 44.3 Test products (in Faber et al 1986)[16]

Group 1		
Marsupial pads and pants	Kanga lady pants and single pads	Kanga Hospital Products Ltd
	Sandralux pants and single pads	Henley's Group Kanga Hospital Products Ltd
Inco roll and pants	Moltexal interliner roll and pants	Brevet Hospital Products
Plastic-backed pads and stretch pants	Dandeliner	Smith and Nephew Medical Ltd
	Tenette Plus Sanitary towel	Molnlycke Ltd Johnson and Johnson (UK) Ltd
	Daisy	LIC Ltd
	Molinea	Paul Hartmann AG
	Tranquility	Henley's Group
	Cumfie, small	Veron Carus Ltd
Group 2		
Plastic-backed pads and stretch pants	Tenaform, normal	Molnlycke Ltd
	Polypad	Undercover Products International Ltd
	Interliner	IPS Hospital Supplies
	Molinea	Paul Hartmann AG
	Inco care	Robinson and Sons Ltd
	Cumfie, large	Veron Carus Ltd
	Cumfie, medium	Veron Carus Ltd
All-in-one nappy	Slipad	Peaudouce (UK) Ltd
Wingfold pads and stretch pants	Doublet	Kanga Hospital Products Ltd
	Incontinette	Ancilla (UK) Ltd
Marsupial pads and pants	Kanga standard	Kanga Hospital Products Ltd
	Urocare	IDC (UK) Ltd
Group 3		
Plastic-backed pads and stretch pants	Tenaform, super	Molnlycke
All-in-one nappy	Tenders	Ancilla (UK) Ltd
Wingfold pads and stretch pants	Diaper	IPS Hospital Supplies Ltd
	Deopad	LIC Ltd

Table 44.4 Patient groupings (Faber et al 1986)[16]

Group 1	Garments for light incontinence	33 female, 1 male
Group 2	Garments for heavy daytime incontinence	79 female, 22 male
Group 3	Garments for heavy night-time incontinence	39 female, 8 male Taken from group 2

previously been graded lightly, moderately or heavily incontinent, according to their degree of urinary leakage over a 3-day period, were then allocated to a group (Table 44.4).

The testers chose the products in their group that they wished to try. The pads were worn in random order for at least 7 days. Comments were then gathered regarding performance of each product. The study found that a pulp-filled pad worn with pouch pants was the most suitable for mobile independent patients (group 1). However, immobile or dependent patients (groups 2 and 3) required highly absorbent shaped pads worn with stretch net pants, so mobility and independence would seem to be the most important factors determining what type of incontinence garment is suitable for a patient. Mobile independent patients require smaller, discreet pads. Immobile or dependent patients require larger, more absorbent pads. A range of garments is necessary to suit the needs of the incontinent patient.

Pad types

Absorbent roll

Not used as often as shaped pads, absorbent roll is really only useful for light incontinence. However, it has the advantage that it can be cut to suit an individual's requirements. A variation of this product worn with pants with a waterproof panel scored highly in Faber's study as the testers preferred to cut their own length of pad. Because the size of pad was adapted by the tester this product was reported to have no effect at all on which clothes the patient chose to wear. The pieces are cut from the roll and can be worn with stretch net or pouch pants or the subject's own underwear.

Plastic-backed pads

These pads are used extensively. Manufactured in varying weights, shapes and sizes, they may or may not contain superabsorbers. Worn with the patient's own underwear, or with mesh pants, they often have a self-adhesive strip to ensure correct placement and prevent movement.

The absorbency of these pads is dependent on the material used in production. One of the major disadvantages with pads is that they can bulk up and the coverstock (outside covering) sheet comes apart if they are not changed appropriately. The inclusion of superabsorbers was felt to hold considerable potential, but the study by Philp et al[13] concluded that superabsorbers do not necessarily improve performance and acceptability of a pad. This study trialed 3 plastic pads with superabsorbers and 3 plastic pads without; a breakdown of products is shown in Table 44.5.

Pouch pads

This type of pad is not plastic-backed, and is designed for use with the marsupial or pouch pants system. Size is dependent on the pouch used and the degree of incontinence. This system has proved popular with patients with light to moderate incontinence. However, the disadvantage of this system is that the soiled garment remains in contact with the skin even when the pad is removed, and is therefore not recommended in those patients who suffer from fecal incontinence.

Table 44.5 Products used in the study by Philp et al 1986

Cumfie, small (Vernon Carus Ltd)	
Size:	31.5 × 11.0 × 1.0
Weight:	30 g
Core:	Fluff pulp
Coverstock:	Viscose
Backing:	Polyethylene film
Features:	Core embossed in cross-hatch pattern

Tennette, extra (Molnlycke Ltd)	
Size:	33.5 × 9.0 (centre) and 15.0 (ends) × 0.8(centre) and 0.2 (ends) cm
Weight:	29 g
Core:	Fluff pulp
Coverstock:	Polypropylene
Backing:	Polyethylene film
Features:	Shaped

Serenity, regular (Johnson and Johnson)	
Size:	21.5 × 6.5 (centre) × 11.0 (end) × 2.0 (centre) and 0.3 (ends) cm
Weight:	16 g
Core:	Powdered superabsorber beneath corrugated polyester web
Coverstock:	Polyethylene polyester
Backing:	Polyethylene vinylacetate foam
Features:	Shaped and cupped

Restful 200 (International Disposables Corporation)	
Size:	29.5 × 11.0 × 1.0 cm
Weight:	22 g
Core:	Fluff pulp
Coverstock:	Polypropylene
Backing:	Polyethylene film
Features:	Core embossed in cross-hatch pattern

Conveen, regular (Colopast Ltd)	
Size:	21.0 × 9.0 × 0.8 cm
Weight:	18 g
Core:	Fluff pulp + powdered superabsorber + thermoplastic fibers
Coverstock:	Polypropylene
Backing:	Polyethylene film
Features:	Core longitudinally grooved; pad end curved

Super Strola, large (IPS Hospital Supplies Ltd)	
Size:	30.5 × 12.0 × 0.5 cm
Weight:	Approx 20 g
Core:	Fluff pulp + powdered superabsorbers + thermoplastic fibers
Coverstock:	Polyester
Backing:	Polyethylene film
Features:	Core longitudinally embossed

Washable pads

Some pads are reusable and are made from an absorbent polyester. They have a waterproof backing and can be worn with normal underwear or stretch pants, but are unsuitable for double incontinence. Recent trials have been undertaken to assess the suitability and acceptability of this type of product.

All-in-one pads

These are similar to babies' nappies and are worn without additional pants. Because of their easy side fastenings they are particularly suitable for disabled patients. They can be used for both heavy urinary incontinence and fecal incontinence.

Bed protectors

Bed-bound patients and those with nocturnal enuresis may find that even well-fitted incontinence systems cannot prevent some degree of leakage. They require the additional protection of a bed pad. These can be disposable or reusable, and comparative trials have been carried out to assess performance. Clancy[17] concluded in a trial of 6 bed protectors that in the absence of a substantially improved disposable pad, washable bed protectors should be considered for a heavily incontinent adult, but with the proviso that this would have implications for appropriate washing and drying facilities.

Clancy[17] also stressed the need for individual assessment and careful selection of the most appropriate products for each patient. More recently, Norris et al[18] carried out a multicenter controlled crossover trial to compare 6 reusable bed pads. The pads were evaluated in community, nursing home and hospital patients and were assessed on their performance and laundering durability. The study concluded that the decision whether or not to use reusable incontinence products is a complex one dependent on individual needs and preferences. The availability of suitable laundry facilities is also paramount, as are financial constraints. Another factor in the choice concerns organization and convenience.

PANTS

There are numerous designs of pants available (Fig. 44.1) which can be adapted to suit the severity and type of incontinence. When considering pants it is important to assess mobility and possible spasticity of the limbs. Manual dexterity is also an important factor. Pants should be well fitting without being too tight. Care needs to be taken to ensure that the fabric does not damage skin at the waist or groin. Most products are designed to be reusable, and therefore laundry facilities and possible allergies to detergents need to be taken into consideration.

Skin which will be in contact with urine needs to be treated carefully. Thick layers of barrier cream should not be applied as this will affect the absorption of the pads or pants used. Barrier cream should therefore only be used in a thin layer applied to dry unbroken skin. Vaseline is perhaps the simplest and cheapest product available. Broken skin needs closer nursing management to effect healing and may require a more specific topical cream.

Stretch pants

There are lightweight garments made from washable nylon net. They are used with varying sizes of plastic-backed pads. This style of pants has been extensively trial led, but it is normally the pad that is analyzed, not the pants.

Marsupial pants

These pants are manufactured from a one-way fabric with a pouch into which a pad can be fitted, thus keeping all plastic away from the skin.

The advantage of this type of appliance is that the pad can be changed without changing pants. This type of garment is not suitable for heavy urinary incontinence or double incontinence. Pants with a plastic gusset should not be used with plastic-backed pads as a double layer of plastic will encourage skin irritation and chaffing. The main disadvantage is that the soiled pouch remains in contact with the skin when the pad is changed.

Waterproof pants

Waterproof pants are not recommended, but can still be purchased at commercial outlets. They look like babies' plastic pants, and their main disadvantage is the skin excoriation leading to chaffing, irritation and local infection.

Washable pants

This type of underwear is useful for light incontinence. The pants have a special absorbent gusset which will soak up urine, and can therefore be used without a pad. These pants can be washed in the normal way. They avoid the need for bulky products and are therefore useful on holidays.

SUMMARY

The main aim of pads and pants is to provide an acceptable form of urinary control which will ensure the dignity and self-confidence of the consumer. It has been demonstrated by almost every recent study that no one product is suitable for all. Individual assessment is therefore mandatory in order to ensure that the correct systems are allocated.

Only a small selection of products available have been subjected to clinical trial. There is a need for more comprehensive studies comparing classes of pads and pants systems as opposed to specific products.

Having selected the most suitable products for the incontinent patient, it is important to assess compliance and to change the incontinence aids as necessary to suit different needs and maintain optimum efficacy and acceptability.

NOTE

In the studies of products presented in the tables in this chapter, it is important to note that it is the *system* of incontinence protection used rather than the product that is of relevance. Up-to-date information on products currently available with price guides can be found in the Directory of Continence and Toileting Aids.[2] The directory also provides addresses of companies who can be contacted directly for product details.

REFERENCES

1 Health Services Supplies Council. A market appraisal of the supply of incontinence pads to the National Health Service. 1984.
2 Association of Continence Advisors. Directory of continence and toileting aids. London, 1992.
3 Philp J, Cottenden A. Picking and choosing. Nursing Times 1993; 89(30).
4 Cottenden A, Ledger D, Phlip J. A study of reusable body worn absorbent incontinence from the UK consumer's perspective. London: Continence Advisory Service, 1992.
5 Cottenden A, Ledger D, Philp J. The reuser's guide. Nursing Times 1992; 88(44): 66–72.
6 Cottenden A, Ledger D, Philp J. A testing time. Nursing Times 1993; 89(14): 59–62.
7 Cottenden A, Ledger D, Philp J. Well disposed. Nursing Times 1993: 89(16): 65–68.
8 Cottenden A, Ledger D, Philp J. Mix and match. Nursing Times 1993; 89(16): 70–74.
9 Cottenden A, Ledger D, Philp J. Wash and wear. Nursing Times 1993; 21: 63–66.
10 Roper N, Logan W, Tierney A. The elements of nursing, 4th edn. Edinburgh: Churchill Livingstone, 1990.
11 Duffin H. Assessment of urinary incontinence. Clinical nursing practice: the promotion and management of continence. Prentice-Hall, 1992.
12 Cottenden A. Incontinence pads: clinical performance, design, and technical properties. J of biomedical engineering 1988; 10(6): 506–514.
13 Philp J, Butchers D, Cottenden A. Are you sitting comfortably? Nursing Times 1989; 85(7): 68–73.
14 Jornet C. DHSS aids assessment programme: incontinence aids for handicapped children. HMSO, 1981.
15 Malone-Lee J, McCreery M, Exton-Smith A. A community study of the performance of incontinence garments. DHSS aids assessment programme. HMSO, 1982.
16 Faber M, Barnes E, Malone-Lee J, Cottenden A. Incontinence garments: results of a DHSS study. Health Equipment Information 156, 1986.
17 Clancy B. Bed protectors no easy choice. Nursing Times 1989; 85(33): 20–23.
18 Norris C, Cottenden A, Ledger D. Underpad overview. Nursing Times 1993; 89(21).

45 Aids and appliances

The female anatomy does not allow easy application of aids and appliances to maintain dryness. For this reason the number of devices available for women with incontinence is far more limited than it is for men. In this chapter we will first describe those aids that help keep the patient dry followed by those aids that inform the patient when she is being incontinent. The latter may help teach certain groups of women toilet training. Finally, we will describe those aids that are available for women who have intractable incontinence, either due to lack of treatment or failure of treatment, and which will prevent long-term skin reaction from exposure to urine.

MAINTAINING CONTINENCE

In women with proven genuine stress incontinence, where pelvic floor exercises and operative techniques have failed, or in those women who have chosen not to have an operation or are unfit for surgery, there are certain devices that may help in maintaining continence. Vaginal plugs work by causing a relative outflow obstruction, thus raising the urethral pressure. They are useful for women who merely leak during strenuous exercise.[1] Normal commercial sanitary tampons may be suitable but alternatively there are available specific tampons designed for this purpose. Femcare produce a tampon known as the Contrelle; however, these are not available on prescription. The tampon can be washed and reused to reduce costs.

Other devices that may be of benefit are vaginal rings and Hodge pessaries that are used for prolapse, as again these cause relative outflow obstruction. These are usually worn continuously by women with prolapse and genuine stress incontinence, but there is no reason why they cannot be taught how to insert these themselves, enabling intermittent use. The physician must, however, be aware that occasionally ring pessaries can lead to urinary retention. Another potentially useful device is the contraceptive diaphragm. All vaginal plugs may be of benefit in cases of mild genuine stress incontinence but in more severe cases they are unlikely to be suitable. As they are all effective because of the relative outflow obstruction that they cause, those that are left in place for long periods of time may result in incomplete bladder emptying and urinary tract infections.

A new vaginal device, specifically designed for women with incontinence, the introl, has two bladder neck supports to avoid the problem of outflow obstruction during voiding. It can easily be removed, washed and re-used.

A further device that has been studied but which is not available in the United Kingdom is the urethral plug.[2] This consists of a urethral plate, a soft stalk and one or two spheres along the stalk. The plug is inserted into the end of the urethra preventing leakage of urine. It is removed to enable voiding. Urethral plugs have not gained much popularity and at the moment are not used in clinical practice.

Another device that is not yet available on the market is the foam barrier.[3] It consists of a small triangular foam pad with a layer of hydrophilic adhesive on one side. It is placed within the vulva and the adhesive covers the urethral meatus preventing leakage of urine. Preliminary data suggest that it may have a use in clinical practice.

Recently, Staskin et al[4] have reported the results of an expandable occlusion device for maintenance of continence in women with stress incontinence. The silicone device is inserted into the urethra with the aid of an attached syringe and a small balloon is inflated to maintain it in place. The device is removed for voiding and when not needed by pulling a short string which deflates the balloon. The data suggest a high degree of satisfaction and continence by users of this continence device.

As an alternative to pads the FemAssist, which occludes the urethral externally by improving the Lernietic Seal, may prove to be useful, but still undergoing clinical triale. It is cheap and can be washed and re-used for up to a week.

TRAINING THE BLADDER

Body-worn (Fig. 45.1) and bed alarms (Fig. 45.2) can be used to alert the patient when she has started to wet herself or the bed. They are particularly useful for those patients with nocturnal enuresis who have failed to improve with pharmacological agents. These devices provide a form of bladder training. When the patient leaks urine, an alarm will go off which will alert or wake her. Therefore, with time she will learn to wake up when she needs to pass urine. Whether a body-worn alarm or a bed alarm is used is determined by doctor and patient preference and the patient will be assessed in order to determine that which best fits her lifestyle. Obviously, the bed alarm is only used for nocturnal enuresis but the body-worn alarm can also be used for daytime bladder training. The alarm can be on a remote device so that when it wakes her, she has to get up and got to the bathroom to turn it off. Alarms are available with various modifications such as a vibrating device to wake the patient rather than a sonic alarm. This could be used when a couple are sharing a bed to prevent the alarm also waking her partner. Alternatively, for use in a double bed, a body-worn alarm would be more sensible than a bed one.

Another aid available for bladder training, particularly for children or adults with learning difficulties, is the musical toilet (Fig. 45.3). Every

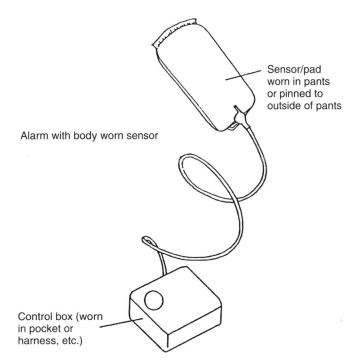

Sensor/pad
worn in pants
or pinned to
outside of pants

Alarm with body worn sensor

Fig. 45.1   A body-worn alarm
(With permission, Directory
of Continence and Toileting
Aids from Association
Continence Advisers 1988)

Control box (worn
in pocket or
harness, etc.)

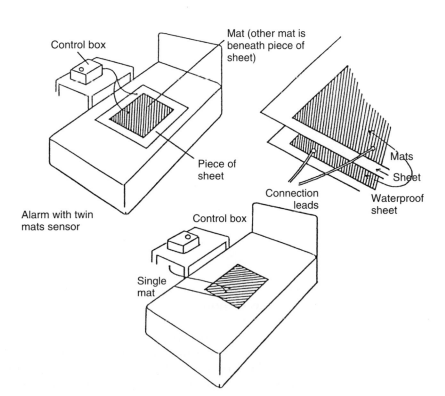

Control box

Mat (other mat is
beneath piece of
sheet)

Piece of
sheet

Mats

Sheet

Connection
leads

Waterproof
sheet

Alarm with twin
mats sensor

Control box

Single
mat

Fig. 45.2   A bed alarm
(With permission, Directory
of Continence and Toileting
Aids from Association
Continence Advisers 1988)

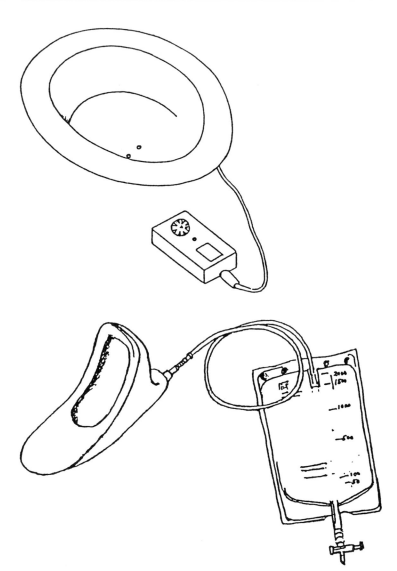

Fig. 45.3 A musical toilet
(With permission, Directory
of Continence and Toileting
Aids from Association
Continence Advisers 1988)

Fig. 45.4 The Bridge urinal
(With permission, Directory
of Continence and Toileting
Aids from Association
Continence Advisers 1988)

time urine passes into the toilet, a tune is played. This is obviously of limited use in adults and is of more benefit for toilet training children.

INTRACTABLE INCONTINENCE

Collecting devices Some women are unable to get to the toilet in time and this results in leakage of urine. This is the case, for example, with in women with intractable detrusor instability (i.e. in whom treatment with anticholinergic drugs or bladder drill has failed) and those women with mobility problems.[5] Collecting devices are merely portable toilets. They are all hand-held collecting devices but are designed so that they fit over the vulva and can be kept at the bedside, chairside or in the car to be used at a moment's notice. Examples include the Bridge urinal (Fig. 45.4), the St Peter's boat, the Pantype female urinal and the swan-necked female urinal. To aid in the use of hand-held voiding devices, various cushions are available and are especially useful for the wheelchair-bound patient.

Commodes

For those women who are mobile but not able to get to the toilet in time, a commode is useful. There are many varieties of commode and some of the more attractive ones look like normal furniture, where the lid can be lifted to reveal a commode seat. There are many commercially available types; some are collapsible so that they can travel with the patient; others have adjustable legs, backs and sides so that the dimensions fit the particular person. Health authorities will have a selection of different commodes that can be ordered to suit everyone.

Chemical toilets

Some commodes are chemical toilets, and this avoids the need for emptying after each use. They can be used by an elderly or disabled person on her own as they only need to be emptied once a day or even every other day.

Toilet adaptation

Some people need to have their existing toilet adapted so that it is easier to use. Adaptations include raising the toilet seat if the existing toilet is at too low a level, or adding handlebars to allow steadying during voiding.

Aiding easy toileting

Pads and pants have already been described in a previous chapter, but in addition to these, special items of clothing are available. Articles of clothing are designed such that toileting is quicker and easier and include open-

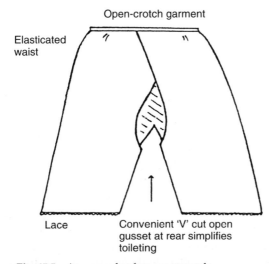

Open-crotch garment

Elasticated waist

Lace

Convenient 'V' cut open gusset at rear simplifies toileting

Fig. 45.5 An example of an open-crotch garment
(With permission, Directory of Continence and Toileting Aids from Association Continence Advisers 1988)

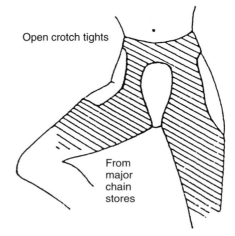

Open crotch tights

From major chain stores

Fig. 45.6 An example of open-crotch tights (obtainable from major chain stores)
(With permission, Directory of Continence and Toileting Aids from Association Continence Advisers 1988)

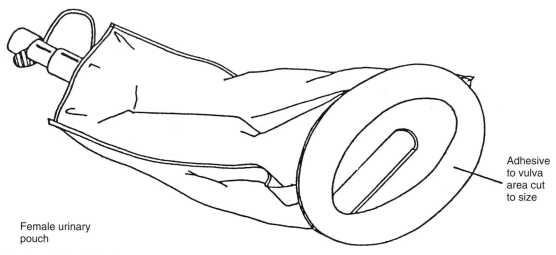

Female urinary pouch

Adhesive to vulva area cut to size

Fig. 45.7 A female body-worn device with adhesive backing
(With permission, Directory of Continence and Toileting Aids from Association Continence Advisers 1988)

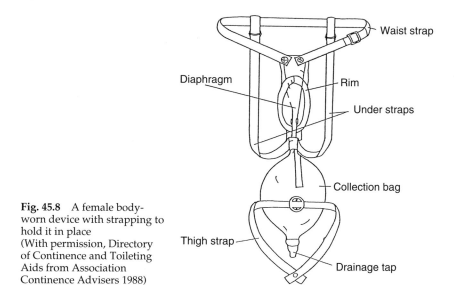

Waist strap

Diaphragm

Rim

Under straps

Collection bag

Thigh strap

Drainage tap

Fig. 45.8 A female body-worn device with strapping to hold it in place
(With permission, Directory of Continence and Toileting Aids from Association Continence Advisers 1988)

backed skirts. These save time as there is no need to pull up a skirt prior to sitting on the commode. Other designs such as open-crotch garments allow the patient to wear tights or underwear but still enable them to get to the toilet rapidly (Fig. 45.5 and 45.6). Furthermore, clothing can be adapted with Velcro and loose-fitting waists to allow ease of toileting.

Collection of leakage

The male anatomy is suitable for sheaths to prevent leakage of urine. Although the female anatomy is more limiting, there are certain devices worn against the body to collect leaked urine. These are known as female body-worn urinals. An example is shown in Fig. 45.7. The part that sticks on to the vulva has adhesive backing and is regularly changed but can be attached to a drainage bag for overnight use. More complex devices, involving strapping to hold them in place, have been produced but are not commonly used (Fig. 45.8).

Furniture protection

For women with intractable incontinence who have nocturnal enuresis, wetting the bed will lead to damage of the mattress and long-term hygienic problems. For this reason waterproof covers are available. These include plastic sheets to cover the mattress which can either be loose-fitting or fitted, to prevent leakage around the side. Also plastic pillow cases and plastic duvet covers can be used. Unfortunately, although plastic helps to keep the mattress and pillows dry, it may result in skin irritation and excoriation.

Odor control

In patients with intractable incontinence, leakage can result in a persistent smell of urine. Various proprietary sprays are available to try and cover up ammoniacal smells. Suitable pads and pants and protective clothing in addition to frequent toileting will limit the need for their use, but they are still essential in certain patients. They are based on traditional air fresheners that are available for general use.

Many of the devices described in this chapter can be obtained through community health services, usually under the direction of the local continence advisor. Although the aim of treatment is to achieve continence, this is not always possible, and these devices will at least improve the lifestyle of this group of patients.

REFERENCES

1 Nygaard IE. Treatment of exercise incontinence with mechanical devices. Neurourol Urodyn 1992; 11: 367–368.
2 Nielsen KK, Kromann-Andersen B, Jacobsen H et al. The urethral plug: a new treatment for genuine stress incontinence in women. J Urol 1990; 144: 1199–1202.
3 Newman DK, Smith DA, Harris T, Diokno A. An external female barrier device in the management of urinary incontinence. Neurourol Urodyn 1992; 11: 368–369.
4 Staskin D, Bevendam T, Davila G et al. A multicentre experience using an expandable urethral occlusion device for management of urinary stress incontinence. Neurourol Urodyn 1994; 13: 380–381.
5 Wyman JF, Elswick RK Jr, Ory MG, Wilson MS, Fantl JA. Influence of functional, urological and environmental characteristics on urinary incontinence in community dwelling older women. Nurs Res 1993; 42(5): 270–275.

Section 9 Quality of Life

46

Quality of life

INTRODUCTION

Urinary incontinence is a distressing and disabling condition causing significant morbidity within society. It affects the social, psychological, occupational, domestic, physical and sexual lives of 15–30% of women of all ages.[1] Sufferers give up many aspects of their usual lifestyle with obvious detriment to their social interactions, interpersonal and sexual relationships, careers and psychological wellbeing. Activities such as household chores, physical recreation and hobbies are particularly affected and a new way of life organized around the location of toilets and the avoidance of potentially embarrassing situations developing.

Disappointingly, although incontinence is the source of considerable morbidity, over 50% of incontinent women never seek help for their condition or do so only after many years of misery.[2] An equally distressing finding is that many women who do tell their doctor about their urinary symptoms are either told to live with them, briefly instructed to do pelvic floor exercises without training or explanation, or prescribed anticholinergic drugs. Often patients do not benefit from this advice, which reinforcing the belief that little can be done to help their incontinence, and spreading this pessimistic outlook to their friends and relatives.

Research has until recently concentrated on the prevalence, etiology, diagnosis and management of incontinence, and relatively little was known about the effects of this chronic condition or indeed its management on quality of life and psychosocial functioning.

Over the last few decades interest in the incorporation of patient-assessed health status or quality of life (QoL) measures into the evaluation of medical care has increased.[3] Studies have shown that clinicians' and patients' judgements of QoL and the effects of clinical interventions differ substantially, which has increased recognition of the patient's view as central to the assessment of disease severity and evaluation of medical care.

This view has brought with it a multitude of approaches for the measurement of QoL. Unfortunately, although clinicians often find the information from QoL assessment useful and informative, trials have shown that it rarely alters clinical decision-making.[4,5] Many feel that the concepts of QoL or health, especially if self-assessed by a patient or member of the public, are too subjective, vague or imprecise to be of any clinical value. In addition, QoL data are often inappropriate to the clinical context, or presented in an uninterpretable manner.

As part of our attempt to understand the plight of the incontinent population and the efficacy of our therapeutic interventions, QoL assessment is appealing. Not only would it allow us to quantify distress and evaluate treatment efficacy, but it would also enable us to understand how lives are affected, how adaptive changes are made and what finally makes women ask for help.

WHAT IS QUALITY OF LIFE?

There is no consensus definition of QoL or indeed subjective health status, although it has come to mean a combination of patient-assessed measures of health, including physical function, role function, social function, emotional or mental state, burden of symptoms and sense of wellbeing.[6]

Quality of life is highly subjective, mediated by personal and cultural values, beliefs, self-concepts, goals and life expectancy. The term is influenced by a broad spectrum of human experiences including diseases, accidents, treatments, interpersonal relationships and social support. The World Health Organization (WHO) has defined health as 'not merely the absence of disease, but complete physical, mental and social wellbeing'.[7]

It is now recognized that a patient's QoL and psychosocial adjustment to illness are both equally as important as the status of their physical disease,[8,9,10] and the success of treatment can no longer be measured purely in terms of clinical parameters alone.

HOW TO MEASURE QUALITY OF LIFE

Quality of life is usually measured by the use of questionnaires completed by the patient herself, or as part of a structured clinical interview. Although many different questionnaires are now available each conforms to the same basic structure. The questionnaires consist of a variable number of domains (or sections), usually 1–7, which gather information focused on particular aspects of health and QoL. The commonly listed dimensions of QoL are as follows:

- physical function, e.g. mobility, self care, exercise
- emotional function, e.g. depression, anxiety, worry
- social function, e.g. intimacy, social support, social contact, leisure activities
- role performance, e.g. work, housework, shopping
- pain
- sleep/nausea
- disease-specific symptoms.

APPLICATIONS OF QOL MEASURES IN UROGYNECOLOGY

Quality of life questionnaires have many different applications:

- screening and monitoring for psychosocial problems in individual patient care
- population surveys of perceived health problems
- medical audit
- outcome measures in health services or evaluation research
- clinical trials
- cost–utility analyses
- an adjunct to the clinical interview.

Perhaps the most obvious use for standardized health measurement profiles is as outcome measures in clinical trials.

For the purpose of clinical trials urinary symptoms and/or urodynamic parameters are usually assessed before and after treatment, but these measurements convey little information regarding the impact of urinary incontinence on the QoL of urinary incontinent women. Quality of life measures would be of great benefit for the initial evaluation of the impact of urinary incontinence and of improvement following treatment. They would be of particular value for the comparison of treatments with little apparent objective or subjective difference in clinical outcome, but where, by methodology or limitation of side effects, they confer QoL benefit over standard and accepted techniques.

An example would be the comparison of laparoscopic colposuspension with that performed via a transverse suprapubic incision, although the technique and objective success of the former has yet to be formally evaluated in long-term clinical trials.[11]

Of particular interest would be the use of QoL assessment in the evaluation of treatment for detrusor instability (DI). Although clinical trials often report significant improvements in objective urodynamic parameters following the treatment of this condition, it is often difficult to evaluate improvement in the QoL of the women treated.

The standard treatment for DI usually includes the prescription of anticholinergic drugs, which themselves produce side effects and may adversely affect QoL. Follow-up studies have reported disappointing long-term results of treatment with anticholinergic therapy,[12,13] and clinical trials have often found little difference in the efficacy of active and placebo treatments.

In addition to these obvious clinical applications, QoL assessment may prove to be important for the allocation of financial resources in an already overutilized and underfunded health service. The economic impact of continence care is considerable but difficult to quantify accurately. Research in the United States estimated the cost of continence care in 1984 to be $8.8 billion.[14] Allocating resources amongst competing clinical specialties requires a common aspect of health care output to be measured, and subsequent assessment of need.

An extreme example is the American Medicaid Oregon experiment, in which 714 condition–treatment pairs were placed in rank order by a consumer survey, in order to determine funding from the Medicaid budget. Consumer opinion differed widely from the accepted medical viewpoint and cosmetic breast surgery was ranked higher than treatment for a compound femoral fracture, casting doubt on the whole ranking process.[15]

Inevitably, some degree of rationing of resources is unavoidable, and methods of comparing the need for, and the treatment outcome of, different medical conditions are required.

QUALITY OF LIFE QUESTIONNAIRES

Two major types of QoL questionnaires are available, namely generic and disease-specific. Generic QoL assessment is the standard approach adopted in the majority of studies, and this form of assessment is simplified by the availability of a large number of validated questionnaires from which the researcher can choose. In addition, extensive previous research using these questionnaires provides comparative data and normative values both of which are of value in QoL studies.

Generic questionnaires (e.g. Nottingham Health Profile,[16] Short Form 36,[17] Psychosocial Adjustment to Illness Scale[18]) are designed as general measures of QoL, are applicable to a wide range of different populations and clinical conditions and are not specific to a particular disease, treatment or age group. Such measures therefore allow broad comparisons to be made between different patient groups, and between women with and without medical complaints. Normal values are available for each questionnaire stratified by the age, social class and sex.

Many different generic questionnaires are available and not all are equally applicable for the assessment of urinary incontinent women. The Short Form 36, for example, is widely used in clinical practice, but has no questions covering sexual function or sleep, both of which are pertinent to women with urinary incontinence.

Unfortunately, generic questionnaires necessitate non-specific questioning, and scoring systems applicable to widely differing states of health. Such questionnaires are also restricted in length and complexity in order to improve the response rate to questioning. Generic questionnaires therefore lack sensitivity when applied to women with urinary incontinence, and this may be particularly important in respect of their inability to detect clinically important improvement in urinary incontinence when incorporated into clinical trials.

Disease-specific questionnaires aim to overcome this problem and are designed to assess with greater complexity and accuracy the impact of certain medical or surgical complaints. Not only can the questions be designed to concentrate on those aspects of QoL which are more likely to be affected by urinary incontinence, but the scoring system can be designed in such a way that it is likely to detect clinically relevant improvement following treatment.

The major disadvantage of disease-specific questionnaires is that the questionnaire must be carefully designed to maintain the multidimensional approach to QoL assessment and be extensively validated prior to use. In addition the questionnaire should preferably be universally accepted as a valid measure of the QoL of the chosen condition.

All the disease-specific and generic questionnaires discussed in this chapter were designed and validated in isolation, and therefore results on one questionnaire are not comparable with those obtained using a different instrument, even though the two may appear to measure the same basic concepts.

A sensible approach for clinical trials would include use of both a disease-specific and a generic questionnaire, preferably both of which have previously been validated and used in similar studies.

Unfortunately, many studies which attempt to measure QoL do so in a haphazard manner. In a recent critical appraisal of the 'quality of QoL research', Gill & Feinstein[19] randomly selected 75 articles from 579 referenced in a QoL bibliography.[20] A total of 159 different QoL questionnaires were used in these papers, although in only 15% was QoL defined, and in only 36% was the reason for using the selected questionnaire(s) stated.

Although several published studies have attempted to measure the QoL of urinary incontinent women, the majority do so in an equally heterogeneous fashion, rendering the comparison of studies and their collective interpretation difficult.

PREDICTORS OF QUALITY OF LIFE IMPAIRMENT FOR INCONTINENT WOMEN

Urinary incontinence results in impairment of many aspects of the QoL of sufferers, yet it is impossible to predict, on the basis of urinary symptoms and urodynamic diagnosis alone, the degree of this impairment.

Many factors affect the perception of incontinence as a significant health problem and no study to date has analyzed the use of urinary symptoms or urodynamic parameters as a valid assessment of the impact of urinary incontinence on QoL. It is clear that different women vary greatly in their tolerance of urinary symptoms, and in order to measure the impact of this condition, QoL should be measured.

Little is known about the effect of age on the subjective severity of urinary incontinence. Gjorp et al[21] found that 72% of a sample of 79 elderly women with genitourinary symptoms felt them to be normal for elderly people. In addition Norton et al[2] have shown that elderly women tend to present later for the assessment and treatment of urinary incontinence, although there is insufficient evidence to support the assumption that their urinary symptoms are less troublesome.

It is possible that in the study by Norton[2] the earlier presentation of younger women reflects a greater knowledge about incontinence and its treatment, as neither symptom severity nor diagnosis affected presentation to the same degree. It is also possible that urinary incontinence may affect the young and old differently. Incontinence, for example, often results in sexual dysfunction and exercise restriction which may be more problematic for younger women.

Unfortunately, many assumptions are made regarding the impact of urinary incontinence in the elderly despite insufficient research. Our own studies have shown that QoL is often significantly improved by bladder neck surgery in elderly women, yet age itself is a major factor upon which surgery may be denied to such patients.

Undoubtedly, cultural beliefs and social pressure affect women's perception of their urinary symptoms. In August 1983, the popular USA columnist Abigail Von Buren ('Dear Abbey') discussed incontinence, and advised her readers to write to the 'Help for Incontinent People' organization for further help. Within a few weeks over 50 000 readers responded expressing embarrassment, loneliness, isolation, and depressive symptoms as a result of their urinary problems. Although never intended as a prevalence study due to the biased selection of the study population, this survey demonstrated that selected groups of women can be influenced by many factors to regard their urinary symptoms as a significant health problem.

In our own catchment area of south-east London, a large proportion of the population is West Indian yet few of these people are seen in the urodynamic clinic for the assessment of urinary incontinence. Although there are reasons to suppose that urinary incontinence is seen less frequently in these women, Bump[22] found that interracial variations in prolapse and possibly also incontinence do not exist. It is possible that racial differences are major determinants of QoL impairment, although large community-based studies are still awaited to clarify this issue.

Although it would be expected that the duration of symptoms and severity of leakage are major predictors of QoL impairment, symptom duration and severity of urinary incontinence per se do not appear to correlate well with loss of QoL.[18]

The urodynamic diagnosis appears to be a major factor predicting QoL impairment. It has been shown by a number of studies that women with DI have a greater QoL impairment than those with genuine stress incontinence (GSI). Wyman[23] attributed this to the fact that women with DI are less able to predict incontinent episodes, have more precipitating factors and more severe leakage and therefore have less feeling of control over their bladder symptoms than those with GSI. In addition, interpersonal and sexual problems appear to be particularly common amongst urinary incontinent women, and are greater for women with DI than for those with GSI.[24]

Undoubtedly, targeting treatment towards women with greater QoL impairment and isolating particular problem areas in the management of urinary incontinence would be of great benefit to continence carers, and ultimately improve our treatment of incontinent women.

QUALITY OF LIFE STUDIES ON URINARY INCONTINENT WOMEN

A number of studies have attempted to measure the QoL of incontinent women (Table 46.1). They vary in their design and methodology and the criteria used for the diagnosis of urinary incontinence. The majority of studies have made no attempt objectively to diagnose the cause or presence of incontinence at all, despite the fact that urinary symptoms and objective urodynamic diagnoses correlate poorly.[25,26]

Table 46.1

Author	Sample	Assessment	Method	Results
Yarnell et al 1981[27]	441 incontinent women, aged 17 and older	History, stress 22%. urge 10%, mixed 14%	Interview	8% social/domestic impairment
Vetter et al 1981[28]	254 incontinent men and women (aged > 70)	N.A.	Interview	Depression, anxiety, social restriction
McGrother et al 1987[29]	8% of community survey (n = 1097) aged > 75 years	N.A.	Interview	Limited social contact
Thomas et al 1980[1]	158 incontinent men and women, not previously treated	N.A.	Interview (pad use, expense, activity restriction, laundry)	Activity restriction financial burden
Iosif et al 1981[30]	321 incontinent women aged 20–70	History, stress 13%, urge 11%, mixed 27%	Question: social activities/social contact.	19% restricted for stress and 38% for urge incontinence
Harris 1986[31]	498 incontinent women and men aged > 75 years.	N.A.	Interview	Social and recreational restrictions
Sutherst 1979[32]	103 women aged 20–68 attending a urodynamic clinic	Urodynamics	Sexual function interview	48% sexual difficulty. 7% GSI, 28% DI
Catanzaro 1982[33]	42 subjects with multiple sclerosis	Urodynamics	Interview	52% social restriction, 14% employment problems
Norton 1982[34]	53 women aged 22–78	Unstated	10-item questionnaire	49% affected in 70% of items
Kujansuu 1984[35]	45 women attending for urodynamics (aged 44–53)	Urodynamics (all GSI)	3-item social restriction score	95% with higher scores had lower urethral closure pressures
Burns et al 1986[36]	40 women with incontinence (mean age 62)	Urodynamics	Incontinence Impact Questionnaire	Higher scores associated with poor treatment outcome
Macauley et al 1987[37]	211 women attending for urodynamics (aged 15–79)	Urodynamics (GSI 37%, DI 15%)	'How troubled are you by your bladder problem?' (vis analog)	45% rated at scale midpoint, 22% at upper end
Wyman et al 1987[38]	69 incontinent women (aged 55–86)	Urodynamics	Incontinence Impact Questionnaire	22% mod–severe impact.
Brink et al 1987[39]	197 incontinent women	Not stated	Questionnaire	12% social/activity restriction
Frazer et al 1987[40]	110 women attending a urodynamic clinic	Urodynamics	Symptom severity visual analog scale	DI worse severity than GSI
Breakwell & Walker 1988[41]	17 incontinent women	Not stated	Questionnaire	Social impairment
Abelson & Ouslander 1988[42]	164 incontinent women (mean age 78.5)	Not stated	Interview	42% interference with daily life
Norton et al 1988[2]	133 incontinent women attending for urodynamics	History	Questionnaire	60% avoid travel, 58% work affected, 40% sexual problems
Mitteness 1987[43]	23 incontinent women in subsidized housing (aged 41–97)	N A	Interview	80% cope with UI by social isolation
Hunskaar & Vinsnes 1991[44]	76 incontinent women (aged 40–60, and >70)	History	Sickness Impact	Urge incontinence resulted in higher scores
Kondo et al 1992[45]	85 women following Stamey procedure	Urodynamics	4-items questionnaire	Everyday life improved by surgery
Grimby et al 1993[46]	120 incontinent Swedish women (mean age 75.4 years)	History + pad test	Nottingham Health Profile	Emotional and social problems common
Wyman et al 1993[47]	69 incontinent women (mean age 67.8 years)	Urodynamics	Incontinence Distress and Incontinence Impact Inventory	QoL impaired for incontinent women
Renck Hopper & McKenna 1994[48]	25 women with urge incontinence (aged 32–82 years)	History	Urge incontinence disease-specific measure	Questionnaire reliable and validity tested

GENERIC QUALITY OF LIFE ASSESSMENT

Few studies in the literature have used generic, validated QoL instruments to assess women with urinary incontinence. Hunskaar & Vinsnes[44] used the Norwegian language version of the Sickness Impact Profile (SIP),[49] a validated 136-item questionnaire. Seventy women attending a self-referral center for incontinent women were divided on the basis of age into two groups (middle-aged, 40–60 years; and elderly, > 70 years), and on the basis of symptom questionnaires into stress and urge symptom subgroups. Women were asked to respond to SIP items only if they considered them attributable to their bladder symptoms. Mean scores on the SIP were low for both groups, but the study concluded that the impact of urinary incontinence on QoL was both age- and symptom-dependent. Younger women scored significantly higher on the SIP as did women with urge symptoms. Sleep, rest, emotional behavior, mobility, social interaction and recreational activities were most commonly affected.

The study unfortunately lacked objective urodynamic assessment, the sample sizes were small and no account was taken of the women's age in the comparison of QoL scores. Similarly, the practice of encouraging women to respond to questionnaire items only if attributable to their urinary symptoms may introduce inaccuracies in both the scoring and interpretation of QoL measures. This is particularly problematic in an elderly population, who may be unsure as to the cause of their QoL impairment, and which problems are attributable to urinary incontinence and which to other causes.

Grimby et al[46] recently published the results of a study comparing Nottingham Health Profile (NHP) scores from 120 elderly women (65–84 years) with urinary incontinence with those of 313 76-year-old women without urinary symptoms. Their data were obtained from a large population study of 6000 women living in the city of Göteborg in Sweden and the overall response rate to this parent study was 70.1%. Elderly women (> 70 years of age) with subjectively reported urinary incontinence were subdivided into those with urge incontinence (48 women, 40%), stress incontinence (34 women, 28.3%) or both (38 women, 31.7%) on the basis of a pad test, urinary diary, a cough provocation test and a clinical history, but without the benefit of urodynamic investigations. The mean age of the incontinent group was 75.4 years and that of the continent control group 76 years.

Unfortunately, the total number of incontinent women in the parent study was not stated and the women included in this study were merely the first 120 women in whom incontinence could be demonstrated by either a pad or cough provocation test. No attempt was made to determine incontinence in the control group by similar tests and continence was assumed on the basis of their lack of admission to this symptom. Ideally, for a true control group a cough provocation test and pad test should also have been performed on these women, and the number of women in the test and control groups matched.

Using the NHP Grimby et al[46] showed a significantly higher level of both emotional impairment and social isolation amongst the incontinent women. They also showed a higher level of emotional disturbance amongst women with urge and mixed incontinence than amongst those with stress incontinence. Women with urge incontinence had significantly greater sleep disturbance than the control women.

Sand et al[50] used the Short Form 36 health status questionnaire to assess the efficacy of treatment for women with GSI entered into a prospective randomized double-blind placebo-controlled trial comparing the use of an active pelvic floor stimulator to a sham device. Thirty-five women used the active device and 17 the sham device, the latter acting as controls. A significant benefit of the active device was demonstrated by both objective (pad testing, urinary diary, vaginal muscle strength) and subjective (urinary symptom questionnaire, severity of urinary incontinence on visual analog scale) measures, although no significant improvement was seen in Short Form 36 scores. It is highly likely that this result was attributable to the small number of women entered into the study, and that results would have been different had a disease-specific measure been used.

DISEASE-SPECIFIC QUALITY OF LIFE ASSESSMENT OF URINARY INCONTINENCE

One of the first incontinence-specific QoL questionnaires to be developed was the Incontinence Impact Questionnaire, designed by Wyman et al[38] for an American patient population. The questionnaire consists of 26 items in which subjects are asked to rate the extent to which their urinary leakage affects their daily functioning in three main areas: activities of daily living, social interactions and self-perception. These items are listed below:

1. Daily activities
   a. Cooking
   b. House cleaning
   c. Laundry
   d. Household repair work
   e. Shopping
   f. Hobbies
   g. Physical recreation
   h. Entertainment
   i. Travel (< 30 min)
   j. Travel (> 30 min)
   k. Visits to places with unknown rest rooms
   l. Vacation
   m. Church or temple attendance
   n. Volunteer activity or work
2. Social interactions
   a. Having friends visit
   b. Visiting friends or relatives
   c. Participating in social activities outside the home
   d. Relationships with friends
   e. Relationship with family

    f. Relationship with husband
    g. Sexual relations
    h. Way you dress
3. Self perceptions
    a. Physical health
    b. Mental health
    c. Fear of odor
    d. Fear of embarrassment.

The scoring system for the Incontinence Impact Questionnaire[38] is as follows:

- Not at all = 0
- Slightly = 1
- Moderately = 2
- Greatly = 3
- Not applicable = 4

Shumaker et al[51] extended this early work and modified the IIQ to a 30-item questionnaire measuring impairment in the domains of physical activity, travel, social/relationships and emotional health. A urogenital distress symptom inventory consisting of 19 items was also developed, measuring obstructive discomfort, irritative and stress symptoms. As yet there are no published intervention studies using these scales.

In order to make these scales even easier to use, Uerbersax et al[52] have recently published short form versions of both questionnaires consisting of 7 and 6 items respectively. These provide a rapid assessment and approximation of scores generated by the long versions of the questionnaires.

A more complex system of analyzing the multidimensional impact of urinary incontinence was proposed by Raz & Erikson[53] and called the SEAPI QMM Incontinence Classification System. Each letter in the questionnaire title refers to a single domain, namely: S = stress related leakage; E = emptying ability; A = anatomy (female); P = protection; I = inhibition; Q = quality of life; M = mobility; and M = mental status. The authors suggested that the system be analogous to the TNM system for tumor staging with each of the above aspects being scored as follows:

- 0 = not present
- 1 = minimal
- 2 = moderate
- 3 = severe

- U = unknown
- N = not tested.

The QoL section of this fairly complex system includes 15 questions concerning emotional wellbeing, interpersonal relationships, work, financial situation, physical health, recreation and overall life satisfaction. These questions are further divided into three groups, namely those concerning mostly individual satisfaction, those concerning mostly interpersonal relationships and those concerning both. All 15 questions are listed as follows:

1. How much does your bladder problem affect your ability to perform your usual daily tasks?
2. How much does your incontinence interfere with your ability to engage in physical recreation (sports, dancing, etc.)?
3. How much does your bladder problem affect your ability to engage in non-strenuous recreation (movie, dining out, etc.)?
4. How much does your incontinence affect your relationship with your friends?
5. How much does your incontinence affect your relationship with your spouse/companion?
6. How much does your incontinence interfere with your sexual activity?
7. Does your incontinence make it difficult for you to establish new relationships with other people (friends, business associates, etc.)?
8. How does your incontinence affect your financial situation?
9. How does your incontinence affect your overall health?
10. Do you feel increased nervousness or anxiety because of your incontinence?
11. How much does your incontinence affect your overall level of energy?
12. Does your incontinence make you feel less useful?
13. How would you rate your overall quality of life?
14. How would you rate the overall quality of your life if you did not leak urine?
15. How much does your incontinence affect your overall satisfaction with your life?

Further refinement of the condition-specific questionnaire was recently reported by Renck Hooper and McKenna,[48] who proposed a questionnaire for the assessment of women with urge incontinence symptoms alone. This was motivated largely by the need to assess the efficacy of drug treatment of DI and the content of this questionnaire is shown below:

1. General Health status
2. Incontinence symptoms
3. Adverse effects
4. Function
5. Quality of life
   a. Impact on health
   b. Mobility
   c. Work
   d. Housework
   e. Family relations
   f. Partner relations
   g. Sexual function
   h. Social life
   i. Self-esteem
   j. Anxiety
   k. Sleep.

Although full details of this questionnaire are as yet unavailable it would appear that a questionnaire aimed at women with urge incontinence alone is in danger of becoming too condition-specific, particularly when many women present with predominantly mixed symptoms.

Developing a questionnaire is a lengthy process and in 1991 we began development of a disease-specific questionnaire in our own department at Kings College Hospital, London.

Following our analysis of the results of over 1100 completed generic QoL questionnaires, it became apparent that urinary incontinence affected each of the components of QoL to a different degree. In addition, in order to concentrate specifically on the impact of urinary incontinence, it was evident that a condition-specific questionnaire should also include an assessment of urinary symptoms, incontinence coping strategies and subjective severity measures.

Extensive pilot and validation studies were undertaken prior to completion of the questionnaire, which is shown in its entirety below. The scoring system of the questionnaire is similar to that of the Short Form 36 and scores can be presented in the form of a QoL profile with scores out of 100 presented for each domain, or the scores can be summated to produce a total score for each patient.

King's Health Questionnaire   Scale   Score
Part I
General health perception

1. How would you describe your health at present?	Very good	1
	Good	2
	Fair	3
	Poor	4
	Very poor	5

Incontinence impact

2. How much do you think your bladder problem affects your life?	Not at all	1
	A little	2
	Moderately	3
	A lot	4

Part II
Role limitations
3a. To what extent does your bladder problem affect your household tasks (e.g. cleaning, shopping)?
3b. Does your bladder problem affect your job, or your normal daily activities outside the home?

	Not at all	1
Physical limitations	Slightly	2
4a. Does your bladder problem affect your physical	Moderately	3
activities (e.g. going for a walk, run, sport, gym)?	A lot	4
4b. Does your bladder problem affect your ability to travel?		

Social limitations
4c. Does your bladder problem restrict your social life?

4d. Does your bladder problem limit your ability to see/visit friends?

Personal relationships

5a. Does your bladder problem affect your relationship with your partner?	Not applicable	0
5b. Does your bladder problem affect your sex life?	Not at all	1
5c. Does your bladder problem affect your	Slightly	2
family life?	Moderately	3
	A lot	4

Emotions

6a. Does your bladder problem make you feel depressed?	Not at all	1
6b. Does your bladder problem make you feel	Slightly	2
anxious or nervous?	Moderately	3
6c. Does your bladder problem make you feel bad	Very much	4
about yourself?		

Sleep/energy

7a. Does your bladder problem affect your sleep?	Never	1
7b. Do you feel worn out or tired?	Sometimes	2
	Often	3
	All the time	4

Severity measures

Do you do any of the following; if so how much?

8a. Wear pads to keep dry?		
8b. Be careful how much fluid you drink?	Never	1
8c. Change your underclothes when they get wet?	Sometimes	2
8d. Worry in case you smell?	Often	3
8e Get embarrassed because of your bladder	All the time	4
problem?		

To calculate scores

1. General health perceptions

   Score = ((Score to Qu1 − 1)/4) × 100

2. Incontinence impact

   Score = ((Score to Qu 2 − 1)/3) × 100

3. Role limitations

   Scores = (((Scores to Qu 3a + 3b) −2) /6) × 100

4. Physical limitations

   Score = (((Score to Qu 4a + 4b) −2) /6) × 100

5. Social limitations

   Score = (((Score to Qu 4c + 4d + 5c) −3) /9) × 100**

** If score to Qu 5c > = 1, If 0 then. ..−2) /6) × 100

6. Personal relationships

   Score = (((Score to Qu 5a + 5b) −2) /6) × 100***

** If score to Qu 5a + 5b > = 2,

   If Qu 5a + 5b = 1; ... −1) /3) × 100

   If Qu 5a + 5b = 0; ... treat as missing value (not applicable)

7. Emotions

   Score = (((Score to Qu 6a + 6b + 6c) −3) /9) × 100

8. Sleep/energy
Score = (((Score to Qu 7a + 7b) –2) /6) × 100
9. Severity measures
Score = (((Score to Qu 8a + 8b + 8c + 8d + 8e) –5) /15) × 100

Part III
We would like to know what your bladder problems are and how much they affect you. From the list below choose only those problems that you have at present. Leave out those that do not apply to you.

- Frequency: Going to the toilet very often
- Nocturia: Getting up at night to pass urine
- Urgency: A strong and difficult to control desire to pass urine
- Urge incontinence: Urinary leakage associated with strong desire to pass urine
- Stress incontinence: Urinary leakage with physical activity, e.g. coughing, sneezing, running
- Nocturnal enuresis: Wetting the bed at night
- Intercourse incontinence: Urinary leakage with sexual intercourse
- Frequent waterworks infections
- Bladder pain
- Difficulty passing urine
- Other (please specify)

Scale	Score
A little	= 1
Moderately	= 2
A lot	= 3
Omitted	= 0

CONCLUSION

Studies have demonstrated that relatively simple and indeed short QoL questionnaires can be used to measure the impact of urinary incontinence on the lives of urinary incontinent women. These will improve our understanding of the effects of urinary incontinence, and may also improve our clinical management of this condition.

Unfortunately, the heterogeneity of the many different studies performed and the lack of standardization of the QoL questionnaires used has created much confusion. Such confusion is in danger of concealing the enormous potential benefit of QoL assessment of urinary incontinent women.

It remains to be seen whether these measures will be adopted into routine clinical practice, although they certainly have an important role to play in controlled clinical trials.

REFERENCES

1 Thomas TM, Plymat KR, Blannin J, Meade TW. Prevalence of urinary incontinence. Br Med J 1980; 281: 1243–1245.

2 Norton PA, MacDonald LD, Sedgwick PM, Stanton SL. Distress and delay associated with urinary incontinence, frequency and urgency in women. Br Med J 1988; 297: 1187–1189.

3 Fitzpatrick R, Fletcher A, Gore S, Jones D, Spiegelhalter D, Cox D. Quality of life measures in health care. 1: Applications and issues in assessment. Br Med J 1992; 305: 1075–1077.

4 Pearlman R, Uhlmann R. Patient and physician perceptions of quality of life across chronic diseases. J Gerontol 1988; 43: 25–30.

5 Slevin M, Plant H, Lynch D, Drinkwater J, Gregory WM. Who should measure quality of life, the doctor or the patient? Br J Cancer 1988; 57: 109–112.

6 Coulter A. Measuring quality of life. In: Kinmonth AL, Jones R (eds) Critical reading in general practice. Oxford: Oxford University Press, 1993.

7 World Health Organization. Definition of health from preamble to the constitution of the WHO basic documents, 28th edn. Geneva: WHO, 1978: p 1.

8 Kaplan-DeNour A. Social adjustment of chronic dialysis patients. Am J Psychiatr 1982; 139: 97–100.

9 Murawski BJ. Social support in health and illness; the concept and its measurement. Ca Nurs 1978; 1: 365–371.

10 Zyzanski SJ. Medical and social outcomes of survivors of major heart surgery. J Psychosom Res 1981; 23: 213–221.

11 Burton G. A randomised comparison of laparoscopic and open colposuspension. Neurourol Urodyn 1994; 13 (4): 99.

12 Aitchison MA, Carter R, Paterson P, Ferrie B. Is the treatment of urgency incontinence a placebo response? Results of a five year follow up. Br J Urol 1989; 64: 478–480.

13 Kelleher CJ, Cardozo LD, Khullar V. Anticholinergic therapy: the need for continued surveillance. Neurourol Urodyn 1994; 13: 432–433.

14 Hu TW. The economic impact of urinary incontinence. Clin Geriatr Med 1986; 2: 673.

15 Klein R. On the Oregon trail: rationing health care. Br Med J 1991; 302: 1–2.

16 Hunt SM, McEwen J, McKenna SP. Measuring health status. A new tool for clinicians and epidemiologists. J Royal College of General Practitioners 1985; 35: 185–188.

17 Jenkinson C, Coulter A, Wright L. Short Form 36 (SF-36) health survey questionnaire. Normative data for adults of working age. Br Med J 1993; 306: 1437–1440.

18 Derogatis LR, Derogatis MF. The Psychosocial Adjustment to Illness Scale. (PAIS and PAIS SR) Administration, scoring and procedures manual-II. Clinical Psychometric Research, Inc. Towson, Maryland 21204, USA, 1995.

19 Gill TM, Feinstein AR. A critical appraisal of the quality of quality of life measurements. JAMA 1994; 272 (8): 619–626.

20 Spiker B, Molinek FR Jr, Johnson KA, Simpson RL Jr, Tilson HH. Quality of life bibliography and indexes. Med Care 1990; 28 (Suppl 12) DS1–DS77.

21 Gjorp T, Hendriksen C, Lund E, Stromgard E. Is growing old a disease? A study of the attitudes of elderly people to physical symptoms. J Chron Dis 1987; 40 (12): 1095–1098.

22 Bump RC. Racial comparisons and contrasts in urinary incontinence and genital prolapse. Neurourol Urodyn 1992; 11 (4): 357–358.

28 Wyman JF, Harkins S, Choi S, Taylor J, Fantl JA. Psychosocial impact of urinary incontinence in women. Obstet Gynaecol 1987; 70: 378–380.

24 Kelleher CJ, Cardozo LD. Sexual dysfunction and urinary incontinence. The Journal of Sexual Health 1994; 3 (7): 186–191.

25 Bergman A, Bader K. Reliability of the patient's history in the diagnosis of urinary incontinence. Int J Gynaecol Obstet 1990; 32: 255–259.

26 Versi E, Cardozo L, Anand D, Cooper D. Symptoms analysis for the diagnosis of genuine stress incontinence. Br J Obstet Gynaecol 1991; 98 (8): 815–819.

27 Yarnell JWG, St Leger AS. The prevalence, severity, and factors associated with urinary incontinence in a random sample of the elderly. Age Ageing 1979; 8: 81.

28 Vetter NJ, Jones DA, Victor CR. Urinary incontinence in the elderly at home. Lancet 1981; 2: 1275.

29 McGrother CW, Castleden CM, Duffin H et al. Do the elderly need better incontinence services? Community Med 1987; 9: 62.

30 Iosif S, Henriksson L, Ulmsten U. The frequency of disorders of the urinary tract, urinary incontinence in particular, as evaluated by a questionnaire survey in a gynaecological health control population. Acta Obstet Gynaecol Scand 1981; 60: 71.

31 Harris T. Aging in the eighties: prevalence and impact of urinary problems in

individuals age 65 years and over. Supplement on aging to the National Health Interview Survey, United States Jan–June 1984. No 121 DHSS publication number (PHS). 86–1250, 1986.

32 Sutherst JR. Sexual dysfunction and urinary incontinence. Br J Obstet Gynaecol 1979; 86: 387.

33 Catanzaro M. Urinary bladder dysfunction as a remedial disability in multiple sclerosis. A sociologic perspective. Arch Phys Med Rehab 1982; 63: 472.

34 Norton C. The effects of urinary incontinence in women. Int Rehab Med 1982; 4: 9.

35 Kujansuu E. Degree of female stress urinary incontinence: an objective classification by simultaneous urethrocystometry. Gynaecol Obstet Invest 1984; 18: 66.

36 Burns P, Reis J, Pranikoff K. An analysis of perceived impact versus objective measures of incontinence. Proceedings of the Third Joint Meeting of the International Continence Society and Urodynamic Society 1986; p 87.

37 Macauley AJ, Stern RS, Holmes DM, Stanton SL. Micturition and the mind: psychological factors in the aetiology and treatment of urinary symptoms in women. Br Med J 1987; 294: 540–543.

38 Wyman JF, Harkins S, Choi S, Taylor J, Fantl JA. Psychosocial impact of urinary incontinence in women. Obstet Gynaecol 1987; 70: 378–380.

39 Brink CA, Wells TJ, Diokno AC. Urinary incontinence in women. Public Health Nurs 1987; 4: 114.

40 Frazer MI, Sutherst JR, Holland EFN. Visual analogue scores and urinary incontinence. Br Med J 1987; 295: 582.

41 Breakwell SL, Walker SN. Differences in physical health, social interaction, and personal adjustment between continent and incontinent homebound aged women. J Community Health 1988; 5: 19.

42 Abelson S, Ouslander J. Perceptions of urinary incontinence among elderly outpatients. Gerontologist 1988; 28: 4A.

43 Mitteness LS. So what do you expect when you're 85? Urinary incontinence in later life. Research in the sociology of health care: vol 6. The experience and management of chronic illness. Greenwich, Conn: JAI Press, 1987; pp 177–219.

44 Hunskaar S, Vinsnes A. The quality of life in women with urinary incontinence as measured by the sickness impact profile. JAGS 1991; 39: 378–382.

45 Kondo A, Itoh Y, Yamada M, Saito M, Kato K. Effects of urinary incontinence on quality of life. Int Urogynecol J 1992; 3: 121–123.

46 Grimby A, Milstrom I, Molander U, Wiklund I, Ekelund P. The influence of urinary incontinence on the quality of life of women. Age and Ageing 1993; 22: 82–89.

47 Wyman JF, Shumaker S, McClish D, Uebersax J, Fantl JA. Health related quality of life in women with urinary incontinence. Non presentation poster. International Continence Society 23rd Annual Meeting, Rome. Abstract book pp 144–145.

48 Renck Hooper U, McKenna SP. Quality of life in urge incontinent women: translation and validation of a condition specific measure. (Non presentation poster) International Continence Society 24th Annual Meeting, Prague, Czech Republic, Abstract publications pp 140–141.

49 Bergner M, Bobbitt R, Carter W, Gibson B. The sickness impact profile: development and final revision of a health status measure. Med Care 1981; 19: 787–805.

50 Sand PK, Richardson DA, Staskin DR et al. Pelvic floor stimulation in the treatment of genuine stress incontinence: a multicentre placebo controlled trial. Neurourol Urodyn 13: 356–357.

51 Shumaker SA, Wyman JF, Uerbersax JS, McClish D, Fantl JA. Health related quality of life measures for women with urinary incontinence. The Urogenital Distress Inventory and the Incontinence Impact Questionnaire. Quality Life Res 1994; 3: 291–306.

52 Uerbersax JS, Wyman JF, Shumaker SA, McClish DK, Fantl JA. Short forms to assess life quality and symptom distress for urinary incontinence in women. The Incontinence Impact Questionnaire and Urogenital Distress Inventory. Neurourol Urodyn 1995; 14: 131–139.

53 Raz S, Erikson DR. SEAPI QMM Incontinence Classification system. Neurourol Urodyn 1992; 11: 187–199.

Appendix 1: Special contribution

The Standardization of Terminology of Lower Urinary Tract Function Recommended by the International Continence Society

P. Abrams, J. G. Blaivas, S. L. Stanton and J. T. Andersen (Chairman)
ICS Committee on Standardization of Terminology

Reprinted with permission from Int Urogynecol J (1990) 1: 45–58, Springer Verlag London Limited, UK and the International Continence Society.

Contents

Keywords: Lower urinary tract function; Terminology; Definitions; Urinary incontinence; Urodynamics

1 Introduction

The International Continence Society (ICS) established a committee for the standardization of terminology of lower urinary tract function in 1973. Five of the six reports from this committee, approved by the Society, have been published [1–5]. The fifth report, on quantification of urine loss, was an internal ICS document but appears, in part, in this document.

These reports are revised, extended and collated in this monograph. The standards are recommended to facilitate comparison of results by investigators who use urodynamic methods. These standards are recommended not only for urodynamic investigations carried out on human patients but also during animal studies. When using urodynamic studies in animals the type of any anesthesia used should be stated. It is suggested that acknowledgement of these standards in written publications be indicated by a footnote to the section 'Methods and Materials' or its equivalent, to read as follows: 'Methods, definitions and units conform to the standards recommended by the International Continence Society, except where specifically noted.'

Urodynamic studies involve the assessment of the function and dysfunction of the urinary tract by any appropriate method. Aspects of urinary tract morphology, physiology, biochemistry, and hydro-dynamics affect urine transport and storage. Other methods of investigation such as the radiographic visualization of the lower urinary tract is a useful adjunct to conventional urodynamics. This monograph concerns the urodynamics of the lower urinary tract.

2 Clinical assessment

The clinical assessment of patients with lower urinary tract dysfunction should consist of a detailed history, a frequency/volume chart, and a physical examination. In urinary incontinence, leakage should be demonstrated objectively.

2.1. History

The general history should include questions relevant to neurological and congenital abnormalities as well as information on previous urinary infections and relevant surgery. Information must be obtained on medication with known or possible effects on the lower urinary tract. The general history should also include assessment of menstrual, sexual and bowel function, and obstetric history.

The urinary history must consist of symptoms related to both the storage and the evacuation functions of the lower urinary tract.

2.2 Frequency/Volume Chart

The frequency/volume chart is a specific urodynamic investigation recording fluid intake and urine output per 24-hour period. The chart gives objective information on the number of voidings, the distribution of voidings between daytime and nighttime and each voided volume. The chart can also be used to record episodes of urgency and leakage and the number of incontinence pads used. The frequency/volume chart is very useful in the assessment of voiding disorders, and in the follow-up of treatment.

2.3. Physical Examination

Besides a general urologic and, when appropriate, gynecologic examination, the physical examination should include the assessment of perineal sensation, the perineal reflexes supplied by the sacral segments S2–S4, and anal sphincter tone and control.

3 Procedures Related to the Evaluation of Urine Storage

3.1. Cystometry

Cystometry is the method by which the pressure/volume relationship of the bladder is measured. All systems are zeroed at atmospheric pressure. For external transducers the reference point is the level of the superior edge of the symphysis pubis. For catheter-mounted transducers the reference point is the transducer itself. Cystometry is used to assess detrusor activity, sensation, capacity, and compliance.

Before starting to fill the bladder the residual urine may be measured. However, the removal of a large volume of residual urine may alter detrusor function, especially in neuropathic disorders. Certain cystometric parameters may be significantly altered by the speed of bladder filling (see Compliance, 6.2.1).

During cystometry it is taken for granted that the patient is awake, unanesthetized and neither sedated nor taking drugs that affect bladder function. Any variations should be specified.

3.1.1. General Information. The following details should be given:

1. Access (transurethral or percutaneous).
2. Fluid medium (liquid or gas).
3. Temperature of fluid (state in degrees Celsius).
4. Position of patient (e.g., supine, sitting, or standing).
5. Filling method – may be by diuresis or catheter. Filling by catheter may be continuous or incremental; the precise filling rate should be stated. When the incremental method is used the volume increment should be stated. For general discussion, the following terms for the range of filling rate may be used:

   a. Up to 10 ml/min is *slow fill cystometry* ('physiological' filling).
   b. 10–100 ml/min is *medium fill cystometry*.
   c. Over 100 ml/min is *rapid fill cystometry*.

3.1.2.   Technical Information. The following details should be given:

1. Fluid-filled catheter – specify number of catheters, single or multiple lumens, type of catheter (manufacturer), size of catheter.
2. Catheter tip transducer – list specifications.
3. Other catheters – list specifications.
4. Measuring equipment.

3.1.3.   Definitions. Cystometric terminology is defined as follows:

Intravesical pressure is the pressure within the bladder.

Abdominal pressure is taken to be the pressure surrounding the bladder. In current practice it is estimated from rectal, or less commonly, extraperitoneal pressure.

Detrusor pressure is that component of intravesical pressure that is created by forces in the bladder wall (passive and active). It is estimated by subtracting abdominal pressure from intravesical pressure. The simultaneous measurement of abdominal pressure is essential for interpretation of the intravesical pressure trace. However, artifacts on the detrusor pressure trace may be produced by intrinsic rectal contractions.

Bladder sensation. Sensation is difficult to evaluate because of its subjective nature. It is usually assessed by questioning the patient in relation to the fullness of the bladder during cystometry.

Commonly used descriptive terms include:

First desire to void.

Normal desire to void – defined as the feeling that leads the patient to pass urine at the next convenient moment, but voiding can be delayed if necessary.

Strong desire to void – defined as a persistent desire to void without the fear of leakage.

Urgency – defined as a strong desire to void accompanied by fear of leakage or fear of pain.

Pain. The site and character of pain should be specified. Pain during bladder filling or micturition is abnormal.

The use of objective or semi-objective tests for sensory function, such as electrical threshold studies (sensory testing), is discussed in detail under Sensory Testing (see 5.6).

The term 'Capacity' must be qualified as follows:

Maximum cystometric capacity, in patients with normal sensation, is the volume at which the patient feels he/she can no longer delay micturition. In the absence of sensation the maximum cystometric capacity cannot be defined in the same terms and is the volume at which the clinician decides to terminate filling. In the presence of sphincter incompetence the maximum cystometric capacity may be significantly increased by occlusion of the urethra, e.g., by Foley catheter.

The *functional bladder capacity,* or voided volume, is more relevant and is assessed from a frequency/volume chart (urinary diary).

The *maximum (anesthetic) bladder capacity* is the volume measured after filling during a deep general or spinal/epidural anesthetic, specifying fluid temperature, filling pressure, and filling time.

Compliance indicates the change in volume for a change in pressure. Compliance is calculated by dividing the volume change (ΔV) by the change in detrusor pressure (ΔP_{det}) during that change in bladder volume ($\Delta V / \Delta P_{det}$). Compliance is expressed as milliliters per centimeters of water pressure. (See also Compliance, 6.2.1.)

3.2.   Urethral Pressure Measurement

It should be noted that the urethral pressure and the urethral closure pressure are idealized concepts which represent the ability of the urethra to prevent leakage (see Urinary Incontinence, 6.2.3). In current urodynamic practice the urethral pressure is measured by a number of different techniques which do not always yield consistent values. Not only do the values differ with the method of measurement, but there is often lack of consistency for a single method; for example, the affect of catheter rotation when urethral pressure is measured by a catheter-mounted transducer.

Intraluminal urethral pressure may be measured:

At rest, with the bladder at any given volume.
During coughing or straining.
During the process of voiding (see section on voiding urethral pressure profile, 4.4).

Measurements may be made at one point in the urethra over a period of time, or at several points along the urethra consecutively forming a *urethral pressure profile* (UPP).

Two types of UPP may be measured in the *storage phase*:

1. Resting urethral pressure profile – with the bladder and subject at rest.
2. Stress urethral pressure profile – with a defined applied stress (e.g., cough, strain, valsalva).

In the storage phase the *urethral pressure profile* denotes the intraluminal pressure along the length of the urethra. All systems are zeroed at atmospheric pressure. For external transducers the reference point is the superior edge of the symphysis pubis. For catheter-mounted transducers the reference point is the transducer itself. Intravesical pressure should be measured to exclude a simultaneous detrusor contraction. The subtraction of intravesical pressure from urethral pressure produces the *urethral closure pressure profile*.

It is essential to record both intravesical and intraurethral pressures simultaneously during stress urethral profilometry.

3.2.1.   General Information. The following details should be given:

1. Infusion medium (liquid or gas).
2. Rate of infusion.
3. Stationary, continuous, or intermittent withdrawal.

4. Rate of withdrawal.
5. Bladder volume.
6. Position of patient (supine, sitting, or standing).

3.2.2.   Technical Information. The following details should be given:
1. Open catheter: Specify type (manufacturer), size, number, position, and orientation of side or end hole.
2. Catheter-mounted transducers: Specify manufacturer; number of transducers; spacing of transducers along the catheter; orientation with respect to one another; transducer design, e.g., transducer face depressed or flush with catheter surface; catheter diameter; and material. The orientation of the transducer(s) in the urethra should be stated.
3. Other catheters, e.g., membrane, fiberoptic: Specify type (manufacturer), size, and number of channels as for microtransducer catheter.
4. Measurement technique: For stress profiles the particular stress employed should be stated, e.g., cough or valsalva.
5. Recording apparatus: Describe type of recording apparatus. The frequency response of the total system should be stated. The frequency response of the catheter in the perfusion method can be assessed by blocking the eyeholes and recording the consequent rate of change of pressure.

3.2.3.   Definitions. Terminology referring to profiles measured in storage phase (see Fig. 1) is defined as follows:
Maximum urethral pressure is the maximum pressure of the measured profile.
Maximum urethral closure pressure is the maximum difference between the urethral pressure and the intravesical pressure.
Functional profile length is the length of the urethra along which the urethral pressure exceeds intravesical pressure.
Functional profile length (on stress) is the length over which the urethral pressure exceeds the intravesical pressure on stress.
Pressure 'transmission' ratio is the increment in urethral pressure on stress as a percentage of the simultaneously recorded increment in intravesical pressure. For stress profiles obtained during coughing, pressure transmission ratios can be obtained at any point along the urethra. If single values are given, the position in the urethra should be stated. If several pressure transmission ratios are defined at different points along the urethra, a pressure 'transmission' profile is obtained. During 'cough profiles' the amplitude of the cough should be stated if possible. *Note:* The term 'transmission' is in common usage and cannot be changed. However, 'transmission' implies a completely passive process. Such an assumption is not yet justified by scientific evidence. A role for muscular activity cannot be excluded.
Total profile length is not generally regarded as a useful parameter.

The information gained from urethral pressure measurements in the storage phase is of limited value in the assessment of voiding disorders.

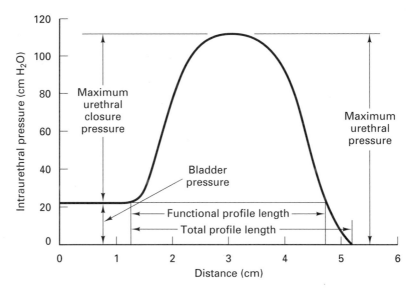

Figure 1. Diagram of a female urethral pressure profile (static) with ICS recommended nomenclature.

3.3. Quantification of Urine Loss

Subjective grading of incontinence may not indicate reliably the degree of abnormality. However, it is important to relate the management of the individual patients to their complaints and personal circumstances, as well as to objective measurements.

In order to assess and compare the results of the treatment of different types of incontinence in different centers, a simple standard test can be used to measure urine loss objectively in any subject. In order to obtain a representative result, especially in subjects with variable or intermittent urinary incontinence, the test should occupy as long a period as possible; yet it must be practical. The circumstances should approximate to those of everyday life, yet be similar for all subjects to allow meaningful comparison. On the basis of pilot studies performed in various centers, an internal report of the ICS [6] recommended a test occupying a 1-hour period during which a series of standard activities was carried out. This test *can* be extended by further 1-hour periods if the result of the first 1-hour test were not considered representative by either the patient or the investigator. Alternatively, the test can be repeated, after filling the bladder to a defined volume.

The total amount of urine lost during the test period is determined by weighing a collecting device such as a nappy, absorbent pad, or condom appliance. A nappy or pad should be worn inside waterproof under-pants or should have a waterproof backing. Care should be taken to use a collecting device of adequate capacity. Immediately before the test begins the collecting device is weighed to the nearest gram.

3.3.1. Typical Test Schedule:
1. Test is started without the patient voiding.
2. Preweighed collecting device is put on and first 1-hour test period begins.
3. Subject drinks 500 ml sodium-free liquid within a short period (max. 15 min), then sits or rests.

4. Half-hour period: subject walks, including stair climbing equivalent to one flight up and down.
5. During the remaining period the subject performs the following activities:
   a) Standing up from sitting, 10 times.
   b) Coughing vigorously, 10 times.
   c) Running on the spot for 1 min.
   d) Bending to pick up small object from floor, 5 times.
   e) Washing hands in running water for 1 min.
6. At the end of the 1-hour test the collecting device is removed and weighed.
7. If the test is regarded as representative, the subject voids and the volume is recorded.
8. Otherwise the test is repeated, preferably without voiding.

If the collecting device becomes saturated or filled during the test it should be removed and weighed, and replaced by a fresh device. The total weight of urine lost during the test period is taken to be equal to the gain in weight of the collecting device(s). In interpreting the results of the test it should be borne in mind that a weight gain of up to 1 g may be due to weighing errors, sweating, or vaginal discharge.

The activity program may be modified according to the subject's physical ability. If substantial variations from the usual test schedule occur, these should be recorded so that the same schedule can be used on subsequent occasions.

In principle the subject should not void during the test period. If the patient experiences urgency, then he/she should be persuaded to postpone voiding and to perform as many of the activities in section 5 as possible in order to detect leakage. Before voiding the collection device is removed for weighing. If voiding cannot be postponed, then the test is terminated. The voided volume and the duration of the test should be recorded. For subjects not completing the full test the results may require separate analysis, or the test may be repeated after rehydration.

The test result is given as grams urine lost in the 1-hour test period in which the greatest urine loss is recorded.

3.3.2. Additional Procedures. Provided that there is no interference with the basic test, additional procedures intended to give information of diagnostic value are permissible. For example, additional changes and weighing of the collecting device can give information about the timing of urine loss; the absorbent nappy may be an electronic recording nappy so that the timing is recorded directly.

3.3.3. Presentation of Results. The following details should be given:

1. Collecting device.
2. Physical condition of subject (ambulant, chairbound, bedridden).
3. Relevant medical condition of subject.
4. Relevant drug treatments.
5. Test schedule.

In some situations the timing of the test (e.g., in relation to the menstrual cycle) may be relevant.

Findings: A record should be made of the weight of urine lost during the test (in the case of repeated tests, greatest weight in any stated period). A loss of less than 1 g is within experimental error and the patient should be regarded as essentially dry. Urine loss should be measured and recorded in grams.

Statistics: When performing statistical analysis of urine loss in a group of subjects, nonparametric statistics should be employed, since the values are not normally distributed.

4 Procedures Related to the Evaluation of Micturition

4.1. Measurement of Urinary Flow

Urinary flow may be described in terms of *rate* and *pattern* and may be *continuous* or *intermittent*. *Flow rate* is defined as the volume of fluid expelled via the urethra per unit time. It is expressed in milliliters per second.

4.1.1. General Information.   The following details should be given:

1. Voided volume.
2. Patient environment and position (supine, sitting, or standing).
3. Filling:
   a) By diuresis (spontaneous or forced: specify regimen).
   b) By catheter (transurethral or suprapubic).
4. Type of fluid.

4.1.2. Technical Information.   The following details should be given:

1. Measuring equipment
2. Solitary procedure or combined with other measurements.

4.1.3. Definitions.   The terminology referring to urinary flow is defined as follows:

1. *Continuous flow* (Fig. 2):
   Voided volume is the total volume expelled via the urethra.
   Maximum flow rate is the maximum measured value of the flow rate.
   Average flow rate is voided volume divided by flow time. The calculation of average flow rate is only meaningful if flow is continuous and without terminal dribbling.
   Flow time is the time over which measurable flow actually occurs.
   Time to maximum flow is the elapsed time from onset of flow to maximum flow.
   The flow pattern must be described when flow time and average flow rate are measured.
2. *Intermittent Flow* (Fig. 3):

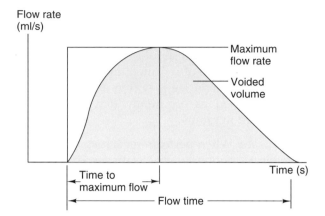

Figure 2. Diagram of a continuous urine flow recording with ICS recommended nomenclature.

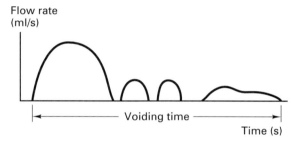

Figure 3. Diagram of an interrupted urine flow recording with ICS recommended nomenclature.

The same parameters used to characterize continuous flow may be applicable, if care is exercised, in patients with intermittent flow. In measuring flow time the time intervals between flow episodes are disregarded.

Voiding time is total duration of micturition, i.e., includes interruptions. When voiding is completed without interruption, voiding time is equal to flow time.

4.2. Bladder Pressure Measurements During Micturition

The specification of patient position, access for pressure measurement, catheter type, and measuring equipment are as for cystometry (see 3.1).

4.2.1. Definitions. The terminology referring to bladder-pressure during micturition is defined as follows (Fig. 4):

Opening time is the elapsed time from initial rise in detrusor pressure to onset of flow. This is the initial isovolumetric contraction period of micturition. Time lags should be taken into account. In most urodynamic systems a time lag occurs equal to the time taken for the urine to pass from the point of pressure measurement to the uroflow transducer.

The following parameters are applicable to measurements of each of the pressure curves – intravesical, abdominal, and detrusor pressure:

Premicturition pressure is the pressure recorded immediately before the initial isovolumetric contraction.

Opening pressure is the pressure recorded at the onset of measured flow.
Maximum pressure is the maximum value of the measured pressure.
Pressure at maximum flow is the pressure recorded at maximum measured flow rate.
Contraction pressure at maximum flow is the difference between pressure at maximum flow and premicturition pressure. Postmicturition events (e.g., after contraction) are not well understood and so cannot be defined as yet.

4.3. Pressure Flow Relationships

In the early days of urodynamics the flow rate and voiding pressure were related as a 'urethral resistance factor.' The concept of a resistance factor originates from rigid tube hydrodynamics. The urethra does not generally behave as a rigid tube; it is an irregular and distensible conduit and its walls and surroundings have active and passive elements which influence the flow through it. Therefore a resistance factor cannot provide a valid comparison between patients.

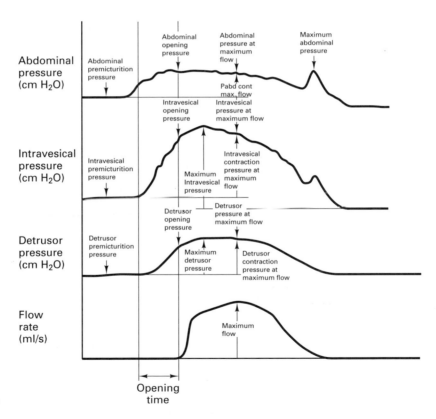

Figure 4. Diagram of a pressure-flow recording of micturition with ICS recommended nomenclature.

There are many ways of displaying the relationships between flow and pressure during micturition. An example is suggested in the third ICS report [3] (Fig. 5). As yet, available data do not permit a standard presentation of pressure/flow parameters.

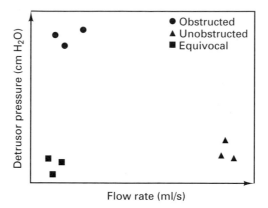

Figure 5. Diagram illustrating the presentation of pressure flow data on individual patients in three groups of 3 patients: obstructed, unobstructed, and equivocal.

When data from a group of patients are presented, pressure flow relationships may be shown on a graph, as illustrated in Fig. 5. This form of presentation allows lines of demarcation to be drawn on the graph to separate the results according to the problem being studied. The points shown in Fig. 5 are purely illustrative to indicate how the data might fall into groups. The group of equivocal results might include either an unrepresentative micturition in an obstructed or an unobstructed patient, or underactive detrusor function with or without obstruction. This is the group which invalidates the use of the term 'urethral resistance factors.'

4.4. Urethral Pressure Measurements During Voiding

The voiding urethral pressure profile (VUPP) is used to determine the pressure and site of urethral obstruction. Pressure is recorded in the urethra during voiding. The technique is similar to that used in the UPP measured during storage (the resting and stress profiles; see 3.2).

General and technical information should be recorded as for UPP during storage (see 3.2.).

Accurate interpretation of VUPP depends on the simultaneous measurement of intravesical pressure and the measurement of pressure at a precisely localized point in the urethra. Localization may be achieved by radiopaque marker on the catheter, which allows the pressure measurements to be related to a visualized point in the urethra. This technique is not fully developed, and a number of technical as well as clinical problems need to be solved before the VUPP is widely used.

4.5. Residual Urine

Residual urine is defined as the volume of fluid remaining in the bladder immediately following the completion of micturition. The measurement of residual urine forms an integral part of the study of micturition. However, voiding in unfamiliar surroundings may lead to unrepresentative results, as may voiding on command with a partially filled or overfilled bladder. Residual urine is commonly estimated by the following methods:

1. Catheter or cystoscope (transurethral, suprapubic).
2. Radiography (excretion urography, micturition cystography).
3. Ultrasonics.
4. Radioisotopes (clearance, gamma camera).

When estimating residual urine the measurement of voided volume and the time interval between voiding and residual urine estimation should be recorded. This is particularly important if the patient is in a diuretic phase. In the condition of vesicoureteric reflux, urine may re-enter the bladder after micturition and may falsely be interpreted as residual urine. The presence of urine in bladder diverticula following micturition presents special problems of interpretation, since a diverticulum may be regarded either as part of the bladder cavity or as outside the functioning bladder.

The various methods of measurement each have limitations as to their applicability and accuracy in the various conditions associated with residual urine. Therefore it is necessary to choose a method appropriate to the clinical problems. The absence of residual urine is usually an observation of clinical value, but does not exclude infravesical obstruction or bladder dysfunction. An isolated finding of residual urine requires confirmation before being considered significant.

5   Procedures Related to Neurophysiological Evaluation of the Urinary Tract During Filling and Voiding

5.1.   Electromyography

Electromyography (EMG) is the study of electrical potentials generated by the depolarization of muscle. The following refers to striated muscle EMG. The functional unit in EMG is the motor unit. This comprises a single motor neuron and the muscle fibers it innervates. A motor unit action potential is the recorded depolarization of muscle fibers which results from activation of a single anterior horn cell. Muscle action potentials may be detected either by needle electrodes or by surface electrodes.

Needle electrodes are placed directly into the muscle mass and permit visualization of the individual motor unit action potentials. Surface electrodes are applied to an epithelial surface as close to the muscle under study as possible. Surface electrodes detect the action potentials from groups of adjacent motor units underlying the recording surface.

EMG potentials may be displayed on an oscilloscope screen or played through audio amplifiers. A permanent record of EMG potentials can only be made using a chart recorder with a high-frequency response (in the range of 10 KHz).

EMG should be interpreted in the light of the patient's symptoms, physical findings, and urologic and urodynamic investigations.

5.1.1.   General Information.   The following details should be given:

1 EMG (solitary procedure, part of urodynamic or other electro-physiological investigation).
2 Patient position (supine, standing, sitting, or other).
3 Electrode placement:
  a) Sampling site – intrinsic striated muscle of the urethra, periurethral striated muscle, bulbocavernosus muscle, external anal sphincter, pubococcygeus, or other. State whether sites are single or multiple, unilateral or bilateral. Also state number of samples per site.
  b) Recording electrode – define the precise anatomical location of the electrode. For needle electrodes, include site of needle entry, angle of entry, and needle depth. For vaginal or urethral surface electrodes, state method of determining position of electrode.
  c) Reference electrode position. *Note:* ensure that there is no electrical interference with any other machines, e.g., x-ray apparatus.

5.1.2. Technical Information.   The following details should be given:

1 Electrodes:
  a) Needle electrodes – design (concentric, bipolar, monopolar, single fiber, other); dimensions (length, diameter, recording area); electrode material (e.g., platinum).
  b) Surface electrodes – type (skin, plug, catheter, other); size and shape; electrode material; mode of fixation to recording surface; conducting medium (e.g., saline, jelly).
2 Amplifier (make and specifications).
3 Signal processing (data: raw, averaged, integrated, or other).
4 Display equipment (make and specifications to include method of calibration, time base, full scale deflection in microvolts and polarity):
  a) Oscilloscope.
  b) Chart recorder.
  c) Loudspeaker.
  d) Other.
5 Storage (make and specifications):
  a) Paper.
  b) Magnetic tape recorder.
  c) Microprocessor.
  d) Other.
6 Hard copy production (make and specifications):
  a) Chart recorder.
  b) Photographic/video reproduction of oscilloscope screen.
  c) Other.

5.2.   EMG Findings

5.2.1. Individual motor unit action potentials. Normal motor unit potentials have a characteristic configuration, amplitude and duration. Abnormalities of the motor unit may include an increase in the amplitude, duration, and complexity of waveform (polyphasicity) of the potentials. A polyphasic potential is defined as one having more than five deflections. The EMG findings of fibrillations, positive sharp waves, and bizarre high-frequency potentials are thought to be abnormal.

5.2.2. Recruitment patterns. In normal subjects there is a gradual increase in 'pelvic floor' and 'sphincter' EMG activity during bladder filling. At the onset of micturition there is complete absence of activity. Any sphincter EMG activity during voiding is abnormal unless the patient is attempting to inhibit micturition. The finding of increased sphincter EMG activity during voiding, accompanied by characteristic simultaneous detrusor pressure and flow changes is described by the term 'detrusor-sphincter-dyssynergia.' In this condition a detrusor contraction occurs concurrently with an inappropriate contraction of the urethral and/or periurethral striated muscle.

5.3. Nerve Conduction Studies

Nerve conduction studies involve stimulation of a peripheral nerve and recording the time taken for a response to occur in muscle innervated by the nerve under study. The time taken from stimulation of the nerve to the response in the muscle is called the 'latency.' Motor latency is the time taken by the fastest motor fibers in the nerve to conduct impulses to the muscle and it depends on conduction distance and the conduction velocity of the fastest fibers.

5.3.1. General Information.   Also applicable to reflex latencies and evoked potentials (see below). The following details should be given:
1 Type of investigation:
  a) Nerve conduction study (e.g., pudendal nerve).
  b) Reflex latency determination (e.g., bulbocavernosus).
  c) Spinal evoked potential.
  d) Cortical evoked potential.
  e) Other.
2 Is the study a solitary procedure or part of urodynamic or neurophysiological investigations?
3 Patient position and environmental temperature, noise level, and illumination.
4 Electrode placement. Define electrode placement in precise anatomical terms. The exact interelectrode distance is required for nerve conduction velocity calculations.
  a Stimulation site (penis, clitoris, urethra, bladder neck, bladder, or other).
  b Recording sites (external anal sphincter, periurethral striated muscle, bulbocavernosus muscle, spinal cord, cerebral cortex or other).
    When recording spinal evoked responses, the sites of the recording electrodes should be specified according to the bony landmarks (e.g., L4). In cortical evoked responses the sites of the recording electrodes should be specified as in the international 10–20 system [6]. The sampling techniques should be specified (single or multiple, unilateral or bilateral, ipsilateral or contralateral, or other).

c Reference electrode position.

d Grounding electrode site. Ideally this should be between the stimulation and recording sites to reduce stimulus artifact.

5.3.2. Technical Information. Also applicable to reflex latencies and evoked potentials (see 5.4). The following details should be given:

1 Electrodes (make and specifications). Describe separately stimulus and recording electrodes as below:

   a) Design (e.g., needle, plate, ring, and configuration of anode and cathode where applicable).

   b) Dimensions.

   c) Electrode material (e.g., platinum).

   d) Contact medium.

2 Stimulator (make and specifications):

   a) Stimulus parameters (pulse width, frequency, pattern, current density, electrode impedance in Kohms). Also define in terms of threshold (e.g., in case of supramaximal stimulation).

3 Amplifier (make and specifications):

   a) Sensitivity (mV–μV).

   b) Filters – low pass (Hz) or high pass (kHz).

   c) Sampling time (ms).

4 Averager – make and specifications:

   a) Number of stimuli sampled.

5 Display equipment (make and specifications to include method of calibration, time base, full scale deflection in microvolts, and polarity):

   a) Oscilloscope.

6 Storage (make and specifications):

   a) Paper.

   b) Magnetic tape recorder.

   c) Microprocessor.

   d) Other.

7 Hard copy production (make and specification):

   a) Chart recorder.

   b) Photographic/video reproduction of oscilloscope screen.

   c) XY recorder.

   d) Other.

5.3.3. Description of Nerve Conduction Studies. Recordings are made from muscle, and the latency of response of the muscle is measured. The latency is taken as the time to onset of the earliest response.

To ensure that response time can be precisely measured, the gain should be increased to give a clearly defined take-off point (gain setting at least 100 μV/div and using a short time base, e.g., 1–2 ms/div).

Additional information may be obtained from nerve conduction studies, if, when using surface electrodes to record a compound muscle action potential, the amplitude is measured. The gain setting must be reduced so that the whole response is displayed and a longer time base is recommended (e.g., 1 mV/div and 5 ms/div). Since the amplitude is proportional to the number of motor unit potentials within the vicinity of the recording electrodes, a reduction in amplitude indicates loss of motor units and therefore denervation. (*Note:* A prolongation of latency is not necessarily indicative of denervation.)

5.4. Reflex Latencies

Reflex latencies require stimulation of sensory fields and recordings from the muscle which contracts reflexly in response to the stimulation. Such responses are a test of reflex arcs, which comprise both afferent and efferent limbs and a synaptic region within the central nervous system. The reflex latency expresses the nerve conduction velocity in both limbs of the arc and the integrity of the central nervous system at the level of the synapse(s). Increased reflex latency may occur as a result of slowed afferent or efferent nerve conduction or due to central nervous system conduction delays.

5.4.1. General and Technical Information. The same technical and general details apply as discussed above under Nerve Conduction Studies.

5.4.2. Description of Reflex Latency Measurements. Recordings are made from muscle, and the latency of response of the muscle is measured. The latency is taken as the time to onset of the earliest response.

To ensure that response time can be precisely measured, the gain should be increased to give a clearly defined take-off point (gain setting at least 100 μV/div and using a short time base, e.g., 1–2 ms/div).

5.5. Evoked Responses

Evoked responses are potential changes in central nervous system neurons resulting from distant stimulation, usually electrical. They are recorded using averaging techniques. Evoked responses may be used to test the integrity of peripheral, spinal, and central nervous pathways. As with nerve conduction studies, the conduction time (latency) may be measured. In addition, information may be gained from the amplitude and configuration of these responses.

5.5.1. General and Technical Information. See under Nerve Conduction Studies (5.3.).

5.5.2. Description of Evoked Responses. When describing the presence or absence of stimulus evoked responses and their configuration the following details should be given:

1 Single or multiple response.
2 Onset of response – defined as the start of the first reproducible potential. Since the onset of the response may be difficult to ascertain precisely, the criteria used should be stated.
3 Latency to onset – defined as the time (in milliseconds) from the onset of stimulus to the onset of response. The central conduction time relates to cortical evoked potentials and is defined as the difference between the latencies of the cortical and the spinal evoked potentials.

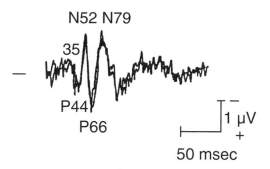

Figure 6. Multiphasic evoked response recorded from the cerebral cortex after stimulation of the dorsal aspect of the penis. The recording shows the conventional labelling of negative (N) and positive (P) deflections, with the latency of each deflection from the point of stimulation in milliseconds.

This parameter may be used to test the integrity of the corticospinal neuraxis.

4 Latencies to peaks of positive and negative deflections in multiphasic response (Fig. 6). P denotes positive deflections, N denotes negative deflections. In multiphasic responses, the peaks are numbered consecutively (e.g., P1, N1, P2, N2 . . .) or according to the latencies to peaks in milliseconds (e.g., P44, N52, P66 . . .).

5 The amplitude of the responses is measured in microvolts.

5.6. *Sensory Testing*

Limited information, of a subjective nature, may be obtained during cystometry by recording such parameters as the first desire to micturate, urgency, or pain. However, sensory function in the lower urinary tract can be assessed by semi-objective tests by the measurement of urethral and/or vesical sensory thresholds to a standard applied stimulus such as a known electrical current.

5.6.1. *General Information.*   The following details should be given:

1 Patient's position (supine, sitting, standing, other).
2 Bladder volume at time of testing.
3 Site of applied stimulus (intravesical, intraurethral).
4 Number of times the stimulus was applied and the response, e.g., the first sensation or the sensation of pulsing.
5 Type of applied stimulus:
   a) Electrical current – is usual to use a constant current stimulator in urethral sensory measurement. State electrode characteristics and placement as in section on EMG (5.2); electrode contact area and distance between electrodes if applicable; impedance characteristics of the system; type of conductive medium used for electrode/epithelial contact. *Note: Topical anesthetic agents should not be used.* Also state stimulator make and specifications; and stimulation parameters (pulse width, frequency, pattern, duration, current density).
   b) Other (e.g., mechanical, chemical).

5.6.2. *Definition of Sensory Thresholds.*   The vesical/urethral sensory threshold is defined as the least current which consistently produces a

sensation perceived by the subject during stimulation at the site under investigation. However, the absolute values will vary in relation to the site of the stimulus, the characteristics of the equipment, and the stimulation parameters. Normal values should be established for each system.

6 Classification of Lower Urinary Tract Dysfunction

The lower urinary tract is composed of the *bladder* and *urethra*. They form a functional unit and their interaction cannot be ignored. Each has two functions, the bladder to store and void, the urethra to control and convey. When a reference is made to the hydrodynamic function or to the whole anatomical unit as a storage organ – the vesica urinaria – the correct term is the *bladder*. When the smooth muscle structure known as the m.detrusor urinae is being discussed, then the correct term is *detrusor*. For simplicity the bladder/detrusor and the urethra will be considered separately so that a classification based on a combination of functional anomalies can be reached. Sensation cannot be precisely evaluated but must be assessed. This classification depends on the results of various objective urodynamic investigations. A complete urodynamic assessment is not necessary in all patients. However, studies of the filling and voiding phases are essential for each patient. As the bladder and urethra may behave differently during the storage and micturition phases of bladder function it is most useful to examine bladder and urethral activity separately in each phase.

Terms used should be objective and definable, and ideally should be applicable to the whole range of abnormality. When authors disagree with the classification presented below, or use terms which have not been defined here, they should ensure that the meaning of their terminology is made clear.

Assuming the absence of inflammation, infection, and neoplasm, *lower urinary tract dysfunction* may be caused by:

1 Disturbance of the pertinent nervous or psychological control system.
2 Disorders of muscle function.
3 Structural abnormalities.

Urodynamic diagnoses based on this classification should correlate with the patient's symptoms and signs. For example, the presence of an unstable contraction in an asymptomatic continent patient does not warrant a diagnosis of detrusor overactivity during storage.

6.1. The Storage Phase

6.1.1. Bladder Function During Storage. This may be described according to:

Detrusor activity
Bladder sensation

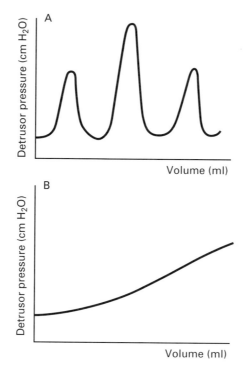

Figure 7. Diagrams of filling cystometry.
Part A: Illustrates typical phasic unstable detrusor contraction.
Part B: Illustrates the gradual increase of detrusor pressure with filling characteristic of reduced bladder compliance.

Bladder capacity
Compliance

6.1.2. Detrusor activity. In this context detrusor activity is interpreted from the measurement of detrusor pressure (P_{det}). Detrusor activity may be:

Normal
Overactive

In normal detrusor function the bladder volume increases during the filling phase without a significant rise in pressure (accommodation). No involuntary contractions occur despite provocation. A normal detrusor so defined may be described as 'stable.'

Overactive detrusor function is characterized by involuntary detrusor contractions during the filling phase, which may be spontaneous or provoked and which the patient cannot completely suppress. Involuntary detrusor contractions may be provoked by rapid filling, alterations of posture, coughing, walking, jumping, and other triggering procedures. Various terms have been used to describe these features and they are defined as follows:

The *unstable detrusor* is one that is shown objectively to contract, spontaneously or on provocation, during the filling phase while the patient is attempting to inhibit micturition. Unstable detrusor contractions may be asymptomatic or may be interpreted as a normal desire to void. The presence of these contractions does not necessarily imply a neurologic disorder. Unstable contractions are usually phasic in type (Fig. 7a). A gradual increase in detrusor pressure without subsequent decrease is best regarded as a change of compliance (Fig. 7b).

Detrusor hyperreflexia is defined as overactivity due to disturbance of the nervous control mechanisms. The term 'detrusor hyperreflexia' should only be used when there is objective evidence of a relevant neurologic disorder. The use of conceptual and undefined terms such as 'hypertonic,' 'systolic,' 'uninhibited,' 'spastic,' and 'automatic' should be avoided.

6.1.3. Bladder sensation. During filling bladder sensation can be classified in qualitative terms (see Cystometry, 3.1.) and by objective measurement (see Sensory Testing, 5.6.). Sensation can be classified broadly as follows:

Normal
Increased (hypersensitive)
Reduced (hyposensitive)
Absent

6.2. Bladder capacity. (See Cystometry, 3.1.)

6.2.1. Compliance. This is defined as: $\Delta V/\Delta P$ (see Cystometry, 3.1.). compliance may change during the cystometric examination and is variably dependent upon a number of factors including:

1 Rate of filling.
2 The part of the cystometrogram curve used for compliance calculation.
3 The volume interval over which compliance is calculated.
4 The geometry (shape) of the bladder.
5 The thickness of the bladder wall.
6 The mechanical properties of the bladder wall.
7 The contractile/relaxant properties of the detrusor.

During normal bladder filling little or no pressure change occurs and this is termed 'normal compliance.' However, at present there is insufficient data to define normal, high and low compliance.

When reporting compliance, specify:

1 The rate of bladder filling.
2 The bladder volume at which compliance is calculated.
3 The volume increment over which compliance is calculated.
4 The part of the cystometrogram curve used for the calculation of compliance.

6.2.2. Urethral Function During Storage. The urethral closure mechanism during storage may be:

Normal
Incompetent

The *normal urethral closure mechanism* maintains a positive urethral closure pressure during filling even in the presence of increased abdominal pressure. Immediately prior to micturition the normal closure pressure decreases to allow flow.

An *incompetent urethral closure mechanism* is defined as one which allows leakage of urine in the absence of a detrusor contraction. Leakage may occur whenever intravesical pressure exceeds intraurethral pressure (genuine stress incontinence) or when there is an involuntary fall in urethral pressure. Terms such as 'the unstable urethra' await further data and precise definition.

6.2.3. Urinary Incontinence. This is defined as involuntary loss of urine which is objectively demonstrable and a social or hygienic problem. Loss of urine through channels other than the urethra is extraurethral incontinence.

Urinary incontinence denotes:

1 A symptom.
2 A sign.
3 A condition.

The symptom indicates the patient's statement of involuntary urine loss, the sign is the objective demonstration of urine loss, and the condition is the urodynamic demonstration of urine loss.

6.2.4. Symptoms. These can be defined as follows:

Urge incontinence – the involuntary loss of urine associated with a strong desire to void (urgency). *Urgency* may be associated with two types of dysfunction:
   Overactive detrusor function (*motor urgency*)
   Hypersensitivity (*sensory urgency*)

Stress incontinence – the symptom indicates the patient's statement of involuntary loss of urine during physical exertion.

'Unconscious' incontinence – incontinence may occur in the absence of urge and without conscious recognition of the urinary loss.

Enuresis – any involuntary loss of urine. If the term is used to denote incontinence during sleep, it should always be qualified with the adjective 'nocturnal.'

Post micturition dribble and *continuous leakage* – denote other symptomatic forms of incontinence.

6.2.5. Signs. The sign stress incontinence denotes the observation of loss of urine from the urethra synchronous with physical exertion (e.g., coughing). Incontinence may also be observed without physical exercise. Post-micturition dribble and continuous leakage denote other signs of incontinence. Symptoms and signs alone may not disclose the cause of urinary incontinence. Accurate diagnosis often requires urodynamic investigation in addition to careful history and physical examination.

6.2.6. Conditions. These can be defined as follows:

Genuine stress incontinence – the involuntary loss of urine occurring when, in the absence of a detrusor contraction, the intravesical pressure exceeds the maximum urethral pressure.
Reflex incontinence – loss of urine due to detrusor hyperreflexia and/or involuntary urethral relaxation in the absence of the sensation usually associated with the desire to micturate. This condition is only seen in patients with neuropathic bladder/urethral disorders.

Overflow incontinence – any involuntary loss of urine associated with overdistension of the bladder.

6.3. The Voiding Phase

6.3.1. The Detrusor During Voiding. During micturition the detrusor may be:

Acontractile
Underactive
Normal

The *acontractile detrusor* is one that cannot be demonstrated to contract during urodynamic studies. *Detrusor areflexia* is defined as acontractility due to an abnormality of nervous control and denotes the complete absence of centrally coordinated contraction. In detrusor areflexia due to a lesion of the conus medullaris or sacral nerve outflow, the detrusor should be described as *decentralized* – not denervated, since the peripheral neurons remain. In such bladders pressure fluctuations of low amplitude, sometimes known as 'autonomous' waves, may occasionally occur. The use of terms such as 'atonic,' 'hypotonic,' 'autonomic,' and 'flaccid' should be avoided.

Detrusor underactivity is defined as a detrusor contraction of inadequate magnitude and/or duration to effect bladder emptying with a normal time span. The term should be reserved as an expression describing detrusor activity during micturition. Patients may have underactivity during micturition and detrusor overactivity during filling.

Normal detrusor contractility. Normal voiding is achieved by a voluntarily initiated detrusor contraction that is sustained and can usually be suppressed voluntarily. A normal detrusor contraction will effect complete bladder emptying in the absence of obstruction. For a given detrusor contraction, the magnitude of the recorded pressure rise will depend on the degree of outlet resistance.

Urethral Function During Micturition. During voiding urethral function may be:

Normal
Obstructive
   overactivity
   mechanical

Normal. The normal urethra opens to allow the bladder to be emptied.

Obstruction. This occurs when the urethral closure mechanism contracts against a detrusor contraction or fails to open at attempted micturition. Synchronous detrusor and urethral contraction is *detrusor/urethral dyssynergia*. This diagnosis should be qualified by stating the location and type of the urethral muscles (striated or smooth) which are involved. Despite the confusion surrounding 'sphincter' terminology, the use of certain terms is so widespread that they are retained and defined here. The term *detrusor/external sphincter dyssynergia* or *detrusor-sphincter-dyssynergia (DSD)* describes a detrusor contraction concurrent with an involuntary contraction of the urethral and/or periurethral striated muscle. In the adult, detrusor sphincter dyssynergia is a feature of neurologic voiding disorders. In the absence of neurologic features the validity of this diagnosis should be questioned. The term *detrusor/bladder neck dyssynergia* is used to denote a detrusor contraction concurrent with an objectively demonstrated failure of bladder neck opening. No parallel term has been elaborated for possible detrusor/distal urethral (smooth muscle) dyssynergia.

Overactivity of the striated urethral sphincter may occur in the absence of detrusor contraction, and may prevent voiding. This is not detrusor/sphincter dyssynergia.

Overactivity of the urethral sphincter may occur during voiding in the absence of neurologic disease and is termed *dysfunctional voiding*. The use of terms such as 'non-neurogenic' and 'occult neuropathic' should be avoided.

Mechanical obstruction. This is most commonly anatomical, e.g., caused by urethral stricture.

Summary

Using the characteristics of detrusor and urethral function during storage and micturition an accurate definition of lower urinary tract behavior in each patient becomes possible.

7   Units of Measurement

In the urodynamic literature pressure is measured in centimeters of water pressure and *not* in millimeters of mercury. When Laplace's law is used to calculate tension in the bladder wall, it is often found that pressure is then measured in $dyne/cm^2$. This lack of uniformity in the systems used leads to confusion when other parameters, which are a function of pressure, are computed – for instance, 'compliance', contraction force, velocity, etc. From these few examples it is evident that standardization is essential for meaningful communication. Many journals now require that the results be given in SI Units. This section is designed to give guidance in the application of the SI system to urodynamics and defines the units involved. The principal units to be used are listed in Table 1.

Table 1. Recommended units of measurement

Quantity	Acceptable unit	Symbol
Volume	milliliter	ml
Time	second	s
Flow rate	milliliters/second	ml/s
Pressure	centimeters of water[a]	cmH_2O
Length	meters or submultiples	m, cm, mm
Velocity	meters/second or submultiples	m/s, cm/s
Temperature	degrees Celsius	°C

[a]The SI Unit is the pascal (Pa), but it is only practical at present to calibrate our instruments in cmH_2O. One centimeter of water pressure is approximately equal to 100 pascals (1 cmH_2O=98.07 Pa=0.098 kPa).

Table 2. List of symbols

Basic symbols		Urologic qualifiers		Value	
Pressure	P	Bladder	ves	Maximum	max
Volume	V	Urethra	ura	Minimum	min
Flow rate	Q	Ureter	ure	Average	ave
Velocity	v	Detrusor	det	Isovolumetric	isv
Time	t	Abdomen	abd	Isotonic	ist
Temperature	T	External		Isobaric	isb
		Stream	ext	Isometric	ism
Length	l				
Area	A				
Diameter	d				
Force	F				
Energy	E				
Power	P				
Compliance	C				
Work	W				
Energy per unit volume	e				

$P_{det, max}$ =maximum detrusor pressure
e_{ext} =kinetic energy per unit volume in the external stream

8   Symbols

It is often helpful to use symbols in a communication. The system in Table 2 has been devised to standardize a code of symbols for use in urodynamics. The rationale of the system is to have a basic symbol representing the physical quantity with qualifying subscripts. The list of basic symbols largely conforms to international usage. The qualifying subscripts relate to the basic symbols for commonly used urodynamic parameters.

References

1. Bates P, Bradley WE, Glen E et al. First report on the standardization of terminology of lower urinary tract function. Urinary incontinence. Procedures related to the evaluation of urine storage – cystometry, urethral closure pressure profile, units of measurement.

Br J Urol 1976; 48:39–42; *Eur Urol 1976*; 2:274–276; *Scand J Urol Nephrol 1976*; 11:193–196; *Urol Int 1976*; 2:81–87

2. Bates P, Glen E, Griffiths D et al. Second report on the standardization of terminology of lower urinary tract function. Procedures related to the evaluation of micturition – flow rate, pressure measurement, symbols. *Acta Urol Jpn 1977*; 27:1563–1566; *Br J Urol 1977*; 49:207–210; *Eur Urol 1977*; 3:168–170; *Scand J Urol Nephrol 1977*; 11:197–199

3. Bates P, Bradley WE, Glen E et al. Third report on the standardization of terminology of lower urinary tract function. Procedures related to the evaluation of micturition: pressure flow relationships, residual urine. *Br J Urol 1980*; 52:348–350; *Eur Urol 1980*; 6:170–171; *Acta Urol Jpn 1980*; 27:1566–1568; *Scand J Urol Nephrol 1980*; 12:191–193

4. Bates P, Bradley WE, Glen E et al. Fourth report on the standardization of terminology of lower urinary tract function. Terminology related to neuromuscular dysfunction of lower urinary tract. *Br J Urol 1981*; 53:333–335; *Urology 1981*; 17:618–620; *Scand J Urol Nephrol 1981*; 15:169–171; *Acta Urol Jpn 1981*; 27:1568–1571

5. Abrams P, Blaivas JG, Stanton SL et al. Sixth report on the standardization of terminology of lower urinary tract function. Procedures related to neurophysiological investigations: Electromyography, nerve conduction studies, reflex latencies, evoked potentials and sensory testing. *World J Urol 1986*; 4:2–5; *Scand J Urol Nephrol 1986*; 20:161–164; *Br J Urol 1987*; 59:300–307

6. Jasper HH. Report to the committee on the methods of clinical examination in electroencephalography. *Electroencephalogr Clin Neurophysiol 1958*; 10:370–375

Appendix 2

**The Standardisation of Terminology of Female Pelvic Organ Prolapse
and Pelvic Floor Dysfunction**

*Reprinted with permission by the International Continence Society Committee
on Standardisation of Terminology,
Anders Mattiasson (chairman)
Subcommittee on Pelvic Organ Prolapse and Pelvic Floor Dysfunction,
Members: Richard Bump (chairman), Kari Bø, Linda Brubaker, John DeLancey,
Peter Klarskov, Bob Shull, Anthony Smith*

Contents

1   INTRODUCTION

The International Continence Society (ICS) has been at the forefront in the standardization of terminology of lower urinary tract function since the establishment of the Committee on Standardization of Terminology in 1973. This committee's efforts over the past two decades have resulted in the world-wide acceptance of terminology standards that allow clinicians and researchers interested in the lower urinary tract to communicate efficiently and precisely. While female pelvic organ prolapse and pelvic floor dysfunction are intimately related to lower urinary tract function, such accurate communication using standard terminology has not been possible for these conditions.

There is no universally accepted system for describing the anatomic position of the pelvic organs. Many reports use terms for the description of pelvic organ prolapse which are undefined; none of the many aspiring grading systems has been adequately validated with respect either to reproducibility or to the clinical significance of different grades. The absence of standard, validated definitions prevents comparisons of published series from different institutions and longitudinal evaluation of an individual patient. A primary goal of this report is to introduce a system that will allow the accurate, quantitative description of pelvic support findings in individual patients.

This document is a first effort toward the establishment of standard, reliable, and validated descriptions of female pelvic anatomy and function. The subcommittee acknowledges a need for well designed reliability studies to evaluate and validate various descriptions and definitions. We have tried to develop guidelines that will promote new insights rather than existing biases. Acknowledgement of these standards in written publications and scientific presentations should be indicated in the Methods Section with the following statement: 'Methods, definitions, and descriptions conform to the standards recommended by the International Continence Society, except where specifically noted.'

2   DESCRIPTION OF PELVIC ORGAN PROLAPSE

The clinical description of pelvic floor anatomy is determined during the physical examination of the external genitalia and vaginal canal. The specifics of the examination technique are not dictated by this document however authors should precisely describe their specific technique. Segments of the lower reproductive tract will replace such terms as 'cystocele, rectocele, enterocele, or urethrovesical junction' because these terms may imply an unrealistic certainty as to the structures on the other side of the reproductive tract bulge particularly in women who have had previous prolapse surgery.

2.1   *Conditions of the Examination*
Many variables of examination technique may influence findings in patients with pelvic organ prolapse. It is critical that the examiner sees and describes the maximum protrusion noted by the individual subject

during her daily activities. Therefore the criteria for the end point of the examination and the full development of the prolapse must be specified in any report.

Suggested criteria for demonstration of maximum prolapse should include one or all of the following:

a Any protrusion of the vaginal wall has become tight during straining by the patient.

b Traction on the prolapse causes no further descent.

c The subject confirms that the size of the prolapse and extent of the protrusion seen by the examiner is as extensive as the most severe protrusion which she has experienced. The means of this confirmation should be specified. For example, the subject may use a small hand-held mirror to visualize the protrusion.

d A standing, straining examination confirms that the full extent of the prolapse was observed in other positions used.

Other variables of technique that should be specified during the quantitative description (Section 2.2) and ordinal staging (Section 2.3) of pelvic organ prolapse include the following:

a the position of the subject (e.g., supine lithotomy, lateral Sims position, specified degrees of upright, erect sitting, standing, etc);

b the type of examination table or chair used;

c the type of standard vaginal specula, retractors, or tractors used;

d diagrams of any customized retraction, traction, or measuring devices used;

e the type (e.g., Valsalva maneuver, cough) and, if measured, intensity (e.g. vesical or rectal pressure rise) of straining used to develop the prolapse maximally;

f fullness of bladder and, if the bladder was empty, whether this was by spontaneous voiding or by catheterization;

g content or rectum;

f the method by which any quantitative measurements were made (e.g., estimation by visualization or palpation, direct measurement with a calibrated device, etc).

There is a critical need to define the importance of all variables of technique as they relate to the ease of assessment and reproducibility of measurements. Researchers should determine the inter-observer and intra-observer reliability of measurements made with their assessment techniques before utilizing them as baseline and outcome variables. Manuscript descriptions of assessment techniques should include sufficient detail to ensure that other researchers can precisely replicate them.

2.2 *Quantitative Description of Pelvic Organ Position*
This descriptive system is a tandem profile in that it contains a series of component measurements grouped together in combination, but listed separately in tandem, without being fused into a distinctive new expression or 'grade'. It allows for the precise description of an

individual woman's pelvic support without assigning a 'severity value'. Second, it allows accurate site-specific observations of the stability or progression of prolapse over time by the same or different observers. Finally, it allows similar judgements as to the outcome of surgical repair of prolapse. For example, noting that a surgical procedure moved the vaginal apex from 0.5 cm beyond the hymeneal ring to 0.5 cm above the hymeneal ring denotes more meager improvement than stating that the prolapse was reduced from Grade 3 to Grade 1 as would be the case using some current grading systems.

2.2.1 *Definition of Anatomic Landmarks*
Prolapse should be evaluated by a standard system relative to clearly defined anatomic points of reference. These are of two types, fixed reference points and defined points for measurement.

a Fixed Point of Reference
Prolapse should be evaluated relative to a fixed anatomic landmark which can be consistently and precisely identified. The hymen will be the fixed point of reference used throughout this system of quantitative prolapse description.

Visually, the hymen provides a precisely identifiable landmark for reference. Although it is recognized that the plane of the hymen is somewhat variable depending upon the degree of levator ani dysfunction, it remains the best landmark available. 'Hymen' is preferable to the ill-defined and imprecise term 'introitus'. The anatomic position of the six defined points for measurement [section 2.2.1(b)] should be centimeters above or proximal to the hymen (negative number) or centimeters below or distal to the hymen (positive number) with the plane of the hymen being defined as zero (0). For example, a cervix that protruded 3 cm distal to the hymen would be +3 cm.

Palpably, the ischial spines provide precisely identifiable landmarks. In the sitting or standing position or in situations with limited viability due to obesity or limited ability for hip abduction, the position of the cervix or the leading point of the prolapse relative to the ischial spines may be measured by palpation. Measurements so obtained should be normalized to the level of the hymen by noting the distance between the ischial spines and the plane of the hymen. For example, a cervix that is 3 cm distal to the ischial spines would be at –2cm if the spines were 5 cm above the plane of the hymen.

b Defined Points for Measurement

Anterior Vaginal Wall. Because the only structure directly visible to the examiner is the surface of the vagina, anterior prolapse should be discussed in terms of a segment of the vaginal wall rather than the organs which lie behind it. Thus, the term 'anterior vaginal wall prolapse' is preferable to 'cystocele' or 'anterior enterocele' unless the organs involved are identified by ancillary tests.

Point Aa   A point located in the midline of the anterior vaginal wall three (3) cm proximal to the external urethral meatus. This corresponds to the approximate location of the 'urethro-vesical crease', a visible landmark of variable prominence that is obliterated in many patients. By definition, the range of position of Point Aa relative to the hymen is –3 to +3 cm.

Point Ba   A point that represents the **most distal (i.e., most dependent)** position of the upper portion of the anterior vaginal wall from the vaginal cuff or anterior vaginal fornix to Point Aa. By definition, Point Ba is at –3 cm in the absence of prolapse and would have a positive value equal to the position of the cuff in women with total post-hysterectomy vaginal eversion.

Vaginal Apex   These points represent the most proximal locations of the normally positioned lower reproductive tract.

Point C   A point that represents either the most distal (i.e., most dependent) edge of the cervix or the leading edge of the vaginal cuff scar in a woman who has undergone total hysterectomy.

Point D   A point that represents the location of the posterior fornix (or pouch of Douglas) in a woman who still has a cervix. It represents the level of uterosacral ligament attachment to the proximal posterior cervix. It is included as a point of measurement to differentiate suspensory failure of the uterosacral-cardinal ligament complex from cervical elongation. When the location of Point C is significantly more positive than the location of Point D, this is indicative of cervical elongation which may be symmetrical or eccentric (e.g., involving only the anterior lip of the cervix due to a prior laceration). Point D is omitted as a point for measurement in the absence of the cervix.

Posterior Vaginal Wall   Analogous to anterior prolapse, posterior prolapse should be discussed in terms of segments of the vaginal wall rather than the organs which lie behind it. Thus, the term 'posterior vaginal wall prolapse' is preferable to 'rectocele' or 'enterocele' unless the organs involved are identified by ancillary tests. If small bowel appears to be present in the rectovaginal space, the examiner should comment on this fact and should clearly describe the basis for this clinical impression (e.g., by observation of peristaltic activity in the distended posterior vagina, by palpation of loops of small bowel between an examining finger in the rectum and one in the vagina, etc). In such cases, a 'pulsion' addendum to the point Bp position should be noted (e.g., Bp = +5 [pulsion]). See sections 3.1(a) and 3.1(b) for further discussion.

Point Bp   A point that represents the **most distal (i.e., most dependent)** position of the upper portion of the posterior vaginal wall from the vaginal cuff or posterior vaginal fornix to Point Ap. By definition, Point Bp is at −3 cm in the absence of prolapse and would have a positive value equal to the position of the cuff in a woman with total post-hysterectomy vaginal eversion.

Point Ap   A point located in the midline of the posterior vaginal wall three (3) cm proximal to the hymen. By definition, the range of position of Point Ap relative to the hymen is −3 to +3 cm.

c   Other Landmarks and Measurements

The *genital hiatus* is measured from the middle of the external urethral meatus to the posterior midline hymen. If the location of the hymen is distorted by a loose band of skin without underlying muscle or connective tissue, the firm palpable tissue of the perineal body should be substituted as the posterior margin for this measurement.

The *perineal body* is measured from the posterior margin of the genital hiatus (as just described) to the mid-anal opening. Measurement of the genital hiatus and perineal body are expressed in centimeters.

The total *vaginal length* is the greatest depth of the vagina in cm when Point C or D is reduced to its full normal position. Note: Eccentric elongation of a prolapsed anterior or posterior vaginal wall should not be included in the measurement of total vaginal length. (See Figure 4.A. and accompanying discussion.) The points and measurements discussed in this section are represented in Figure 1.

2.2.2   *Making and Recording Measurements*

The position of Points Aa, Ba, Ap, Bp, C, and (if applicable) D with reference to the hymen should be measured and recorded. Positions are expressed as centimeters above or proximal to the hymen (negative number) or centimeters below or distal to the hymen (positive number) with the plane of the hymen being defined as zero (0). While an examiner may be able to make measurements to the nearest half (0.5) cm, it is doubtful that further precision is possible. All reports should clearly

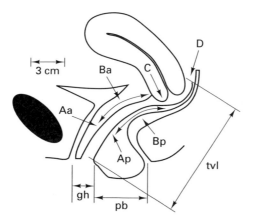

Figure 1.   Six points, genital hiatus (gh), perineal body (pb), and total vaginal length (tvl) used for prolapse quantitation.

specify how measurements were derived. For example, were direct measurements made using a probe, ruler, glove, speculum or other device marked in centimeters, were indirect measurements made with the examiner's fingers and then measured off a centimeter tape, were measurements estimated by the examiner without using a graduated device, or were combinations of techniques used? If customized measuring devices were used, diagrams of such should be included in any manuscript or presentation.

Measurements may be recorded as a simple line of numbers (e.g., –3, –3, –7, –9, –3, –3, 9, 2, 2 for Points Aa, Ba, C, D, Bp, Ap, total vaginal length, genital hiatus, and perineal body respectively). Note that the last three numbers have no sign (i.e., – or +) attached to them because they denote lengths and not positions relative to the hymen. Alternatively, a three by three 'tic-tac-toe' grid can be used to organize concisely the measurements as noted in Figure 2. If point D is not applicable due to a prior hysterectomy, this should be noted as such with 'NA' or '–' in either the line of numbers or in the grid.

Point Aa anterior wall	Point Ba anterior wall	Point C cervix or cuff
Genital hiatus	Perineal body	Total vaginal length
Point Ap posterior wall	Point Bp posterior wall	Point D posterior fornix

Figure 2. A three-by-three grid for recording the quantitative description of pelvic organ prolapse.

Figure 3 is a line diagram contrasting measurements indicating normal support to those of post hysterectomy vaginal eversion.

In the example of normal support (Figure 3.A.), Points Aa and Ba and Points Ap and Bp are all –3 since there is no anterior or posterior wall descent. The lowest point of the cervix is 8 cm above the hymen (–8) and the posterior fornix is 2 cm above this (–10). The vaginal length is 10 cm and the genital hiatus and perineal body measure 2 and 3 cm respectively.

In the example of complete eversion (Figure 3.B.), the most distal point of the anterior wall (Point Ba), the vaginal cuff scar (Point C), and the most distal point of the posterior wall (Point Bp) are all at the same position (+8) and Points Aa and Ap are maximally distal (both at +3). The fact that the total vaginal length equals the maximum protrusion reflects the fact that the eversion is total.

Figure 4 is a line diagram representing predominant anterior and posterior vaginal wall prolapse with partial vault descent.

In the example of a predominant anterior support defect (Figure 4.A.), the leading point of the prolapse is the upper anterior vaginal wall, Point

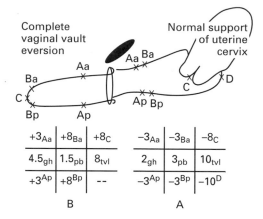

Figure 3. A. (right) normal support; **B.** (left) complete eversion.

+3Aa	+8Ba	+8C		−3Aa	−3Ba	−8C
4.5gh	1.5pb	8tvl		2gh	3pb	10tvl
+3Ap	+8Bp	−−		−3Ap	−3Bp	−10D
	B				A	

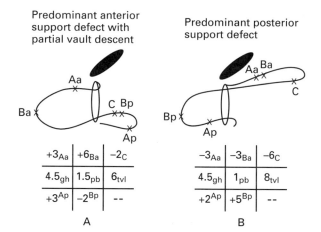

Figure 4. A. (left) predominant anterior prolapse; **B.** (right) predominant posterior prolapse.

+3Aa	+6Ba	−2C		−3Aa	−3Ba	−6C
4.5gh	1.5pb	6tvl		4.5gh	1pb	8tvl
+3Ap	−2Bp	−−		+2Ap	+5Bp	−−
	A				B	

Ba (+6). Note that there is significant elongation of the bulging anterior wall. Point Aa is maximally distal (+3) and the vaginal cuff scar is 2 cm above the hymen (C = −2). The cuff scar has undergone 4 cm of descent since it would be at −6 (the total vaginal length) if it were perfectly supported. In this example, the total vaginal length is not the maximum depth of the vagina with the elongated anterior vaginal wall maximally reduced, but rather the depth of the vagina at the cuff with Point C reduced to its normal full extent as specified in Section 2.2.1(c).

In the example of the predominant posterior support defect (Figure 4.B.), the leading point of the prolapse is the upper posterior vaginal wall, Point Bp (+5). Point Ap is 2 cm distal to the hymen (+2) and the vaginal cuff scar is 6 cm above the hymen (−6). The cuff has undergone only 2 cm of descent since it would be at −8 (the total vaginal length) if it were perfectly supported.

2.3   *Ordinal Staging of Pelvic Organ Prolapse*

The tandem profile for quantifying prolapse just described provides a precise description of anatomy for individual patients. However, because of the many possible combinations, such profiles cannot be directly ranked; the many variations are too numerous to permit useful analysis and comparisons when populations are studied. Consequently they are analogous to other tandem profiles such as the TNM Index for various cancers. For the TNM description of individual patient's cancers to be useful in population studies evaluating prognosis or response to therapy, they are clustered into an ordinal set of stages. Ordinal stages represent adjacent categories that can be ranked in an ascending sequence of magnitude, but the categories are assigned arbitrarily and the intervals between them cannot be actually measured.

While the committee is aware of the arbitrary nature of an ordinal staging system and the possible biases that it introduces, we conclude such a system is necessary if populations are to be described and compared, if symptoms putatively related to prolapse are to be evaluated, and if the results of various treatment options are to be assessed and compared.

Stages are assigned according to the most severe portion of the prolapse when the full extent of the protrusion has been demonstrated according to the criteria in Section 2.1. **In order for a stage to be assigned to an individual subject, it is essential that her quantitative description be completed first**. The 2 cm buffer related to the total vaginal length in Stages 0 and IV is an effort to compensate for vaginal distensibility and the inherent imprecision of the measurement of total vaginal length. The 2 cm buffer around the hymen in Stage II is an effort to avoid confining a stage to a single plane and to acknowledge practical limits of precision in this assessment.

a Stage 0

No prolapse is demonstrated. Points Aa, Ap, Ba, and Bp are all at –3 cm and either Point C or D is between –X cm and – (X–2) cm, where X = the total vaginal length in cm [i.e., the quantitation value of point C or D is $\leq -$ (X–2) cm]. Figure 3.A. represents Stage 0 pelvic organ prolapse.

b Stage I

The criteria for Stage 0 are not met but the most distal portion of the prolapse is more than 1 cm above the level of the hymen (i.e., its quantitation value is < –1 cm). Stage I can be subgrouped according to which portion of the lower reproductive tract is the <u>most distal</u> part of the prolapse using the following letter qualifiers: a = anterior vaginal wall, p = posterior vaginal wall, C = vaginal cuff, Cx = cervix, and Aa, Ap, Ba, Bp, and D for the Points of measurement already defined. (e.g., I-Cx if the cervix is the most distal, I-Bp if the upper posterior wall is most distal, or I- if the junction of the distal and proximal anterior wall is the most distal part of the prolapse.

c Stage II

The most distal portion of the prolapse is 1 cm or less proximal to or distal to the plane of they hymen (i.e., its quantitation value is $\geq$ –1 cm but $\leq$ + 1 cm). Stage II can be subgrouped according to the scheme described under Stage I (e.g., II-a, II-C, or II-Bp).

d Stage III

The most distal portion of the prolapse is more than 1 cm below the plane of the hymen but protrudes no further than two centimeters less than the total vaginal length in cm [i.e., its quantitation value is > +1 cm but < +(X–2) cm where X = total vaginal length]. Stage III can be subgrouped according to the scheme described under Stage I. For example, Figure 4.A. represents Stage III-Ba and Figure 4.B. represents Stage III-Bp prolapse.

e Stage IV

Essentially complete eversion of the total length of the lower genital tract is demonstrated. The distal portion of the prolapse protrudes to at least (X–2) cm where X = the total vaginal length in cm [i.e., it quantitation value is $\geq$ + (X–2) cm]. In most instances, the leading edge of Stage IV prolapse will be the cervix or vaginal cuff scar. Rare exceptions to this can be noted according to the subgrouping scheme described under Stage I. Figure 3.B. represents Stage IV-C prolapse. Table 1 summarizes the staging system.

3   ANCILLARY TECHNIQUES FOR DESCRIBING PELVIC ORGAN PROLAPSE

This series of procedures may help to further characterize pelvic organ prolapse in an individual patient. They are considered ancillary either because they are not yet standardized or validated or because they are not universally available to all patients.

Authors utilizing these procedures should include the following information in their manuscripts:

a Describe the objective information they intended to generate and how it enhanced their ability to evaluate or treat prolapse.
b Describe precisely how the test was performed, any instruments that were used, and the specific testing conditions (see Section 2.1.) so that other authors can reproduce the study.
c Document the reliability of the measurement obtained with the technique.

Stage 0	Points Aa, Ap, Ba, & Bp are all at –3 cm <u>and</u> Either Point C or D is at $\leq$ – (X–2) cm
Stage I	The criteria for Stage 0 are not met <u>and</u> The leading edge of prolapse is < –1 cm
Stage II	Leading edge of prolapse is $\geq$ –1 cm but $\leq$ + 1 cm
Stage III	Leading edge of prolapse is > + 1 cm but < + (X–2) cm
Stage IV	Leading edge of prolapse is $\geq$ + (X–2) cm

X = Total Vaginal Length in centimeters in Stages 0, III, and IV

Stages I through IV can be subgrouped according to which portion of the lower reproductive tract is the leading edge of the prolapse using the following qualifiers: a = anterior vaginal wall, p = posterior vaginal wall, C = vaginal cuff, Cx = cervix, and Aa, Ba, Ap, Bp, and D for the defined points of measurement. (e.g., IV-Cx, II-a, or III-Bp)

Table 1. ICS Pelvic Organ Prolapse Ordinal Staging System.

3.1   *Supplementary Physical Examination Techniques*

Many of these techniques are essential to the adequate pre-operative evaluation of a patient with pelvic organ prolapse. While they do not directly affect either the tandem profile or the ordinal stage, they are important for the selection and performance of an effective surgical repair. These techniques include, but are not necessarily limited to, the following:

a   performance of a digital rectal-vaginal examination while the patient is straining and the prolapse is maximally developed to differentiate between a high rectocele and an enterocele;
b   digital assessment of the contents of the rectal-vaginal septum during the examination noted in 3.1(a) to differentiate between a 'traction' enterocele (the posterior cul-de-sac is pulled down with the prolapsing cervix or vaginal cuff but is not distended by intestines) and a 'pulsion' enterocele (the intestinal contents of the enterocele distend the rectal-vaginal septum and produced a protruding mass);
c   Q-tip testing for the measurement of urethral axial mobility;
d   measurements of perineal descent;
e   measurements of the transverse diameter of the genital hiatus or of the protruding prolapse;
f   measurements of vaginal volume;
g   description and measurement of rectal prolapse;
h   examination techniques for differentiating between various types of defects (e.g., central versus paravaginal defects of the anterior vaginal wall).

3.2   *Endoscopy*

Cystoscopic visualization of bowel peristalsis under the bladder base or trigone may identify an anterior enterocele in some patients. The endoscopic visualization of the bladder base and rectum and observation of the voluntary constriction and dilation of the urethra, vagina, and rectum has, to date, played a minor role in the evaluation of pelvic floor anatomy and function. When such techniques are described, authors should include the type, size, and lens angle of the endoscope used, the doses of any analgesic, sedative, or anesthetic agents used, and a statement of the level of consciousness of the subjects in addition to a description of the other conditions of the examination.

3.3   *Photography*

Still photographic documentation of prolapse beyond Stage II may be utilized both to document serial changes in individual patients and to illustrate findings for manuscripts and presentations. Photographs should contain an internal frame of reference such as a centimeter ruler or tape.

3.4   *Imaging Procedures*

Different imaging techniques have been used to visualize pelvic floor anatomy, support defects, and relationships among adjacent organs.

These techniques may be more accurate than physical examination in determining which organs are involved in pelvic organ prolapse. However, they share the limitations of the other techniques in this section, i.e, a lack of standardisation, validation, and/or availability. For this reason, no specific technique can be recommended but guidelines for reporting various techniques will be considered.

3.4.1   *General Guidelines for Imaging Procedures*

Landmarks should be defined to allow comparisons with other imaging studies and the physical examination. The lower edge of the symphysis pubis should be given high priority as a landmark. Other examples of bony landmarks include the superior edge of the pubic symphysis, the ischial spine, the obturator foramen, and the promontory of the sacrum.

All reports on imaging techniques should specify the following:

a position of the patient including the position of her legs. (Images in manuscripts should be oriented to reflect the patient's position when the study was performed and should not be oriented to suggest an erect position unless the patient was erect.);
b specific verbal instructions given to the patient;
c bladder volume and content and bowel content, including any pre-study preparations;
d the performance and display of simultaneous monitoring such as pressure measurements that might be used to document that exposures were made at the most appropriate moment.

3.4.2   *Ultrasonography*

Continuous visualization of dynamic events is possible. All reports using ultrasound should include the following information:

a transducer type and manufacturer (e.g., sector, linear, MHz);
b transducer size;
c transducer orientation;
d route of scanning (e.g., abdominal, perineal, vaginal, rectal, urethral).

3.4.3   Contrast Radiography

Contrast radiography may be static or dynamic and may include voiding colpo-cysto-urethrography, defecography, peritoneography, and pelvic fluoroscopy among others. All reports of contrast radiography should include the following information:

a projection (e.g., lateral, frontal, horizontal, oblique);
b type and amount of contrast media used and sequence of opacification of the bladder, vagina, rectum and colon, small bowel, and peritoneal cavity;
c any urethral or vaginal appliance used (e.g., tampon, catheter, bead-chain);
d type of exposures (e.g., single exposure, video);
e magnification — an internal reference scale should be included.

3.4.4 *Computed Tomography and Magnetic Resonance Imaging*
These techniques do not allow for continuous imaging under dynamic conditions. Currently available equipment usually dictates supine scanning. Specifics of the technique should be specified including:

a the specific equipment used, including the manufacturer;
b the plane of imaging (e.g., axial, sagittal, coronal, oblique);
c the field of view;
d the thickness of sections and the number of slices;
e the scan time;
f the use and type of contrast;
g the type of image analysis.

3.5 *Surgical Assessment*

Intra-operative evaluation of pelvic support defects is intuitively attractive but as yet of unproven value. The effects of anesthesia, diminished muscle tone, and loss of consciousness are of unknown magnitude and direction. Limitations due to the position of the patient must also be evaluated.

4 PELVIC FLOOR MUSCLE TESTING
Pelvic floor muscles are voluntarily controlled, but selective contraction and relaxation necessitates muscle awareness. Optimal squeezing technique involves contraction of the pelvic floor muscles without contraction of the abdominal wall muscles and without a Valsalva maneuver. Squeezing synergists are the intraurethral and anal sphincteric muscles. In normal voiding, defecation, and optimal abdominal-strain voiding, the pelvic floor is relaxed, while the abdominal wall and the diaphragm may contract. With coughs and sneezes and often when other stresses are applied, the pelvic floor and abdominal wall are contracted simultaneously.

Evaluation and measurement of pelvic floor muscle function includes 1) an assessment of the patient's ability to contract and relax the pelvic muscles selectively (i.e., squeezing without abdominal straining and vice versa) and 2) measurement of the force (strength) of contraction.

There are pitfalls in the measurement of pelvic floor muscle function because the muscles are invisible to the investigator and because patients often simultaneously and erroneously activate other muscles. Contraction of the abdominal, gluteal, and hip adductor muscles, Valsalva maneuver, straining, breath holding, and forced inspirations are typically seen. These factors affect the reliability of available testing modalities and have to be taken into consideration in the interpretation of these tests.

The individual types of tests cited in this report are based both on the scientific literature and current clinical practice. It is the intent of the committee neither to endorse specific tests or techniques nor to restrict evaluations to the examples given. The standards recommended are intended to facilitate comparison of results obtained by different investigators and to allow investigators to replicate studies precisely.

For all types of measuring techniques the following should be specified:

a patient position, including the position of the legs;
b specific instructions given to the patient;
c the status of bladder and bowel fullness;
d techniques of quantification or qualification (estimated, calculated, directly measured);
e the reliability of the technique.

4.1 *Inspection*

A visual assessment of muscle integrity, including a description of scarring and symmetry, should be performed. Pelvic floor contraction causes inward movement of the perineum and straining causes the opposite movement. Perineal movements can be observed directly or assessed indirectly by movement of an externally visible device placed into the vagina or urethra. The abdominal wall and other specified regions might be watched simultaneously. The type, size, and placement of any device used should be specified as should the state of undress of the patient.

4.2 *Palpation*

Palpation may include digital examination of the pelvic floor muscles through the vagina or rectum as well as assessment of the perineum, abdominal wall, and/or other specified regions. The number of fingers and their position should be specified. Scales for the description of the strength of voluntary and reflex (e.g., with coughing) contractions and of the degree of voluntary relaxation should be clearly described and intra- and inter-observer reliability documented. Standardized palpation techniques could also be developed for the semiquantitative estimation of the bulk or thickness of pelvic floor musculature around the circumference of the genital hiatus. These techniques could allow for the localization of any atrophic or asymmetric segments.

4.3 *Electromyography*

Electromyography from the pelvic floor muscles can be recorded alone or in combination with other measurements. Needle electrodes permit visualization of individual motor unit action potentials, while surface or wire electrodes detect action potentials from groups of adjacent motor units underlying or surrounding the electrodes. Interpretation of signals from these latter electrodes must take into consideration that signals from erroneously contracted adjacent muscles may interfere with signals from the muscles of interest. Reports of electromyographic recordings should specify the following:

a type of electrode;
b placement of electrodes;
c placement of reference electrode;

d specifications of signal processing equipment;

e type and specifications of display equipment;

f muscle in which needle electrode is placed;

g description of decision algorithms used by the analytic software.

4.4 *Pressure Recording*

Measurements of urethral, vaginal, and anal pressures may be used to assess pelvic floor muscle control and strength. However, interpretations based on these pressure measurements must be made with a knowledge of their potential for artifact and their unproven or limited reproducibility. Anal sphincter contractions, rectal peristalsis, detrusor contractions, and abdominal straining can affect pressure measurements. Pressures recorded from the proximal vagina accurately mimic fluctuations in abdominal pressure. Therefore it may be important to compare vaginal pressures to simultaneously measured vesical or rectal pressures. Reports using pressure measurements should specify the following:

a the type and size of the measuring device at the recording site (e.g., balloon, open catheter, etc);

b the exact placement of the measuring device;

c the type of pressure transducer;

d the type of display system;

e the display of simultaneous control pressures.

As noted in section 4.1, observation of the perineum is an easy and reliable way to assess for abnormal straining during an attempt at a pelvic muscle contraction. Significant straining or a Valsalva maneuver causes downward/caudal movement of the perineum; a correctly performed pelvic muscle contraction causes inward/cephalad movement of the perineum. Observation for perineal movement should be considered as an additional validation procedure whenever pressure measurements are recorded.

5   DESCRIPTION OF FUNCTIONAL SYMPTOMS

Functional deficits caused by pelvic organ prolapse and pelvic floor dysfunction are not well characterized or absolutely established. There is an ongoing need to develop, standardize, and validate various clinimetric scales such as condition-specific quality of life questionnaires for each of the four functional symptom groups (section 5.1 through 5.4) thought to be related to pelvic organ prolapse.

Researchers in this area should try to use standardized and validated symptom scales whenever possible. **They must always ask precisely the same questions regarding functional symptoms before and after therapeutic intervention**. The description of functional symptoms should be directed toward four primary areas: 1) lower urinary tract, 2) bowel, 3) sexual, and 4) other local symptoms.

5.1 *Urinary Symptoms*

This report does not supplant any currently approved ICS terminology related to lower urinary tract function [1]. However, some important prolapse related symptoms are not included in the current standards (e.g., the need to manually reduce the prolapse or assume an unusual position to initiate or complete micturition). Urinary symptoms that should be considered for dichotomous, ordinal, or visual analog scaling include, but are not limited to, the following:

a stress incontinence
b frequency (diurnal and nocturnal)
c urgency
d urge incontinence
e hesitancy
f weak or prolonged urinary stream
g feeling of incomplete emptying
h reduction to start or complete voiding
i positional changes to start or complete voiding

5.2 *Bowel Symptoms*

Bowel symptoms that should be considered for dichotomous, ordinal, or visual analog scaling include, but are not limited to, the following:

a difficulty with defecation
b incontinence of flatus
c incontinence of liquid stool
d incontinence of solid stool
e fecal staining of underwear
f urgency of defecation
g discomfort with defecation
h digital manipulation or vagina or perineum to complete defecation
i feeling of incomplete evacuation

5.3 *Sexual Symptoms*

Research is needed to attempt to differentiate the complex and multifactorial aspects of 'satisfactory sexual function' as it relates to pelvic organ prolapse and pelvic floor dysfunction. It may be difficult to distinguish between the ability to have vaginal intercourse and normal sexual function. The development of satisfactory tools will require multidisciplinary collaboration. Sexual function symptoms that should be considered for dichotomous, ordinal, or visual analog scaling include, but are not limited to, the following:

a Is the patient sexually active?
b If she is not sexually active, why?
c Does sexual activity include vaginal coitus?
d What is the frequency of vaginal intercourse?
e Does the patient experience pain with coitus?
f Is the patient satisfied with her sexual activity?
h Has there been any change in orgasmic response?

5.4   *Other Local Symptoms*

We currently lack knowledge regarding the precise nature of symptoms that may be caused by the presence of a protrusion or bulge. Possible anatomically based symptoms that should be considered for dichotomous, ordinal, or visual analog scaling include, but are not limited to, the following:

a   vaginal pressure or heaviness;
b   vaginal or perineal pain;
c   sensation or awareness of tissue protrusion from the vagina;
d   low back pain;
e   abdominal pressure or pain;
f   observation or palpation of a mass.

Reference

[1]Abrams P, Blaivas JG, Stanton SL, Andersen JT: The International Continence Society Committee on Standardization of Terminology. The standardization of terminology of lower urinary tract function. Scand J Urol Nephrol 1988; 114S:5–19

Acknowledgements

The subcommittee would like to acknowledge the contributions of the following consultants who contributed to the development and revision of this document:

W. Glenn Hurt, M.D., Richmond, VA, U.S.
Bernhard Schüssler, M.D., Luzern, Switzerland
L. Lewis Wall, M.D. D.Phil., New Orleans, LA, U.S.

Index